Virus Infections and Skin Cancer

Virus Infections and Skin Cancer

Editor: Julio Casey

AMERICAN
MEDICAL PUBLISHERS
www.americanmedicalpublishers.com

AMERICAN
MEDICAL PUBLISHERS
www.americanmedicalpublishers.com

Cataloging-in-Publication Data

Virus infections and skin cancer / edited by Julio Casey.
p. cm.
Includes bibliographical references and index.
ISBN 979-8-88740-559-9
1. Skin--Cancer. 2. Virus diseases. 3. Dermatology. I. Casey, Julio.
RC280.S5 V57 2023
616.994 77--dc23

American Medical Publishers,
41 Flatbush Avenue,
1st Floor, New York,
NY 11217, USA

ISBN 979-8-88740-559-9 (Hardback)

Contents

Preface

This book has been a concerted effort by a group of academicians, researchers and scientists, who have contributed their research works for the realization of the book. This book has materialized in the wake of emerging advancements and innovations in this field. Therefore, the need of the hour was to compile all the required researches and disseminate the knowledge to a broad spectrum of people comprising of students, researchers and specialists of the field.

Cancer refers to a group of diseases that involve abnormal cell growth in one or more parts of a body which may also spread to other parts of the body. Cancers that arise from the skin are called skin cancers. They can be categorized mainly into three types, basal-cell cancer (BCC), squamous-cell cancer (SCC), and melanoma. Basal skin cancer grows gradually and damages the surrounding tissue. It becomes visible as a raised area of skin that appears shiny with small blood vessels running over it. It may also appear as a raised area with an ulcer. The most common form of treatment for skin cancers is surgical excision or reconstructive surgery. Human papillomaviridae (HPVs) are small non-enveloped viruses belonging to the papillomaviridae family. There are five main classes or genera of HPVs namely α, β, γ, ν, and μ. Out of these five, α-HPV and β-HPV are known to play a role in human diseases. α-HPVs play an etiological role in mucosal and skin infections as well as cervical carcinoma and benign viral warts. β-HPVs have been associated with skin infections and SCC. This book presents various researches on the role of viruses in the development of skin cancers. Those in search of information to further their knowledge will be greatly assisted by this book.

At the end of the preface, I would like to thank the authors for their brilliant chapters and the publisher for guiding us all-through the making of the book till its final stage. Also, I would like to thank my family for providing the support and encouragement throughout my academic career and research projects.

Editor

1

Natural History of Cutaneous Human Polyomavirus Infection in Healthy Individuals

Luisa Bopp[1,2†], Ulrike Wieland[1†], Martin Hellmich[3], Alexander Kreuter[4], Herbert Pfister[1] and Steffi Silling[1]*

[1] Institute of Virology, National Reference Center for Papilloma- and Polyomaviruses, University of Cologne, Faculty of Medicine and University Hospital of Cologne, Cologne, Germany, [2] Department of Dermatology and Venereology, University of Cologne, Cologne, Germany, [3] Institute of Medical Statistics and Computational Biology, Faculty of Medicine and University Hospital Cologne, University of Cologne, Cologne, Germany, [4] Department of Dermatology, Venereology and Allergology, Helios St. Elisabeth Hospital Oberhausen, University Witten-Herdecke, Witten, Germany

****Correspondence:***
Steffi Silling
steffi.silling@uk-koeln.de

† These authors have contributed equally to this work

Several human polyomaviruses (HPyVs) were recently discovered. Merkel cell polyomavirus (MCPyV) induces Merkel cell carcinoma. HPyV6, HPyV7, and TSPyV have been associated with rare skin lesions in immunosuppressed patients. HPyV9, HPyV10, and Saint Louis Polyomavirus (STLPyV) have not been convincingly associated with any disease. The aim of this prospective study was to evaluate the cutaneous prevalence, persistence and viral load of HPyVs in healthy individuals. Eight hundred seventy forehead and hand swabs were collected from 109 volunteers 4–6 weeks apart (collection period-1). Fifty-nine participants were available for follow-up a decade later (collection period-2). HPyV-DNA prevalence and viral loads of MCPyV, HPyV6, HPyV7, TSPyV, HPyV9, HPyV10, and STLPyV were determined by virus-specific real-time PCRs. Risk factors for HPyV prevalence, short- and long-term persistence were explored by logistic regression analyses. Baseline prevalence rates were similar for forehead and hand: MCPyV 67.9/67.0%, HPyV6 31.2/25.7%, HPyV7 13.8/11.0%, HPyV10 11.9/15.6%, STLPyV 7.3/8.3%, TSPyV 0.9/0.9%, and HPyV9 0.9/0.9%. Short-term persistence in period-1 was found in 59.6% (MCPyV), 23.9% (HPyV6), 10.1% (HPyV7), 6.4% (HPyV10), 5.5% (STLPyV), and 0% (TSPyV and HPyV9) on the forehead, with similar values for the hand. Long-term persistence for 9–12 years occurred only for MCPyV (forehead/hand 39.0%/44.1% of volunteers), HPyV6 (16.9%/11.9%), and HPyV7 (3.4%/5.1%). Individuals with short-term persistence had significantly higher viral loads at baseline compared to those with transient DNA-positivity ($p < 0.001$ for MCPyV, HPyV6, HPyV7, and HPyV10, respectively). This was also true for median viral loads in period-1 of MCPyV, HPyV6, and HPyV7 of volunteers with long-term persistence. Multiplicity (two or more different HPyVs) was a risk factor for prevalence and persistence for most HPyVs. Further risk factors were older age for HPyV6 and male sex for MCPyV on the forehead. Smoking was not a risk factor. In contrast to MCPyV, HPyV6, HPyV7, and rarely STLPyV, polyomaviruses TSPyV, HPyV9, and HPyV10 do not seem to be long-term constituents of the human skin virome of healthy individuals. Furthermore, this study showed that higher viral loads are associated with both short- and long-term persistence of HPyVs on the skin. HPyV multiplicity is a risk factor for prevalence, short-term and/or long-term persistence of MCPyV, HPyV6, HPyV7, and HPyV10.

Keywords: polyomaviruses, skin, persistence, MCPyV, HPyV, TSPyV, STLPyV

INTRODUCTION

Human polyomaviruses (HPyVs) are small, non-enveloped viruses with a double-stranded circular DNA genome. To date, 15 different HPyVs have been identified, with only some of them being associated with human disease, especially in immunosuppressed patients.

The first two HPyVs, BKPyV, and JCPyV, were discovered in 1971. Primary infection is usually asymptomatic, but reactivation is linked to serious diseases such as JCPyV-induced leukoencephalopathy or BKPyV-induced nephropathy in immunosuppressed patients (Gardner et al., 1971; Padgett et al., 1971). In 2007, KIPyV and WUPyV were discovered in respiratory secretions from patients with acute respiratory tract infections. However, their association with human disease is not well established (Allander et al., 2007; Gaynor et al., 2007). In 2008, Merkel cell polyomavirus (MCPyV) was described as an aetiological agent of Merkel cell carcinoma (MCC), a rare aggressive skin cancer of neuroectodermal origin (Feng et al., 2008). Since 2010, several novel HPyV species have been isolated. Four of them are possibly associated with rare skin lesions in immunosuppressed individuals: the skin-tropic HPyVs 6 and 7 were discovered on healthy human forehead skin in 2010 (Schowalter et al., 2010). Both of them are associated with pruritic and dyskeratotic dermatoses in immunosuppressed patients (Ho et al., 2015; Nguyen et al., 2017). Moreover, HPyV6 was detected in epithelial neoplasms such as keratoacanthomas (Schrama et al., 2014; Beckervordersandforth et al., 2016), while HPyV7 was found in thymomas (Rennspiess et al., 2015). However, their aetiological role in the development of these tumours remains unclear (Scola et al., 2012; Keijzers et al., 2015; Haeggblom et al., 2017; Amorrortu et al., 2021; Klufah et al., 2021). Trichodysplasia spinulosa–associated polyomavirus (TSPyV) was detected in immunosuppressed individuals with the rare skin disease trichodysplasia spinulosa, which is characterised by follicular keratotic papules and spicules in the face (van der Meijden et al., 2010; Kazem et al., 2013). New Jersey PyV (NJPyV-2013) was isolated from a muscle biopsy of a pancreatic transplant patient with vasculitic myopathy and retinal blindness in 2014 (Mishra et al., 2014). Five further HPyVs not associated with any disease have been identified in recent years (Ehlers and Wieland, 2013; Feltkamp et al., 2013; Moens et al., 2017): HPyV9 was discovered in the serum of a renal transplant patient in 2011 (Scuda et al., 2011). In 2012, HPyV10, or Malawi PyV (MWPyV), was detected coincidentally in perianal warts of a immunosuppressed patient as well as in stool samples of healthy children from Malawi (Buck et al., 2012; Siebrasse et al., 2012). Saint Louis PyV (STLPyV) was detected in stool specimens, and HPyV12 was found in liver, caecum, and rectum tissue (Korup et al., 2013; Lim et al., 2013) in 2013. In 2017, Gheit et al. (2017) reported the characterisation of a 14th HPyV, Lyon IARC PyV (LIPyV), from skin and oral gargle samples of healthy individuals. However, it cannot be excluded that HPyV12 and LIPyV may be contaminants from shrew and cat, respectively. Another probable HPyV, Quebec polyomavirus (QPyV), was recently identified in a metagenomic analysis of faecal samples of an elderly man and could also be detected by PCR in urine samples of immunosuppressed patients and pregnant women (Ondov et al., 2019; Prezioso et al., 2021).

Several studies have reported high seroprevalence (60–100%) for the majority of HPyVs in adults (Nicol et al., 2013; Van Der Meijden et al., 2013; Gossai et al., 2016; Kamminga et al., 2018). Lower seroprevalence rates (around 5%) were found for the recently identified HPyV12, NJPyV-2013, and LIPyV (Kamminga et al., 2018). Although serological evidence indicates that most adults have been immunologically exposed to the majority of HPyVs, the natural history of HPyV infections in healthy individuals has not yet been fully elucidated. To date, only a limited number of studies have assessed the prevalence of the recently detected HPyVs on the skin of healthy individuals, with the majority of them limited to men (Wieland et al., 2011, 2014; Hampras et al., 2015; Hashida et al., 2018). To identify individuals at high risk for infection and virus-associated disease, it is important to investigate the natural history of these potentially pathogenic viruses by studying their prevalence and persistence on human skin (Wieland et al., 2014; Hampras et al., 2015). The aim of this prospective study was to evaluate the cutaneous DNA prevalence, short- and long-term persistence and viral load of seven HPyVs with assumed skin tropism – MCPyV, HPyV6, HPyV7, TSPyV, HPyV9, HPyV10, and STLPyV – in healthy men and women.

MATERIALS AND METHODS

Study Participants and Specimen Collection

Within the first collection period (August 2009 to June 2012), 870 non-lesional skin swabs (forehead and back of the left hand) were collected from 109 healthy adult volunteers (**Table 1** and **Figure 1**) at four points in time, each 4–6 weeks apart. For the long-term follow-up analysis, one forehead swab and one hand swab were taken between April and May 2021 (collection period-2) from the still-available volunteers (n = 59, 23 males, 36 females) 9–12 years after the initial collection period (**Figure 1**). Participants had to be free of skin cancer, skin infections, and acute or chronic inflammatory dermatoses. Data

TABLE 1 | Study participants' characteristics at baseline.

No. of participants		109
Sex – No. (%)	Female	63 (57.8)
	Male	46 (42.2)
Age – yr	Mean (range)	41.6 (20–81)
	Median (IQR)	39.0 (32.0–48.5)
Smoking status – No. (%)	Non-smoker	83 (76.1)
	Smoker	26 (23.9)
Acute or chronic dermatosis – No. (%)	No	109 (100)
	Yes	0
Chronic underlying disease* – No. (%)	No	103 (94.5)
	Yes	6 (5.5)
Immunosuppression – No. (%)	No	108 (99.1)
	Yes	1** (0.9)

No., number; yr, year; IQR, interquartile range.
**Diabetes mellitus (n = 3, males), Crohn's disease (n = 1, female), cystic fibrosis (n = 1, female), rheumatoid arthritis (n = 1, female).*
***Iatrogenic immunosuppression (sulfasalazine for rheumatoid arthritis).*

on the participants' underlying diseases, immunosuppression and smoking status was collected. The study was approved by the ethics review board of the faculty of medicine of the University of Cologne (no. 10-230). Written informed consent was obtained from all participants. For sampling, a sterile cotton swab wetted with PBS was forcefully rubbed on the forehead including the eyebrows or on the back of the left hand of the participants.

Human Polyomavirus DNA Detection

DNA isolation from the swab material was performed as previously described using a commercially available DNA extraction kit (QIAamp DNA Mini; Qiagen, Hilden, Germany) (Weissenborn et al., 2010; Wieland et al., 2011). Real-time human beta-globin-gene polymerase chain reaction (PCR) was performed to demonstrate that samples contained adequate DNA and were free of substances inhibitory to PCR [period-1: LightCycler Control Kit DNA; Roche, Mannheim, Germany; period-2: beta-Globin PCR according to the protocol of Van Duin et al. (2002)]. All samples were analysed by virus-specific quantitative real-time PCR (q-PCR) targeting the VP1 gene for the presence of MCPyV, HPyV6, HPyV7, TSPyV, HPyV9, and HPyV10 as previously reported (Weissenborn et al., 2010; Wieland et al., 2014). The same protocol was applied for the detection of STLPyV using primers 5′-GAAAATCTAGATGCACCTCACAGA-3′ and 5′-TTTGGCACGGATCATATTCA-3′ together with UPL-probe no. 63 (Roche, Mannheim, Germany, Cat no.: 04688627001). Viral loads were expressed as viral DNA-copies per beta-globin gene copy.

Definitions

Baseline prevalence was defined as being positive for the respective HPyV in the first swab. Period prevalence was defined as being positive for the respective virus in ≥1 swab in period-1. Short-term persistence was defined as ≥3 of 4 swabs being positive for the respective HPyV in period-1. Long-term persistence was defined by a positive follow-up swab in period-2 in volunteers with previous short-term persistence (**Figure 1**).

Data Analysis

Qualitative data were cross-tabulated and evaluated for association by the exact McNemar test, 2-sided, or the Fisher's exact test, 2-sided. Distributions of HPyV DNA loads (forehead vs. hand) were tested for difference in location using the Wilcoxon signed-rank test. Distributions of HPyV DNA load (no persistence vs. persistence) were tested for difference in location using the non-parametric Mann–Whitney *U* test for two independent samples. The exact Clopper–Pearson approach was used for calculation of 95% confidence intervals (CI). Risk was modelled (explained) using univariable and multivariable logistic regression. Statistical analyses were done using Statistical Package for the Social Sciences (SPSS) Statistics 26 (IBM Corp., Armonk, NY, United States).

RESULTS

Study Participants' Characteristics

The participants' characteristics at baseline are given in **Table 1**. 46 of the 109 volunteers were men, 63 were women. The age range was 20–81 years (mean age 41.6 years). Twenty-three point nine percent (n = 26) were smokers. At the time of sample collection, all participants were free of skin cancer, skin infections and acute or chronic inflammatory dermatoses. Six participants (5.5%) had a chronic underlying disease; one person was receiving immunosuppressive medication (see **Table 1** for details).

Site-Specific Human Polyomaviruses DNA Prevalence, Multiplicity, and Viral DNA Load at Baseline

At baseline, about three-quarters of the 109 participants were positive for any HPyV 73.4% (95%CI 64.1–81.4) on the forehead and 80.7% (95%CI 72.1–87.7) on the back of the hand. Twenty-six point six percent (95%CI 18.6–35.9) of the volunteers did not carry any HPyV on the forehead, and in 19.3% (95%CI 12.3–27.9), no HPyV DNA was found on the hands at baseline. Baseline prevalence on the forehead and on the hand was highest for MCPyV (67.9%, 95%CI 58.3–76.5 and 67.0%, 95%CI 57.3–75.7, respectively), followed by HPyV6 (31.2%, 95%CI 22.7–40.8 and 25.7%, 95%CI 17.8–34.9). HPyV7, HPyV10, and STLPyV were less frequent and had similar baseline prevalence rates around 10% (see **Table 2** for details). TSPyV and HPyV9 were detected in only 0.9% (95%CI 0–5.0) of baseline swabs, respectively (**Table 2**).

Concomitant detection of more than one HPyV was found in 42.2% of baseline forehead swabs and in 31.2% of baseline hand swabs. In baseline forehead and hand swabs, two different HPyVs were detected in 26.6% (95%CI 18.6–35.9) and 19.3% (95%CI 12.3–27.9), three different HPyVs were detected in 12.8% (95%CI 7.2–20.6) and 6.4% (95%CI 2.6–12.8) and four different HPyVs in 2.8% (95%CI 0.6–7.8) and 5.5% (95%CI 2.0–11.6), respectively. Monoinfections occurred more frequently on the hand than on the forehead (p = 0.003; exact McNemar test, two-sided) (**Table 2**).

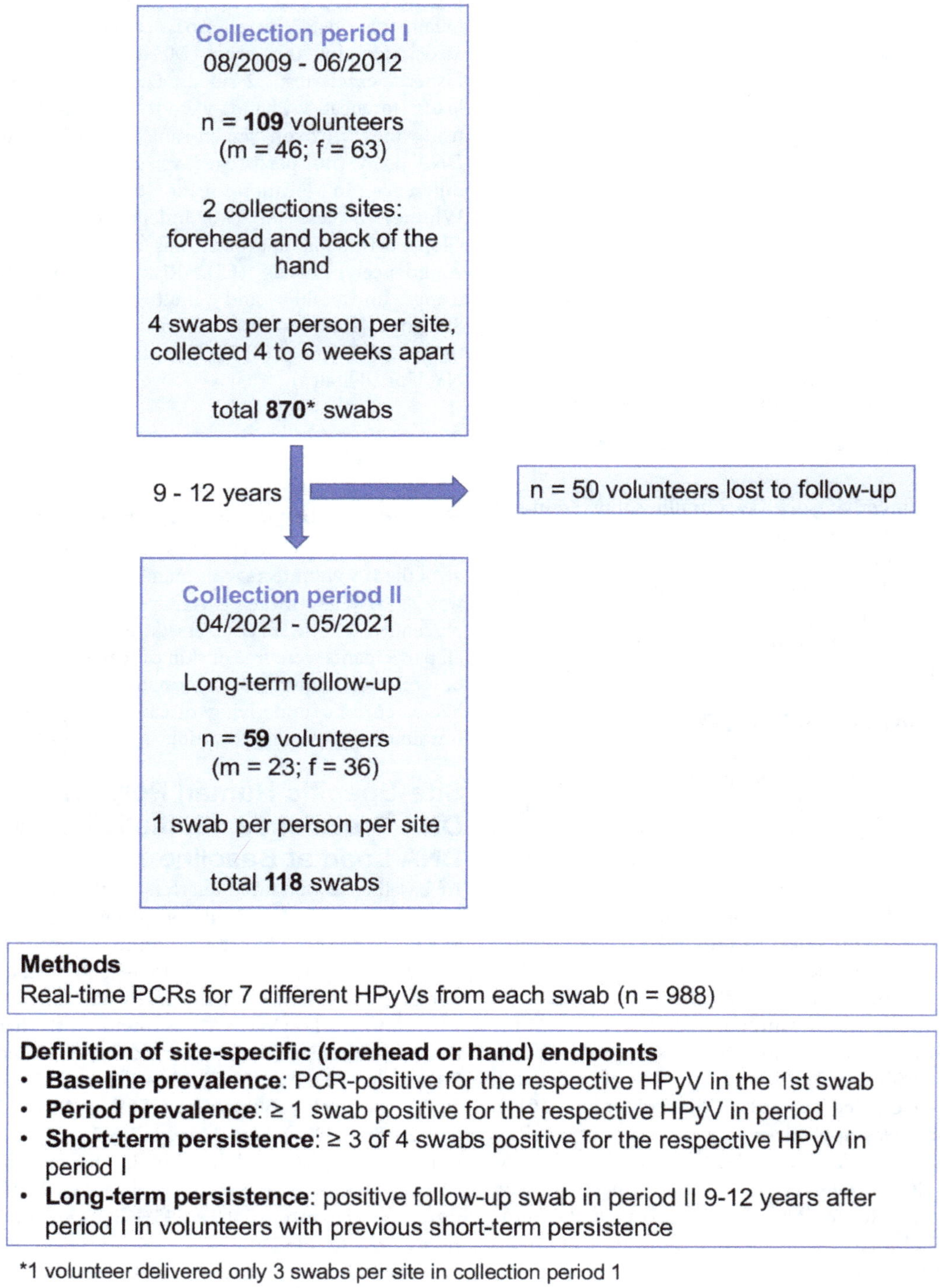

FIGURE 1 | Study design. f, female; m, male; n, number; HPyV, human polyomavirus.

While there were no significant differences in site-specific HPyV detection rates, the median viral load for MCPyV, HPyV10, and STLPyV was significantly higher in hand swabs compared to forehead swabs ($p = 0.002$, $p = 0.001$, and $p = 0.016$, respectively, Wilcoxon signed-rank test) (**Table 2**).

MCPyV DNA prevalence at baseline was higher in forehead swabs of men (80.4%; 95%CI 66.1–90.6) compared to women (58.7%; 95%CI 45.6–71.0; $p = 0.022$). Similar results were observed for hand swabs ($p = 0.013$). For all other HPyVs, no significant differences in baseline

TABLE 2 | Site-specific human polyomavirus (HPyV) prevalence, multiplicity, and viral load at baseline.

	Polyomavirus	Forehead	Hand	*p*-value*,°
HPyV DNA prevalence No. (%, 95%CI#) *n* = 109	MCPyV	74 (67.9, 58.3–76.5)	73 (67.0, 57.3–75.7)	1.000*
	HPyV6	34 (31.2, 22.7–40.8)	28 (25.7, 17.8–34.9)	0.263*
	HPyV7	15 (13.8, 7.9–21.7)	12 (11.0, 5.8–18.4)	0.581*
	TSPyV	1 (0.9, 0–5.0)	1 (0.9, 0–5.0)	1.000*
	HPyV9	1 (0.9, 0–5.0)	1 (0.9, 0–5.0)	1.000*
	HPyV10	13 (11.9, 6.5–19.5)	17 (15.6, 9.4–23.8)	0.289*
	STLPyV	8 (7.3, 3.2–14.0)	9 (8.3, 3.8–15.1)	1.000*
Multiplicity No. of different HPyVs per swab (%, 95%CI#) *n* = 109	All HPyVs negative	29 (26.6, 18.6–35.9)	21 (19.3, 12.3–27.9)	0.152*
	Any HPyV	80 (73.4, 64.1–81.4)	88 (80.7, 72.1–87.7)	0.152*
	Monoinfection	34 (31.2, 22.7–40.8)	54 (49.5, 39.8–59.3)	**0.003***
	2 different HPyVs	29 (26.6, 18.6–35.9)	21 (19.3, 12.3–27.9)	0.215*
	3 different HPyVs	14 (12.8, 7.2–20.6)	7 (6.4, 2.6–12.8)	0.167*
	4 different HPyVs	3 (2.8, 0.6–7.8)	6 (5.5, 2.0–11.6)	0.250*
Median viral DNA load in HPyV-positive swabs (*n*, IQR)	MCPyV	0.37 (74, 0.06–5.00)	2.00 (73, 0.35–7.92)	**0.002°**
	HPyV6	0.06 (34, 0.01–0.29)	0.20 (28, 0.08–0.73)	0.683°
	HPyV7	0.05 (15, 0.01–0.73)	0.14 (12, 0.06–0.52)	0.478°
	TSPyV	0.002 (1)	0.42 (1)	0.655°
	HPyV9	1.43 (1)	0.38 (1)	0.317°
	HPyV10	0.04 (13, 0.02–0.05)	0.11 (17, 0.06–0.31)	**0.001°**
	STLPyV	0.01 (8, 0.01–0.04)	0.10 (9, 0.06–0.12)	**0.016°**

No., number; CI, confidence interval; IQR, interquartile range.
 # Exact Clopper–Pearson confidence intervals.
**Exact McNemar test, two-sided.*
° Wilcoxon signed-rank test.
p-values that indicate statistically significant differences are printed in bold.

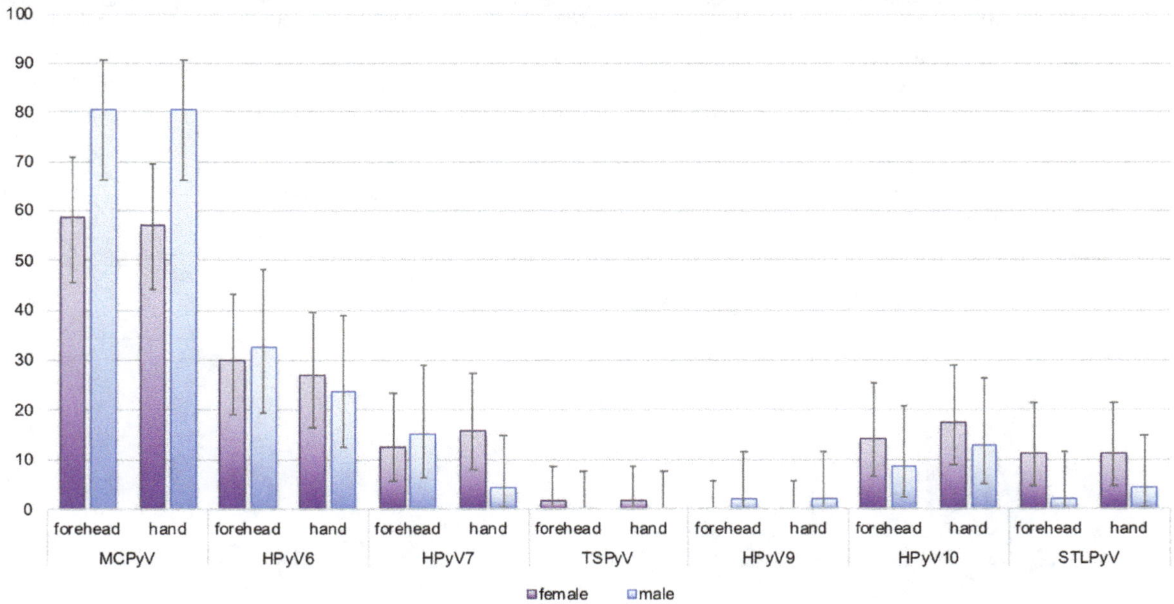

FIGURE 2 | Site-specific human polyomavirus (HPyV) baseline prevalence by sex. Y-axis: prevalence in percentage (%) with error bars. Purple bars: females; blue bars: males. The difference in baseline prevalence between females and males was statistically significant for Merkel cell polyomavirus (MCPyV) (forehead, $p = 0.022$, hand $p = 0.013$; Fisher's exact test, 2-sided).

detection rates in men compared to women were found (**Figure 2** and **Supplementary Table 1**). Looking at age-specific baseline prevalence, detection rates for MCPyV and HPyV10 were comparable in all age groups, while baseline prevalence rates for HPyV6, and less pronounced for HPyV7 and STLPyV, rose at both collection sites in the small group ($n = 13$) of participants aged $\geq$ 60 years (**Supplementary Table 2A**).

Site-Specific Human Polyomavirus Period Prevalence and Persistence

Within collection period-1, MCPyV was the most prevalent HPyV (forehead 92.7%, 95%CI 86.0–96.8; hand 95.4%, 95%CI 89.6–98.5), followed by HPyV6 (forehead 56.9%, 95%CI 47.0–66.3; hand 48.6%, 95%CI 38.9–58.4) and, in decreasing order, by HPyV10, HPyV7, STLPyV, TSPyV, and HPyV9 (**Table 3** and **Figure 3**). MCPyV, TSPyV, and HPyV10 period prevalence rates were comparable in all age groups at both sampling sites, while they tended to be higher in participants aged 60 years and older for HPyV6, HPyV7, and less prominent, in STLPyV (**Supplementary Table 2B**).

Concerning short-term persistence, the highest rate was found for MCPyV with 59.6% (95%CI 49.8–68.9) on the forehead and 67.9% (95%CI 58.3–76.5) on the hand, followed by HPyV6 [forehead 23.9% (95%CI 16.2–33.0); hand 19.3% (95%CI 12.3–27.9)]. Short-term persistence rates at 10% or below were found for HPyV7, HPyV10, and STLPyV. No short-term persistence could be observed for TSPyV and HPyV9 (**Table 3** and **Figure 3**).

Of the 59 volunteers available in collection period-2, around 60% had long-term persistence for any HPyV. Again, MCPyV was the most persistent virus with 39.0% (95%CI 26.5–52.6) on the forehead and 44.1% (95%CI 31.2–57.6) on the hand, followed by HPyV6 (forehead 16.9%, 95%CI 8.4–29.0; hand 11.9%, 95%CI 4.9–22.9) and HPyV7 (forehead 3.4%, 95%CI 0.4–11.7; hand 5.1%, 95%CI 1.1–14.1). Only one person had a long-term persistence for STLPyV on the forehead (1.7%; 95%CI 0.0–9.1). No long-term persistence occurred for TSPyV, HPyV9, and HPyV10 (**Table 4** and **Figure 3**).

TABLE 4 | Site-specific HPyV long-term persistence.

Polyomavirus	Forehead *n* = 59 No. (%, 95%CI[#])	Hand *n* = 59 No. (%, 95%CI[#])
MCPyV	23 (39.0, 26.5–52.6)	26 (44.1, 31.2–57.6)
HPyV6	10 (16.9, 8.4–29.0)	7 (11.9, 4.9–22.9)
HPyV7	2 (3.4, 0.4–11.7)	3 (5.1, 1.1–14.1)
TSPyV	0 (0.0, 0.0–6.1)	0 (0.0, 0.0–6.1)
HPyV9	0 (0.0, 0.0–6.1)	0 (0.0, 0.0–6.1)
HPyV10	0 (0.0, 0.0–6.1)	0 (0.0, 0.0–6.1)
STLPyV	1 (1.7, 0.0–9.1)	0 (0.0, 0.0–6.1)

No., number; CI, confidence interval.
[#]Exact Clopper–Pearson confidence intervals.
Long-term persistence was defined as a positive follow-up swab in collection period-2 in volunteers with previous short-term persistence.

TABLE 3 | Site-specific HPyV period-prevalence and short-term persistence.

Polyoma-virus	Forehead *n* = 109		Hand *n* = 109	
	Period prevalence No. (%, 95%CI[#])	Short-term persistence No. (%, 95%CI[#])	Period prevalence No. (%, 95%CI[#])	Short-term persistence No. (%, 95%CI[#])
MCPyV	101 (92.7, 86.0–96.8)	65 (59.6, 49.8–68.9)	104 (95.4, 89.6–98.5)	74 (67.9, 58.3–76.5)
HPyV6	62 (56.9, 47.0–66.3)	26 (23.9, 16.2–33.0)	53 (48.6, 38.9–58.4)	21 (19.3, 12.3–27.9)
HPyV7	28 (25.7, 17.8–34.9)	11 (10.1, 5.1–17.3)	20 (18.3, 11.6–26.9)	6 (5.5, 2.0–11.6)
TSPyV	8 (7.3, 3.2–14.0)	0 (0.0, 0.0–3.3)	9 (8.3, 3.8–15.1)	0 (0.0, 0.0–3.3)
HPyV9	2 (1.8, 0.2–6.5)	0 (0.0, 0.0–3.3)	1 (0.9, 0.0–5.0)	0 (0.0, 0.0–3.3)
HPyV10	28 (25.7, 17.8–34.9)	7 (6.4, 2.6–12.8)	37 (33.9, 25.1–43.6)	9 (8.3, 3.8–15.1)
STLPyV	21 (19.3, 12.3–27.9)	6 (5.5, 2.0–11.6)	22 (20.2, 13.1–28.0)	6 (5.5, 2.0–11.6)

No., number; CI, confidence interval.
[#]Exact Clopper–Pearson confidence intervals.
Short-term persistence was defined as ≥3 of 4 swabs positive for the respective HPyV in collection period-1.

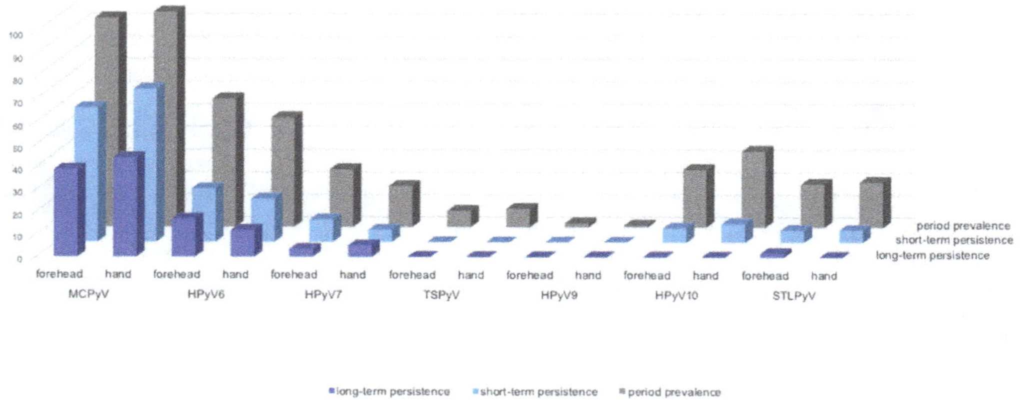

FIGURE 3 | Human polyomavirus period-prevalence, short-, and long-term persistence by collection site. Y-axis: prevalence in percentage (%). Dark-blue bars: long-term persistence; light-blue bars: short-term persistence; grey bars: period prevalence (period-1).

Human Polyomavirus DNA Persistence and Viral Load

Volunteers with short-term persistence of MCPyV, HPyV6, HPyV7, HPyV10, and STLPyV had significantly higher viral DNA loads in the baseline swab compared to those without short-term persistence. This was true for both sampling sites ($p < 0.001$, respectively; **Figures 4A,B** and **Supplementary Figures 1A–C**). Similarly, participants with long-term persistence of MCPyV, HPyV6, and HPyV7 had significantly higher median viral loads in collection period-1 on forehead and hand, compared to those without long-term persistence (**Figures 4C,D** and **Supplementary Figure 2**).

Risk Factors for Human Polyomavirus DNA Prevalence and Persistence

Evaluation of age, sex, smoking, underlying disease, and HPyV multiplicity at baseline as risk factors for prevalence and persistence of the different HPyVs was performed by univariable and multivariable logistic regression analyses. Regarding the forehead, significant risk factors for baseline prevalence were older age for HPyV6, male sex for MCPyV and multiplicity for all HPyVs with the exception of TSPyV and HPyV9 (**Table 5**). Multiplicity turned out to be a risk factor only for HPyV6, 7, and 10 period prevalence (**Table 6**). Risk factors for short-term persistence were older age for HPyV6, male sex for MCPyV and multiplicity for MCPyV, HPyV6, 7 and 10 (**Table 7**). Finally, risk factors for long-term persistence were only older age for HPyV6 and multiplicity for MCPyV and HPyV6 on the forehead (**Table 8**). Similar results were obtained for the hand (**Supplementary Tables 3A–D**). Smoking did not play any role as a risk factor. Underlying disease reduced the risk for MCPyV period prevalence on the forehead (OR 0.12, 95%CI 0.02–0.82, $p = 0.030$), but not on the hand (**Table 6** and **Supplementary Table 3B**).

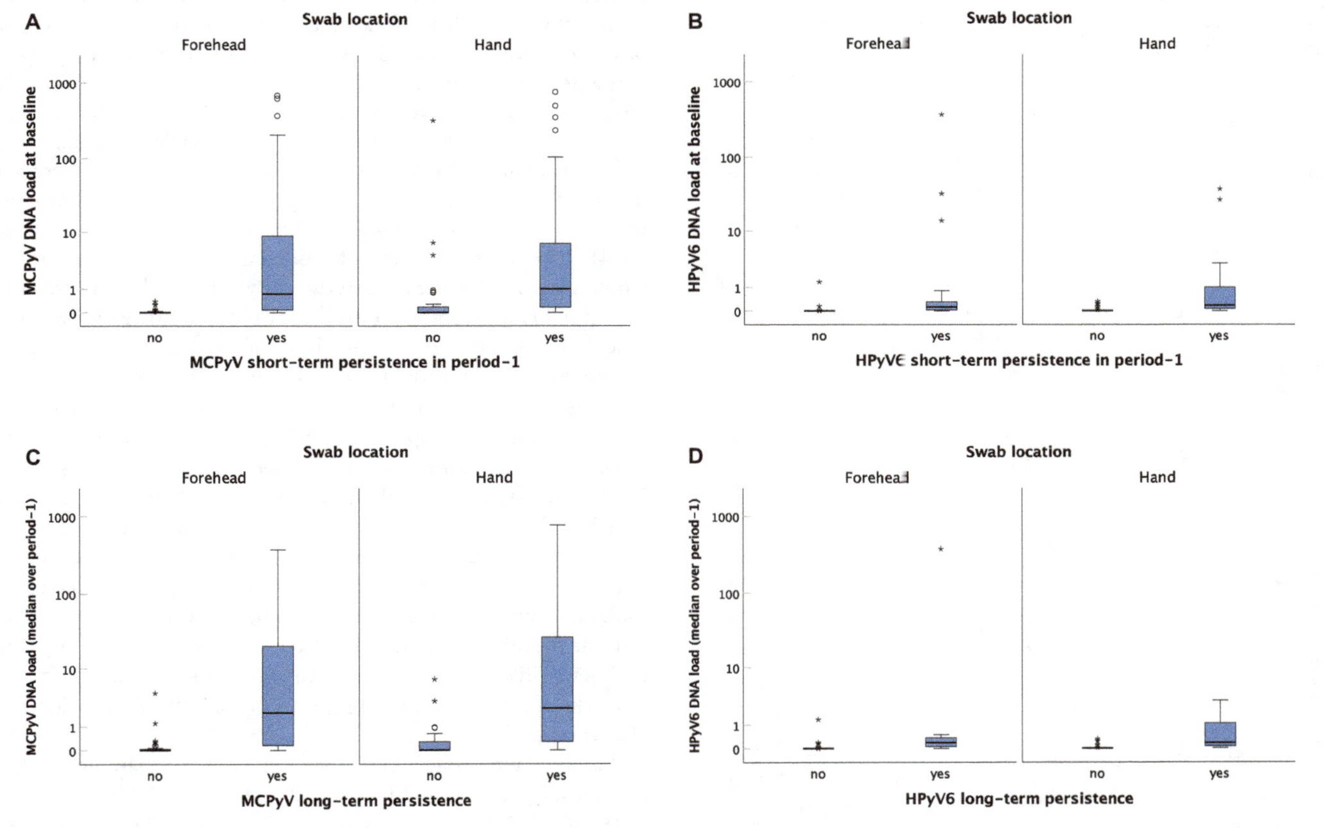

FIGURE 4 | Merkel cell polyomavirus (MCPyV) and HPyV6 DNA loads on the forehead and the hand of individuals without and with short-term **(A,B)** and long-term **(C,D)** persistence. Viral DNA loads (Y-axis) were expressed as viral DNA copies per betaglobin-gene copy. Boxes represent the interquartile range with the median. Whiskers are vertical lines ending in horizontal lines at the largest and smallest observed values that are not statistical outliers, i.e., values more than three IQRs from the end of a box are labelled as extreme, denoted with an asterisk (*) and values more than 1.5 IQRs but less than 3 IQRs from the end of the box are labelled as outliers (o). **(A)** MCPyV and **(B)** HPyV6 baseline viral DNA load distribution of individuals without (left box plot) and with (right box plot) short-term persistence in collection period-1. The differences in viral DNA loads between individuals without and with short-term persistence were significant for both locations and both viruses [$p < 0.001$ for forehead ($n = 109$) and hand ($n = 109$), respectively; independent-samples Mann–Whitney *U* test]. **(C)** MCPyV and **(D)** HPyV6 median DNA loads over collection period-1 of individuals without (left box plot) and with (right box plot) long-term persistence. The differences in viral DNA loads between individuals without and with long-term persistence were significant for both locations and both viruses [$p < 0.001$ for forehead ($n = 59$) and hand ($n = 59$), respectively; independent-samples Mann–Whitney *U* test].

TABLE 5 | Risk factors for HPyVs baseline prevalence on the forehead of healthy individuals found in univariable logistic regression analysis.

Candidate variables	n	MCPyV OR (95% CI#)	MCPyV p-value[1]	HPyV6 OR (95% CI#)	HPyV6 p-value[1]	HPyV7 OR (95% CI#)	HPyV7 p-value[1]	TSPyV OR (95% CI#)	TSPyV p-value[1]	HPyV9 OR (95% CI#)	HPyV9 p-value[1]	HPyV10 OR (95% CI#)	HPyV10 p-value[1]	STLPyV OR (95% CI#)	STLPyV p-value[1]
Age (per decade)	109	1.33 (0.96–1.85)	0.092	**1.91** (1.35–2.70)	**<0.001**	1.34 (0.93–1.93)	0.116	1.13 (0.30–4.31)	0.857	0.16 (0.01–4.95)	0.292	0.92 (0.59–1.43)	0.711	1.36 (0.86–2.17)	0.191
Sex (male vs. female)	109	**2.89** (1.19–7.00)	**0.019**	1.12 (0.49–2.54)	0.785	1.23 (0.41–3.69)	0.706	0 (0)	0.998	>1 (0)	0.997	0.57 (0.17–1.98)	0.378	0.18 (0.02–1.50)	0.112
Smoking (yes vs. no)	109	1.09 (0.42–2.81)	0.867	0.76 (0.29–2.04)	0.591	0.45 (0.09–2.13)	0.314	>1 (0)	0.997	0 (0)	0.998	0.55 (0.11–2.64)	0.451	2.04 (0.45–9.17)	0.355
Underlying disease (yes vs. no)	109	0.45 (0.01–2.36)	0.345	1.11 (0.19–6.37)	0.907	1.27 (0.14–11.70)	0.832	0 (0)	0.999	0 (0)	0.999	1.52 (0.16–14.10)	0.714	2.74 (0.28–26.82)	0.386
Multiplicity[2] (yes vs. no)	109	**52.76** (6.84–406.81)	**<0.001**	**69.71** (14.91–325.88)	**<0.001**	**27.13** (3.41–215.63)	**0.002**	>1 (0)	0.997	>1 (0)	0.997	**21.88** (2.73–175.58)	**0.004**	**11.13** (1.32–93.95)	**0.027**

OR, odds ratio; CI, confidence interval.
#Exact Clopper–Pearson confidence intervals.
[1]p-values < 0.05 are significant and printed in bold.
[2]Defined as ≥two different HPyVs at baseline.
The risk factors found for MCPyV, HPyV6, HPyV7, HPyV10, and STLPyV in univariable regression analysis were included in a multivariable logistic regression model and remained significant after adjustment for the other covariates.

DISCUSSION

In the present study, we have analysed prevalence, short- and long-term persistence of human polyomaviruses MCPyV, HPyV6, HPyV7, TSPyV, HPyV9, HPyV10, and STLPyV on healthy skin. HPyV12, NJPyV-2013, LIPyV, and QPyV were not included in the present study due to their low seroprevalence, the uncertainty that they are genuine HPyVs and/or their unknown pathogenicity in humans (Nicol et al., 2013; Van Der Meijden et al., 2013; Gossai et al., 2016; Moens et al., 2017; Kamminga et al., 2018).

The HPyV DNA detection rates at baseline observed here are basically in line with previous studies. Hampras et al. (2015) detected MCPyV, HPyV6, and HPyV7 in 65.9, 12, and 2.1% of 192 healthy males, respectively. In previous studies from our group MCPyV, HPyV6, HPyV7, TSPyV, HPyV9, and HPyV10 were found in 49.4, 27.6, 13.4, 0.8, 0, and 3.4% of healthy males who underwent skin cancer screening, respectively (Wieland et al., 2011, 2014). A study from Japan reported comparable prevalence rates for MCPyV, HPyV6, and HPyV7 in healthy individuals (Hashida et al., 2016, 2018). The low baseline prevalence for TSPyV and HPyV9 found in the present study is consistent with the results from recent studies, in which both viruses were either undetectable or were detected only sporadically on the skin of adults (Wieland et al., 2014; Hampras et al., 2015; Wang et al., 2019). Interestingly, here, we observed a higher HPyV10 DNA prevalence (11.9%) compared to 3.4% of healthy males in a former study (Wieland et al., 2014). The difference might be related to the inclusion of women, as in the present study, HPyV10 baseline prevalence was higher in women compared to men, however, without reaching significance. To the best of our knowledge, this is the first study to provide data on prevalence of STLPyV in the skin, which was found in 7.3 and 8.3% on forehead and hand at baseline, respectively. STLPyV was first detected in stool specimens (Lim et al., 2013). Recently, STLPyV was found in 2% of palatine tonsil swabs from children with chronic tonsillar disease (Peng et al., 2016), while in another study, it was undetectable in benign and malignant tonsillar tissue of adults (Herberhold et al., 2017). STLPyV was not detected in malignant and non-malignant lung tissue (Csoma et al., 2018) but was found in nose and throat swabs from a kidney transplant recipient (Bialasiewicz et al., 2016) and in skin warts from the buttocks of a patient suffering from a primary immunodeficiency (Pastrana et al., 2013).

Baseline viral loads measured here are comparable to data previously published (Wieland et al., 2011, 2014; Hashida et al., 2016, 2018). With the exception of MCPyV, HPyV DNA loads in non-lesional skin swabs were low, possibly indicating chronic shedding of HPyV from healthy skin with low-level replication, similar to cutaneous human papillomaviruses of the genus beta (Weissenborn et al., 2009, 2010; Schowalter et al., 2010).

In contrast to Foulongne et al. (2010b) who found a significantly higher MCPyV DNA prevalence on the face compared to limbs and Hampras et al. (2015) who found higher MCPyV detection rates in arm swabs compared to eyebrow hair, we could not observe site-specific differences regarding

TABLE 6 | Risk factors for HPyVs period prevalence on the forehead of healthy individuals found in univariable logistic regression analysis.

Candidate variables	*n*	MCPyV		HPyV6		HPyV7		TSPyV		HPyV9		HPyV10		STLPyV	
		OR (95% CI[#])	*p*-value[1]	OR (95% CI[#])	*p*-value[1]	OR (95% CI[#])	*p*-value[1]	OR (95% CI[#])	*p*-value[1]	OR (95% CI[#])	*p*-value[1]	OR (95% CI[#])	*p*-value[1]	OR (95% CI[#])	*p*-value[1]
Age (per decade)	109	0.87 (0.53–1.41)	0.563	**1.44** (1.05–1.97)	**0.024***	1.30 (0.96–1.76)	0.096	0.86 (0.48–1.53)	0.603	0.71 (0.20–2.54)	0.600	0.88 (0.63–1.23)	0.448	1.29 (0.93–1.79)	0.130
Sex (male vs. female)	109	5.63 (0.67–47.42)	0.112	0.72 (0.33–1.55)	0.397	0.69 (0.29–1.69)	0.421	1.41 (0.33–5.94)	0.644	>1 (0)	0.997	**0.36** (0.14–0.94)	**0.036**	0.48 (0.17–1.35)	0.165
Smoking (yes vs. no)	109	0.49 (0.11–2.21)	0.355	2.53 (0.96–6.65)	0.061	0.62 (0.21–1.84)	0.391	2.04 (0.45–9.17)	0.355	0 (0)	0.998	1.40 (0.53–3.70)	0.498	2.39 (0.86–6.65)	0.094
Underlying disease (yes vs. no)	109	**0.12** (0.02–0.82)	**0.030**	0.36 (0.06–2.05)	0.248	0.56 (0.06–5.04)	0.607	0 (0)	0.999	0 (0)	0.999	3.12 (0.59–16.45)	0.180	2.21 (0.38–12.96)	0.379
Multiplicity[2] (yes vs. no)	109	>1 (0)	0.997	**16.40** (5.65–47.62)	**<0.001**	**4.22** (1.69–10.57)	**0.002**	4.58 (0.88–23.80)	0.071	>1 (0)	0.997	**2.77** (1.15–6.71)	**0.024**	1.67 (0.64–4.34)	0.296

OR, odds ratio; CI, confidence interval.
[#]Exact Clopper–Pearson confidence intervals.
[1]p-values < 0.05 are significant and printed in bold.
[2]Defined as ≥2 different HPyVs at baseline.
**Not significant anymore in multivariable modeling.*
The risk factors found for MCPyV, HPyV6, HPyV7, HPyV10, and STLPyV in univariable regression analysis were included in a multivariable logistic regression model and remained significant after adjustment for the other covariates, with the exception of age for HPyV6.

baseline prevalence rates of all HPyVs analysed. This is in line with a study showing that the amount of MCPyV DNA shed from the skin is similar at multiple environmentally exposed and unexposed anatomical sites (Pastrana et al., 2012). However, we observed higher MCPyV, HPyV6, HPyV10, and STLPyV DNA loads at baseline in hand compared to forehead swabs. Possibly, an increased rate of cell division in environmentally exposed areas of the body might favour amplification of commensal viruses.

Investigating consecutive skin swabs showed that above 90% of participants were MCPyV-positive, about half HPyV6-positive and about a quarter HPyV7-positive within the 12–18 weeks of period-1. The higher prevalence rates in period-1 compared to baseline are in line with incident infections of MCPyV, HPyV6, and HPyV7 in follow-up samples as reported by Hampras et al. (2015).

Short-term persistence was observed on both locations in over two-thirds of MCPyV-positive cases, which is in line with persistence rates on healthy skin found by Hashida et al. (2016) in 38 individuals who were reassessed 6 months after baseline sample. Hampras et al. (2015) observed comparable MCPyV persistence rates in normal skin and eyebrow hairs of healthy males, while HPyV6 and HPyV7 persistence were detected more frequently (73.0 and 37.5%, respectively) than in the present work. However, the definition of short-term persistence used here (three of four swabs positive) was stricter than the definition used by Hampras et al. (2015) (two positive consecutive swabs), and both studies differ in terms of population and sampling intervals. So far, no comparable data has been published on persistence of the remaining HPyVs investigated here. While no short-term persistence was observed for TSPyV and HPyV9, polyomaviruses HPyV10 and STLPyV persisted in both locations in 6–8%, which has not yet been shown for STLPyV.

Long-term persistence was observed for MCPyV in 39.0% (forehead) and 44.1% (hand), followed by HPyV6 (16.9 and 11.9%), HPyV7 (3.4 and 5.1%) and, in one case, STLPyV, while it did not occur in the other HPyVs investigated. However, a single negative follow-up swab does not definitely rule out long-term persistence, especially when short-term persistent individuals were lost to follow-up. A reduction of HPyV-positive individuals in collection period-2 (2021) might also be explained by frequent disinfection of the hands and contact reduction due to the COVID-19 pandemic. The finding that persistent infections with TSPyV did not occur supports the assumption that the clinical picture of trichodysplasia spinulosa is the result of primary TSPyV infection (Van Der Meijden et al., 2017; Borgogna et al., 2019).

Elevated HPyV DNA loads were associated both with short- and long-term persistence of the HPyVs investigated in the present study. This is in line with results from Hashida et al. (2016) for MCPyV's 6-month persistence and might be of clinical relevance. Possibly elevated cutaneous MCPyV loads could indicate an increased risk for later MCC development, since higher MCPyV loads are associated with long-term persistence and thus with possibly sustained oncogene expression and more chances for the viral genome to integrate into the host genome.

TABLE 7 | Risk factors for HPyVs short-term persistence on the forehead of healthy individuals found in univariable logistic regression analysis.

Candidate variables	n	MCPyV OR (95% CI[#])	MCPyV p-value[1]	HPyV6 OR (95% CI[#])	HPyV6 p-value[1]	HPyV7 OR (95% CI[#])	HPyV7 p-value[1]	HPyV10 OR (95% CI[#])	HPyV10 p-value[1]	STLPyV OR (95% CI[#])	STLPyV p-value[1]
Age (per decade)	109	1.28 (0.94–1.73)	0.114	**1.88** (1.33–2.67)	**<0.001**	**1.74** (1.15–2.62)	**0.009***	0.99 (0.57–1.74)	0.981	1.64 (0.98–2.74)	0.059
Sex (male vs. female)	109	**2.93** (1.28–6.66)	**0.011**	0.82 (0.33–2.01)	0.658	1.16 (0.33–4.06)	0.818	1.03 (0.22–4.84)	0.971	0.26 (0.03–2.29)	0.223
Smoking (yes vs. no)	109	1.11 (0.45–2.74)	0.821	0.95 (0.33–2.68)	0.915	0.29 (0.04–2.40)	0.252	1.30 (0.24–7.13)	0.763	0 (0)	0.998
Underlying disease (yes vs. no)	109	0.32 (0.06–1.81)	0.197	0.62 (0.07–5.60)	0.674	1.86 (0.20–17.54)	0.588	3.23 (0.32–32.25)	0.317	3.92 (0.38–40.19)	0.250
Multiplicity[2] (yes vs. no)	109	**5.14** (2.13–12.41)	**<0.001**	**33.27** (7.26–152.53)	**<0.001**	**7.42** (1.52–36.22)	**0.013**	**9.30** (1.08–80.16)	**0.042**	2.91 (0.51–16.59)	0.230

OR, odds ratio; CI, confidence interval.
[#]Exact Clopper–Pearson confidence intervals.
[1]p-values < 0.05 are significant and printed in bold.
[2]Defined as ≥2 different HPyVs at baseline.
**Not significant anymore in multivariable modeling.*
Short-term persistence did not occur in TSPyV and HPyV9. The risk factors found for MCPyV, HPyV6, HPyV7 and HPyV10 in univariable regression analysis were included in a multivariable logistic regression model and remained significant after adjustment for the other covariates, with the exception of age for HPyV7.

TABLE 8 | Risk factors for HPyVs long-term persistence on the forehead of healthy individuals found in univariable logistic regression analysis.

Candidate variables	n	MCPyV OR (95% CI[#])	MCPyV p-value[1]	HPyV6 OR (95% CI[#])	HPyV6 p-value[1]	HPyV7 OR (95% CI[#])	HPyV7 p-value[1]	STLPyV OR (95% CI[#])	STLPyV p-value[1]
Age (per decade)	109	1.34 (0.87–2.07)	0.186	**3.37** (1.64–6.92)	**0.001**	2.57 (0.91–7.22)	0.074	4.72 (0.55–40.81)	0.159
Sex (male vs. female)	109	2.48 (0.84–7.32)	0.100	1.05 (0.26–4.22)	0.942	0 (0)	0.998	0 (0)	0.998
Smoking (yes vs. no)	109	0.53 (0.12–2.23)	0.382	0.43 (0.05–3.83)	0.452	0 (0)	0.999	0 (0)	0.999
Underlying disease (yes vs. no)	109	0 (0)	1.000	>1 (0)	1.000	0 (0)	1.000	0 (0)	1.000
Multiplicity[2] (yes vs. no)	109	**3.75** (1.25–11.30)	**0.019**	**15.50** (1.81–132.54)	**0.012**	>1 (0)	0.998	>1 (0)	0.998

OR, odds ratio; CI, confidence interval.
[#]Exact Clopper–Pearson confidence intervals.
[1]p-values < 0.05 are significant.
[2]Defined as ≥2 different HPyVs at baseline.
Long-term persistence did not occur in TSPyV, HPyV9, and HPyV10. The risk factors found for MCPyV and HPyV6 in univariable regression analysis were included in a multivariable logistic regression model and remained significant after adjustment for the other covariates.

The major risk factor for baseline prevalence and short-term persistence of MCPyV, HPyV6, HPyV7, and HPyV10, as well as for long-term persistence of MCPyV and HPyV6 DNA found in multivariable regression analysis, was the detection of two or more HPyVs per swab (multiplicity) at baseline. Waning immunity in aging people may lead to enhanced viral replication. Concordantly, baseline prevalence for HPyV6, HPyV7, and STLPyV rose in participants aged 60 years and older. However, in multivariable regression analyses, older age remained only a risk factor for baseline prevalence, short- and long-term persistence of HPyV6. Increasing MCPyV, HPyV6, and HPyV7 prevalence with age has been described by other groups in eyebrow hairs but not in normal skin (Hampras et al., 2015; Hashida et al., 2016, 2018).

Male sex was an independent risk factor for MCPyV baseline prevalence and short-term persistence. According to literature, men are more likely to develop MCC than women (Stang et al., 2018). However, considering the widespread distribution of MCPyV, MCC development seems to be a rare multifactorial event with several risk factors such as UV radiation, older age and immunosuppression and is probably not solely due to the persistence of MCPyV in the skin (Foulongne et al., 2010a). Smoking was shown to be a risk factor for persistent human papillomavirus infections and subsequent development of anogenital warts, precancer, and cancer (Arcavi and Benowitz, 2004; Kaderli et al., 2014; Wieland et al., 2015). In contrast, current smoking was not associated with MCPyV prevalence in previous studies (Wieland et al., 2011; Hampras et al., 2015). This is in line with the present study showing that smoking was not a risk factor for prevalence or persistence of any HPyV.

Our results on prevalence and persistence of MCPyV, HPyV6, and HPyV7 are in concordance with serological studies in healthy individuals that found antibodies against MCPyV, HPyV6, and HPyV7 capsid proteins in 81.9, 83.8, and 71.7% of healthy blood donors, respectively (Kamminga et al., 2018). TSPyV- and HPyV9-specific antibodies were detected in 80–90% and >30–70%, respectively, and primary infection seems to occur during early childhood and adolescence (Foulongne et al., 2012; Nicol et al., 2013; Kamminga et al., 2018). Hence, it is possible that the skin is not the only tissue infected by these viruses. This notion is supported by several studies, in which TSPyV and HPyV9 were detected sporadically in tonsil tissue, faeces, respiratory samples, urine or peripheral blood, mainly in immunosuppressed persons (Rockett et al., 2013; Herberhold et al., 2017; Kourieh et al., 2018; Borgogna et al., 2019; Kamminga et al., 2019). In our study, short-term persistence rates of HPyV10 were low and long-term persistence did not occur, although HPyV10 reaches a seroprevalence rate of nearly 100% in adults (Kamminga et al., 2018). This indicates that the skin is only transiently infected and does not represent a permanent viral reservoir of HPyV10. HPyV10/MWPyV has been found in respiratory specimens, in 18.4% of tonsil cancer samples and in 5–7% of stool specimens from children and adults (Rockett et al., 2013; Herberhold et al., 2017; Pinheiro et al., 2020). The relatively high overall seroprevalence of STLPyV (64.8%) compared to the low DNA prevalence and persistence rate detected in our study also suggests sites of infection other than the skin, particularly the gut (Lim et al., 2013; Kamminga et al., 2018).

Limitations of our study are the high number of participants lost to long-term follow-up, and the fact that only a single swab pair was sampled in collection period-2. Furthermore, the number of participants 60 years and older was smaller than the number of participants in the other age groups and the sample was not representative of the German general population. We have not performed sequence analysis of the viral isolates and thus cannot exclude that persistent detection of the same HPyV represents new infections with different isolates instead of persistence of the same isolate. To corroborate our findings, future studies should include a larger number of participants of all ages and sexes, more frequent swab sampling during long-term follow-up and next-generation sequencing of individual samples. A strength of this study is that in contrast to previous studies (Wieland et al., 2011, 2014; Hampras et al., 2015), not only swabs from men but also from healthy women were included. Furthermore, the present study allowed comparison of HPyV prevalence, persistence and viral load in paired skin samples from two different body sites. To the best of our knowledge, this is the first study to collect long-term data over a decade on cutaneous HPyVs.

In summary, long-term persistence on the skin was shown for MCPyV, HPyV6, and HPyV7 on both forehead and hand. Higher viral loads and HPyV multiplicity were associated with short- and long-term persistence for several of the analysed HPyVs. In contrast to MCPyV, HPyV6, and HPyV7 and to a lesser extent STLPyV, polyomaviruses TSPyV and HPyV9 do not seem to be a regular part of the human skin virome in healthy individuals.

ETHICS STATEMENT

The studies involving human participants were reviewed and approved by Ethics review board of the faculty of medicine of the University of Cologne. The participants provided their written informed consent to participate in this study.

AUTHOR CONTRIBUTIONS

LB wrote the manuscript and made contributions to the analysis and interpretation of data. MH performed the statistical analyses. AK and HP made substantial contributions to sampling and critically revising the manuscript for important intellectual content. UW and SS designed the study, performed sampling, analysis and interpretation of data, and drafted the manuscript. All authors contributed to the article and approved the submitted version.

ACKNOWLEDGMENTS

Our expressed gratitude goes to all the volunteers without whose participation this study would not have been possible. We would like to thank Monika Junk, Nabila Ristow, and Jacqueline Frohnert for excellent technical assistance.

REFERENCES

Allander, T., Andreasson, K., Gupta, S., Bjerkner, A., Bogdanovic, G., Persson, M. A. A., et al. (2007). Identification of a third human Polyomavirus. *J. Virol.* 81, 4130–4136. doi: 10.1128/jvi.00028-07

Amorrortu, R. P., Zhao, Y., Messina, J. L., Schell, M. J., Fenske, N. A., Cherpelis, B. S., et al. (2021). Association between human polyomaviruses and keratinocyte carcinomas: a prospective cohort study. *Cancer Epidemiol. Biomarkers Prev.* 32:ceb0332. doi: 10.1158/1055-9965.epi-21-0332

Arcavi, L., and Benowitz, N. L. (2004). Cigarette smoking and infection. *Arch. Intern. Med.* 164, 2206–2216. doi: 10.1001/archinte.164.20.2206

Beckervordersandforth, J., Pujari, S., Rennspiess, D., Speel, E. J. M., Winnepenninckx, V., Diaz, C., et al. (2016). Frequent detection of human polyomavirus 6 in keratoacanthomas. *Diagn. Pathol.* 11, 10–16. doi: 10.1186/s13000-016-0509-z

Bialasiewicz, S., Rockett, R. J., Barraclough, K. A., Leary, D., Dudley, K. J., Isbel, N. M., et al. (2016). Detection of recently discovered human polyomaviruses in a longitudinal kidney transplant cohort. *Am. J. Transplant.* 16, 2734–2740. doi: 10.1111/ajt.13799

Borgogna, C., Albertini, S., Zavattaro, E., Veronese, F., Peruzzi, L., van der Meijden, E., et al. (2019). Primary trichodysplasia spinulosa polyomavirus infection in a kidney transplant child displaying virus-infected decoy cells in the urine. *J. Med. Virol.* 91, 1896–1900. doi: 10.1002/jmv.25519

Buck, C. B., Phan, G. Q., Raiji, M. T., Murphy, P. M., McDermott, D. H., and McBride, A. A. (2012). Complete genome sequence of a tenth human polyomavirus. *J. Virol.* 86:10887. doi: 10.1128/jvi.01690-12

Csoma, E., Bidiga, L., Méhes, G., Katona, M., and Gergely, L. (2018). Survey of KI. WU, MW, and STL Polyomavirus in cancerous and non-cancerous lung tissues. *Pathobiology* 85, 179–185. doi: 10.1159/000481174

Ehlers, B., and Wieland, U. (2013). The novel human polyomaviruses HPyV6, 7, 9 and beyond. *APMIS* 121, 783–795. doi: 10.1111/apm.12104

Feltkamp, M. C. W., Kazem, S., van der Meijden, E., Lauber, C., and Gorbalenya, A. E. (2013). From stockholm to malawi: recent developments in studying human polyomaviruses. *J. Gen. Virol.* 94, 482–496. doi: 10.1099/vir.0.048462-0

Feng, H., Shuda, M., Chang, Y., and Moore, P. S. (2008). Clonal integration of a polyomavirus in human Merkel cell carcinoma. *Science* 319, 1096–1100. doi: 10.1126/science.1152586

Foulongne, V., Kluger, N., Dereure, O., Mercier, G., Molès, J. P., Guillot, B., et al. (2010b). Merkel cell polyomavirus in cutaneous swabs. *Emerg. Infect. Dis.* 16, 685–687. doi: 10.3201/eid1604.091278

Foulongne, V., Dereure, O., Kluger, N., Molès, J. P., Guillot, B., and Segondy, M. (2010a). Merkel cell polyomavirus DNA detection in lesional and nonlesional skin from patients with Merkel cell carcinoma or other skin diseases. *Br. J. Dermatol.* 162, 59–63. doi: 10.1111/j.1365-2133.2009.09381.x

Foulongne, V., Sauvage, V., Hebert, C., Dereure, O., Cheval, J., Gouilh, M. A., et al. (2012). Human skin Microbiota: high diversity of DNA viruses identified on the human skin by high throughput sequencing. *PLoS One* 7:e38499. doi: 10.1371/journal.pone.0038499

Gardner, S. D., Field, A. M., Coleman, D. V., and Hulme, B. (1971). New human papovavirus (B.K.) isolated from urine after renal transplantation. *Lancet* 1, 1253–1257.

Gaynor, A. M., Nissen, M. D., Whiley, D. M., Mackay, I. M., Lambert, S. B., Wu, G., et al. (2007). Identification of a novel polyomavirus from patients with acute respiratory tract infections. *PLoS Pathog.* 3, 0595–0604. doi: 10.1371/journal.ppat.0030064

Gheit, T., Dutta, S., Oliver, J., Robitaille, A., Hampras, S., Combes, J. D., et al. (2017). Isolation and characterization of a novel putative human polyomavirus. *Virology* 506, 45–54. doi: 10.1016/j.virol.2017.03.007

Gossai, A., Waterboer, T., Nelson, H. H., Michel, A., Willhauck-Fleckenstein, M., Farzan, S. F., et al. (2016). Seroepidemiology of human polyomaviruses in a US population. *Am. J. Epidemiol.* 183, 61–69. doi: 10.1093/aje/kwv155

Haeggblom, L., Franzén, J., and Näsman, A. (2017). Human polyomavirus DNA detection in keratoacanthoma and Spitz naevus: no evidence for a causal role. *J. Clin. Pathol.* 70, 451–453. doi: 10.1136/jclinpath-2016-204197

Hampras, S. S., Giuliano, A. R., Lin, H. Y., Fisher, K. J., Abrahamsen, M. E., McKay-Chopin, S., et al. (2015). Natural history of polyomaviruses in men: the HPV infection in Men (HIM) study. *J. Infect. Dis.* 211, 1437–1446. doi: 10.1093/infdis/jiu626

Hashida, Y., Higuchi, T., Matsuzaki, S., Nakajima, K., Sano, S., and Daibata, M. (2018). Prevalence and genetic variability of human polyomaviruses 6 and 7 in healthy skin among asymptomatic individuals. *J. Infect. Dis.* 217, 483–493. doi: 10.1093/infdis/jix516

Hashida, Y., Kamioka, M., Tanaka, M., Hosokawa, S., Murakami, M., Nakajima, K., et al. (2016). Ecology of merkel cell polyomavirus in healthy skin among individuals in an asian cohort. *J. Infect. Dis.* 213, 1708–1716. doi: 10.1093/infdis/jiw040

Herberhold, S., Hellmich, M., Panning, M., Bartok, E., Silling, S., Akgül, B., et al. (2017). Human polyomavirus and human papillomavirus prevalence and viral load in non-malignant tonsillar tissue and tonsillar carcinoma. *Med. Microbiol. Immunol.* 206, 93–103. doi: 10.1007/s00430-016-0486-6

Ho, J., Jedrych, J. J., Feng, H., Natalie, A. A., Grandinetti, L., Mirvish, E., et al. (2015). Human polyomavirus 7-associated pruritic rash and viremia in transplant recipients. *J. Infect. Dis.* 211, 1560–1565. doi: 10.1093/infdis/jiu524

Kaderli, R., Schnüriger, B., and Brügger, L. E. (2014). The impact of smoking on HPV infection and the development of anogenital warts. *Int. J. Colorectal Dis.* 29, 899–908. doi: 10.1007/s00384-014-1922-y

Kamminga, S., van der Meijden, E., de Brouwer, C., Feltkamp, M., and Zaaijer, H. (2019). Prevalence of DNA of fourteen human polyomaviruses determined in blood donors. *Transfusion* 59, 3689–3697. doi: 10.1111/trf.15557

Kamminga, S., van der Meijden, E., Feltkamp, M. C. W., and Zaaijer, H. L. (2018). Seroprevalence of fourteen human polyomaviruses determined in blood donors. *bioRxiv* [Preprint]. doi: 10.1101/357350

Kazem, S., van der Meijden, E., and Feltkamp, M. C. W. (2013). The trichodysplasia spinulosa-associated polyomavirus: virological background and clinical implications. *APMIS* 121, 770–782. doi: 10.1111/apm.12092

Keijzers, M., Rensspiess, D., Pujari, S., Abdul-Hamid, M. A., Hochstenbag, M., Dingemans, A. M., et al. (2015). Expression of pRb and p16INK4 in human thymic epithelial tumors in relation to the presence of human polyomavirus 7. *Diagn. Pathol.* 10, 6–11. doi: 10.1186/s13000-015-0418-6

Klufah, F., Mobaraki, G., Liu, D., Alharbi, R. A., Kurz, A. K., Speel, E. J. M., et al. (2021). Emerging role of human polyomaviruses 6 and 7 in human cancers. *Infect. Agent. Cancer* 16:35. doi: 10.1186/s13027-021-00374-3

Korup, S., Rietscher, J., Calvignac-Spencer, S., Trusch, F., Hofmann, J., Moens, U., et al. (2013). Identification of a novel human polyomavirus in organs of the gastrointestinal tract. *PLoS One* 8:e58021. doi: 10.1371/journal.pone.0058021

Kourieh, A., Combes, J. D., Tommasino, M., Dalstein, V., Clifford, G. M., St Guily, J. L., et al. (2018). Prevalence and risk factors of human polyomavirus infections in non-malignant tonsils and gargles: the SPLIT study. *J. Gen. Virol.* 99, 1686–1698. doi: 10.1099/jgv.0.001156

Lim, E. S., Reyes, A., Antonio, M., Saha, D., Ikumapayi, U. N., Adeyemi, M., et al. (2013). Discovery of STL polyomavirus, a polyomavirus of ancestral recombinant origin that encodes a unique T antigen by alternative splicing. *Virology* 436, 295–303. doi: 10.1016/j.virol.2012.12.005

Mishra, N., Pereira, M., Rhodes, R. H., An, P., Pipas, J. M., Jain, K., et al. (2014). Identification of a novel Polyomavirus in a pancreatic transplant recipient with retinal blindness and Vasculitic Myopathy. *J. Infect. Dis.* 210, 1595–1599. doi: 10.1093/infdis/jiu250

Moens, U., Krumbholz, A., Ehlers, B., Zell, R., Johne, R., Calvignac-Spencer, S., et al. (2017). Biology, evolution, and medical importance of polyomaviruses: an update. *Infect. Genet. Evol.* 54, 18–38. doi: 10.1016/j.meegid.2017.06.011

Nguyen, K. D., Lee, E. E., Yue, Y., Stork, J., Pock, L., North, J. P., et al. (2017). Human polyomavirus 6 and 7 are associated with pruritic and dyskeratotic dermatoses. *J. Am. Acad. Dermatol.* 76, 932.e–940.e. doi: 10.1016/j.jaad.2016.11.035

Nicol, J. T. J., Robinot, R., Carpentier, A., Carandina, G., Mazzoni, E., Tognon, M., et al. (2013). Age-specific seroprevalences of merkel cell polyomavirus, human polyomaviruses 6, 7, and 9, and trichodysplasia spinulosa-associated polyomavirus. *Clin. Vaccine Immunol.* 20, 363–368. doi: 10.1128/CVI.00438-12

Ondov, B. D., Starrett, G. J., Sappington, A., Kostic, A., Koren, S., Buck, C. B., et al. (2019). Mash Screen: high-throughput sequence containment estimation for genome discovery. *Genome Biol.* 20:232. doi: 10.1186/s13059-019-1841-x

Padgett, B. L., Zurhein, G. M., Walker, D. L., Eckroade, R. J., and Dessel, B. H. (1971). Case of progressive multifocal leucoencephalopathy (P.M. L.) complicating Case-report. *Lancet* 297, 1257–1260.

Pastrana, D. V., FitzGerald, P. C., Phan, G. Q., Raiji, M. T., Murphy, P. M., McDermott, D. H., et al. (2013). A divergent variant of the eleventh human polyomavirus species, Saint Louis polyomavirus. *Genome Announc.* 1, e00812–e00813. doi: 10.1128/genomeA.e00812-13

Pastrana, D. V., Wieland, U., Silling, S., Buck, C. B., and Pfister, H. (2012). Positive correlation between Merkel cell polyomavirus viral load and capsid-specific antibody titer. *Med. Microbiol. Immunol.* 201, 17–23. doi: 10.1007/s00430-011-0200-7

Peng, J., Li, K., Zhang, C., and Jin, Q. (2016). MW polyomavirus and STL polyomavirus present in tonsillar tissues from children with chronic tonsillar disease. *Clin. Microbiol. Infect* 22, e1–e97. doi: 10.1016/j.cmi.2015.08.028

Pinheiro, M. S., Mendes, G. S., and Santos, N. (2020). Human polyomaviruses 10 and 11 in faecal samples from Brazilian children. *Brazilian J. Microbiol.* 51, 585–591. doi: 10.1007/s42770-019-00166-3

Prezioso, C., Van Ghelue, M., Pietropaolo, V., and Moens, U. (2021). Detection of quebec polyomavirus dna in samples from different patient groups. *Microorganisms* 9:1082. doi: 10.3390/microorganisms9051082

Rennspiess, D., Pujari, S., Keijzers, M., Abdul-Hamid, M. A., Hochstenbag, M., Dingemans, A. M., et al. (2015). Detection of human polyomavirus 7 in human thymic epithelial tumors. *J. Thorac. Oncol.* 10, 360–366. doi: 10.1097/JTO.0000000000000390

Rockett, R. J., Sloots, T. P., Bowes, S., O'Neill, N., Ye, S., Robson, J., et al. (2013). Detection of Novel Polyomaviruses. TSPyV, HPyV6, HPyV7, HPyV9 and MWPyV in feces, urine, blood, respiratory swabs and cerebrospinal fluid. *PLoS One* 8:e62764. doi: 10.1371/journal.pone.0062764

Schowalter, R. M., Pastrana, D. V., Pumphrey, K. A., Moyer, A. L., and Buck, C. B. (2010). Merkel cell polyomavirus and two previously unknown polyomaviruses are chronically shed from human skin. *Cell Host Microbe* 7, 509–515. doi: 10.1016/j.chom.2010.05.006

Schrama, D., Groesser, L., Ugurel, S., Hafner, C., Pastrana, D. V., Buck, C. B., et al. (2014). Presence of human polyomavirus 6 in mutation-Specific braf inhibitor-Induced epithelial proliferations. *JAMA Dermatol.* 150, 1180–1186. doi: 10.1001/jamadermatol.2014.1116

Scola, N., Wieland, U., Silling, S., Altmeyer, P., Stücker, M., and Kreuter, A. (2012). Prevalence of human polyomaviruses in common and rare types of non-Merkel cell carcinoma skin cancer. *Br. J. Dermatol.* 167, 1315–1320. doi: 10.1111/j.1365-2133.2012.11141.x

Scuda, N., Hofmann, J., Calvignac-Spencer, S., Ruprecht, K., Liman, P., Kuhn, J., et al. (2011). A novel human polyomavirus closely related to the african green monkey-derived lymphotropic polyomavirus. *J. Virol.* 85, 4586–4590. doi: 10.1128/jvi.02602-10

Siebrasse, E. A., Reyes, A., Lim, E. S., Zhao, G., Mkakosya, R. S., Manary, M. J., et al. (2012). Identification of MW polyomavirus, a novel polyomavirus in human stool. *J. Virol.* 86, 10321–10326. doi: 10.1128/jvi.01210-12

Stang, A., Becker, J. C., Nghiem, P., and Ferlay, J. (2018). The association between geographic location and incidence of Merkel cell carcinoma in comparison to melanoma: an international assessment. *Eur. J. Cancer* 94, 47–60. doi: 10.1016/j.ejca.2018.02.003

Van Der Meijden, E., Bialasiewicz, S., Rockett, R. J., Tozer, S. J., Sloots, T. P., and Feltkamp, M. C. W. (2013). Different serologic behavior of MCPyV. TSPyV, HPyV6, HPyV7 and HPyV9 polyomaviruses found on the skin. *PLoS One* 8:e81078. doi: 10.1371/journal.pone.0081078

Van Der Meijden, E., Horváth, B., Nijland, M., De Vries, K., Rácz, E., Diercks, G. F., et al. (2017). Primary polyomavirus infection, not reactivation, as the cause of trichodysplasia spinulosa in immunocompromised patients. *J. Infect. Dis.* 215, 1080–1084. doi: 10.1093/infdis/jiw403

van der Meijden, E., Janssens, R. W. A., Lauber, C., Bavinck, J. N. B., Gorbalenya, A. E., and Feltkamp, M. C. W. (2010). Discovery of a new human polyomavirus associated with Trichodysplasia Spinulosa in an immunocompromized patient. *PLoS Pathog.* 6:e1001024. doi: 10.1371/journal.ppat.1001024

Van Duin, M., Snijders, P. J. F., Schrijnemakers, H. F. J., Voorhorst, F. J., Rozendaal, L., Nobbenhuis, M. A. E., et al. (2002). Human papillomavirus 16 load in normal and abnormal cervical scrapes: an indicator of CIN II/III and viral clearance. *Int. J. Cancer* 98, 590–595. doi: 10.1002/ijc.10232

Wang, Y., Keinonen, A., Koskenmies, S., Pitkänen, S., Fyhrquist, N., Sadeghi, M., et al. (2019). Occurrence of newly discovered human polyomaviruses in skin of liver transplant recipients and their relation with squamous cell carcinoma in situ and actinic keratosis – a single-center cohort study. *Transpl. Int.* 32, 516–522. doi: 10.1111/tri.13397

Weissenborn, S. J., De Koning, M. N. C., Wieland, U., Quint, W. G. V., and Pfister, H. J. (2009). Intrafamilial transmission and family-specific spectra of cutaneous betapapillomaviruses. *J. Virol.* 83, 811–816. doi: 10.1128/jvi.01338-08

Weissenborn, S. J., Wieland, U., Junk, M., and Pfister, H. (2010). Quantification of beta-human papillomavirus DNA by real-time PCR. *Nat. Protoc.* 5, 1–13. doi: 10.1038/nprot.2009.153

Wieland, U., Hellmich, M., Wetendorf, J., Potthoff, A., Höfler, D., Swoboda, J., et al. (2015). Smoking and anal high-risk human papillomavirus DNA loads in HIV-positive men who have sex with men. *Int. J. Med. Microbiol.* 305, 689–696. doi: 10.1016/j.ijmm.2015.08.019

Wieland, U., Silling, S., Hellmich, M., Potthoff, A., Pfister, H., and Kreuter, A. (2014). Human polyomaviruses 6, 7, 9, 10 and trichodysplasia spinulosa-associated polyomavirus in HIV-infected men. *J. Gen. Virol.* 95, 928–932. doi: 10.1099/vir.0.061259-0

Wieland, U., Silling, S., Scola, N., Potthoff, A., Gambichler, T., Brockmeyer, N. H., et al. (2011). Merkel cell polyomavirus infection in HIV-positive men. *Arch. Dermatol.* 147, 401–406. doi: 10.1001/archdermatol.2011.42

2

Detection of Merkel Cell Polyomavirus in Seborrheic Keratosis

*Lisa M. Hillen[1], Dorit Rennspiess[1], Ernst-Jan Speel[1], Anke M. Haugg[2], Véronique Winnepenninckx[1] and Axel zur Hausen[1]**

[1] *Department of Pathology and GROW-School for Oncology and Developmental Biology, Maastricht University Medical Center, Maastricht, Netherlands,* [2] *Department of Gynaecology, University Hospital RWTH Aachen, Aachen, Germany*

Correspondence:
Axel zur Hausen
axel.zurhausen@mumc.nl

Seborrheic keratosis (SK) is the most common benign cutaneous neoplasm. A subset shows increased p16 expression. Since SK shares several features with verruca vulgaris, e.g., increased p16 expression, human papillomaviruses (HPV) have been suggested as possible causal agents. However, a relevant association could not be established between HPV and SK. In the present study we aimed to investigate the presence of Merkel cell polyomavirus (MCPyV) in relation to p16 expression in SK. P16 expression was investigated using immunohistochemistry (IHC). Presence of MCPyV was assessed in 23 formalin-fixed paraffin-embedded tissue samples of SK by molecular techniques (i.e., PCR and FISH) and IHC. 16/23 SK showed strong to moderate p16 expression. 6/23 of SK were MCPyV positive by PCR which was confirmed by FISH. Of interest, two samples with strong FISH signals also showed MCPyV expression as tested by IHC. Samples with weaker signal intensity were negative in IHC. P16 expression was not associated with the presence of MCPyV. Concluding, the detection of MCPyV DNA by PCR and FISH in SK reflects the widespread prevalence of MCPyV in the skin. However, low detection rates exclude MCPyV as a major pathogenic factor in SK, most likely representing a coincidental infection. P16 IHC does not appear as useful adjunctive surrogate marker for the presence of MCPyV in SK.

Keywords: seborrheic keratosis, Merkel cell polyomavirus, MCPyV, p16, fluorescence *in situ* hybridization, FISH, immunohistochemistry, IHC

INTRODUCTION

Seborrheic keratosis (SK) is the most frequent benign human skin proliferation, with increasing incidence in the elderly. The preferential localization is on the chest, interscapular region, waistline, and forehead (Yeatman et al., 1997; Kyriakis et al., 2012). SK shares several clinical and histopathological features with verruca vulgaris and condyloma acuminatum including increased p16 expression which is a tumor-suppressor protein and cyclin-dependent kinase (cdk) inhibitor (Chazal et al., 2002; Hodges and Smoller, 2002; Nakamura and Nishioka, 2003; Genders et al., 2017). Assessment of p16 protein expression by immunohistochemistry (IHC) is frequently used as a surrogate marker for human papillomavirus (HPV) infection in genital and oropharyngeal cancers (Dehn et al., 2007; Shelton et al., 2017). HPV infection has been suggested as a possible causative agent in SK, however a higher prevalence of HPV was only detected in subgroups of genital SK in comparison to non-genital SK, thereby excluding HPV to play a major pathogenic role (Zhu et al., 1991, 1992; Gushi et al., 2003; Nakamura and Nishioka, 2003; Tardío et al., 2012). Limited data is available concerning a possible role of p16 expression in SK and association with Merkel cell polyomavirus (MCPyV; Andres et al., 2010; Mertz et al., 2010). Similar to HPV, MCPyV is composed of a circular double-stranded DNA genome, possesses an icosahedral capsid symmetry, a homologous LxCxE motive in the encoded Retinoblastoma (Rb) binding site (Felsani et al., 2006; Shuda et al., 2008), and has a similar genome size (approximately 5,600 bp for MCPyV and 8,000 bp for HPV). In high risk HPV infection the Rb protein is inactivated resulting in cell cycle progression. As a consequence p16 expression is upregulated. Approximately 80% of Merkel cell carcinomas (MCC), a rare highly aggressive neuroendocrine skin cancer, are associated with MCPyV infection (Feng et al., 2008; Kassem et al., 2008). Interestingly, MCC and SK share several risk factors, such as long-term sun exposure, older age, and immunosuppression. Based on these findings we investigated p16 IHC expression in SK and tested for the presence of MCPyV using IHC and molecular methods (FISH and PCR).

MATERIALS AND METHODS

Patients and Tissues

Formalin-fixed and paraffin-embedded (FFPE) tissues of 23 skin specimens were included in this study. All respective samples had been excised for diagnostic and therapeutic reasons and were obtained from the Maastricht Pathology Tissue Collection (MPTC). All use of tissue and patient data was in agreement with the Dutch Code of Conduct for Observational Research with Personal Data (2004) and Tissue (Federatie van Medisch Wetenschappelijke Verenigingen, FMWV, https://www.federa.org/) with written informed consent from all subjects in accordance with the Declaration of Helsinki. The protocol was approved by the Maastricht Ethic Committee (MEC) group. Diagnoses were previously defined by histology in routine diagnostics and have been reviewed by 3 experienced dermatopathologists (VW, AzH, LMH). The patient group consisted of 9 men and 13 women (ages 34–79; mean 58.8). Further details of the clinicopathologic parameters are included in **Table 1**. Serial sections of the specimens were used for hematoxylin and eosin (H.E.) staining, IHC, fluorescence *in situ* hybridization (FISH) and DNA isolation. In addition 16 non-neoplastic skin specimens originating from patients undergoing plastic surgery were tested (ages 18–63 year; mean 41.4 year).

Immunohistochemistry (IHC)

The following antibodies and dilutions were used in this study: anti-LT MCPyV (clone: CM2B4, dilution 1:50, Santa Cruz, Inc.), anti-p16 (clone: JCS, dilution 1:400, Santa Cruz, Inc.). Immunohistochemical stainings were conducted on a Dako Autostainer Link 48 using the EnVision FLEX Visualization Kit K8008 DAKO according to standard diagnostic routine protocols and manufacturers' instructions. P16 expression was correlated with the results obtained by MCPyV FISH and PCR data as described earlier (Hopman et al., 2005; Mertz et al., 2013; Haugg et al., 2014). P16 expression was evaluated by 4 experienced investigators (AzH, VW, DR, LH) with − as negative, + as moderate and ++ as strong positive score (**Figure 1**).

Five consecutive 10 μm thick sections were cut from each FFPE tissue. After deparaffinization, the tissues were lysed with proteinase K overnight (56°C) until complete tissue lysis, and DNA was extracted using a DNA Isolation QIAamp minikit (Qiagen, Hilden, Germany). Purified DNA was measured in a spectrophotometer (Nanodrop, 2000; Thermo Scientific). DNA quality and integrity were assessed by a specimen control size (SCS) ladder (**Table 1**) as described earlier (van Dongen et al., 2003). Inadequate samples were excluded from further study.

Polymerase Chain Reaction (PCR)

PCR was performed with 150 ng of genomic DNA using the AmpliTaq Gold (Roche) DNA polymerase in a final volume of 50 μl. For MCPyV detection we used the VP1 and M1M2 primer sets and PCR conditions as published earlier (Feng et al., 2008; Kassem et al., 2008). Negative controls with water instead of patient samples were included in each amplification series.

Sequence Analysis

PCR products were submitted to automated nucleotide sequencing in an ABI 3130XL genetic analyser (ABI). DNA sequences were compared and analyzed with the reference sequences of the National Center for Biotechnology Information (NCBI) Entrez Nucleotide database gb EU375803.1 (MCC isolate 350) and gb EU375804.1 (MCC isolate 339) using the NCBI Blast program. Multiple sequence alignments were performed with Clustal W2 (EMBL-EBI-2015).

MCPyV Fluorescence *in situ* Hybridization (FISH) Probe

FISH was optimized and performed as described earlier (Hopman et al., 2005; Haugg et al., 2011, 2014). In brief, full length (5104 bp) MCPyV DNA was cloned into a StrataClone PCR Cloning Vector (pSC-A-amp/kan; Stratagene, Santa Clara, CA). The Plasmid DNA Purification Kit NucleoBond® PC 2000 (Macherey-Nagel, Dueren, Germany) was used to extract MCPyV plasmid DNA and sequenced using T7 and T3 primers. Labeling of the DNA was performed by standard nick translation with Biotin-Nick Translation Mix (Roche, Mannheim, Germany) containing biotin (Bio)-16-dUTPs. The final concentration of the labeled DNA was 2 ng/μl in 50% formamide, 20% dextran sulfate, 2x SSC pH 7.0, 50x excess carrier DNA from salmon sperm (Sigma Chemical, St. Louis, MO) and 50x tRNA from S. cerevisiae (Sigma Chemical, St. Louis, MO).

Detection of MCPyV by FISH MCPyV

Deparaffinized 3 μm thick sections were pretreated for 20 min with 0.2 M HCl, incubated with 1 M NaSCN for 30 min at 80°C, washed in dH_2O and 2x SCC and digested with 1 mg/ml pepsin (2,500–3,500 U/mg, Sigma Chemical, St. Louis, MO) in 0.14 M NaCl solution, pH2. The biotin labeled full length MCPyV DNA probe was added to the samples at a concentration of 5 ng/μl followed by denaturation of DNA (5 min, 80°C) and hybridization overnight (37°C, humid chamber, Thermobrite, Abbott, IL). Unbound MCPyV DNA probe was stringently washed away in 2x SSC, pH7

TABLE 1 | Summary of clinicopathological data, immunohistochemical staining and molecular results.

Lab ID	Age	G	Localization	P16 IHC	SCS	PCR MCPyV M1M2	PCR MCPyV VP1	FISH MCPyV	IHC MCPyV
VS1.1	55	f	Breast	+	+	+	+	+	−
VS2.2	79	f	Back	++	+	−	−	NA	−
VS4.1	58	f	Head	++	+	−	−	−	−
VS5.1	49	f	Back	−	+	+	+	+	−
VS6.1	70	f	Back	−	+	−	−	−	−
VS8.1	52	f	Head	++	+	+	−	+	−
VS10.1	65	f	Breast	+	+	+	−	+	−
VS11.1	56	m	Head	+	+	+	−	++	+
VS12.1	34	f	Axilla	−	+	−	−	−	−
VS13.1	59	f	Head	++	+	+	−	++	+
VS14.1	58	m	NA	−	+	−	−	NA	NA
VS15.2	59	m	Back	+	+	−	−	NA	NA
VS16.2	68	f	Head	+	+	−	−	NA	NA
VS17.2	47	f	Head	++	+	−	−	NA	NA
VS19.2	49	f	Head	−	+	−	−	NA	NA
VS20.2	73	m	Back	−	+	−	−	NA	NA
VS25.2	60	f	Breast	+	+	−	−	NA	NA
VS30.2	73	m	Back	+	+	−	−	NA	NA
VS37.2	58	f	Breast	++	+	−	−	NA	NA
VS38.2	73	m	Back	++	+	−	−	NA	NA
VS53.2	58	m	Head	++	+	−	−	NA	NA
VS54.2	54	m	Back	−	+	−	−	NA	NA
VS56.2	45	m	Back	+	+	−	−	NA	NA
Total: 23 samples	Mean: 58.8 year, SD 10.6 year	f (n = 14, 60.9%) m (n = 9, 39.1%)		++ 8/23 (34.8%) + 8/23 (34.8%) − 7/23 (30.4%)		6/23 26.1%	2/23 8.7%	6/23 26.1%	2/23 8.7%

f, female; FISH, fluorescence in situ hybridization using full length MCPyV as probe with ++, strong, +, moderate, and −, negative nuclear signal pattern; G, gender; p16 IHC, immunohistochemistry using p16 with ++, strong; +; moderate; −, negative staining pattern; Lab ID, laboratory identification; m, Male; M1M2 PCR, PCR amplifying the M1M2 PCR product (178 bp); NA, not applicable; SCS ladder, specimen control size ladder; SD, standard deviation; VP1, PCR amplifying the viral capsid protein 1 (VP1) gen (315 bp); y, years.

at 70°C for 2 min. Bound probe was detected by sequential incubation in a combination of fluorescein isothiocyanate (FITC) biotinylated avidin (AvFITC; 1:500; Vector, Brunswig Chemie, Amsterdam, The Netherlands) and biotin conjugated goat antiavidin (BioGaA; 1:100; Vector). Prior to incubation aspecific binding sites were blocked with Boehringer Blocking reagent. Cell nuclei were counterstained and coverslipped with 4,6-diamidino-2-phenylindole dihydrochloride (DAPI; 0.2 μg/ml, Vectashield, Vector Laboratories, CA). Samples were visualized using a DM 5000B fluorescence microscope (Leica, Wetzlar, Germany) coupled to an online digital camera (Leica DC 300 Fx) for independent evaluation of FISH signals by 3 investigators (AzH, DR, LH) according to criteria described earlier (Hafkamp et al., 2008; Haugg et al., 2014).

Statistics

Data analysis was performed by SPSS statistical software (SPSS for windows, release 23.0; SPSS Inc., Chicago, IL, USA). Dichotomous variables were compared using the Pearson's chi-square test or Fisher's exact test as appropriate. The Spearman's rank correlation was used in nonparametric data to study the associations between different variables. A two-sided *P-value* less than 0.05 was considered statistically significant.

RESULTS

P16 Expression in SK

In total 16/23 (69.6%) of SK samples showed increased p16 expression in comparison to normal adjacent perilesional skin in all 16 samples. 8/23 (34.8%) showed strong (++) nuclear as well as cytoplasmatic p16 expression of the keratinocytes patchy scattered throughout the lesions. 8/23 (34.8%) showed a moderate (+) patchy p16 staining profile. 7/23 (30.4%) samples were negative for p16 expression (**Figure 1** and **Table 1**).

MCPyV Detection in SK by PCR, FISH, and IHC

PCR directed against diverse regions of the viral genome revealed that 6/23 (26.1%) of SK were MCPyV positive, including the viral M1M2 PCR product and in two cases the VP1 PCR product (**Table 1**). Sequence analyses of the PCR amplicons identified all PCR products as MCPyV DNA sequences. In the non-neoplastic

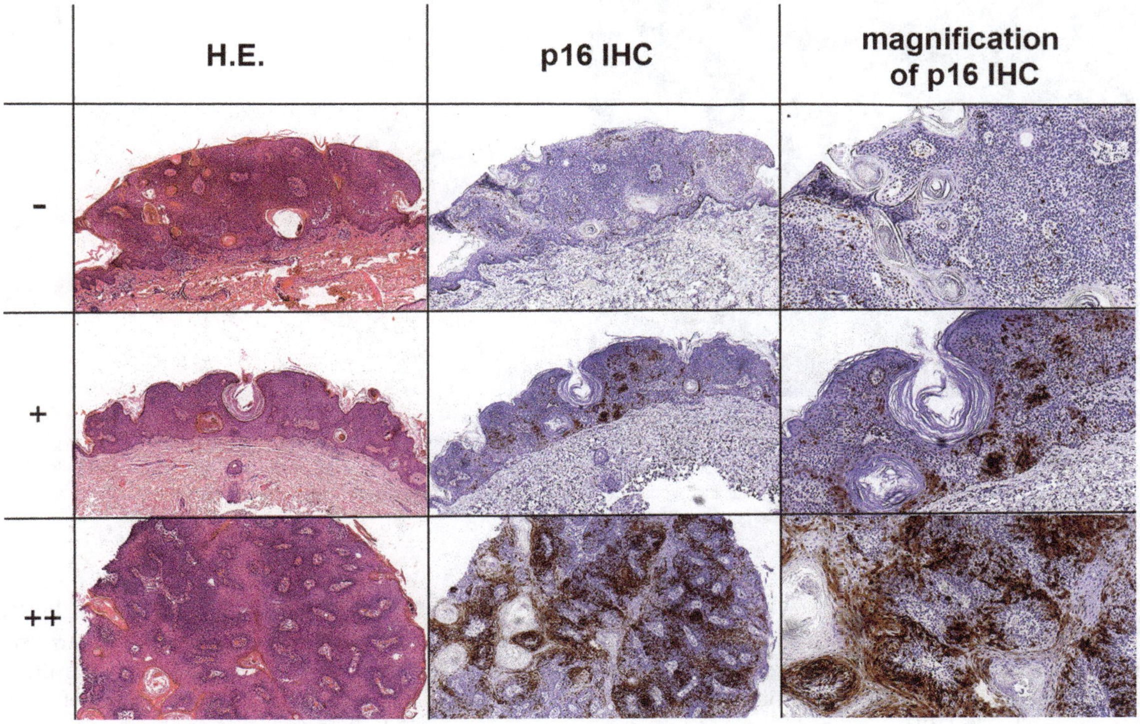

FIGURE 1 | P16 IHC expression in SK. Three representative SK samples with H.E. staining and p16 IHC. The top images show a negative (–) score, center images a moderate (+) positive score, and bottom images a strong (++) positive score with nuclear and cytoplasmic staining for p16 in SK. The magnification of all pictures is 10x, with exception of the pictures in the very right row (top and center plot magnification: 20x; bottom plot magnification: 40x).

skin specimens the presence of MCPyV PCR products was detected in 3/16 (18.8%) cases (data not shown). Results from PCR analyses could be confirmed by MCPyV FISH revealing nuclear hybridization with a punctual signal pattern in 6/23 (26.1%) of SK (**Figure 2A** and **Table 1**). In sample 11 and 13 there was a strong (++) nuclear signal pattern with FISH analyses. In sample 1, 5, 8, and 10 FISH signal intensity was moderate (+) and presence of MCPyV could be confirmed on PCR level, but was not detected by IHC. By IHC sample 11 and 13 (2/23, 8.7%) showed nuclear positivity for MCPyV large T (LT) antigen. The nuclear staining was seen in keratinocytes of SK and partly in surrounding intracapillary blood cells that resembled lymphocytes (**Figure 2B**). Molecular analyses with PCR and FISH were in good agreement (MCPyV M1M2 PCR vs. FISH with $p = 0.03$ and MCPyV VP1 PCR vs. FISH with $p = 0.6$). Importantly, specific nuclear hybridization signals of MCPyV were in several samples not only restricted to intralesional keratinocytes, but also seen in the adjacent preexistent skin. Thoroughly tested MCPyV-PCR negative cases subjected to FISH analyses and IHC staining remained negative for MCPyV.

No Correlation of p16 Expression with MCPyV in SK

P16 expression was neither associated with presence of MCPyV on the DNA level ($p = 0.69$ for the M1M2 PCR product, $p = 0.34$ for the VP1 PCR product) nor on the translational level ($p = 0.91$). Furthermore there was no significant correlation of p16 expression with clinicopathological data (i.e., age, gender or localization of the lesions, **Table 1**).

DISCUSSION

In this study, we systematically evaluated p16 expression and the presence of MCPyV in SK and normal skin on the DNA and on the translational level by IHC. We were able to correlate molecular PCR results with the presence of viral DNA at a single cell level visualized by FISH analyses.

In our study 16/23 (69.6%) of SK showed a patchy moderate to strong p16 expression, and 7/23 (30.4%) of SK were negative for p16 in IHC. These findings are consistent with previous observations reporting 65% of SK with a patchy p16 expression profile and 35% of SK to be negative for p16 (Harvey et al., 2013). In another study 75% of benign keratotic lesions (including 11 SK and 5 verruca vulgaris) showed p16 staining including two SK lesions with intense p16 staining profile (Genders et al., 2017). Since the discovery of p16 in 1993 (Serrano et al., 1993), there has been an ongoing, controversial discussion concerning the meaning of increased p16 expression, which acts as a cyclin dependent kinase (CDK) inhibitor and specifically blocks CDK4 and CDK6. This blockade leads to decreased phosphorylation of Rb protein with subsequent arrest in the G1 phase of the cell cycle (Sharpless and DePinho, 1999). In general three major

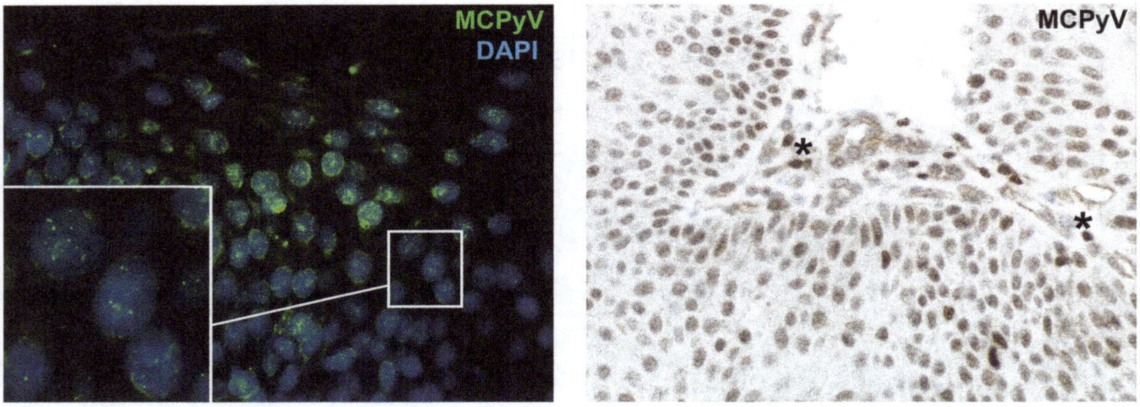

FIGURE 2 | Presence of MCPyV detected by FISH and IHC in SK. **(A)** MCPyV DNA sequence nuclear hybridization signals visualized by FISH in the keratinocytes of the lesion (green); DAPI staining depicts the nuclei of the keratinocytes (blue) with a magnification of 63x. The white square shows a high magnification of nuclei to better illustrate the punctuate hybridization pattern. **(B)** IHC staining directed against MCPyV-LT antigen shows nuclear signals in the keratinocytes as well as in intracapillary blood cells, resembling lymphocytes (see *) with a magnification of 40x.

interpretational lines are followed in case of increased p16 expression in human epithelial cells: (i) p16 and its role as tumor progression marker (Nilsson et al., 2004; Conscience et al., 2006; Bagazgoitia et al., 2010; Harvey et al., 2013), (ii) p16 expression as virus surrogate marker in HPV associated lesions (Klaes et al., 2002; Nilsson et al., 2004; Horn et al., 2008; Schache et al., 2011), and (iii) p16 as a marker for cell senescence (Pavey et al., 1999, 2001; Nakamura and Nishioka, 2003; Vun et al., 2006; Liu et al., 2009; Donati et al., 2013; Shelton et al., 2017). In SK enhanced p16 expression has been mainly attributed to cell senescence and UV-exposure related photo-aging (Pavey et al., 1999, 2001; Nakamura and Nishioka, 2003; Liu et al., 2009; Donati et al., 2013). In the background of cutaneous lesions increased p16 expression has also been associated with malignant progression in actinic keratosis and Bowen's disease (Hodges and Smoller, 2002; Nilsson et al., 2004; Conscience et al., 2006; Bagazgoitia et al., 2010; Harvey et al., 2013). However, this interpretational approach seems not to account for increased p16 expression in SK, in which malignant transformation remains an extremely rare event (Vun et al., 2006; Rajabi et al., 2012; Conic et al., 2017). In the background of virus infection p16 IHC is a well-established surrogate marker for the diagnosis of HPV associated squamous cell neoplasms of the female genital tract and the oropharynx and the nasopharynx (Klaes et al., 2002; Horn et al., 2008; Schache et al., 2011; Vent et al., 2013). In line with this we hypothesized that the increased p16 in SK is possibly associated with a MCPyV infection in SK. However, in this study p16 expression did not correlate with presence of MCPyV.

To date there are only few data available on the prevalence of MCPyV in SK. Sample sizes of SK in other studies included at maximum 12 patients (Andres et al., 2010). Although the present study contains the largest sample number of SK ($n = 23$) and normal skin ($n = 16$) testing for the presence of MCPyV, the study number remains small and might represent a limitation. Designing this study, we aimed for a sample size of $n = 20$ for both groups. This number is statistically sufficient to screen if there is increased presence of MCPyV in relation to normal skin and if this correlates with p16 expression. A positive correlation was not identified such that the sample size has not been enlarged. Since normal skin by definition does not constitute an indication for a diagnostic procedure the number $n = 20$ could unfortunately not be sustained completely ($n = 16$).

Andres et al. reported an overall presence of MCPyV in 6% of sun-exposed non-MCC lesions. Interestingly both MCPyV positive non-MCC samples belonged to the SK-group (2 of 12 samples, 17%) while all lentigo maligna melanoma and basal cell carcinomas were negative for MCPyV (Andres et al., 2010). Concerning SK, this is in line with the findings in this study detecting the presence of MCPyV in 6 out of 23 samples (26.1%). Other reported data about presence of MCPyV in SK represent a case report of one patient with 3 SK samples. The patient was immunosuppressed with a MCPyV positive MCC. Mertz et al. found MCPyV sequences in all of this patients common warts (4/4), half of his carcinoma *in situ* lesions (3/6) and two SK (2/3; Mertz et al., 2010). Depending on the detection method, we found MCPyV in 8.7% of samples via IHC and in 26.1% by molecular analyses by PCR and FISH in SK. We could not demonstrate an increased prevalence of MCPyV in SK compared to the tested normal non-neoplastic skin samples ($n = 16$), thereby most likely excluding MCPyV from playing a major pathogenic role in SK.

In this study MCPyV PCR sequences were detected in 3/16 (18.8%) of normal skin samples. Data from the literature show high variability of MCPyV in normal skin with percentages between 0% (Garneski et al., 2009; Kassem et al., 2009; Mangana et al., 2010) and 78% (Loyo et al., 2010) with most data ranging from 17 to 24% (Wieland et al., 2009; Foulongne et al., 2010; Mertz et al., 2010). The differences in the reported prevalence between the studies may be caused by heterogeneity of the study population (immune status, age-, and gender distribution), as well as heterogeneity in performed methods for detection of viral load (i.e., primer selection, viral-DNA copy number, etc. Dworkin et al., 2009; Garneski et al., 2009; Wieland et al., 2012).

In case of PCR as screening method, multiple factors may account for the variable MCPyV detection rates including tissue quality, quantity and fixation, DNA extraction method, PCR technique, choice of viral gene targets, and primer selection. A further limitation is the relatively low number of investigated samples from studies which have addressed normal, non-neoplastic, skin samples.

In line with other studies, the used MCPyV primer sets yielded partially heterogeneous results. Differences in detection frequency might be caused by changes due to the viral integration process (Andres et al., 2010; Kassem et al., 2010). In this study we were able to correlate molecular results from PCR to a single cell level and visualize MCPyV nucleic acids with FISH, thereby studying infected cells within the histological context. The two samples with strong punctual nuclear signal pattern in FISH analyses also showed IHC MCPyV expression on the translational level. PCR positive samples with weak signal intensity in FISH analyses were negative in IHC. This observation is in line with findings of several other studies which detected MCPyV on the IHC level to a lesser extent than by PCR (Katano et al., 2009; Shuda et al., 2009; Mertz et al., 2010; Ly et al., 2012). Discrepancies in MCPyV detection rates may be attributed to the enhanced sensitivity of PCR and FISH to detect low viral loads in contrast to IHC. Although unlikely, another reason for the lower detection rate with IHC might be a putative mutational loss of the antibody epitope. Indeed, the discrepancy in PCR and FISH compared to IHC is partly because PCR can target other viral components such as structural proteins VP1, VP2, and VP3, small T antigen and large T (LT) antigen, whereas the IHC derived from clone CM2B4 only targets the MCPyV LT antigen. Finally, although PCR effectively detects viral DNA, it does not distinguish incidental presence of virus from a causal infection. Comparatively, MCPyV FISH enables direct visualization of MCPyV DNA on a single cell level, while IHC allows the direct visualization of nuclear LT antigen expression only in the setting of relatively high viral load which may be more indicative of a causal infection (Ly et al., 2012; Haugg et al., 2014). Summarizing these findings indicate that MCPyV infection with low viral amplification rate (i.e., viral load) yields positive in FISH and PCR analyses but negative in IHC results.

Molecular analyses with FISH and observations in IHC revealed that in several samples MCPyV was not only restricted to intralesional keratinocytes and adjacent skin but also present in some intracapillary blood cells with a lymphocytic morphology. These observations indicate MCPyV to be ubiquitously present in diverse human tissue independently of malignant or benign histological status (Feng et al., 2008; Shuda et al., 2008).

The interpretation of the IHC stain for p16 may have been affected by pigmentation in the SKs. Therefore, substitution of the brownish dye for red as secondary antibody was used in strongly pigmented lesions to rule out the possibility of false-positive interpretations.

CONCLUSION

The frequent detection of the MCPyV genome by PCR and FISH reflects ubiquitous spread of the virus. However, the low rate of MCPyV detection by IHC most likely excludes a major pathogenic association of MCPyV in SK development, similar to the lack of evidence for a role of MCPyV in other non-melanoma skin neoplasm. The sporadic detection most likely represents a coincidental infection with a ubiquitous virus (Loyo et al., 2010; Wieland et al., 2012; Mertz et al., 2013; Peretti et al., 2014). Our data indicate that p16 IHC is unlikely to be a helpful adjunctive biomarker in the detection of MCPyV infection.

AUTHOR CONTRIBUTIONS

Designed the experiments: AzH, VW, and LH. Conceived and supervised the study: AzH, AMH, and VW. Performed the experiments: LH and DR. Contributed reagents, materials: E-JS and AMH. Data analyzed: LH, DR, AzH, and VW. Wrote the manuscript: LH and AzH. All authors read and approved the final manuscript.

REFERENCES

Andres, C., Belloni, B., Puchta, U., Sander, C. A., and Flaig, M. J. (2010). Prevalence of MCPyV in Merkel cell carcinoma and non-MCC tumors. *J. Cutan. Pathol.* 37, 28–34. doi: 10.1111/j.1600-0560.2009.01352.x

Bagazgoitia, L., Cuevas, J., and Juarranz, A. (2010). Expression of p53 and p16 in actinic keratosis, bowenoid actinic keratosis and Bowen's disease. *J. Eur. Acad. Dermatol. Venereol.* 24, 228–230. doi: 10.1111/j.1468-3083.2009.03337.x

Chazal, M., Marionnet, C., Michel, L., Mollier, K., Dazard, J. E., Della Valle, V., et al. (2002). P16(INK4A) is implicated in both the immediate and adaptative response of human keratinocytes to UVB irradiation. *Oncogene* 21, 2652–2661. doi: 10.1038/sj.onc.1205349

Conic, R. Z., Napekoski, K., Schuetz, H., Piliang, M., Bergfeld, W., and Atanaskova Mesinkovska, N. (2017). The role of immunosuppression in squamous cell carcinomas arising in seborrheic keratosis. *J. Am. Acad. Dermatol.* 76, 1146–1150. doi: 10.1016/j.jaad.2016.12.002

Conscience, I., Jovenin, N., Coissard, C., Lorenzato, M., Durlach, A., Grange, F., et al. (2006). P16 is overexpressed in cutaneous carcinomas located on sun-exposed areas. *Eur. J. Dermatol.* 16, 518–522.

Dehn, D., Torkko, K. C., and Shroyer, K. R. (2007). Human papillomavirus testing and molecular markers of cervical dysplasia and carcinoma. *Cancer* 111, 1–14. doi: 10.1002/cncr.22425

Donati, P., Paolino, G., Panetta, C., Cota, C., Zaccarini, M., and Muscardin, L. (2013). Another point of view on p16 and Ki67 expression in melanocytic and non-melanocytic cutaneous lesions. *Acta Dermatovenerol. Croat.* 21, 149–154.

Dworkin, A. M., Tseng, S. Y., Allain, D. C., Iwenofu, O. H., Peters, S. B., and Toland, A. E. (2009). Merkel cell polyomavirus in cutaneous squamous cell carcinoma of immunocompetent individuals. *J. Invest. Dermatol.* 129, 2868–2874. doi: 10.1038/jid.2009.183

Felsani, A., Mileo, A. M., and Paggi, M. G. (2006). Retinoblastoma family proteins as key targets of the small DNA virus oncoproteins. *Oncogene* 25, 5277–5285. doi: 10.1038/sj.onc.1209621

Feng, H., Shuda, M., Chang, Y., and Moore, P. S. (2008). Clonal integration of a polyomavirus in human Merkel cell carcinoma. *Science* 319, 1096–1100. doi: 10.1126/science.1152586

Foulongne, V., Dereure, O., Kluger, N., Moles, J. P., Guillot, B., and Segondy, M. (2010). Merkel cell polyomavirus DNA detection in lesional and nonlesional skin from patients with Merkel cell carcinoma or other skin diseases. *Br. J. Dermatol.* 162, 59–63. doi: 10.1111/j.1365-2133.2009.09381.x

Garneski, K. M., Warcola, A. H., Feng, Q., Kiviat, N. B., Leonard, J. H., and Nghiem, P. (2009). Merkel cell polyomavirus is more frequently present in North American than Australian Merkel cell carcinoma tumors. *J. Invest. Dermatol.* 129, 246–248. doi: 10.1038/jid.2008.229

Genders, R. E., Beck, S., Bouwes Bavinck, J. N., van den Munckhof, H. A., Kouwenhoven, S. T., de Koning, M. N., et al. (2017). p16 immunostaining in keratinocytic neoplasia in organ transplant recipients: Bowen's disease shows a characteristic pattern. *J. Cutan. Pathol.* 44, 28–33. doi: 10.1111/cup.12840

Gushi, A., Kanekura, T., Kanzaki, T., and Eizuru, Y. (2003). Detection and sequences of human papillomavirus DNA in nongenital seborrhoeic keratosis of immunopotent individuals. *J. Dermatol. Sci.* 31, 143–149. doi: 10.1016/S0923-1811(03)00002-1

Hafkamp, H. C., Manni, J. J., Haesevoets, A., Voogd, A. C., Schepers, M., Bot, F. J., et al. (2008). Marked differences in survival rate between smokers and nonsmokers with HPV 16-associated tonsillar carcinomas. *Int. J. Cancer* 122, 2656–2664. doi: 10.1002/ijc.23458

Harvey, N. T., Leecy, T., and Wood, B. A. (2013). Immunohistochemical staining for p16 is a useful adjunctive test in the diagnosis of Bowen's disease. *Pathology* 45, 402–407. doi: 10.1097/PAT.0b013e328360c064

Haugg, A. M., Rennspiess, D., zur Hausen, A., Speel, E. J., Cathomas, G., Becker, J. C., et al. (2014). Fluorescence *in situ* hybridization and qPCR to detect Merkel cell polyomavirus physical status and load in Merkel cell carcinomas. *Int. J. Cancer* 135, 2804–2815. doi: 10.1002/ijc.28931

Haugg, A. M., Speel, E. J., Pantulu, N. D., Pallasch, C., Kurz, A. K., Kvasnicka, H. M., et al. (2011). Fluorescence *in situ* hybridization confirms the presence of Merkel cell polyomavirus in chronic lymphocytic leukemia cells. *Blood* 117, 5776–5777. doi: 10.1182/blood-2011-03-339895

Hodges, A., and Smoller, B. R. (2002). Immunohistochemical comparison of p16 expression in actinic keratoses and squamous cell carcinomas of the skin. *Mod. Pathol.* 15, 1121–1125. doi: 10.1097/01.MP.0000032536.48264.D1

Hopman, A. H., Kamps, M. A., Smedts, F., Speel, E. J., Herrington, C. S., and Ramaekers, F. C. (2005). HPV *in situ* hybridization: impact of different protocols on the detection of integrated HPV. *Int. J. Cancer* 115, 419–428. doi: 10.1002/ijc.20862

Horn, L. C., Reichert, A., Oster, A., Arndal, S. F., Trunk, M. J., Ridder, R., et al. (2008). Immunostaining for p16INK4a used as a conjunctive tool improves interobserver agreement of the histologic diagnosis of cervical intraepithelial neoplasia. *Am. J. Surg. Pathol.* 32, 502–512. doi: 10.1097/PAS.0b013e31815ac420

Kassem, A., Pantulu, D., Technau, K., Kurz, A. K., Diaz, C., Hörster, S., et al. (2010). Merkel cell polyomavirus in naevoid basal cell carcinoma syndrome-associated basal cell carcinomas and sporadic trichoblastomas. *J. Dermatol. Sci.* 59, 140–142. doi: 10.1016/j.jdermsci.2010.06.005

Kassem, A., Schöpflin, A., Diaz, C., Weyers, W., Stickeler, E., Werner, M., et al. (2008). Frequent detection of Merkel cell polyomavirus in human Merkel cell carcinomas and identification of a unique deletion in the VP1 gene. *Cancer Res.* 68, 5009–5013. doi: 10.1158/0008-5472.CAN-08-0949

Kassem, A., Technau, K., Kurz, A. K., Pantulu, D., Löning, M., Kayser, G., et al. (2009). Merkel cell polyomavirus sequences are frequently detected in nonmelanoma skin cancer of immunosuppressed patients. *Int. J. Cancer* 125, 356–361. doi: 10.1002/ijc.24323

Katano, H., Ito, H., Suzuki, Y., Nakamura, T., Sato, Y., Tsuji, T., et al. (2009). Detection of Merkel cell polyomavirus in Merkel cell carcinoma and Kaposi's sarcoma. *J. Med. Virol.* 81, 1951–1958. doi: 10.1002/jmv.21608

Klaes, R., Benner, A., Friedrich, T., Ridder, R., Herrington, S., Jenkins, D., et al. (2002). p16INK4a immunohistochemistry improves interobserver agreement in the diagnosis of cervical intraepithelial neoplasia. *Am. J. Surg. Pathol.* 26, 1389–1399.

Kyriakis, K. P., Alexoudi, I., Askoxylaki, K., Vrani, F., and Kosma, E. (2012). Epidemiologic aspects of seborrheic keratoses. *Int. J. Dermatol.* 51, 233–234. doi: 10.1111/j.1365-4632.2010.04560.x

Liu, Y., Sanoff, H. K., Cho, H., Burd, C. E., Torrice, C., Ibrahim, J. G., et al. (2009). Expression of p16(INK4a) in peripheral blood T-cells is a biomarker of human aging. *Aging Cell* 8, 439–448. doi: 10.1111/j.1474-9726.2009.00489.x

Loyo, M., Guerrero-Preston, R., Brait, M., Hoque, M. O., Chuang, A., Kim, M. S., et al. (2010). Quantitative detection of Merkel cell virus in human tissues and possible mode of transmission. *Int. J. Cancer* 126, 2991–2996. doi: 10.1002/ijc.24737

Ly, T. Y., Walsh, N. M., and Pasternak, S. (2012). The spectrum of Merkel cell polyomavirus expression in Merkel cell carcinoma, in a variety of cutaneous neoplasms, and in neuroendocrine carcinomas from different anatomical sites. *Hum. Pathol.* 43, 557–566. doi: 10.1016/j.humpath.2011.06.005

Mangana, J., Dziunycz, P., Kerl, K., Dummer, R., and Cozzio, A. (2010). Prevalence of Merkel cell polyomavirus among Swiss Merkel cell carcinoma patients. *Dermatology* 221, 184–188. doi: 10.1159/000315067

Mertz, K. D., Paasinen, A., Arnold, A., Baumann, M., Offner, F., Willi, N., et al. (2013). Merkel cell polyomavirus large T antigen is detected in rare cases of nonmelanoma skin cancer. *J. Cutan. Pathol.* 40, 543–549. doi: 10.1111/cup.12129

Mertz, K. D., Pfaltz, M., Junt, T., Schmid, M., Fernandez Figueras, M. T., Pfaltz, K., et al. (2010). Merkel cell polyomavirus is present in common warts and carcinoma *in situ* of the skin. *Hum. Pathol.* 41, 1369–1379. doi: 10.1016/j.humpath.2010.01.023

Nakamura, S., and Nishioka, K. (2003). Enhanced expression of p16 in seborrhoeic keratosis; a lesion of accumulated senescent epidermal cells in G1 arrest. *Br. J. Dermatol.* 149, 560–565. doi: 10.1046/j.1365-2133.2003.05589.x

Nilsson, K., Svensson, S., and Landberg, G. (2004). Retinoblastoma protein function and p16INK4a expression in actinic keratosis, squamous cell carcinoma *in situ* and invasive squamous cell carcinoma of the skin and links between p16INK4a expression and infiltrative behavior. *Mod. Pathol.* 17, 1464–1474. doi: 10.1038/modpathol.3800220

Pavey, S., Conroy, S., Russell, T., and Gabrielli, B. (1999). Ultraviolet radiation induces p16CDKN2A expression in human skin. *Cancer Res.* 59, 4185–4189.

Pavey, S., Russell, T., and Gabrielli, B. (2001). G2 phase cell cycle arrest in human skin following UV irradiation. *Oncogene* 20, 6103–6110. doi: 10.1038/sj.onc.1204707

Peretti, A., Borgogna, C., Rossi, D., De Paoli, L., Bawadekar, M., Zavattaro, E., et al. (2014). Analysis of human beta-papillomavirus and Merkel cell polyomavirus infection in skin lesions and eyebrow hair bulbs from a cohort of patients with chronic lymphocytic leukaemia. *Br. J. Dermatol.* 171, 1525–1528. doi: 10.1111/bjd.13215

Rajabi, P., Adibi, N., Nematollahi, P., Heidarpour, M., Eftekhari, M., and Siadat, A. H. (2012). Bowenoid transformation in seborrheic keratosis: a retrospective analysis of 429 patients. *J. Res. Med. Sci.* 17, 217–221.

Schache, A. G., Liloglou, T., Risk, J. M., Filia, A., Jones, T. M., Sheard, J., et al. (2011). Evaluation of human papilloma virus diagnostic testing in oropharyngeal squamous cell carcinoma: sensitivity, specificity, and prognostic discrimination. *Clin. Cancer Res.* 17, 6262–6271. doi: 10.1158/1078-0432.CCR-11-0388

Serrano, M., Hannon, G. J., and Beach, D. (1993). A new regulatory motif in cell-cycle control causing specific inhibition of cyclin D/CDK4. *Nature* 366, 704–707.

Sharpless, N. E., and DePinho, R. A. (1999). The INK4A/ARF locus and its two gene products. *Curr. Opin. Genet. Dev.* 9, 22–30. doi: 10.1016/S0959-437X(99)80004-5

Shelton, J., Purgina, B. M., Cipriani, N. A., Dupont, W. D., Plummer, D., and Lewis, J. S. Jr. (2017). p16 immunohistochemistry in oropharyngeal squamous cell carcinoma: a comparison of antibody clones using patient outcomes and high-risk human papillomavirus RNA status. *Mod. Pathol.* 30, 1194–1203. doi: 10.1038/modpathol.2017.31

Shuda, M., Arora, R., Kwun, H. J., Feng, H., Sarid, R., Fernández-Figueras, M. T., et al. (2009). Human Merkel cell polyomavirus infection I. MCV T antigen expression in Merkel cell carcinoma, lymphoid tissues and lymphoid tumors. *Int. J. Cancer* 125, 1243–1249. doi: 10.1002/ijc.24510

Shuda, M., Feng, H., Kwun, H. J., Rosen, S. T., Gjoerup, O., Moore, P. S., et al. (2008). T antigen mutations are a human tumor-specific signature for Merkel cell polyomavirus. *Proc. Natl. Acad. Sci. U.S.A.* 105, 16272–16277. doi: 10.1073/pnas.0806526105

Tardío, J. C., Bancalari, E., Moreno, A., and Martin-Fragueiro, L. M. (2012). Genital seborrheic keratoses are human papillomavirus-related lesions. A linear array genotyping test study. *APMIS* 120, 477–483. doi: 10.1111/j.1600-0463.2011.02853.x

van Dongen, J. J., Langerak, A. W., Brüggemann, M., Evans, P. A., Hummel, M., Lavender, F. L., et al. (2003). Design and standardization of PCR primers and protocols for detection of clonal immunoglobulin and T-cell receptor gene recombinations in suspect lymphoproliferations: report of the

BIOMED-2 Concerted Action BMH4-CT98-3936. *Leukemia* 17, 2257–2317. doi: 10.1038/sj.leu.2403202

Vent, J., Haidle, B., Wedemeyer, I., Huebbers, C., Siefer, O., Semrau, R., et al. (2013). p16 expression in carcinoma of unknown primary: diagnostic indicator and prognostic marker. *Head Neck* 35, 1521–1526. doi: 10.1002/hed.23190

Vun, Y., De'Ambrosis, B., Spelman, L., Muir, J. B., Yong-Gee, S., Wagner, G., et al. (2006). Seborrhoeic keratosis and malignancy: collision tumour or malignant transformation? *Australas. J. Dermatol.* 47, 106–108. doi: 10.1111/j.1440-0960.2006.00242.x

Wieland, U., Mauch, C., Kreuter, A., Krieg, T., and Pfister, H. (2009). Merkel cell polyomavirus DNA in persons without merkel cell carcinoma. *Emerg. Infect. Dis.* 15, 1496–1498. doi: 10.3201/eid1509.081575

Wieland, U., Scola, N., Stolte, B., Stücker, M., Silling, S., and Kreuter, A. (2012). No evidence for a causal role of Merkel cell polyomavirus in keratoacanthoma. *J. Am. Acad. Dermatol.* 67, 41–46. doi: 10.1016/j.jaad.2011.07.026

Yeatman, J. M., Kilkenny, M., and Marks, R. (1997). The prevalence of seborrhoeic keratoses in an Australian population: does exposure to sunlight play a part in their frequency? *Br. J. Dermatol.* 137, 411–414.

Zhu, W. Y., Leonardi, C., Kinsey, W., and Penneys, N. S. (1991). Irritated seborrheic keratoses and benign verrucous acanthomas do not contain papillomavirus DNA. *J. Cutan. Pathol.* 18, 449–452. doi: 10.1111/j.1600-0560.1991.tb01383.x

Zhu, W. Y., Leonardi, C., and Penneys, N. S. (1992). Detection of human papillomavirus DNA in seborrheic keratosis by polymerase chain reaction. *J. Dermatol. Sci.* 4, 166–171. doi: 10.1016/0923-1811(92)90015-4

3

Cutaneous Papillomaviruses and Non-melanoma Skin Cancer: Causal Agents or Innocent Bystanders?

*Daniel Hasche[1], Sabrina E. Vinzón[2] and Frank Rösl[1]**

[1] *Division of Viral Transformation Mechanisms, Research Program "Infection, Inflammation and Cancer", German Cancer Research Center, Heidelberg, Germany,* [2] *Laboratory of Molecular and Cellular Therapy, Fundación Instituto Leloir, IIBBA-CONICET, Buenos Aires, Argentina*

Correspondence:
Frank Rösl
f.roesl@dkfz.de

There is still controversy in the scientific field about whether certain types of cutaneous human papillomaviruses (HPVs) are causally involved in the development of non-melanoma skin cancer (NMSC). Deciphering the etiological role of cutaneous HPVs requires – besides tissue culture systems – appropriate preclinical models to match the obtained results with clinical data from affected patients. Clear scientific evidence about the etiology and underlying mechanisms involved in NMSC development is fundamental to provide reasonable arguments for public health institutions to classify at least certain cutaneous HPVs as group 1 carcinogens. This in turn would have implications on fundraising institutions and health care decision makers to force – similarly as for anogenital cancer – the implementation of a broad vaccination program against "high-risk" cutaneous HPVs to prevent NMSC as the most frequent cancer worldwide. Precise knowledge of the multi-step progression from normal cells to cancer is a prerequisite to understand the functional and clinical impact of cofactors that affect the individual outcome and the personalized treatment of a disease. This overview summarizes not only recent arguments that favor the acceptance of a viral etiology in NMSC development but also reflects aspects of causality in medicine, the use of empirically meaningful model systems and strategies for prevention.

Keywords: cutaneous papillomaviruses, hit-and-run mechanism, *Mastomys coucha*, causality, skin cancer, animal models, NMSC

Abbreviations: AK, actinic keratosis; ALK, ALK Receptor Tyrosine Kinase; ATM, ataxia telangiectasia mutated; ATR, ataxia telangiectasia and Rad3-related protein; BPV1, bovine papillomavirus 1; BRAFi, Inhibitors of the B-Raf Proto-Oncogene; CDKN2A, cyclin-dependent kinase inhibitor 2A; cGMP, current good manufacturing practice; CKIT, KIT proto-oncogene receptor tyrosine kinase; CREBBP, CREB binding protein (CREB, CAMP responsive element binding protein 1); DDR, DNA damage response; E6AP, Ubiquitin Protein Ligase E3A; EGFR, epidermal growth factor receptor; FAT1, FAT atypical cadherin 1; FGFR3, fibroblast growth factor receptor 3; HIPK2, homeodomain-interacting protein kinase 2; HRAS, Harvey rat sarcoma virus oncogene; KA, Keratoacanthoma; KRAS, Kirsten rat sarcoma viral oncogene homolog; MAML1, mastermind like transcriptional coactivator 1; McPV2, *Mastomys coucha* papillomavirus 2; MHC, major histocompatibility complex; MmuPV1, Mus musculus papillomavirus type 1; MnPV, *Mastomys natalensis* papillomavirus; NMSC, non-melanoma skin cancer; OTRs, organ transplant recipients; PIK3CA, Phosphatidylinositol-4,5-Bisphosphate 3-Kinase Catalytic Subunit Alpha; pRb, RB transcriptional corepressor 1; Pten, phosphatase and tensin homolog; SCC, squamous cell carcinoma; TLR, Toll-like receptor; TP53, tumor protein P53 (human); *Trp53*, transformation related protein 53 (mouse).

THE PROBLEM – A SERIOUS AND COMMON DISEASE: NON-MELANOMA SKIN CANCER

Non-melanoma skin cancer is the most frequent cancer in fair-skinned individuals worldwide and its incidence has increased during the last three decades (Welsh et al., 2011; Lomas et al., 2012). There are up to 3 million new cases every year, whereby women below 45 years are even more affected (Al-Dujaili et al., 2017). Based on different UV exposure rates, there are also geographical variations, with the highest incidence of NMSC in Australia (Lomas et al., 2012). Although the metastatic potential and the mortality rates in immunocompetent individuals are low in comparison to malignant melanomas, NMSC has a strong impact on the quality of life of the affected persons and the financial burden on health care systems. Taking the United States as an example, total annual expenses for NMSC medical care amounts to 650 million dollars (Apalla et al., 2017). Hence, there should be a quite obvious public health interest to understand and to prevent this cancer entity.

Non-melanoma skin cancer principally refers to cancer derived from keratinocytes (Small et al., 2016) and can be further divided into basal cell carcinomas (BCCs) and squamous cell carcinomas (SCCs), with relative frequencies of 80 and 20%, respectively (Eisemann et al., 2014). While BCCs are not very different in their biological behaviors, SCCs show broad histopathological diversities that are associated with markedly different clinical outcomes. Depending on the immune status of the patient, these may range from indolent tumors with low metastatic capacity to aggressive tumors with high invasive potential. Approximately 97% of invasive SCCs are found in association with malignant progression of an actinic keratosis (AK), considered as a precursor of SCCs. These lesions can display erythematous, scaling, and rough patches. They can either spontaneously regress, persist as a benign AK or progress to an invasive SCC where cells infiltrate the basement membrane into the dermis (reviewed in Yanofsky et al., 2011). TP53 is found to be mutated in dysplastic AKs, indicating that functional loss is a very early event, connected with loss of chromosomes including the cell cycle regulator p16INK4A (Ratushny et al., 2012). To define some general histopathological features, a committee of European dermatologists has recently identified telangiectasia, atrophy, and pigmentation disorders as the most reliable markers for AKs (Dreno et al., 2017).

Other clinically common lesions are keratoacanthomas (KAs) which can form spontaneously but, after a proliferative and subsequent resting phase, have the tendency to regress, apparently due to apoptosis. Histologically, a KA is an exo-/endophytic growing squamous proliferative tumor with a characteristic central keratin plug, surrounded by epidermal lips, forming a relatively well-defined symmetrical structure (Takai, 2017). Of note, approximately 25% of KAs can develop into SCCs (Sanchez Yus et al., 2000). Although still controversially discussed in terms of whether a KA is a variant of SCC, other dermatologists believe it represents a self-resolving benign epidermal lesion (reviewed in Savage and Maize, 2014). This illustrates the current discrepancies between histopathological phenotypes and deep sequencing DNA profiles of respective specimens, since KAs and SCCs are distinct entities at least by their unique molecular gene signatures (Ra et al., 2015). Nonetheless, according to the "World Health Organization Classification of Tumors" as a guideline for pathologists in diagnostics, KAs are still regarded as a well-differentiated SCC (LeBoit et al., 2006).

Another thought-provoking inquiry that has clinical significance in the context of NMSC pathogenesis emerged during the last years, when patients with advanced metastatic melanomas were treated with BRAF inhibitors (BRAFi) (e.g., vemurafenib or dabrafenib) (reviewed in Gibney et al., 2013). The off-target outcome of such drugs results in deleterious dermatological side effects, histopathologically ranging from *verrucal keratosis,* hair follicle changes, plantar hyperkeratosis, KAs and finally cutaneous SCCs (Anforth et al., 2013). Vemurafenib also has a photosensitizing activity (Boussemart et al., 2013), consistent with the finding that most SCCs can be detected at chronically sun-damaged skin regions (Hassel et al., 2015).

ENDOGENOUS AND ENVIRONMENTAL RISK FACTORS FOR NMSC

The Individual Genotype

Cancer in general is a multi-factorial disease and as individual as the patient, a reasonable concept that is culminating in the contemporary discourse of personalized medicine (reviewed in Mavropoulos et al., 2014; Harwood et al., 2016). Referring to this notion, meta-analyses of the current literature have deciphered several risk factors that are either distinct in terms of an inherent genetic predisposition of an individual patient and/or caused by environmental factors (reviewed in Wang et al., 2014; Belbasis et al., 2016). Individual risk factors for NMSC are age, family history, pigmentation, polymorphisms within genes encoding IL10, IL4R, TNF, or TNFR2 (Welsh et al., 2011), several inborn genetic disorders like *Xeroderma pigmentosum* (Black, 2016), the basal cell nevus syndrome (reviewed in Bresler et al., 2016) or the WHIM (Wart, Hypogammaglobulinemia, Infection, and Myelokathexis) syndrome, an autosomal dominant inheritance immune deficiency, harboring mutations in the chemokine receptor CXCR4 (Chow et al., 2010; Meuris et al., 2016). Such patients show a high susceptibility for both cutaneous and mucosal HPVs. Multiple warts can occur on hands and feet, but also genital condylomata acuminata can be found (Leiding and Holland, 2012). In the case of patients suffering from the rare hereditary disease *Epidermodysplasia verruciformis* (EV), mutations within at least two genes of homologous transmembrane channel-like (TMC) proteins, TMC6 (EVER1) and TMC8 (EVER2) were described (Lazarczyk et al., 2009, 2012). These proteins are involved in zinc homeostasis and are not only expressed in keratinocytes, but also in lymphocytes, suggesting additional functions in the immune response (reviewed in Kalinska-Bienias et al., 2016). Due to their interaction with the Zn^{2+} transporter protein ZnT-1, TMC6/8 can further modulate MAP kinases and in turn AP-1, a transcription factor involved in many signal transduction pathways (reviewed in Lazarczyk and Favre, 2008).

Immune Status

Another important risk factor is iatrogenic immunosuppression as SCCs appear 65–250 times more frequently in OTRs compared to the general population (reviewed in Nindl and Rösl, 2008; Vinzón and Rösl, 2015). Moreover, the frequency of tumor formation correlates with the extent and duration of immunosuppression (reviewed in Euvrard et al., 2003; Hampton, 2005). It is estimated that up to 40% of OTRs will develop skin cancers within the first 10 years of transplantation and up to 80% after 20 years (Rangwala and Tsai, 2011). Although early detection of NMSC evidently improves the overall survival rate, a 20 year follow-up study including more than 85,000 patients showed that OTRs have a much worse prognosis and a higher mortality rate as compared to immunocompetent individuals (Acuna et al., 2016). The exact physiological reason is still unexplained, but it is assumed that tumors are simply more aggressive in an immunosuppressive environment since substances like cyclosporine both promote tumor invasion and favor neovascularization (reviewed in Geissler, 2015). Immunosuppressive drugs apparently also impair the DDR and counteract p53-dependent cellular senescence (Wu et al., 2010; Kuschal et al., 2012). Since SCCs develop mostly within sun-exposed areas, UV exposure is immune compromising (reviewed in Nakad and Schumacher, 2016). Despite the obvious increase of NMSC, population-based studies of skin cancer mortality after organ transplantation and in immunocompetent individuals are still scant (John et al., 2016). This is mainly due to geographic variability of incidence rates and, most importantly, the exclusion of NMSC from central cancer registries records (reviewed in Apalla et al., 2017) as recently noticed in the "*European Code against Cancer: Infection and Cancer*" (Villain et al., 2015). Such an obvious gap in cancer documentation should be filled as exemplified by initiatives such as the "Keratinocyte Carcinoma Consortium" (Madeleine et al., 2017), because NMSC incidence is increasing worldwide and caused by daily and life-long risk factors such as UV exposure and skin infections (Garrett et al., 2016; Prasad and Katiyar, 2017).

Sun Exposure

Another major environmental risk factor that has to be taken into account for the development of NMSC is the cumulative lifelong exposure to UV light, as well as sunburns in youth (Kennedy et al., 2003). UV light is divided into three categories according to its energy (wave length), which are UVA (320–400 nm), UVB (290–320 nm), and UVC (100–290 nm). UVC is almost completely filtered by the atmospheric ozone layer, which also shields up to 90% of UVB radiation. Thus, only UVA and UVB play roles as risk factors. Although not penetrating in the skin as deep as UVA, due to its higher energy output, UVB is more harmful and can damage cells heavily (reviewed in Seebode et al., 2016). UVB has also additional deleterious side-effects on the immune system, for example, by perturbing the function of antigen-presenting cells and in turn increasing a local immunodeficiency (reviewed in Prasad and Katiyar, 2017). Thus, cumulative UV exposure can contribute to skin tumor development by impairing immune surveillance of the skin (Maglennon et al., 2014). UV has also direct effects on the DNA, leading to a covalent joining of adjacent pyrimidines to form cyclobutane pyrimidine dimers (CPDs). Due to the misincorporation of an adenine at the position complementary to the UV DNA damage, CPDs predominantly lead to C→T transitions (≥60%) and rarely to CC→TT transitions (5%), leaving characteristic signatures within the DNA that can be detected in the landscape of SCCs upon whole genome sequencing (reviewed in Brash, 2015).

However, it is still not clear how to functionally rank the significance and frequencies of such mutations since the appearance of NMSC is, like other forms of cancer, the result of a multi-step process in which the temporal/spatial order and the impact on tumor formation cannot retrospectively be defined. Moreover, comparatively little is known about the temporal combinatory linkage of altered gene expression within a cellular network, thus contributing to the individual manifestation of a tumor (Krogan et al., 2015). Notably, deep-sequencing analyses of normal skin sections of persons with different histories of sun exposures even revealed identical UV specific signatures in their genome with exactly the same genes affected as later found in SCCs or BCCs (Martincorena et al., 2015). The reasons why such mutations are tolerated in normal cells suggest a counter-selective environment consisting of stromal, endothelial, and inflammatory components that prevent the outgrowth of clones finally forming a tumor. Considering recent concepts, cancer is not simply a linear route, but a highly flexible and emergent adaptation process of certain cells where clonal expansion is following according to evolutionary principles that limit the predictability of therapeutic outcomes (reviewed in Greaves, 2015; Lipinski et al., 2016; Davis et al., 2017).

Cutaneous Papillomaviruses

Since individuals are "open systems," the most critical exogenous risk factor for NMSC is not only UV exposure, but also infections with papillomaviruses. These target keratinocytes of the skin and mucosa of different vertebrate species, including humans. Up to date more than 200 human papillomavirus (HPV) types are known according to the PaVE database[1] (Van Doorslaer et al., 2017), which are associated with different clinical manifestations. Genital HPVs cause diverse lesions ranging from benign warts (for "low-risk" HPV types) to different malignancies (for "high-risk" types) of which cervical cancer is the most prominent (zur Hausen, 2002; McLaughlin-Drubin et al., 2012).

On the other hand, there is also a wide range of cutaneous HPV types that have been associated with diverse skin diseases (reviewed in Grce and Mravak-Stipetic, 2014). Including more than 100 healthy human volunteers in a broad study of meta-genomic analyses, whole-genome shotgun sequencing revealed an overall HPV prevalence of 69% in the skin, followed by the vagina (42%), the mouth (30%), and the gut (17%) (Ma et al., 2014). Another study even demonstrated that more

[1]https://pave.niaid.nih.gov

than 95% of all viral sequences detected in skin samples belong to the papillomavirus family, mostly to the beta-and gamma genera. Here, also co-infections could be discerned, which leads to speculation about potential temporal inclusion/exclusion interaction mechanisms between different HPV types in the same cell that may modulate the immune response and in turn viral persistence (Bzhalava et al., 2014).

High prevalence of cutaneous HPV can be already detected in skin of infants and young children, indicating that viral exposure occurs very early in life (Antonsson et al., 2003). Recurrent types are HPV2, 7, 27, 57 (alpha genus), HPV23 and 75 (beta genus), HPV4 and 65 (gamma genus) and HPV1 (mu genus) that typically cause only benign lesions such as common warts (*verrucae vulgaris*), plantar warts (*verrucae plantaris*), and flat warts (*verruca plana*) (Jablonska et al., 1997; Cardoso and Calonje, 2011; Bruggink et al., 2012) which usually spontaneously regress (van Haalen et al., 2009). However, they can represent a serious problem for immunocompromised individuals, especially OTRs, who frequently suffer from confluent wart formation all over the body. The prevalence within this population ranged from 48 to 92% in the first 5 years after immunosuppression (Jablonska et al., 1997; Wang et al., 2014). The HIM study ("cutaneous HPV infection in healthy men") reported a different median time of incidence (=newly diagnosed in skin) and duration of persistence of beta and gamma HPV infections ranging between 6–8 and 6–11 months, respectively. Older volunteers showed a significant higher association with prevalent and persistent HPV infections (Hampras et al., 2014). However, merely monitoring the skin for the presence of a viral DNA does not allow any conclusions about an ongoing infection and the exposure of viral antigens to the immune system. Such questions can only be answered when combined with immunological studies to get estimations about the rates of seroconversion and the serodynamics of cutaneous HPV infections (Rahman et al., 2016), an important criteria when preclinical models are used (see below).

"High Risk" Cutaneous HPVs?

The term "infection" indicates the presence of a microbe which can be pathogenic, commensal or opportunistic (reviewed in Casadevall and Pirofski, 2000). Hence, considering the individual complexity of the human skin virome that in turn also represents an interactome with a defined microbial environment (Hannigan et al., 2015), it is a huge challenge of modern biomedicine to dissect such networks in terms of functionality and causality. Indeed, the skin is an open ecosystem, colonized by a broad spectrum of bacteria and viruses whose landscape and impact on local immunity change during their individual life span and by environmental factors (Belkaid and Segre, 2014). We still do not understand how these different constituents dynamically interact with other microorganisms colonizing the skin, what the selective advantage of such a commensalism is, how the virome in turn affects the transcriptome of the skin (Edqvist et al., 2015), form the individual immunophenotype and how these properties vary with respect of individual skin types, under immunosuppression or UV exposure (Virgin, 2014). The categories commensal, pathogenic or opportunistic are helpful notions in the context of tumor viruses (Moore and Chang, 2017). Accordingly, commensal tumor viruses (e.g., EBV or cutaneous HPVs), are almost ubiquitously spread and usually do not cause symptoms. Contrarily, pathogenic tumor viruses are not so frequent and acquired, for instance via sexual intercourse or blood transfusion (e.g., high-risk mucosal types of HPV or Hepatitis B virus, HBV). Due to their ubiquitous prevalence in the general healthy population, there is still skepticism whether cutaneous HPVs are causally involved in NMSC development. However, there are many epidemiological and mechanistic *in vitro/in vivo* data showing increasing evidence that at least some commensal HPVs represent an essential, if not even a decisive factor for this type of skin cancer, especially for SCC (Madeleine et al., 2013; Wang et al., 2014; Chahoud et al., 2016).

Historically, the oncogenic potential of beta-type HPV infection (e.g., HPV5 and HPV8) in NMSC has been originally identified in patients suffering from EV, characterized by an increased susceptibility to viral infection (Orth, 2006). The oncogenic and transforming capacity of the EV-HPVs has not only been shown in transgenic mouse models (Schaper et al., 2005; Pfefferle et al., 2008; Viarisio et al., 2011), but also in organotypic raft cultures under *in vitro* conditions (Borgogna et al., 2012; Heuser et al., 2016b; Marthaler et al., 2017). Beta-type papillomaviruses were also detected in NMSCs of non-EV patients, although the viral loads are usually very low. It is assumed that the reservoirs for latent infection are hair follicle stem cells (Hufbauer et al., 2013). Different studies have reported HPV DNA in 30–50% of NMSCs from immunocompetent persons (Harwood et al., 2006), whereas in immunosuppressed patients this figure goes up to 90% (Harwood et al., 2000; Arnold and Hofbauer, 2012). Transcriptionally active beta-type HPVs can be found in premalignant lesions such as AKs (Borgogna et al., 2014) but also in normal skin and plucked eyebrow hairs suggesting a functional correlation between the presence of viral DNA and an increased risk of NMSC (Neale et al., 2013). UV exposure *per se* can also directly stimulate viral transcription of the EV-types HPV5 and HPV8 (Akgül et al., 2005b), while other cutaneous types such as HPV38 E6/E7, for instance, can block UV-induced expression of the toll-like receptor 9 (TLR9), normally responsible for endosomal sensoring of exogenic DNA (Pacini et al., 2017). This shows the complexity of a virus–host interaction, demonstrating several modes of action by different HPV types to interfere with signal transduction pathways of the host cell. Moreover, in contrast to anogenital tumors, there are also SCCs that either completely lack HPV or not all cells are virus-positive (Neale et al., 2013), indicating that viral oncoprotein expression is not necessary to maintain a malignant phenotype (reviewed in Arron et al., 2011; Hufbauer and Akgül, 2017).

SOME REFLECTIONS ABOUT THE "CAUSALITY" OF INFECTIONS

The lack of HPV in cancerous skin lesions is in apparent contradiction to the so-called Henle-Koch's postulates that were traditionally used as criteria for "causality" of an infection (reviewed in Inglis, 2007). However, one should keep in mind that the conception of causality is a term historically referring to physical properties of the inanimate matter and not to living systems. Physicists deal with reproducible regular events and experimental settings, while cancer research is investigating "anomalous" scenarios, sometimes rare disorders in terms of cancer development which are, as aforementioned, multi-factorial and individually shaped. Hence, the simple detection of an infection or frequent mutations found in genetically non-predisposed persons cannot be considered as "causal," because they are only contingent and the individual clinical outcome is determined by many additional factors (reviewed in Greaves, 2015). More correct in an epistemic sense is the word "etiology," since this term has a more suitable connotation, reflecting more the complexity of an organism and not implying necessarily a direct and quite obvious causal relationship.

Nonetheless, in principle the Henle-Koch's postulates state that an infectious agent should be consistently detected in the respective lesions, it should be isolated and its re-inoculation should induce the same symptoms or clinical manifestations. However, these postulates have their limitations, because they are not considering multi-factorial events in the development of a disease (reviewed in Edwards and Rohwer, 2005; Virgin, 2014; O'Malley, 2016). Moreover, they also do not reflect asymptomatic, latent or persistent infections, all states in which HPV DNA can exist (Sudenga and Shrestha, 2013). Anecdotally, Robert J. Huebner, Chief of the Laboratory of RNA Tumor Viruses (NCI) recognized this inadequacy by referring it as the "The Virologist's Dilemma" (Huebner, 1957). As a consequence, he paved the way for the inclusion and particularly the acceptance of epidemiological data to corroborate the involvement of a virus as a cause for a specific disease (Vonka, 2000).

The progress in molecular technologies and immunological methods (Falkow, 2004) therefore led to a revision of these criteria, by both including epidemiological and molecular data as well as terminologies like "plausibility" (=whether a causal relationship makes biological sense) and "coherence" (=asking whether causality is compatible with present knowledge of the disease), respectively (Fredricks and Relman, 1996). Such an extension avoids an important category of empiricism, namely the notion of "falsification" and the consequential dump of a theory in favor of another (Buchanan et al., 2006). Revised criteria rather allow the inclusion of other scenarios to explain the absence of viral sequences in some SCCs. For instance, considering the importance of cell–cell communication in a tumor microenvironment, it is also conceivable that a small fraction of HPV-positive cancer cells secrete paracrine acting vesicles (e.g., exosomes) that may stimulate abnormal proliferation of surrounding virus-negative cells and in turn tumor growth (Dalla Pozza et al., 2017; Harden and Munger, 2017). However, the strongest arguments for at least an obligatory initial function of certain viruses in cancer development are vaccination strategies where the prevention of tumor formation is the most stringent read-out criteria for the success of a vaccine (Moore and Chang, 2017).

Hence, the question of an etiological or merely an opportunistic role of beta-HPV types in skin cancer development is accomplished in a concept, referred as the "hit-and-run" mechanism of microbe/virus induced carcinogenesis (reviewed in Galloway and McDougall, 1983; Iwasaka et al., 1992; Niller et al., 2011; Hufbauer and Akgül, 2017). Alternatively, the term "indirect carcinogen" was suggested (Mossman et al., 2004), but this semantically points more toward a substance or an irradiation event as environmental carcinogen than to an infectious agent and confuses the notion of prophylactic vaccination to prevent tumor formation induced by an "indirect" carcinogen. However, a "hit-and run" model of gene regulation is not without precedent. As already suggested several decades ago (Schaffner, 1988), recent experiments indeed showed that certain transcription factors (e.g., bZIP1) epigenetically change the histone code after transient binding ("hit") that allows the assembly of transcription complexes to continue gene expression after its dissociation ("run") (reviewed in Varala et al., 2015). Whether certain HPV types also use this mechanism remains to be elucidated.

Nevertheless, numerous seroepidemiological reports support the notion of an association between beta-HPV infection and SCC or its precursors (Andersson et al., 2012; Chahoud et al., 2016), despite the occasional absence of the viral DNA within malignant lesions. Here, another distinct property between mucosal and cutaneous HPV types may account for the occasional loss of viral DNA during skin carcinogenesis, namely the physical state. In contrast to anogenital cancer, cutaneous HPVs do not integrate into the host genome and persist as extrachromosomal elements in a defined copy number. Since HPVs completely depend on the host cell replication machinery, UV-induced DNA damage and the mode of accompanying repair mechanisms may disrupt the maintenance of episomal DNA during viral persistence (reviewed in Doorbar, 2016; Bristol et al., 2017; Wendel and Wallace, 2017).

HOW CAN A "HIT-AND-RUN" MECHANISM BE EXPLAINED?

Accepting tentatively an etiological function of beta-HPV in conjunction with UV exposure in NMSC development, several studies have identified different mechanisms that may reasonably explain a viral contribution to a "hit-and-run" mode of carcinogenesis. Cutaneous HPVs infect and persist as extrachromosomal genomes in basal keratinocytes especially around hair follicles (Weissenborn et al., 2012) which are a reservoir for stem cells with different properties (Jaks et al., 2010). During wound healing (Donati et al., 2017) and skin cancer development in transgenic mice expressing the complete early region of HPV8 (Lanfredini et al., 2017), these cells become activated and start to proliferate.

The main targets of mucosal HPVs are p53 and pRB, which is sufficient to transform the host cell and initiate uncontrolled proliferation (see Doorbar et al., 2012 and references herein), by impairing many downstream pathways such as cell cycle arrest, metabolism, apoptosis, and cross-talks to the immune system

(Harris and Levine, 2005; Rozan and El-Deiry, 2007; Moody and Laimins, 2010). In contrast, cutaneous papillomaviruses developed several alternative strategies to interfere with their host cells: instead of binding E6AP to facilitate p53 degradation as alpha type HPVs, E6 of most other HPV genera, amongst them the cutaneous types HPV1 and HPV8, binds to MAML1 to inhibit NOTCH signaling, a feature also shared by animal PVs (e.g., BPV1, MmuPV1, and MnPV) (Brimer et al., 2012, 2017; Meyers et al., 2017). MAML1 together with the histone acetyltransferases p300 and CREBBP can form a transcription complex that activates this pathway (Rozenblatt-Rosen et al., 2012). Amongst its function as a tumor suppressor, NOTCH drives differentiation of keratinocytes and is therefore found to be frequently mutated in cutaneous SCCs (Pickering et al., 2014; South et al., 2014). An impairment of this pathway either by mutations or by intervention of HPV keeps the cell in a proliferative state and promotes tumorigenesis. HPV5 and HPV8 additionally interfere with host cell differentiation by an E6-mediated degradation of p300, which in turn decreases the expression of keratin 1 and 10 and involucrin (Howie et al., 2011).

Furthermore, HPV38 E6 binds p300 thereby preventing p53 acetylation at lysine 382 and blocking p53-mediated apoptosis (Muench et al., 2010). HPV38 E6 can also increase the expression of the N-truncated isoform of p73, lacking a transactivation domain. ΔNp73 in turn competes with p53 activity that may perturb apoptosis and the eradication of damaged HPV-positive cells (Caldeira et al., 2003). A recent study further showed that by targeting p300, HPV8 E6 maintains a proliferating state of the host cell by downregulating the CCAAT/enhancer-binding protein (C/EBPα) and decreasing the expression of microRNA-203, a repressor of ΔNp63 expression (Marthaler et al., 2017). While p63, the master regulator of epithelial stemness, can induce cell cycle arrest and apoptosis like p53 and p73, ΔNp63 can act in a dominant-negative manner and maintain proliferation (reviewed in Candi et al., 2015). Indeed, certain beta-HPVs target central hubs within the cellular network that control differentiation, senescence as well as apoptosis, which reasonably explains the capacity of these viruses to stimulate proliferation of undifferentiated cells. Such effects on tissue homeostasis are of profound importance in NMSC development, particularly when HPV-infected skin is cumulatively exposed to UV.

UV exposure under physiological circumstances induces p53 stabilization and activation that leads to a cell cycle arrest and DNA repair or – at higher dosages – to apoptosis (reviewed in Zuckerman et al., 2009). Perturbed p53 function in turn leads to a gradual accumulation of genetically altered cells, thereby promoting the development of NMSC (Feltkamp et al., 2008). While high-risk mucosal types directly target p53 itself after DNA damage, cutaneous beta-HPVs affect a plethora of DDR proteins downstream of p53 (White et al., 2014; Wendel and Wallace, 2017). An important protein that links the ATM/ATR pathway to p53-induced apoptosis is the conserved Ser/Thr kinase HIPK2 (Matt and Hofmann, 2016). Upon severe UV damage, HIPK2 forms a complex with p53 and the CBP acetyltransferase leading to HIPK2-mediated p53 phosphorylation at serine 46 and CBP-mediated p53 acetylation at lysine 382 and finally a strong p53 activation with induction of pro-apoptotic gene expression (reviewed in Bitomsky and Hofmann, 2009; Matt and Hofmann, 2016). As shown for one of the most prevalent HPV types found in skin (de Koning et al., 2009), HPV23 E6 can inhibit HIPK2-mediated phosphorylation of p53 in response to UV damage (Muschik et al., 2011). Intriguingly, HIPK2 also controls the number of stem and progenitor cells in the skin (Wei et al., 2007), the reservoir for cutaneous HPVs (reviewed in Egawa et al., 2015). Moreover, HIPK2-deficient mice show an enhanced susceptibility to develop SCCs (Wei et al., 2007) consistent with decreased levels HIPK2 expression in KAs and SCCs compared to AK (Kwon et al., 2015). Additionally, beta-HPVs can abrogate UV-induced pyrimidine dimer excision (Giampieri and Storey, 2004) or target the pro-apoptotic protein Bak for proteolytic degradation (Jackson et al., 2000; Underbrink et al., 2008; Holloway et al., 2015). In any case, the interference with the DDR and pro-apoptotic pathways can promote long-lasting effects on genomic instability and favors the accumulation of damaged cells (reviewed in Wendel and Wallace, 2017).

Moreover, UV-activated EGFR signaling which causes keratinocyte hyperproliferation and hyperplasia of the skin (El-Abaseri et al., 2006) is enhanced by HPV8 E6, thereby contributing to SCC formation (Taute et al., 2017). Furthermore, HPV5 and 8 E7 alter beta-catenin and zona occludens-1 anchor proteins which disturb cellular adherence and tight junctions (Heuser et al., 2016a). Their reorganization imbalances tissue homeostasis and lead to epithelial-mesenchymal transition (EMT) (Polette et al., 2007), also suggesting a role in NMSC development (reviewed in Chen et al., 2016). This is in line with an HPV8 E7-mediated upregulation of metalloproteases that remodel the extracellular matrix (Akgül et al., 2006) to facilitate migration and invasion of HPV8-positive cells (Akgül et al., 2005a). Furthermore, HPV8 E7 upregulates fibronectin, another EMT marker (Lee et al., 2006), by inducing a switch from E-cadherin to N-cadherin expression in suprabasal cell layers of organotypic skin cultures, considered to be a primary event in invasion of carcinoma cells (Heuser et al., 2016b).

As soon as HPV-infected altered squamous cells invade deeper layers and undergo EMT, it is likely that HPV replication, known to be highly dependent on cell differentiation, cannot be maintained (reviewed in Doorbar et al., 2012). Consequently, viral presence is no longer necessary for malignant progression, since the tumor becomes heterogeneous in terms of acquiring additional mutations. Despite different modes of action for mucosal and cutaneous HPVs, the outcome is similar: in the case of cervical carcinoma, HPV is integrated into the host cell genome but maintains the transformed phenotype by continuous E6/E7 expression (reviewed in Doorbar et al., 2012). Conversely, cutaneous HPVs interfere with their host cell apparently in the beginning of the multi-step process of carcinogenesis, finally leading to an intracellular environment counteracting episomal DNA replication. This may explain why lower or no viral loads are detected in SCCs as compared to pre-malignant lesions (Weissenborn et al., 2012). In any case, this is a "dead end" for both mucosal and cutaneous HPVs, since the permissive cycle is interrupted and no new virus progenies can be formed.

THE IMPORTANCE OF PRECLINICAL MODELS FOR INFECTIOUS AGENTS – SOME GENERAL CONSIDERATIONS

Models in bioscience are indispensable to reduce the complexity of a disease manifested in patients, but of course they also have their inherent limitations (Anisimov et al., 2005; Mazzocchi, 2008; Dougherty and Shmulevich, 2012). Moreover, in contrast to the empirical supposition of a working hypothesis as "right" or "wrong," models can also be tentatively categorized as "relevant" or "irrelevant" for the investigation of a particular scientific question or even a multifactorial disease. Since there is a strong social pressure on basic research to bring reproducible laboratory results into the clinic (Begley and Ellis, 2012), there are indeed many recent initiatives to improve this transfer by validating the relevance and impact of *in vitro* and *in vivo* models with respect of their translational applicability (Denayer et al., 2014; Day et al., 2015; Dolgos et al., 2016; Horvath et al., 2016).

Animal experiments for infectious agents like papillomaviruses are also indispensable (Doorbar, 2016; Christensen et al., 2017) and should reflect as much as possible the molecular and histological key features of a disease as found in patients (reviewed in Greek and Menache, 2013). Nevertheless, besides pragmatic reasons in working with easily managing laboratory animals (e.g., rodents) (reviewed in Hu et al., 2017; Uberoi and Lambert, 2017), there are several other important criteria for validation and predictability to guarantee a successful clinical translation. They can be summarized as follows (Kern, 1982; Greek and Menache, 2013; Denayer et al., 2014):

1. The infectious agents should have the same species specificity, tissue tropism and genome organization as their human etiological counterparts.
2. The natural infection mode should be similar. This is of particular importance with respect of the extent and spread of an infection since it may affect both the time course of seroconversion as well as the pathological outcome of the disease.
3. The infectious agent should accomplish the revised Henle-Koch criteria in terms of etiology (Fredricks and Relman, 1996; Falkow, 2004; Mossman et al., 2004). Here, some restrictions have to be considered, especially in the light of novel insights into the organization of individual human virome that can be changed in a time-dependent manner (Virgin, 2014; Gentile and Micozzi, 2016; Vouga and Greub, 2016).
4. The viral inoculum in an experimental infection should not over stimulate the immune system (Kern, 1982).
5. The animal should be immunocompetent and specific antibodies to the respective agents normally absent before exposure. Although especially inbred rodent systems do not necessarily completely mirror human immunology (reviewed in Mestas and Hughes, 2004), they still allow dissecting virus–host interactions in terms of acute and chronic/persistent infections in correlation with the serological response.
6. Depending on immune surveillance in the case of tumor formation, the same lesions should appear, ideally in the same time frame relative to the median life time of the animals ("face validity").
7. Since cancer is a multi-factorial process, the animal model should also allow the inclusion of additional non-genetic risk factors for a disease (e.g., immunosuppression, UV exposure), leading to an enhanced tumor formation.
8. Having identified a potential infectious agent, subsequent vaccination of animals should prevent the disease. Hence, preclinical models ideally should develop the same clinical manifestations as found in patients, an important read-out criterion for the success of a vaccine to be transferred into the clinic (Moore and Chang, 2017).
9. To be valid as a preclinical model, a scoring system should be applied that includes the careful selection of the animal species, the degree of reflecting a disease, face validity, complexity, and predictability (Denayer et al., 2014).

HOW DO THE CURRENT RODENT MODELS FOR CUTANEOUS HPVS FIT TO THESE CRITERIA?

Transgenic Mice

Transgenic mice are suitable model systems for most research fields and have also contributed enormously to our mechanistic knowledge about mucosal and cutaneous PVs (reviewed in Doorbar et al., 2015; Lambert, 2016; Santos et al., 2017). Current genome editing technologies make them relatively easy to generate and to manipulate (Rocha-Martins et al., 2015). The transgene, regularly containing the open reading frames (ORFs) of E6, E6/E7 or the complete early region of the selected HPV type is typically expressed under control of the keratin 14 promoter which facilitates constitutive oncogenic expression in cycling epithelial cells. The composition of the ORFs and the varying oncogenic potential of cutaneous HPVs significantly influence the outcome of experiments, e.g., the tumor induction. For example, mice harboring the complete early region of HPV8 spontaneously develop papillomatosis, acanthosis and hyperkeratosis, epidermal dysplasia and, to lower frequency, SCC formation (Schaper et al., 2005). Here, overexpression of the early region leads to a clonal expansion of a population of Lrig1^{+} keratinocyte stem cells in the hair-follicles that is accompanied by a switch of p63 to its ΔNp63 isoform, lacking the N-terminal transactivation domain (Lanfredini et al., 2017). This in turn interferes with the function of p63 and p73 to induce cell cycle arrest and apoptosis. It also impairs the cellular differentiation program and drives proliferation (reviewed in Candi et al., 2015). Due to the involvement of Lrig1^{+} stem cells in wound healing (Donati et al.,

2017), it is not surprising that development of papillomatosis could be also accelerated after UV exposure, further suggesting a synergistic effect between HPV8 and exogenous factors (Marcuzzi et al., 2009). Furthermore, via targeting of C/EBPβ, HPV8 E7 also suppresses the expression of the CC chemokine ligand 20 (CCL20), which plays a pivotal role in the recruitment of Langerhans cell precursors into the epidermis (Sperling et al., 2012). Hence, considering all these scenarios, the impact of HPV8 on cell differentiation and innate immunity can reasonably explain how a viral infection commits cells to malignant transformation.

The mechanisms by which cutaneous HPVs interfere with their host cell, e.g., by disturbing p53-connected pathways (White et al., 2014) or the DDR to UV, can lead to different outcomes of experiments (Dong et al., 2008; Hufbauer et al., 2011; Viarisio et al., 2011; Holderfield et al., 2014). For instance, as shown recently for HPV49 E6/E7 transgenic mice, these animals are less susceptible to form UV-induced tumors as compared to mice expressing other beta-HPVs, but are prone to chemically induced carcinogenesis of the upper digestive tract (Viarisio et al., 2016). Moreover, in contrast to the HPV8 model where one UV dose was sufficient to induce skin lesions (Marcuzzi et al., 2009), HPV38 E6/E7 transgenic mice require an extended irradiation protocol (Viarisio et al., 2011), mimicking a more natural situation as found in humans after life-long UV exposure (Maglennon et al., 2014). Tumors obtained in the HPV8 model after a single UV dose lack mutations in the *Trp53* and *Notch1* loci, but these were present after cumulative UV exposure in HPV38 mice. Notably, SCCs appeared much earlier in the latter model when UV irradiation and BRAFi treatment were combined. Intriguingly, although no HRAS and KRAS mutations were found in these tumors, the mitogen-activated protein kinase pathway was activated (Viarisio et al., 2017). Monitoring clinical SCC samples obtained from melanoma patients, it seems that HRAS mutations and the presence of HPV is mutually exclusive (Holderfield et al., 2014), a constellation that is reminiscent of transgenic mice expressing HPV38 E6/E7 constitutively.

Considering the concept of a "hit-and-run" mechanism during tumorigenesis, transgenic models are obviously not fully suitable when used in a conventional way by constitutive transgene expression. However, Viarisio et al. (2018) recently were able to overcome this problem by knocking out the HPV38 E6/E7 cassette via Cre-lox recombination as soon as UV-induced lesions appeared. After this, SCCs continued growing even without oncogene expression, clearly demonstrating that viral presence was no longer required to maintain the tumorigenic phenotype. Moreover, these SCCs acquired a large panel of potential "driver" mutations within *Trp53*, *Notch1*, and other genes (Viarisio et al., 2018) that can also be observed in human and murine SCCs (Pickering et al., 2014; Chitsazzadeh et al., 2016).

Although transgenic and knock-out models definitely have their justification when investigating potential principles of an *in vivo* virus–host interaction, concerns may be raised as they only reflect parts of the whole picture and do only partially, if at all, fulfill the above mentioned criteria to guarantee a successful clinical translation. The described examples are mostly typical "gain-of-function" studies, where the viral transgene is integrated and controlled by a heterologous promoter, thereby not mimicking the physiological gene dosage and the physical state of the viral DNA which normally persists extrachromosomally in the host cell. Additionally, the encoded transgenic proteins, provided there is no conditional gene expression, are self-tolerant and do not mirror a proper immune response against the corresponding genuine antigens expressed during a natural infection (Walrath et al., 2010). Moreover, according to quantitative trait locus (QTL) mapping analysis for cancer susceptibility loci, inbred strains of mice tremendously vary in their ability to develop tumors (Fleming et al., 2013). Hence, although being extremely helpful, experiments with transgenic mice have to be complemented with natural infection models to get also insight in immunological aspects, particularly allowing the production of appropriate vaccines to prevent NMSC (Vinzón and Rösl 2015).

Natural Model Systems

Restricting this overview only to rodent systems, and also considering the above mentioned criteria for a relevant preclinical model, the MmuPV1/ mouse model (reviewed in Hu et al., 2017) is one of the most attractive, since the mouse is not only the best-characterized laboratory animal, but can also be infected by a virus isolated from the same species. Although just discovered in 2011, Xue et al. (2017) recently published a full transcription map of MmuPV1, providing a basis for a further characterization of viral proteins and their function in skin tumor formation. Moreover, first vaccination studies have been carried out in this system (Jiang et al., 2017). However, even with the MmuPV1/mouse model, the setup of a natural infection followed by a complete viral life cycle in a normal and immunocompetent host is unfortunately still not completely fulfilled. In this model, for instance, lesions appear only when infecting mice with high and, in comparison to humans, non-physiological amounts of virus particles at certain sites like the tail and muzzle, while the back skin is relatively resistant (Handisurya et al., 2013, 2014; Wang et al., 2015). This may be attributed to differential expression of MHC molecules, the presence of Langerhans cells and variations in the keratin network (Sundberg et al., 2014; Quigley et al., 2016), supporting the importance of the local immune surveillance (Da Silva et al., 2014) at the region of infection. These differences may also cause inappropriate conditions for virus particle formation that have to be overcome by a high infection rate, since fewer progenies could be detected in back skin than in mucosal tissue, despite equal viral DNA loads in both regions (Cladel et al., 2017). Cutaneous MmuPV1-induced tail papillomas contained high amounts of viral DNA (Uberoi et al., 2016), but no SCCs lacking MmuPV1 DNA are formed in immunocompetent animals that allow to study a "hit-and-run" mechanism as proposed.

Another preclinical model that is used to explore the impact of cutaneous papillomaviruses on skin carcinogenesis is the African multimammate mouse *Mastomys coucha*, formerly taxonomically classified as *Mastomys natalensis* (**Figure 1**; Kruppa et al., 1990). These animals belong to the Muridae family and are naturally infected with MnPV and McPV2, which – like cutaneous and genital HPVs – infect epidermal and mucosal tissues, respectively (Muller and Gissmann, 1978; Nafz et al., 2008). MnPV can spontaneously induce epithelial lesions of the skin (mainly papillomas and KAs), while McPV2 causes anogenital lesions like condylomata at the anus, vulva, and penis, respectively. Similar to cutaneous HPVs, MnPV and McPV2 persist as episomes without any indication of integration but – depending on the type of lesion – in different copy numbers (Nafz et al., 2008). Considering the natural infection mode, *M. coucha* acquire the virus early after birth, as MnPV DNA is found in the skin of four-week-old animals where at the same time seroconversion is taking place (Schäfer et al., 2011).

Similar to cutaneous HPVs, the MnPV genome lacks an ORF for E5 (de Villiers et al., 2004) while parts of the E6, E1, and L1 genes are phylogenetically related to HPV types associated with EV (Tan et al., 1994). MnPV-induced benign lesions do not spontaneously regress but have the capacity to transform to SCCs (Reinacher et al., 1978; Vinzón et al., 2014). The exo-/endophytic keratinized lesions contain high numbers of episomal virus genomes (**Figures 1B–D**) and – similar to cutaneous HPVs – do not show any sign for integration (Amtmann et al., 1984; Hasche et al., 2017). As the animals are immunocompetent, E2-specific antibodies serve as an early infection marker found already in four-week-old animals, while L1-specific antibodies appear later, correlating with the appearance of skin lesions (Schäfer et al., 2011). Having a virus-free colony of *M. coucha* as control, the animals also served as preclinical model for the development of MnPV-specific vaccination strategies both under normal and immunosuppressed conditions (Vinzón et al., 2014). According to the relevance criteria for animal systems summarized above, *M. coucha* permits the follow-up of the complete infection cycle, starting from primary infection until the development of lesions that are not restricted to a certain body area (Nafz et al., 2007). Transcriptome analysis of skin tumors lead to the identification of various mRNA isoforms of MnPV (Salvermoser et al., 2016). Moreover, *M. coucha*-derived cell lines (Hasche et al., 2016) can be used to test the effects of additional factors on viral transcription and replication, making previous drawbacks compared to mouse systems more and more negligible.

Notably, the *M. coucha* model resembles in many characteristics UV-induced NMSC development in humans. In a large long-term study, the animals were irradiated with UV doses that are comparable to different areas of the world (Hasche et al., 2017). Naturally infected animals developed SCCs significantly more often than virus-free controls. Some of these SCCs were well differentiated and keratinizing (KSCCs), containing high amounts of extrachromosomal and transcriptionally active MnPV genomes as observed previously in spontaneous MnPV-induced tumors (Amtmann et al., 1984; Vinzón et al., 2014), whereas poorly differentiated and non-keratinizing SCCs (nKSCCs) only contained low amounts or even lacked viral DNA. Histologically KSCCs were similar to human AKs and Bowen's disease (Majores and Bierhoff, 2015) which also contain high viral loads whereas SCCs usually lack HPV DNA (Weissenborn et al., 2005). However, irrespective of the tumor type, all tumor-bearing animals developed antibody responses against the viral L1 capsid protein, providing evidence for preceding infections, which again is seen in SCC patients (Andersson et al., 2008). Notably, although showing the same time course of induction, the histology of UV-induced SCCs was profoundly influenced by the dose, with KSCCs mostly developing in the lowest dose group and nKSCCs preferentially under higher doses, pointing to the cumulative effect of UV causing human

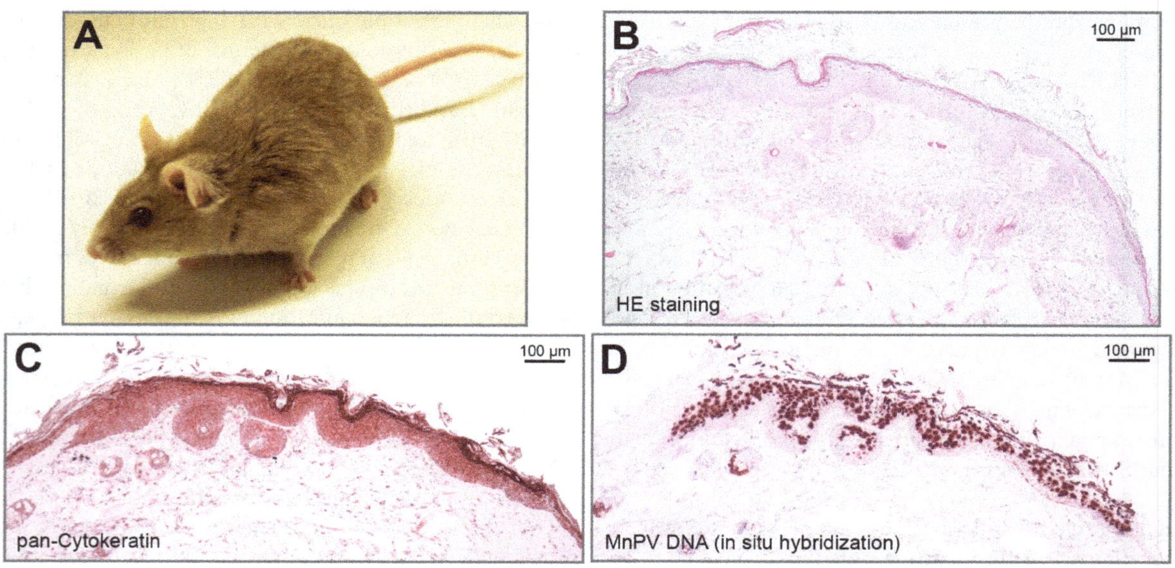

FIGURE 1 | The preclinical animal model *Mastomys coucha* develops MnPV-induced skin lesions. **(A)** A young *Mastomys coucha*. **(B)** HE staining of a dysplastic epithelium at the edge of a spontaneously emerging skin lesion. **(C)** Pan-cytokeratin staining shows the dysplasia of the epithelium. **(D)** *In situ* hybridization reveals squamous cells positive for MnPV DNA.

SCCs (Leiter and Garbe, 2008). Consequently, nKSCCs more often harbored p53 mutants, especially at two hot-spots also known from human SCCs (Pickering et al., 2014) and incapable of activating expression of downstream targets. As shown in mice before, a loss of functional p53 leads to less differentiated tumors (Flores et al., 2016; Page et al., 2016) and induces cell migration and degradation of the extracellular matrix (reviewed in Muller et al., 2011). Since MnPV replication depends – like cutaneous HPVs – on cell differentiation (reviewed in Doorbar et al., 2012), this constellation can explain the loss of viral genomes in these tumors by acquiring additional "driver" mutations (e.g., *Trp53*) (**Figure 2**). Moreover, taking into account that more DNA damages have been detected in MnPV-positive skin compared to MnPV-negative skin, this model provided for the first time evidence for a "hit-and-run mechanism" in a natural infection system (Hasche et al., 2017).

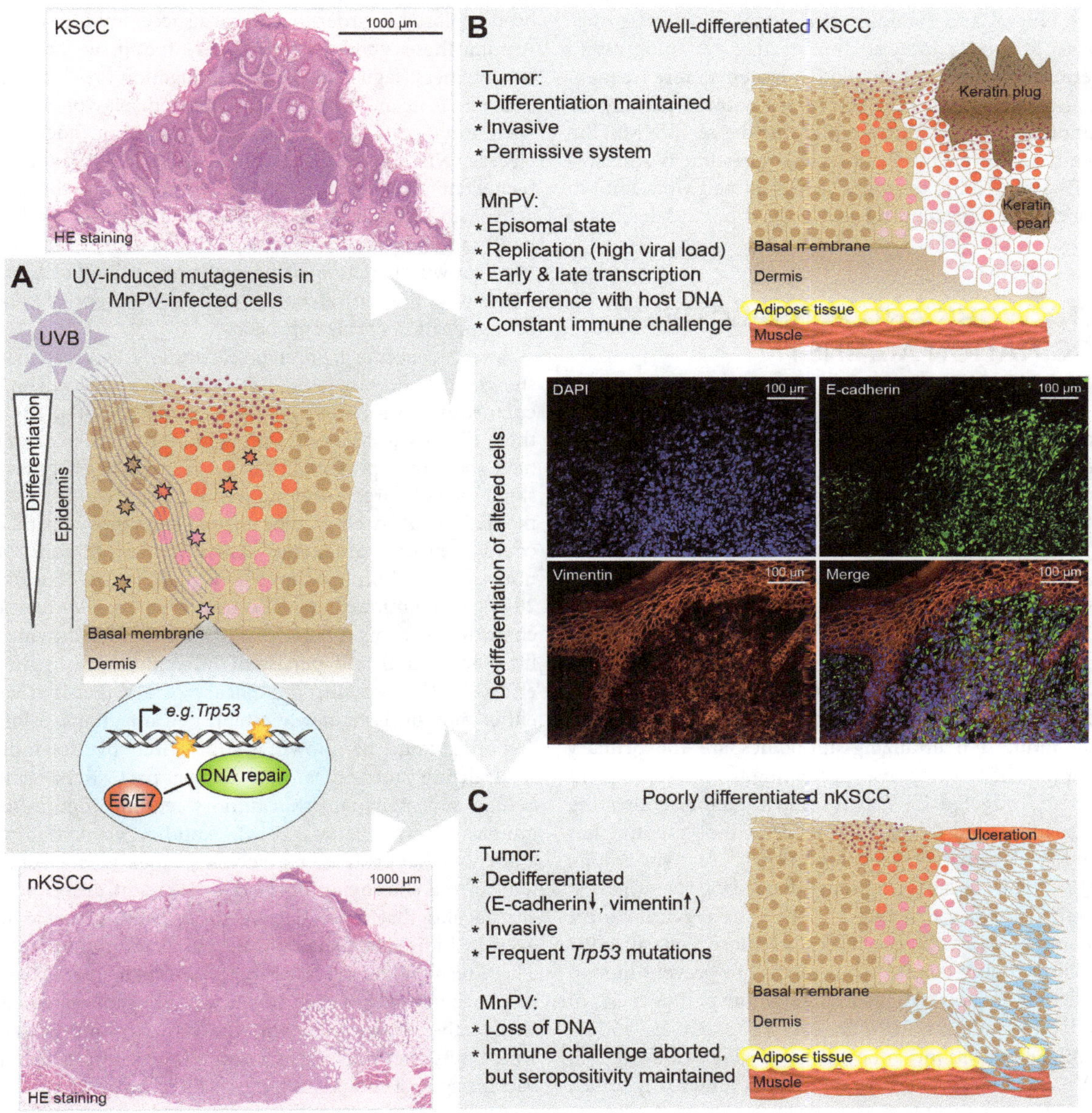

FIGURE 2 | Suggested "hit-and-run" model based on experiments with *Mastomys coucha*. **(A)** Virus replication and virion formation depend on differentiating squamous cells and are favored by UV-induced hyperproliferation. UV induces photoproducts, e.g., in *Trp53*. In uninfected cells, damages are repaired. In infected cells, MnPV reduces chromosomal stability and inhibits DNA repair leading to an accumulation of mutations. **(B)** Altered squamous cells become neoplastic (light blue) and start forming a well-differentiated keratinizing SCC, still representing a permissive system that allows viral replication and formation of virions. **(C)** When neoplastic squamous cells accumulate further mutations (dark blue), a dedifferentiated phenotype (characterized by a switch from E-cadherin to vimentin expression) is acquired, forming a poorly differentiated, non-keratinizing SCC (nKSCC). MnPV cannot replicate in this intracellular environment, resulting in a loss of viral DNA. (Scheme modified from Hasche et al., 2017).

Notably, a recent *in vitro* study showed that MnPV E6 does not interact with E6AP, a prerequisite for p53 degradation, but – like other cutaneous human and animal PVs – interacts with MAML1 to inhibit NOTCH signaling (Brimer et al., 2017). The same was reported for MmuPV1 E6, which also inhibits differentiation of keratinocytes to keep the host cell in a proliferative state (Meyers et al., 2017). However, to examine the effect of UV exposure in the context of a cutaneous PV infection requires more systematic studies, particularly to understand how a single UV dose, shown to have immunosuppressive effects (reviewed in Norval and Halliday, 2011), makes wildtype mice susceptible to MmuPV1-induced tumors that can progress to SCCs (Uberoi et al., 2016), while in other systems more frequent exposure is necessary. This is an important point, especially for immunosuppressed OTRs and the high incidence of NMSC in these patients. However, the fundamental question is still how cutaneous PVs contribute to tumor initiation and what kind of selection mechanisms account for SCC formation and the loss of viral DNA.

CURRENT WORK AND PERSPECTIVES ON VACCINATION AGAINST CUTANEOUS HPVS

The strongest argument for an etiological role of a virus in cancer development is the application of a prophylactic vaccine that prevents tumor formation. In the case of anogenital tumors, three HPV vaccines (Cervarix, Gardasil, and Gardasil 9), consisting of L1 (the major papillomavirus virion protein)-based virus-like particles (VLPs) are currently licensed (Pogoda et al., 2016). They are targeted against two, four, or nine mucosal HPV types (HPV6, 11, 16, 18, 31, 33, 45, 52, and 58), respectively, and – regardless of being very effective – they present limitations, making the development of broad protective second-generation HPV vaccines necessary. Most of the mechanistic studies showed that vaccine-induced neutralizing antibodies are the primary mediators of the elicited response, protecting from a subsequent infection by the targeted HPV types and therefore conferring immunity (Schiller and Lowy, 2012). Since the response has been shown to be largely type-specific and cross-reactivity among different HPV types is almost absent, these vaccines target, at best, the high risk types that cause 90% of the cervical cancer and no cutaneous types. Indeed, there are more than 40 HPV types plausible of being targeted by a vaccine to prevent human diseases: mucosal high-risk HPVs implied in the pathogenesis of cervical and other cancers (HPV16, 18, 31, 33, 35, 39, 45, 51, 52, 56, 58, 59, 68), additional mucosal types which cause genital warts (HPV6 and 11), several beta HPV types potentially linked to NMSC (HPV5, 8, 9, 12, 14, 15, 17, 19, 20, 21, 22, 23, 24, 25, 36, 37, 38, 47, 49) and the different alpha (HPV2, 3, 10, 27, 28, 57), gamma (HPV4, 60, 65), mu (HPV1, 63), and nu (HPV41) types that induce different lesions, being a special burden in children and immunocompromised patients. Given the potential benefits of covering so many different HPV types, a broad-protecting prophylactic HPV vaccine is a rational goal for second-generation vaccine development.

In this context, the papillomavirus minor capsid protein L2 contains a region with a major cross-neutralizing epitope that has been the main immunogen for second-generation vaccines (Gambhira et al., 2007). The goal of developing an L2-based vaccine is to generate a single- or oligo-valent antigen with a distinctively larger spectrum of protection against genital and cutaneous HPVs than the current formulations (Pouyanfard and Muller, 2017). Given that L2-derived linear peptides induce antibody levels which are several orders of magnitude lower that those induced by L1 VLP vaccines, different strategies had been explored in order to achieve a successful immune response. Among these, good responses were found by formation of L2 concatemers (Jagu et al., 2009), conjugation to a T-helper epitope and a TLR ligand (Alphs et al., 2008), display on structures like bacteriophages (Tumban et al., 2011) or on adeno-associated viruses (Nieto et al., 2012), chimeric HPV L2 peptide/L1-VLPs (Schellenbacher et al., 2009), integration into the thioredoxin active site (Rubio et al., 2009) or lipidation and fusion to FcγR-targeting scaffold (Zhang et al., 2016). These approaches have shown elicitation of neutralizing antibodies with a broad range of cross-neutralization, setting the proof-of-principle for the application of this approach.

Several vaccine formulations, either L1- or L2-based, have shown the development of antibodies neutralizing to PV cutaneous types (summarized in **Table 1**), either by targeting them directly or as a cross-protection. In particular, two studies have shown the potential of these vaccines to effectively prevent skin lesions in preclinical models. When *M. coucha* was used as a model, a VLP-based vaccine against a cutaneous papillomavirus could prevent spontaneous skin tumor formation both under normal and immunosuppressed conditions (Vinzón et al., 2014). As mentioned, MnPV-infected *M. coucha* resemble many characteristics of cutaneous HPVs and the human situation, like the natural and persistent infection early in life (Schäfer et al., 2011). Assessing the efficacy of a VLP-based vaccine on either previously or newly established infections, a long-lasting response could be shown, characterized by the induction of neutralizing antibodies that confer protection against both benign and malignant skin tumors even in immunosuppressed animals (Vinzón et al., 2014). Another novel finding of this study was that protection involves the maintenance of a low viral load in the skin by an antibody-dependent prevention of virus spread and that it is effective in preventing tumor formation even in individuals already infected at the time of vaccination. These results offer evidence that VLPs elicit an effective immune response in the skin even under immunosuppressed conditions, irrespective of the infection status at the time of vaccination, which sets the basis for a future clinical implementation of a vaccine against cutaneous HPV-induced tumors to prevent SCCs, especially in OTRs.

DNA vaccines were also explored in the context of cutaneous HPV infection. A recent study (Marcuzzi et al., 2014) showed that a vaccine consisting of HPV8 E6 DNA can generate a specific cellular response in roughly half of the vaccinated animals and partially prevent papilloma formation in those which developed HPV8-E6-specific T cell immunity as demonstrated by ELISPOT. Regarding L2 vaccines, a simple HPV16-L2 DNA

TABLE 1 | Preclinical studies showing reactivity of HPV vaccines to cutaneous types/challenge.

Immunogen scaffold/type	PV immunogen	Cutaneous HPV types neutralized by the vaccine *in vitro*	HPV types neutralized by cutaneous challenge	Projected vaccine development	Reference
VLPs	L1 from HPV 5, 8, and 92	HPV 5	ND	Unknown	Handisurya et al., 2009
Capsomers/VLPs	L1 from HPV 2, 27, and 57	HPV 2, 27, and 57	ND	Unknown	Senger et al., 2010
VLPs	L1 from MnPV	MnPV	MnPV	No	Vinzón et al., 2014
Lipopeptide (P25-P2C-HPV)	HPV16 L2(17–36)	HPV 5, BPV 1	HPV 16 and 45	Unknown	Alphs et al., 2008
L2 concatemers	Fusion of the L2(11-88) region of HPV types 6, 16, 18, 31, 39, 51, 56, and 73	HPV 3, 5, 8, 23, 27, 38, 57, 76	ND	Unknown	Kwak et al., 2014
Lipidated L2-repeat fusioned to an anti-hFcγRI scFv	HPV16 L2(17–36)	HPV 2 and 5	ND	Unknown	Zhang et al., 2016
Chimeric VLPs	HPV16 L2(17–36)	HPV 2, 3, 5, 27, 76	ND	Being produced under cGMP for clinical trials by the NCI PREVENT program (Shi et al., 2001).	Schellenbacher et al., 2009, 2013
Chimeric VLPs	HPV17 L2(17–36)	HPV 5, 20, 24, 38 and 96	HPV 5	Unknown	Huber et al., 2017
Chimeric VLPs	HPV 58 L2(16–37)	HPV 2, 5, 27 and 57	ND	Unknown	Chen et al., 2017
Fusion to bacterial flagellin	L2(11–200), L2(11–88) and/or L2(17–38) of HPV 6, 16, 18, 31, 39 and 52	ND	HPV 6, 16, 18, 31, 39, 52 and CRPV	Unknown	Kalnin et al., 2014, 2017
Pyrococcus furiosus thiorecoxin with L2 octamer	L2(20–38) from HPV 6, 16, 18, 31, 33, 35, 51, and 59	HPV 3, 4, 5, 10, 38, 63, 76, 92, 95, and 96	ND	Close to cGMP production for a planned human trial (Pouyanfard and Muller, 2017).	Pouyanfard et al., 2017; Spagnoli et al., 2017
PP7/MS2 bacteriophage VLPs	HPV16 L2(20–29), (17–31), (14–40) and (14–65)	ND	HPV5	Being developed by the company Agilvax with DMID/NIAID/NIH support (Pouyanfard and Muller, 2017).	Tumban et al., 2012
Naked-DNA, fusion to calreticulin	MmuPV1 E6 and E7 and L2(11–200)	ND	ND	Being produced under cGMP for clinical trials by the NCI PREVENT program (Shi et al., 2001).	Jiang et al., 2017

vaccine showed no induction of neutralizing antibodies and therefore no cross-reactivity potential (Hitzeroth et al., 2009). In contrast, another vaccine composed of HPV16-L2/E6/E7 fused to human calreticulin (hCRT) as a strategy to enhance MHC class I presentation, induced both E6/E7-specific T-cell responses and L2-specific neutralizing antibodies, showing both therapeutic and prophylactic potential (Kim et al., 2008). hCRT-E6E7L2 conferred partial protection in an *in vivo* neutralization assay (Jiang et al., 2017), but its cross-neutralization activity has not been yet reported. Furthermore, when exploring the vaccine in an immunosuppressed setting, hCRT-E6E7L2 vaccination maintained cellular immune reactivity in $CD4^+$ T cell-depleted mice but lost the ability to induce a humoral response (Peng et al., 2014). hCRT-E6E7L2 is currently produced under cGMP for clinical trials by the NCI PREVENT program (Schellenbacher et al., 2017).

The recent development in the MmuPV1 model allowed vaccination studies also in this animal system (Jiang et al., 2017). An hCRT-MmuPV1E6E7L2 DNA vaccine induced strong mE6 and mE7 $CD8^+$ T cell responses and anti-L2 antibodies. In addition to the vaccine-induced antibody titers, also a robust anti-L1 response could be detected regardless of the papilloma status of the animals, probably due to the inoculum used for the experimental infection. Remarkably, persistent papillomas disappeared within 2 months after treatment and the virus could no longer be detected. Given the design of the vaccine, the importance of neutralizing anti-L2 antibodies cannot be dissected, as the anti-L2 response is concomitant to the E6 and E7 responses.

Therefore, the effectivity of pure L2 vaccines in preventing skin tumors is yet to be studied in a complete preclinical model. One important issue to be answered is whether L2 vaccination can elicit enough neutralizing antibodies to confer protection against tumor formation, especially against non-cognate HPV types, since L2 responses are known to be lower than their L1 counterparts. In that context, even when sera display titers below detection limit by *in vitro* neutralization assays and *in vivo* neutralization assays after passive transfer, vaccinated animals still show complete protection against infection, which points to the fact that very low titers are indeed sufficient to confer immunity (Kalnin et al., 2017).

CONCLUSION

Current data strongly support an involvement of cutaneous HPVs in the pathogenesis of NMSC. It is clear that a vaccine targeting a broader spectrum, including mucosal and cutaneous HPVs would be beneficial for certain patients, especially those who are immunosuppressed. Since cutaneous HPV infections are acquired very early in life, vaccination in infancy seems to be most appropriate. The other option would be the vaccination of immunocompromised individuals, for example patients awaiting organ transplantation. By eliminating one of the main risk factors (HPV infection), the incidence of NMSC should be reduced. Clinical development of vaccines that could achieve this goal is currently being pursued.

AUTHOR CONTRIBUTIONS

All authors listed, have made substantial, direct and intellectual contribution to the work, and approved it for publication.

REFERENCES

Acuna, S. A., Fernandes, K. A., Daly, C., Hicks, L. K., Sutradhar, R., Kim, S. J., et al. (2016). Cancer mortality among recipients of solid-organ transplantation in Ontario, Canada. *JAMA Oncol.* 2, 463–469. doi: 10.1001/jamaoncol.2015.5137

Akgül, B., Garcia-Escudero, R., Ghali, L., Pfister, H. J., Fuchs, P. G., Navsaria, H., et al. (2005a). The E7 protein of cutaneous human papillomavirus type 8 causes invasion of human keratinocytes into the dermis in organotypic cultures of skin. *Cancer Res.* 65, 2216–2223. doi: 10.1158/0008-5472.CAN-04-1952

Akgül, B., Lemme, W., Garcia-Escudero, R., Storey, A., and Pfister, H. J. (2005b). UV-B irradiation stimulates the promoter activity of the high-risk, cutaneous human papillomavirus 5 and 8 in primary keratinocytes. *Arch. Virol.* 150, 145–151. doi: 10.1007/s00705-004-0398-4

Akgül, B., Pfefferle, R., Marcuzzi, G. P., Zigrino, P., Krieg, T., Pfister, H., et al. (2006). Expression of matrix metalloproteinase (MMP)-2, MMP-9, MMP-13, and MT1-MMP in skin tumors of human papillomavirus type 8 transgenic mice. *Exp. Dermatol.* 15, 35–42. doi: 10.1111/j.0906-6705.2005.00387.x

Al-Dujaili, Z., Henry, M., Dorizas, A. S., and Sadick, N. S. (2017). Skin cancer concerns particular to women. *Int. J. Womens Dermatol.* 3 1, S49–S51. doi: 10.1016/j.ijwd.2017.02.009

Alphs, H. H., Gambhira, R., Karanam, B., Roberts, J. N., Jagu, S., Schiller, J. T., et al. (2008). Protection against heterologous human papillomavirus challenge by a synthetic lipopeptide vaccine containing a broadly cross-neutralizing epitope of L2. *Proc. Natl. Acad. Sci. U.S.A.* 105, 5850–5855. doi: 10.1073/pnas.0800868105

Amtmann, E., Volm, M., and Wayss, K. (1984). Tumour induction in the rodent *Mastomys natalensis* by activation of endogenous papilloma virus genomes. *Nature* 308, 291–292. doi: 10.1038/308291a0

Andersson, K., Michael, K. M., Luostarinen, T., Waterboer, T., Gislefoss, R., Hakulinen, T., et al. (2012). Prospective study of human papillomavirus seropositivity and risk of nonmelanoma skin cancer. *Am. J. Epidemiol.* 175, 685–695. doi: 10.1093/aje/kwr373

Andersson, K., Waterboer, T., Kirnbauer, R., Slupetzky, K., Iftner, T., de Villiers, E. M., et al. (2008). Seroreactivity to cutaneous human papillomaviruses among patients with nonmelanoma skin cancer or benign skin lesions. *Cancer Epidemiol. Biomarkers Prev.* 17, 189–195. doi: 10.1158/1055-9965.EPI-07-0405

Anforth, R., Fernandez-Penas, P., and Long, G. V. (2013). Cutaneous toxicities of RAF inhibitors. *Lancet Oncol.* 14, e11–e18. doi: 10.1016/S1470-2045(12)70413-8

Anisimov, V. N., Ukraintseva, S. V., and Yashin, A. I. (2005). Cancer in rodents: does it tell us about cancer in humans? *Nat. Rev. Cancer* 5, 807–819. doi: 10.1038/nrc1715

Antonsson, A., Karanfilovska, S., Lindqvist, P. G., and Hansson, B. G. (2003). General acquisition of human papillomavirus infections of skin occurs in early infancy. *J. Clin. Microbiol.* 41, 2509–2514. doi: 10.1128/JCM.41.6.2509-2514.2003

Apalla, Z., Lallas, A., Sotiriou, E., Lazaridou, E., and Ioannides, D. (2017). Epidemiological trends in skin cancer. *Dermatol. Pract. Concept.* 7, 1–6. doi: 10.5826/dpc.0702a01

Arnold, A. W., and Hofbauer, G. F. (2012). Human papillomavirus and squamous cell cancer of the skin–epidermodysplasia verruciformis-associated human papillomavirus revisited. *Curr. Probl. Dermatol.* 43, 49–56. doi: 10.1159/000335151

Arron, S. T., Ruby, J. G., Dybbro, E., Ganem, D., and Derisi, J. L. (2011). Transcriptome sequencing demonstrates that human papillomavirus is not active in cutaneous squamous cell carcinoma. *J. Invest. Dermatol.* 131, 1745–1753. doi: 10.1038/jid.2011.91

Begley, C. G., and Ellis, L. M. (2012). Drug development: raise standards for preclinical cancer research. *Nature* 483, 531–533. doi: 10.1038/483531a

Belbasis, L., Stefanaki, I., Stratigos, A. J., and Evangelou, E. (2016). Non-genetic risk factors for cutaneous melanoma and keratinocyte skin cancers: an umbrella review of meta-analyses. *J. Dermatol. Sci.* 84, 330–339. doi: 10.1016/j.jdermsci.2016.09.003

Belkaid, Y., and Segre, J. A. (2014). Dialogue between skin microbiota and immunity. *Science* 346, 954–959. doi: 10.1126/science.1260144

Bitomsky, N., and Hofmann, T. G. (2009). Apoptosis and autophagy: Regulation of apoptosis by DNA damage signalling - roles of p53, p73 and HIPK2. *FEBS J.* 276, 6074–6083. doi: 10.1111/j.1742-4658.2009.07331.x

Black, J. O. (2016). Xeroderma pigmentosum. *Head Neck Pathol.* 10, 139–144. doi: 10.1007/s12105-016-0707-8

Borgogna, C., Lanfredini, S., Peretti, A., De Andrea, M., Zavattaro, E., Colombo, E., et al. (2014). Improved detection reveals active beta-papillomavirus infection in skin lesions from kidney transplant recipients. *Mod. Pathol.* 27, 1101–1115. doi: 10.1038/modpathol.2013.240

Borgogna, C., Zavattaro, E., De Andrea, M., Griffin, H. M., Dell'Oste, V., Azzimonti, B., et al. (2012). Characterization of beta papillomavirus E4 expression in tumours from Epidermodysplasia Verruciformis patients and in experimental models. *Virology* 423, 195–204. doi: 10.1016/j.virol.2011.11.029

Boussemart, L., Boivin, C., Claveau, J., Tao, Y. G., Tomasic, G., Routier, E., et al. (2013). Vemurafenib and radiosensitization. *JAMA Dermatol.* 149, 855–857. doi: 10.1001/jamadermatol.2013.4200

Brash, D. E. (2015). UV signature mutations. *Photochem. Photobiol.* 91, 15–26. doi: 10.1111/php.12377

Bresler, S. C., Padwa, B. L., and Granter, S. R. (2016). Nevoid basal cell carcinoma syndrome (Gorlin syndrome). *Head Neck Pathol.* 10, 119–124. doi: 10.1007/s12105-016-0706-9

Brimer, N., Drews, C. M., and Vande Pol, S. B. (2017). Association of papillomavirus E6 proteins with either MAML1 or E6AP clusters E6 proteins by structure, function, and evolutionary relatedness. *PLoS Pathog.* 13:e1006781. doi: 10.1371/journal.ppat.1006781

Brimer, N., Lyons, C., Wallberg, A. E., and Vande Pol, S. B. (2012). Cutaneous papillomavirus E6 oncoproteins associate with MAML1 to repress transactivation and NOTCH signaling. *Oncogene* 31, 4639–4646. doi: 10.1038/onc.2011.589

Bristol, M. L., Das, D., and Morgan, I. M. (2017). Why human papillomaviruses activate the DNA damage response (DDR) and how cellular and viral replication persists in the presence of DDR signaling. *Viruses* 9:E268. doi: 10.3390/v9100268

Bruggink, S. C., de Koning, M. N., Gussekloo, J., Egberts, P. F., Ter Schegget, J., Feltkamp, M. C., et al. (2012). Cutaneous wart-associated HPV types: prevalence and relation with patient characteristics. *J. Clin. Virol.* 55, 250–255. doi: 10.1016/j.jcv.2012.07.014

Buchanan, A. V., Weiss, K. M., and Fullerton, S. M. (2006). Dissecting complex disease: the quest for the Philosopher's Stone? *Int. J. Epidemiol.* 35, 562–571. doi: 10.1093/ije/dyl001

Bzhalava, D., Muhr, L. S., Lagheden, C., Ekstrom, J., Forslund, O., Dillner, J., et al. (2014). Deep sequencing extends the diversity of human papillomaviruses in human skin. *Sci. Rep.* 4:5807. doi: 10.1038/srep05807

Caldeira, S., Zehbe, I., Accardi, R., Malanchi, I., Dong, W., Giarre, M., et al. (2003). The E6 and E7 proteins of the cutaneous human papillomavirus type 38 display transforming properties. *J. Virol.* 77, 2195–2206. doi: 10.1128/JVI.77.3.2195-2206.2003

Candi, E., Amelio, I., Agostini, M., and Melino, G. (2015). MicroRNAs and p63 in epithelial stemness. *Cell Death Differ.* 22, 12–21. doi: 10.1038/cdd.2014.113

Cardoso, J. C., and Calonje, E. (2011). Cutaneous manifestations of human papillomaviruses: a review. *Acta Dermatovenerol. Alp. Pannonica Adriat.* 20, 145–154.

Casadevall, A., and Pirofski, L. A. (2000). Host-pathogen interactions: basic concepts of microbial commensalism, colonization, infection, and disease. *Infect. Immun.* 68, 6511–6518. doi: 10.1128/IAI.68.12.6511-6518.2000

Chahoud, J., Semaan, A., Chen, Y., Cao, M., Rieber, A. G., Rady, P., et al. (2016). Association between beta-genus human papillomavirus and cutaneous squamous cell carcinoma in immunocompetent individuals-A meta-analysis. *JAMA Dermatol.* 152, 1354–1364. doi: 10.1001/jamadermatol.2015.4530

Chen, X., Bode, A. M., Dong, Z., and Cao, Y. (2016). The epithelial-mesenchymal transition (EMT) is regulated by oncoviruses in cancer. *FASEB J.* 30, 3001–3010 doi: 10.1096/fj.201600388R

Chen, X., Liu, H., Wang, Z., Wang, S., Zhang, T., Hu, M., et al. (2017). Human papillomavirus 16L1-58L2 chimeric virus-like particles elicit durable neutralizing antibody responses against a broad-spectrum of human papillomavirus types. *Oncotarget* 8, 63333–63344. doi: 10.18632/oncotarget.19327

Chitsazzadeh, V., Coarfa, C., Drummond, J. A., Nguyen, T., Joseph, A., Chilukuri, S., et al. (2016). Cross-species identification of genomic drivers of squamous cell carcinoma development across preneoplastic intermediates. *Nat. Commun.* 7:12601. doi: 10.1038/ncomms12601

Chow, K. Y., Brotin, E., Ben Khalifa, Y., Carthagena, L., Teissier, S., Danckaert, A., et al. (2010). A pivotal role for CXCL12 signaling in HPV-mediated transformation of keratinocytes: clues to understanding HPV-pathogenesis in WHIM syndrome. *Cell Host Microbe* 8, 523–533. doi: 10.1016/j.chom.2010.11.006

Christensen, N. D., Budgeon, L. R., Cladel, N. M., and Hu, J. (2017). Recent advances in preclinical model systems for papillomaviruses. *Virus Res.* 231, 108–118. doi: 10.1016/j.virusres.2016.12.004

Cladel, N. M., Budgeon, L. R., Cooper, T. K., Balogh, K. K., Christensen, N. D., Myers, R., et al. (2017). Mouse papillomavirus infections spread to cutaneous sites with progression to malignancy. *J. Gen. Virol.* doi: 10.1099/jgv.0.000926 [Epub ahead of print].

Da Silva, D. M., Movius, C. A., Raff, A. B., Brand, H. E., Skeate, J. G., Wong, M. K., et al. (2014). Suppression of Langerhans cell activation is conserved amongst human papillomavirus alpha and beta genotypes, but not a micro genotype. *Virology* 45, 279–286. doi: 10.1016/j.virol.2014.01.031

Dalla Pozza, E., Forciniti, S., Palmieri, M., and Dando, I. (2017). Secreted molecules inducing epithelial-to-mesenchymal transition in cancer development. *Semin. Cell Dev. Biol.* doi: 10.1016/j.semcdb.2017.06.027 [Epub ahead of print].

Davis, A., Gao, R., and Navin, N. (2017). Tumor evolution: Linear, branching, neutral or punctuated? *Biochim. Biophys. Acta* 1867, 151–161. doi: 10.1016/j.bbcan.2017.01.003

Day, C. P., Merlino, G., and Van Dyke, T. (2015). Preclinical mouse cancer models: a maze of opportunities and challenges. *Cell* 163, 39–53. doi: 10.1016/j.cell.2015.08.068

de Koning, M. N., Weissenborn, S. J., Abeni, D., Bouwes Bavinck, J. N., Euvrard, S., Green, A. C., et al. (2009). Prevalence and associated factors of betapapillomavirus infections in individuals without cutaneous squamous cell carcinoma. *J. Gen. Virol.* 90(Pt 7), 1611–1621. doi: 10.1099/vir.0.010017-0

de Villiers, E. M., Fauquet, C., Broker, T. R., Bernard, H. U., and zur Hausen, H. (2004). Classification of papillomaviruses. *Virology* 324, 17–27. doi: 10.1016/j.virol.2004.03.033

Denayer, T., Stöhr, T., and Van Roy, M. (2014). Animal models in translational medicine: Validation and prediction. *New Horiz. Transl. Med.* 2, 5–11. doi: 10.1016/j.nhtm.2014.08.001

Dolgos, H., Trusheim, M., Gross, D., Halle, J. P., Ogden, J., Osterwalder, B., et al. (2016). Translational medicine guide transforms drug development processes: the recent Merck experience. *Drug Discov. Today* 21, 517–526. doi: 10.1016/j.drudis.2016.01.003

Donati, G., Rognoni, E., Hiratsuka, T., Liakath-Ali, K., Hoste, E., Kar, G., et al. (2017). Wounding induces dedifferentiation of epidermal Gata6(+) cells and acquisition of stem cell properties. *Nat. Cell Biol.* 19, 603–613. doi: 10.1038/ncb3532

Dong, W., Arpin, C., Accardi, R., Gissmann, L., Sylla, B. S., Marvel, J., et al. (2008). Loss of p53 or p73 in human papillomavirus type 38 E6 and E7 transgenic mice partially restores the UV-activated cell cycle checkpoints. *Oncogene* 27, 2923–2928. doi: 10.1038/sj.onc.1210944

Doorbar, J. (2016). Model systems of human papillomavirus-associated disease. *J. Pathol.* 238, 166–179. doi: 10.1002/path.4656

Doorbar, J., Egawa, N., Griffin, H., Kranjec, C., and Murakami, I. (2015). Human papillomavirus molecular biology and disease association. *Rev. Med. Virol.* 25(Suppl. 1), 2–23. doi: 10.1002/rmv.1822

Doorbar, J., Quint, W., Banks, L., Bravo, I. G., Stoler, M., Broker, T. R., et al. (2012). The biology and life-cycle of human papillomaviruses. *Vaccine* 30(Suppl. 5), F55–F70. doi: 10.1016/j.vaccine.2012.06.083

Dougherty, E. R., and Shmulevich, I. (2012). On the limitations of biological knowledge. *Curr. Genomics* 13, 574–587. doi: 10.2174/138920212803251445

Dreno, B., Cerio, R., Dirschka, T., Nart, I. F., Lear, J. T., Peris, K., et al. (2017). A novel actinic keratosis field assessment scale for grading actinic keratosis disease severity. *Acta Derm. Venereol.* 97, 1108–1113. doi: 10.2340/00015555-2710

Edqvist, P. H., Fagerberg, L., Hallstrom, B. M., Danielsson, A., Edlund, K., Uhlen, M., et al. (2015). Expression of human skin-specific genes defined by transcriptomics and antibody-based profiling. *J. Histochem. Cytochem.* 63, 129–141. doi: 10.1369/0022155414562646

Edwards, R. A., and Rohwer, F. (2005). Viral metagenomics. *Nat. Rev. Microbiol.* 3, 504–510. doi: 10.1038/nrmicro1163

Egawa, N., Egawa, K., Griffin, H., and Doorbar, J. (2015). Human papillomaviruses; epithelial tropisms, and the development of neoplasia. *Viruses* 7, 3863–3890. doi: 10.3390/v7072802

Eisemann, N., Waldmann, A., Geller, A. C., Weinstock, M. A., Volkmer, B., Greinert, R., et al. (2014). Non-melanoma skin cancer incidence and impact of skin cancer screening on incidence. *J. Invest. Dermatol.* 134, 43–50. doi: 10.1038/jid.2013.304

El-Abaseri, T. B., Putta, S., and Hansen, L. A. (2006). Ultraviolet irradiation induces keratinocyte proliferation and epidermal hyperplasia through the activation of the epidermal growth factor receptor. *Carcinogenesis* 27, 225–231. doi: 10.1093/carcin/bgi220

Euvrard, S., Kanitakis, J., and Claudy, A. (2003). Skin cancers after organ transplantation. *N. Engl. J. Med.* 348, 1681–1691. doi: 10.1056/NEJMra022137

Falkow, S. (2004). Molecular Koch's postulates applied to bacterial pathogenicity–a personal recollection 15 years later. *Nat. Rev. Microbiol.* 2, 67–72. doi: 10.1038/nrmicro799

Feltkamp, M. C., de Koning, M. N., Bavinck, J. N., and Ter Schegget, J. (2008). Betapapillomaviruses: innocent bystanders or causes of skin cancer. *J. Clin. Virol.* 43, 353–360. doi: 10.1016/j.jcv.2008.09.009

Fleming, J. L., Gable, D. L., Samadzadeh-Tarighat, S., Cheng, L., Yu, L., Gillespie, J. L., et al. (2013). Differential expression of miR-1, a putative tumor suppressing microRNA, in cancer resistant and cancer susceptible mice. *PeerJ* 1:e68. doi: 10.7717/peerj.68

Flores, A., Grant, W., White, A. C., Scumpia, P., Takahashi, R., and Lowry, W. E. (2016). Tumor suppressor identity can contribute to heterogeneity of phenotype in hair follicle stem cell induced squamous cell carcinoma. *Exp. Dermatol.* 25, 733–735. doi: 10.1111/exd.13037

Fredricks, D. N., and Relman, D. A. (1996). Sequence-based identification of microbial pathogens: a reconsideration of Koch's postulates. *Clin. Microbiol. Rev.* 9, 18–33.

Galloway, D. A., and McDougall, J. K. (1983). The oncogenic potential of herpes simplex viruses: evidence for a 'hit-and-run' mechanism. *Nature* 302, 21–24. doi: 10.1038/302021a0

Gambhira, R., Karanam, B., Jagu, S., Roberts, J. N., Buck, C. B., Bossis, I., et al. (2007). A protective and broadly cross-neutralizing epitope of human papillomavirus L2. *J. Virol.* 81, 13927–13931. doi: 10.1128/JVI.00936-07

Garrett, G. L., Lowenstein, S. E., Singer, J. P., He, S. Y., and Arron, S. T. (2016). Trends of skin cancer mortality after transplantation in the United States: 1987 to 2013. *J. Am. Acad. Dermatol.* 75, 106–112. doi: 10.1016/j.jaad.2016.02.1155

Geissler, E. K. (2015). Skin cancer in solid organ transplant recipients: are mTOR inhibitors a game changer? *Transplant. Res.* 4:1. doi: 10.1186/s13737-014-0022-4

Gentile, G., and Micozzi, A. (2016). Speculations on the clinical significance of asymptomatic viral infections. *Clin. Microbiol. Infect.* 22, 585–588. doi: 10.1016/j.cmi.2016.07.016

Giampieri, S., and Storey, A. (2004). Repair of UV-induced thymine dimers is compromised in cells expressing the E6 protein from human papillomaviruses types 5 and 18. *Br. J. Cancer* 90, 2203–2209. doi: 10.1038/sj.bjc.6601829

Gibney, G. T., Messina, J. L., Fedorenko, I. V., Sondak, V. K., and Smalley, K. S. (2013). Paradoxical oncogenesis–the long-term effects of BRAF inhibition in melanoma. *Nat. Rev. Clin. Oncol.* 10, 390–399. doi: 10.1038/nrclinonc.2013.83

Grce, M., and Mravak-Stipetic, M. (2014). Human papillomavirus-associated diseases. *Clin. Dermatol.* 32, 253–258. doi: 10.1016/j.clindermatol.2013.10.006

Greaves, M. (2015). Evolutionary determinants of cancer. *Cancer Discov.* 5, 806–820. doi: 10.1158/2159-8290.CD-15-0439

Greek, R., and Menache, A. (2013). Systematic reviews of animal models: methodology versus epistemology. *Int. J. Med. Sci.* 10, 206–221. doi: 10.7150/ijms.5529

Hampras, S. S., Giuliano, A. R., Lin, H. Y., Fisher, K. J., Abrahamsen, M. E., Sirak, B. A., et al. (2014). Natural history of cutaneous human papillomavirus (HPV) infection in men: the HIM study. *PLoS One* 9:e104843. doi: 10.1371/journal.pone.0104843

Hampton, T. (2005). Skin cancer's ranks rise: immunosuppression to blame. *JAMA* 294, 1476–1480. doi: 10.1001/jama.294.12.1476

Handisurya, A., Day, P. M., Thompson, C. D., Bonelli, M., Lowy, D. R., and Schiller, J. T. (2014). Strain-specific properties and T cells regulate the susceptibility to papilloma induction by Mus musculus papillomavirus 1. *PLoS Pathog.* 10:e1004314. doi: 10.1371/journal.ppat.1004314

Handisurya, A., Day, P. M., Thompson, C. D., Buck, C. B., Pang, Y. Y., Lowy, D. R., et al. (2013). Characterization of Mus musculus papillomavirus 1 infection in situ reveals an unusual pattern of late gene expression and capsid protein localization. *J. Virol.* 87, 13214–13225. doi: 10.1128/JVI.02162-13

Handisurya, A., Gambhira, R., Schellenbacher, C., Shafti-Keramat, S., Forslund, O., Favre, M., et al. (2009). Serological relationship between cutaneous human papillomavirus types 5, 8 and 92. *J. Gen. Virol.* 90(Pt 1), 136–143. doi: 10.1099/vir.0.006189-0

Hannigan, G. D., Meisel, J. S., Tyldsley, A. S., Zheng, Q., Hodkinson, B. P., SanMiguel, A. J., et al. (2015). The human skin double-stranded DNA virome: topographical and temporal diversity, genetic enrichment, and dynamic associations with the host microbiome. *mBio* 6:e01578-15. doi: 10.1128/mBio.01578-15

Harden, M. E., and Munger, K. (2017). Human papillomavirus 16 E6 and E7 oncoprotein expression alters microRNA expression in extracellular vesicles. *Virology* 508, 63–69. doi: 10.1016/j.virol.2017.05.005

Harris, S. L., and Levine, A. J. (2005). The p53 pathway: positive and negative feedback loops. *Oncogene* 24, 2899–2908. doi: 10.1038/sj.onc.1208615

Harwood, C. A., Proby, C. M., Inman, G. J., and Leigh, I. M. (2016). The promise of genomics and the development of targeted therapies for cutaneous squamous cell carcinoma. *Acta Derm. Venereol.* 96, 3–16. doi: 10.2340/00015555-2181

Harwood, C. A., Proby, C. M., McGregor, J. M., Sheaff, M. T., Leigh, I. M., and Cerio, R. (2006). Clinicopathologic features of skin cancer in organ transplant recipients: a retrospective case-control series. *J. Am. Acad. Dermatol.* 54, 290–300. doi: 10.1016/j.jaad.2005.10.049

Harwood, C. A., Surentheran, T., McGregor, J. M., Spink, P. J., Leigh, I. M., Breuer, J., et al. (2000). Human papillomavirus infection and non-melanoma skin cancer in immunosuppressed and immunocompetent individuals. *J. Med. Virol.* 61, 289–297. doi: 10.1002/1096-9071(200007)61:3<289::AID-JMV2>3.0.CO;2-Z

Hasche, D., Stephan, S., Braspenning-Wesch, I., Mikulec, J., Niebler, M., Gröne, H. J., et al. (2017). The interplay of UV and cutaneous papillomavirus infection in skin cancer development. *PLoS Pathog.* 13:e1006723. doi: 10.1371/journal.ppat.1006723

Hasche, D., Stephan, S., Savelyeva, L., Westermann, F., Rösl, F., and Vinzón, S. E. (2016). Establishment of an immortalized skin keratinocyte cell line derived from the animal model *Mastomys coucha*. *PLoS One* 11:e0161283. doi: 10.1371/journal.pone.0161283

Hassel, J. C., Groesser, L., Herschberger, E., Weichert, W., and Hafner, C. (2015). RAS mutations in benign epithelial tumors associated with BRAF inhibitor treatment of melanoma. *J. Invest. Dermatol.* 135, 636–639. doi: 10.1038/jid.2014.360

Heuser, S., Hufbauer, M., Marx, B., Tok, A., Majewski, S., Pfister, H., et al. (2016a). The levels of epithelial anchor proteins beta-catenin and zona occludens-1 are altered by E7 of human papillomaviruses 5 and 8. *J. Gen. Virol.* 97, 463–472. doi: 10.1099/jgv.0.000363

Heuser, S., Hufbauer, M., Steiger, J., Marshall, J., Sterner-Kock, A., Mauch, C., et al. (2016b). The fibronectin/alpha3beta1 integrin axis serves as molecular basis for keratinocyte invasion induced by betaHPV. *Oncogene* 35, 4529–4539. doi: 10.1038/onc.2015.512

Hitzeroth, I. I., Passmore, J. A., Shephard, E., Stewart, D., Muller, M., Williamson, A. L., et al. (2009). Immunogenicity of an HPV-16 L2 DNA vaccine. *Vaccine* 27, 6432–6434. doi: 10.1016/j.vaccine.2009.06.015

Holderfield, M., Lorenzana, E., Weisburd, B., Lomovasky, L., Boussemart, L., Lacroix, L., et al. (2014). Vemurafenib cooperates with HPV to promote initiation of cutaneous tumors. *Cancer Res.* 74, 2238–2245. doi: 10.1158/0008-5472.CAN-13-1065-T

Holloway, A., Simmonds, M., Azad, A., Fox, J. L., and Storey, A. (2015). Resistance to UV-induced apoptosis by beta-HPV5 E6 involves targeting of activated BAK for proteolysis by recruitment of the HERC1 ubiquitin ligase. *Int. J. Cancer* 136, 2831–2843. doi: 10.1002/ijc.29350

Horvath, P., Aulner, N., Bickle, M., Davies, A. M., Nery, E. D., Ebner, D., et al. (2016). Screening out irrelevant cell-based models of disease. *Nat. Rev. Drug Discov.* 15, 751–769. doi: 10.1038/nrd.2016.175

Howie, H. L., Koop, J. I., Weese, J., Robinson, K., Wipf, G., Kim, L., et al. (2011). Beta-HPV 5 and 8 E6 promote p300 degradation by blocking AKT/p300 association. *PLoS Pathog.* 7:e1002211. doi: 10.1371/journal.ppat.1002211

Hu, J., Cladel, N. M., Budgeon, L. R., Balogh, K. K., and Christensen, N. D. (2017). The mouse papillomavirus infection model. *Viruses* 9:E246. doi: 10.3390/v9090246

Huber, B., Schellenbacher, C., Shafti-Keramat, S., Jindra, C., Christensen, N., and Kirnbauer, R. (2017). Chimeric L2-based virus-like particle (VLP) vaccines targeting cutaneous human papillomaviruses (HPV). *PLoS One* 12:e0169533. doi: 10.1371/journal.pone.0169533

Huebner, R. J. (1957). Criteria for etiologic association of prevalent viruses with prevalent diseases; the virologist's dilemma. *Ann. N. Y. Acad. Sci.* 67, 430–438. doi: 10.1111/j.1749-6632.1957.tb46066.x

Hufbauer, M., and Akgül, B. (2017). Molecular mechanisms of human papillomavirus induced skin carcinogenesis. *Viruses* 9:E187. doi: 10.3390/v9070187

Hufbauer, M., Biddle, A., Borgogna, C., Gariglio, M., Doorbar, J., Storey, A., et al. (2013). Expression of betapapillomavirus oncogenes increases the number of keratinocytes with stem cell-like properties. *J. Virol.* 87, 12158–12165. doi: 10.1128/JVI.01510-13

Hufbauer, M., Lazic, D., Reinartz, M., Akgul, B., Pfister, H., and Weissenborn, S. J. (2011). Skin tumor formation in human papillomavirus 8 transgenic mice is associated with a deregulation of oncogenic miRNAs and their tumor suppressive targets. *J. Dermatol. Sci.* 64, 7–15. doi: 10.1016/j.jdermsci.2011.06.008

Inglis, T. J. (2007). Principia aetiologica: taking causality beyond Koch's postulates. *J. Med. Microbiol.* 56(Pt 11), 1419–1422. doi: 10.1099/jmm.0.47179-0

Iwasaka, T., Hayashi, Y., Yokoyama, M., Hara, K., Matsuo, N., and Sugimori, H. (1992). 'Hit and run' oncogenesis by human papillomavirus type 18 DNA. *Acta Obstet. Gynecol. Scand.* 71, 219–223. doi: 10.3109/00016349209009922

Jablonska, S., Majewski, S., Obalek, S., and Orth, G. (1997). Cutaneous warts. *Clin. Dermatol.* 15, 309–319. doi: 10.1016/S0738-081X(96)00170-8

Jackson, S., Harwood, C., Thomas, M., Banks, L., and Storey, A. (2000). Role of Bak in UV-induced apoptosis in skin cancer and abrogation by HPV E6 proteins. *Genes Dev.* 14, 3065–3073. doi: 10.1101/gad.182100

Jagu, S., Karanam, B., Gambhira, R., Chivukula, S. V., Chaganti, R. J., Lowy, D. R., et al. (2009). Concatenated multitype L2 fusion proteins as candidate prophylactic pan-human papillomavirus vaccines. *J. Natl. Cancer Inst.* 101, 782–792. doi: 10.1093/jnci/djp106

Jaks, V., Kasper, M., and Toftgard, R. (2010). The hair follicle-a stem cell zoo. *Exp. Cell Res.* 316, 1422–1428. doi: 10.1016/j.yexcr.2010.03.014

Jiang, R. T., Wang, J. W., Peng, S., Huang, T. C., Wang, C., Cannella, F., et al. (2017). Spontaneous and vaccine-induced clearance of Mus musculus papillomavirus 1 infection. *J. Virol.* 91:e00699-17. doi: 10.1128/JVI.00699-17

John, S. M., Trakatelli, M., Gehring, R., Finlay, K., Fionda, C., Wittlich, M., et al. (2016). CONSENSUS REPORT: recognizing non-melanoma skin cancer, including actinic keratosis, as an occupational disease - A Call to Action. *J. Eur. Acad. Dermatol. Venereol.* 30(Suppl. 3), 38–45. doi: 10.1111/jdv.13608

Kalinska-Bienias, A., Kowalewski, C., and Majewski, S. (2016). The EVER genes - the genetic etiology of carcinogenesis in epidermodysplasia verruciformis and a possible role in non-epidermodysplasia verruciformis patients. *Postepy Dermatol. Alergol.* 33, 75–80. doi: 10.5114/ada.2016.59145

Kalnin, K., Chivukula, S., Tibbitts, T., Yan, Y., Stegalkina, S., Shen, L., et al. (2017). Incorporation of RG1 epitope concatemers into a self-adjuvanting Flagellin-L2 vaccine broaden durable protection against cutaneous challenge with diverse human papillomavirus genotypes. *Vaccine* 35, 4942–4951. doi: 10.1016/j.vaccine.2017.07.086

Kalnin, K., Tibbitts, T., Yan, Y., Stegalkina, S., Shen, L., Costa, V., et al. (2014). Low doses of flagellin-L2 multimer vaccines protect against challenge with diverse papillomavirus genotypes. *Vaccine* 32, 3540–3547. doi: 10.1016/j.vaccine.2014.04.032

Kennedy, C., Bajdik, C. D., Willemze, R., De Gruijl, F. R., Bouwes Bavinck, J. N., and Leiden Skin Cancer Study. (2003). The influence of painful sunburns and lifetime sun exposure on the risk of actinic keratoses, seborrheic warts, melanocytic nevi, atypical nevi, and skin cancer. *J. Invest. Dermatol.* 120, 1087–1093. doi: 10.1046/j.1523-1747.2003.12246.x

Kern, E. R. (1982). Use of viral infections in animal models to assess changes in the immune system. *Environ. Health Perspect.* 43, 71–79. doi: 10.1289/ehp.824371

Kim, D., Gambhira, R., Karanam, B., Monie, A., Hung, C. F., Roden, R., et al. (2008). Generation and characterization of a preventive and therapeutic HPV DNA vaccine. *Vaccine* 26, 351–360. doi: 10.1016/j.vaccine.2007.11.019

Krogan, N. J., Lippman, S., Agard, D. A., Ashworth, A., and Ideker, T. (2015). The cancer cell map initiative: defining the hallmark networks of cancer. *Mol. Cell* 58, 690–698. doi: 10.1016/j.molcel.2015.05.008

Kruppa, T. F., Iglauer, F., Ihnen, E., Miller, K., and Kunstyr, I. (1990). *Mastomys natalensis* or *Mastomys coucha*, Correct species designation in animal experiments. *Trop. Med. Parasitol.* 41, 219–220.

Kuschal, C., Thoms, K. M., Schubert, S., Schafer, A., Boeckmann, L., Schon, M. P., et al. (2012). Skin cancer in organ transplant recipients: effects of immunosuppressive medications on DNA repair. *Exp. Dermatol.* 21, 2–6. doi: 10.1111/j.1600-0625.2011.01413.x

Kwak, K., Jiang, R., Wang, J. W., Jagu, S., Kirnbauer, R., and Roden, R. B. (2014). Impact of inhibitors and L2 antibodies upon the infectivity of diverse alpha and beta human papillomavirus types. *PLoS One* 9:e97232. doi: 10.1371/journal.pone.0097232

Kwon, M. J., Min, S. K., Seo, J., Kim, D. H., Sung, C. O., Lim, M. S., et al. (2015). HIPK2 expression in progression of cutaneous epithelial neoplasm. *Int. J. Dermatol.* 54, 347–354. doi: 10.1111/ijd.12664

Lambert, P. F. (2016). Transgenic mouse models of tumor virus action. *Annu. Rev. Virol.* 3, 473–489. doi: 10.1146/annurev-virology-100114-054908

Lanfredini, S., Olivero, C., Borgogna, C., Calati, F., Powell, K., Davies, K. J., et al. (2017). HPV8 field cancerization in a transgenic mouse model is due to Lrig1+ Keratinocyte stem cell expansion. *J. Invest. Dermatol.* 137, 2208–2216. doi: 10.1016/j.jid.2017.04.039

Lazarczyk, M., Cassonnet, P., Pons, C., Jacob, Y., and Favre, M. (2009). The EVER proteins as a natural barrier against papillomaviruses: a new insight into the pathogenesis of human papillomavirus infections. *Microbiol. Mol. Biol. Rev.* 73, 348–370. doi: 10.1128/MMBR.00033-08

Lazarczyk, M., Dalard, C., Hayder, M., Dupre, L., Pignolet, B., Majewski, S., et al. (2012). EVER proteins, key elements of the natural anti-human papillomavirus barrier, are regulated upon T-cell activation. *PLoS One* 7:e39995. doi: 10.1371/journal.pone.0039995

Lazarczyk, M., and Favre, M. (2008). Role of Zn2+ ions in host-virus interactions. *J. Virol.* 82, 11486–11494. doi: 10.1128/JVI.01314-08

LeBoit, P. E., Burg, G., Weedon, D., and Sarasain, A. (eds) (2006). *World Health Organization Classification of Tumours. Pathology and Genetics of Skin Tumours.* Lyon: IARC Press.

Lee, J. M., Dedhar, S., Kalluri, R., and Thompson, E. W. (2006). The epithelial-mesenchymal transition: new insights in signaling, development, and disease. *J. Cell Biol.* 172, 973–981. doi: 10.1083/jcb.200601018

Leiding, J. W., and Holland, S. M. (2012). Warts and all: human papillomavirus in primary immunodeficiencies. *J. Allergy Clin. Immunol.* 130, 1030–1048. doi: 10.1016/j.jaci.2012.07.049

Leiter, U., and Garbe, C. (2008). Epidemiology of melanoma and nonmelanoma skin cancer–the role of sunlight. *Adv. Exp. Med. Biol.* 624, 89–103. doi: 10.1007/978-0-387-77574-6_8

Lipinski, K. A., Barber, L. J., Davies, M. N., Ashenden, M., Sottoriva, A., and Gerlinger, M. (2016). Cancer evolution and the limits of predictability in precision cancer medicine. *Trends Cancer* 2, 49–63. doi: 10.1016/j.trecan.2015.11.003

Lomas, A., Leonardi-Bee, J., and Bath-Hextall, F. (2012). A systematic review of worldwide incidence of nonmelanoma skin cancer. *Br. J. Dermatol.* 166, 1069–1080. doi: 10.1111/j.1365-2133.2012.10830.x

Ma, Y., Madupu, R., Karaoz, U., Nossa, C. W., Yang, L., Yooseph, S., et al. (2014). Human papillomavirus community in healthy persons, defined by metagenomics analysis of human microbiome project shotgun sequencing data sets. *J. Virol.* 88, 4786–4797. doi: 10.1128/JVI.00093-14

Madeleine, M. M., Johnson, L. G., Daling, J. R., Schwartz, S. M., Carter, J. J., Berg, D., et al. (2013). Cohort profile: the skin cancer after organ transplant study. *Int. J. Epidemiol.* 42, 1669–1677. doi: 10.1093/ije/dys179

Madeleine, M. M., Patel, N. S., Plasmeijer, E. I., Engels, E. A., Bouwes Bavinck, J. N., Toland, A. E., et al. (2017). Epidemiology of keratinocyte carcinomas after organ transplantation. *Br. J. Dermatol.* 177, 1208–1216. doi: 10.1111/bjd.15931

Maglennon, G. A., McIntosh, P. B., and Doorbar, J. (2014). Immunosuppression facilitates the reactivation of latent papillomavirus infections. *J. Virol.* 88, 710–716. doi: 10.1128/JVI.02589-13

Majores, M., and Bierhoff, E. (2015). Actinic keratosis, Bowen's disease, keratoacanthoma and squamous cell carcinoma of the skin]. *Pathologe* 36, 16–29. doi: 10.1007/s00292-014-2063-3

Marcuzzi, G. P., Awerkiew, S., Hufbauer, M., Schadlich, L., Gissmann, L., Eming, S., et al. (2014). Tumor prevention in HPV8 transgenic mice by HPV8-E6 DNA vaccination. *Med. Microbiol. Immunol.* 203, 155–163. doi: 10.1007/s00430-014-0327-4

Marcuzzi, G. P., Hufbauer, M., Kasper, H. U., Weissenborn, S. J., Smola, S., and Pfister, H. (2009). Spontaneous tumour development in human papillomavirus type 8 E6 transgenic mice and rapid induction by UV-light exposure and wounding. *J. Gen. Virol.* 90(Pt 12), 2855–2864. doi: 10.1099/vir.0.012872-0

Marthaler, A. M., Podgorska, M., Feld, P., Fingerle, A., Knerr-Rupp, K., Grasser, F., et al. (2017). Identification of C/EBPalpha as a novel target of the HPV8 E6 protein regulating miR-203 in human keratinocytes. *PLoS Pathog.* 13:e1006406. doi: 10.1371/journal.ppat.1006406

Martincorena, I., Roshan, A., Gerstung, M., Ellis, P., Van Loo, P., McLaren, S., et al. (2015). Tumor evolution. High burden and pervasive positive selection of somatic mutations in normal human skin. *Science* 348, 880–886. doi: 10.1126/science.aaa6806

Matt, S., and Hofmann, T. G. (2016). The DNA damage-induced cell death response: a roadmap to kill cancer cells. *Cell. Mol. Life Sci.* 73, 2829–2850. doi: 10.1007/s00018-016-2130-4

Mavropoulos, J. C., Aldabagh, B., and Arron, S. T. (2014). Prospects for personalized targeted therapies for cutaneous squamous cell carcinoma. *Semin. Cutan. Med. Surg.* 33, 72–75. doi: 10.12788/j.sder.0083

Mazzocchi, F. (2008). Complexity in biology. Exceeding the limits of reductionism and determinism using complexity theory. *EMBO Rep.* 9, 10–14. doi: 10.1038/sj.embor.7401147

McLaughlin-Drubin, M. E., Meyers, J., and Munger, K. (2012). Cancer associated human papillomaviruses. *Curr. Opin. Virol.* 2, 459–466. doi: 10.1016/j.coviro.2012.05.004

Mestas, J., and Hughes, C. C. (2004). Of mice and not men: differences between mouse and human immunology. *J. Immunol.* 172, 2731–2738. doi: 10.4049/jimmunol.172.5.2731

Meuris, F., Carthagena, L., Jaracz-Ros, A., Gaudin, F., Cutolo, P., Deback, C., et al. (2016). The CXCL12/CXCR4 signaling pathway: a new susceptibility factor in human papillomavirus pathogenesis. *PLoS Pathog.* 12:e1006039. doi: 10.1371/journal.ppat.1006039

Meyers, J. M., Uberoi, A., Grace, M., Lambert, P. F., and Munger, K. (2017). Cutaneous HPV8 and MmuPV1 E6 proteins target the NOTCH and TGF-beta tumor suppressors to inhibit differentiation and sustain keratinocyte proliferation. *PLoS Pathog.* 13:e1006171. doi: 10.1371/journal.ppat.1006171

Moody, C. A., and Laimins, L. A. (2010). Human papillomavirus oncoproteins: pathways to transformation. *Nat. Rev. Cancer* 10, 550–560. doi: 10.1038/nrc2886

Moore, P. S., and Chang, Y. (2017). Common commensal cancer viruses. *PLoS Pathog.* 13:e1006078. doi: 10.1371/journal.ppat.1006078

Mossman, B. T., Klein, G., and Zur Hausen, H. (2004). Modern criteria to determine the etiology of human carcinogens. *Semin. Cancer Biol.* 14, 449–452. doi: 10.1016/j.semcancer.2004.06.008

Muench, P., Probst, S., Schuetz, J., Leiprecht, N., Busch, M., Wesselborg, S., et al. (2010). Cutaneous papillomavirus E6 proteins must interact with p300 and block p53-mediated apoptosis for cellular immortalization and tumorigenesis. *Cancer Res.* 70, 6913–6924. doi: 10.1158/0008-5472.CAN-10-1307

Muller, H., and Gissmann, L. (1978). *Mastomys natalensis* papilloma virus (MnPV), the causative agent of epithelial proliferations: characterization of the virus particle. *J. Gen. Virol.* 41, 315–323. doi: 10.1099/0022-1317-41-2-315

Muller, P. A., Vousden, K. H., and Norman, J. C. (2011). p53 and its mutants in tumor cell migration and invasion. *J. Cell Biol.* 192, 209–218. doi: 10.1083/jcb.201009059

Muschik, D., Braspenning-Wesch, I., Stockfleth, E., Rösl, F., Hofmann, T. G., and Nindl, I. (2011). Cutaneous HPV23 E6 prevents p53 phosphorylation through interaction with HIPK2. *PLoS One* 6:e27655. doi: 10.1371/journal.pone.0027655

Nafz, J., Kohler, A., Ohnesorge, M., Nindl, I., Stockfleth, E., and Rösl, F. (2007). Persistence of *Mastomys natalensis* papillomavirus in multiple organs identifies novel targets for infection. *J. Gen. Virol.* 88(Pt 10), 2670–2678. doi: 10.1099/vir.0.82955-0

Nafz, J., Schäfer, K., Chen, S. F., Bravo, I. G., Ibberson, M., Nindl, I., et al. (2008). A novel rodent papillomavirus isolated from anogenital lesions in its natural host. *Virology* 374, 186–197. doi: 10.1016/j.virol.2007.12.012

Nakad, R., and Schumacher, B. (2016). DNA damage response and immune defense: links and mechanisms. *Front. Genet.* 7:147. doi: 10.3389/fgene.2016.00147

Neale, R. E., Weissenborn, S., Abeni, D., Bavinck, J. N., Euvrard, S., Feltkamp, M. C., et al. (2013). Human papillomavirus load in eyebrow hair follicles and risk of cutaneous squamous cell carcinoma. *Cancer Epidemiol. Biomarkers Prev.* 22, 719–727. doi: 10.1158/1055-9965.EPI-12-0917-T

Nieto, K., Weghofer, M., Sehr, P., Ritter, M., Sedlmeier, S., Karanam, B., et al. (2012). Development of AAVLP (HPV16/31L2) particles as broadly protective HPV vaccine candidate. *PLoS One* 7:e39741. doi: 10.1371/journal.pone.0039741

Niller, H. H., Wolf, H., and Minarovits, J. (2011). Viral hit and run-oncogenesis: genetic and epigenetic scenarios. *Cancer Lett.* 305, 200–217. doi: 10.1016/j.canlet.2010.08.007

Nindl, I., and Rösl, F. (2008). Molecular concepts of virus infections causing skin cancer in organ transplant recipients. *Am. J. Transplant.* 8, 2199–2204. doi: 10.1111/j.1600-6143.2008.02392.x

Norval, M., and Halliday, G. M. (2011). The consequences of UV-induced immunosuppression for human health. *Photochem. Photobiol.* 87, 965–977. doi: 10.1111/j.1751-1097.2011.00969.x

O'Malley, M. A. (2016). Microbiology, philosophy and education. *FEMS Microbiol. Lett.* 363:fnw182. doi: 10.1093/femsle/fnw182

Orth, G. (2006). Genetics of epidermodysplasia verruciformis: insights into host defense against papillomaviruses. *Semin. Immunol.* 18, 362–374. doi: 10.1016/j.smim.2006.07.008

Pacini, L., Ceraolo, M. G., Venuti, A., Melita, G., Hasan, U. A., Accardi, R., et al. (2017). UV radiation activates toll-like receptor 9 expression in primary human keratinocytes, an event inhibited by human papillomavirus type 38 E6 and E7 oncoproteins. *J. Virol.* 91:JVI.1123-17. doi: 10.1128/JVI.01123-17

Page, A., Navarro, M., Suarez-Cabrera, C., Alameda, J. P., Casanova, M. L., Paramio, J. M., et al. (2016). Protective role of p53 in skin cancer: carcinogenesis studies in mice lacking epidermal p53. *Oncotarget* 7, 20902–20918. doi: 10.18632/oncotarget.7897

Peng, S., Song, L., Knoff, J., Wang, J. W., Chang, Y. N., Hannaman, D., et al. (2014). Control of HPV-associated tumors by innovative therapeutic HPV DNA vaccine in the absence of CD4+ T cells. *Cell Biosci.* 4:11. doi: 10.1186/2045-3701-4-11

Pfefferle, R., Marcuzzi, G. P., Akgül, B., Kasper, H. U., Schulze, F., Haase, I., et al. (2008). The human papillomavirus type 8 E2 protein induces skin tumors in transgenic mice. *J. Invest. Dermatol.* 128, 2310–2315. doi: 10.1038/jid.2008.73

Pickering, C. R., Zhou, J. H., Lee, J. J., Drummond, J. A., Peng, S. A., Saade, R. E., et al. (2014). Mutational landscape of aggressive cutaneous squamous cell carcinoma. *Clin. Cancer Res.* 20, 6582–6592. doi: 10.1158/1078-0432.CCR-14-1768

Pogoda, C. S., Roden, R. B., and Garcea, R. L. (2016). Immunizing against anogenital cancer: HPV vaccines. *PLoS Pathog.* 12:e1005587. doi: 10.1371/journal.ppat.1005587

Polette, M., Mestdagt, M., Bindels, S., Nawrocki-Raby, B., Hunziker, W., Foidart, J. M., et al. (2007). Beta-catenin and ZO-1: shuttle molecules involved in tumor invasion-associated epithelial-mesenchymal transition processes. *Cells Tissues Organs* 185, 61–65. doi: 10.1159/000101304

Pouyanfard, S., and Muller, M. (2017). Human papillomavirus first and second generation vaccines-current status and future directions. *Biol. Chem.* 398, 871–889. doi: 10.1515/hsz-2017-0105

Pouyanfard, S., Spagnoli, G., Bulli, L., Balz, K., Yang, F., Odenwald, C., et al. (2017). Minor capsid protein L2 polytope induces broad protection against oncogenic and mucosal human papillomaviruses. *J. Virol.* 92:e01930-17. doi: 10.1128/JVI.01930-17

Prasad, R., and Katiyar, S. K. (2017). Crosstalk among UV-induced inflammatory mediators, DNA damage and epigenetic regulators facilitates suppression of the immune system. *Photochem. Photobiol.* 93, 930–936. doi: 10.1111/php.12687

Quigley, D. A., Kandyba, E., Huang, P., Halliwill, K. D., Sjolund, J., Pelorosso, F., et al. (2016). Gene expression architecture of mouse dorsal and tail skin reveals functional differences in inflammation and cancer. *Cell Rep.* 16, 1153–1165. doi: 10.1016/j.celrep.2016.06.061

Ra, S. H., Su, A., Li, X., Zhou, J., Cochran, A. J., Kulkarni, R. P., et al. (2015). Keratoacanthoma and squamous cell carcinoma are distinct from a molecular perspective. *Mod. Pathol.* 28, 799–806. doi: 10.1038/modpathol.2015.5

Rahman, S., Pierce Campbell, C. M., Waterboer, T., Rollison, D. E., Ingles, D. J., Torres, B. N., et al. (2016). Seroprevalence of cutaneous human papillomaviruses (HPVs) among men in the multinational HPV Infection in Men study. *J. Gen. Virol.* 97, 3291–3301. doi: 10.1099/jgv.0.000620

Rangwala, S., and Tsai, K. Y. (2011). Roles of the immune system in skin cancer. *Br. J. Dermatol.* 165, 953–965. doi: 10.1111/j.1365-2133.2011.10507.x

Ratushny, V., Gober, M. D., Hick, R., Ridky, T. W., and Seykora, J. T. (2012). From keratinocyte to cancer: the pathogenesis and modeling of cutaneous squamous cell carcinoma. *J. Clin. Invest.* 122, 464–472. doi: 10.1172/JCI57415

Reinacher, M., Muller, H., Thiel, W., and Rudolph, R. L. (1978). Localization of papillomavirus and virus-specific antigens in the skin of tumor-bearing *Mastomys natalensis* (GRA Giessen). *Med. Microbiol. Immunol.* 165, 93–99. doi: 10.1007/BF02122744

Rocha-Martins, M., Cavalheiro, G. R., Matos-Rodrigues, G. E., and Martins, R. A. (2015). From gene targeting to genome editing: transgenic animals applications and beyond. *An. Acad. Bras. Cienc.* 87, 1323–1348. doi: 10.1590/0001-3765201520140710

Rozan, L. M., and El-Deiry, W. S. (2007). p53 downstream target genes and tumor suppression: a classical view in evolution. *Cell Death Differ.* 14, 3–9. doi: 10.1038/sj.cdd.4402058

Rozenblatt-Rosen, O., Deo, R. C., Padi, M., Adelmant, G., Calderwood, M. A., Rolland, T., et al. (2012). Interpreting cancer genomes using systematic host network perturbations by tumour virus proteins. *Nature* 487, 491–495. doi: 10.1038/nature11288

Rubio, I., Bolchi, A., Moretto, N., Canali, E., Gissmann, L., Tommasino, M., et al. (2009). Potent anti-HPV immune responses induced by tandem repeats of the

HPV16 L2 (20 - 38) peptide displayed on bacterial thioredoxin. *Vaccine* 27, 1949–1956. doi: 10.1016/j.vaccine.2009.01.102

Salvermoser, M., Chotewutmontri, S., Braspenning-Wesch, I., Hasche, D., Rösl, F., and Vinzon, S. E. (2016). Transcriptome analysis of *Mastomys natalensis* papillomavirus in productive lesions after natural infection. *J. Gen. Virol.* 97, 1658–1669. doi: 10.1099/jgv.0.000471

Sanchez Yus, E., Simon, P., Requena, L., Ambrojo, P., and de Eusebio, E. (2000). Solitary keratoacanthoma: a self-healing proliferation that frequently becomes malignant. *Am. J. Dermatopathol.* 22, 305–310. doi: 10.1097/00000372-200008000-00002

Santos, C., Vilanova, M., Medeiros, R., and Gil da Costa, R. M. (2017). HPV-transgenic mouse models: tools for studying the cancer-associated immune response. *Virus Res.* 235, 49–57. doi: 10.1016/j.virusres.2017.04.001

Savage, J. A., and Maize, J. C. Sr. (2014). Keratoacanthoma clinical behavior: a systematic review. *Am. J. Dermatopathol.* 36, 422–429. doi: 10.1097/DAD.0000000000000031

Schäfer, K., Neumann, J., Waterboer, T., and Rösl, F. (2011). Serological markers for papillomavirus infection and skin tumour development in the rodent model *Mastomys coucha. J. Gen. Virol.* 92, 383–394. doi: 10.1099/vir.0.023515-0

Schaffner, W. (1988). Gene regulation. A hit-and-run mechanism for transcriptional activation? *Nature* 336, 427–428. doi: 10.1038/336427a0

Schaper, I. D., Marcuzzi, G. P., Weissenborn, S. J., Kasper, H. U., Dries, V., Smyth, N., et al. (2005). Development of skin tumors in mice transgenic for early genes of human papillomavirus type 8. *Cancer Res.* 65, 1394–1400. doi: 10.1158/0008-5472.CAN-04-3263

Schellenbacher, C., Kwak, K., Fink, D., Shafti-Keramat, S., Huber, B., Jindra, C., et al. (2013). Efficacy of RG1-VLP vaccination against infections with genital and cutaneous human papillomaviruses. *J. Invest. Dermatol.* 133, 2706–2713. doi: 10.1038/jid.2013.253

Schellenbacher, C., Roden, R., and Kirnbauer, R. (2009). Chimeric L1-L2 virus-like particles as potential broad-spectrum human papillomavirus vaccines. *J. Virol.* 83, 10085–10095. doi: 10.1128/JVI.01088-09

Schellenbacher, C., Roden, R. B. S., and Kirnbauer, R. (2017). Developments in L2-based human papillomavirus (HPV) vaccines. *Virus Res.* 231, 166–175. doi: 10.1016/j.virusres.2016.11.020

Schiller, J. T., and Lowy, D. R. (2012). Understanding and learning from the success of prophylactic human papillomavirus vaccines. *Nat. Rev. Microbiol.* 10, 681–692. doi: 10.1038/nrmicro2872

Seebode, C., Lehmann, J., and Emmert, S. (2016). Photocarcinogenesis and skin cancer prevention strategies. *Anticancer Res.* 36, 1371–1378.

Senger, T., Schadlich, L., Textor, S., Klein, C., Michael, K. M., Buck, C. B., et al. (2010). Virus-like particles and capsomeres are potent vaccines against cutaneous alpha HPVs. *Vaccine* 28, 1583–1593. doi: 10.1016/j.vaccine.2009.11.048

Shi, W., Liu, J., Huang, Y., and Qiao, L. (2001). Papillomavirus pseudovirus: a novel vaccine to induce mucosal and systemic cytotoxic T-lymphocyte responses. *J. Virol.* 75, 10139–10148. doi: 10.1128/JVI.75.21.10139-10148.2001

Small, J., Barton, V., Peterson, B., and Alberg, A. J. (2016). Keratinocyte carcinoma as a marker of a high cancer-risk phenotype. *Adv. Cancer Res.* 130, 257–291. doi: 10.1016/bs.acr.2016.01.003

South, A. P., Purdie, K. J., Watt, S. A., Haldenby, S., den Breems, N. Y., Dimon, M., et al. (2014). NOTCH1 mutations occur early during cutaneous squamous cell carcinogenesis. *J. Invest. Dermatol.* 134, 2630–2638. doi: 10.1038/jid.2014.154

Spagnoli, G., Bolchi, A., Cavazzini, D., Pouyanfard, S., Muller, M., and Ottonello, S. (2017). Secretory production of designed multipeptides displayed on a thermostable bacterial thioredoxin scaffold in Pichia pastoris. *Protein Expr. Purif.* 129, 150–157. doi: 10.1016/j.pep.2016.04.012

Sperling, T., Oldak, M., Walch-Ruckheim, B., Wickenhauser, C., Doorbar, J., Pfister, H., et al. (2012). Human papillomavirus type 8 interferes with a novel C/EBPbeta-mediated mechanism of keratinocyte CCL20 chemokine expression and Langerhans cell migration. *PLoS Pathog.* 8:e1002833. doi: 10.1371/journal.ppat.1002833

Sudenga, S. L., and Shrestha, S. (2013). Key considerations and current perspectives of epidemiological studies on human papillomavirus persistence, the intermediate phenotype to cervical cancer. *Int. J. Infect. Dis.* 17, e216–e220. doi: 10.1016/j.ijid.2012.12.027

Sundberg, J. P., Stearns, T. M., Joh, J., Proctor, M., Ingle, A., Silva, K. A., et al. (2014). Immune status, strain background, and anatomic site of inoculation affect mouse papillomavirus (MmuPV1) induction of exophytic papillomas or endophytic trichoblastomas. *PLoS One* 9:e113582. doi: 10.1371/journal.pone.0113582

Takai, T. (2017). Advances in histopathological diagnosis of keratoacanthoma. *J. Dermatol.* 44, 304–314. doi: 10.1111/1346-8138.13696

Tan, C. H., Tachezy, R., Van Ranst, M., Chan, S. Y., Bernard, H. U., and Burk, R. D. (1994). The *Mastomys natalensis* papillomavirus: nucleotide sequence, genome organization, and phylogenetic relationship of a rodent papillomavirus involved in tumorigenesis of cutaneous epithelia. *Virology* 198, 534–541. doi: 10.1006/viro.1994.1064

Taute, S., Pfister, H. J., and Steger, G. (2017). Induction of tyrosine phosphorylation of UV-activated EGFR by the beta-human papillomavirus type 8 E6 leads to papillomatosis. *Front. Microbiol.* 8:2197. doi: 10.3389/fmicb.2017.02197

Tumban, E., Peabody, J., Peabody, D. S., and Chackerian, B. (2011). A pan-HPV vaccine based on bacteriophage PP7 VLPs displaying broadly cross-neutralizing epitopes from the HPV minor capsid protein. L2. *PLoS One* 6:e23310. doi: 10.1371/journal.pone.0023310

Tumban, E., Peabody, J., Tyler, M., Peabody, D. S., and Chackerian, B. (2012). VLPs displaying a single L2 epitope induce broadly cross-neutralizing antibodies against human papillomavirus. *PLoS One* 7:e49751. doi: 10.1371/journal.pone.0049751

Uberoi, A., and Lambert, P. F. (2017). Rodent Papillomaviruses. *Viruses* 9:362. doi: 10.3390/v9120362

Uberoi, A., Yoshida, S., Frazer, I. H., Pitot, H. C., and Lambert, P. F. (2016). Role of ultraviolet radiation in papillomavirus-induced disease. *PLoS Pathog.* 12:e1005664. doi: 10.1371/journal.ppat.1005664

Underbrink, M. P., Howie, H. L., Bedard, K. M., Koop, J. I., and Galloway, D. A. (2008). E6 proteins from multiple human betapapillomavirus types degrade Bak and protect keratinocytes from apoptosis after UVB irradiation. *J. Virol.* 82, 10408–10417. doi: 10.1128/JVI.00902-08

Van Doorslaer, K., Li, Z., Xirasagar, S., Maes, P., Kaminsky, D., Liou, D., et al. (2017). The papillomavirus episteme: a major update to the papillomavirus sequence database. *Nucleic Acids Res.* 45, D499–D506. doi: 10.1093/nar/gkw879

van Haalen, F. M., Bruggink, S C., Gussekloo, J., Assendelft, W. J., and Eekhof, J. A. (2009). Warts in primary schoolchildren: prevalence and relation with environmental factors. *Br. J. Dermatol.* 161, 148–152. doi: 10.1111/j.1365-2133.2009.09160.x

Varala, K., Li, Y., Marshall-Colon, A., Para, A., and Coruzzi, G. M. (2015). "Hit-and-Run" leaves its mark: catalyst transcription factors and chromatin modification. *Bioessays* 37, 851–856. doi: 10.1002/bies.201400205

Viarisio, D., Mueller-Decker, K., Kloz, U., Aengeneyndt, B., Kopp-Schneider, A., Gröne, H.-J., et al. (2011). E6 and E7 from Beta Hpv38 cooperate with ultraviolet light in the development of actinic keratosis-like lesions and squamous cell carcinoma in mice. *PLoS Pathog.* 7:e1002125. doi: 10.1371/journal.ppat.1002125

Viarisio, D., Muller-Decker, K., Accardi, R., Robitaille, A., Durst, M., Beer, K., et al. (2018). Beta HPV38 oncoproteins act with a hit-and-run mechanism in ultraviolet radiation-induced skin carcinogenesis in mice. *PLoS Pathog.* 14:e1006783. doi: 10.1371/journal.ppat.1006783

Viarisio, D., Muller-Decker, K. Hassel, J. C., Alvarez, J. C., Flechtenmacher, C., Pawlita, M., et al. (2017). The BRAF Inhibitor vemurafenib enhances UV-induced skin carcinogenesis in beta HPV38 E6 and E7 transgenic mice. *J. Invest. Dermatol.* 137, 261–264. doi: 10.1016/j.jid.2016.08.030

Viarisio, D., Muller-Decker, K., Zanna, P., Kloz, U., Aengeneyndt, B., Accardi, R., et al. (2016). Novel ss-HPV49 transgenic mouse model of upper digestive tract cancer. *Cancer Res.* 76, 4216–4225. doi: 10.1158/0008-5472.CAN-16-0370

Villain, P., Gonzalez, P., Almonte, M., Franceschi, S., Dillner, J., Anttila, A., et al. (2015). European code against cancer 4th edition: infections and cancer. *Cancer Epidemiol.* 39(Suppl. 1), S120–S138. doi: 10.1016/j.canep.2015.10.006

Vinzón, S. E., Braspenning-Wesch, I., Muller, M., Geissler, E. K., Nindl, I., Grone, H. J., et al. (2014). Protective vaccination against papillomavirus-induced skin tumors under immunocompetent and immunosuppressive conditions: a preclinical study using a natural outbred animal model. *PLoS Pathog.* 10:e1003924. doi: 10.1371/journal.ppat.1003924

Vinzón, S. E., and Rösl, F. (2015). HPV vaccination for prevention of skin cancer. *Hum. Vaccin. Immunother.* 11, 353–357. doi: 10.4161/21645515.2014.983858

Virgin, H. W. (2014). The virome in mammalian physiology and disease. *Cell* 157, 142–150. doi: 10.1016/j.cell.2014.02.032

Vonka, V. (2000). Causality in medicine: the case of tumours and viruses. *Philos. Trans. R. Soc. Lond. B Biol. Sci.* 355, 1831–1841. doi: 10.1098/rstb.2000.0738

Vouga, M., and Greub, G. (2016). Emerging bacterial pathogens: the past and beyond. *Clin. Microbiol. Infect.* 22, 12–21. doi: 10.1016/j.cmi.2015.10.010

Walrath, J. C., Hawes, J. J., Van Dyke, T., and Reilly, K. M. (2010). Genetically engineered mouse models in cancer research. *Adv. Cancer Res.* 106, 113–164. doi: 10.1016/S0065-230X(10)06004-5

Wang, J., Aldabagh, B., Yu, J., and Arron, S. T. (2014). Role of human papillomavirus in cutaneous squamous cell carcinoma: a meta-analysis. *J. Am. Acad. Dermatol.* 70, 621–629. doi: 10.1016/j.jaad.2014.01.857

Wang, J. W., Jiang, R., Peng, S., Chang, Y. N., Hung, C. F., and Roden, R. B. (2015). Immunologic control of Mus musculus papillomavirus type 1. *PLoS Pathog.* 11:e1005243. doi: 10.1371/journal.ppat.1005243

Wei, G., Ku, S., Ma, G. K., Saito, S., Tang, A. A., Zhang, J., et al. (2007). HIPK2 represses beta-catenin-mediated transcription, epidermal stem cell expansion, and skin tumorigenesis. *Proc. Natl. Acad. Sci. U.S.A.* 104, 13040–13045. doi: 10.1073/pnas.0703213104

Weissenborn, S., Neale, R. E., Waterboer, T., Abeni, D., Bavinck, J. N., Green, A. C., et al. (2012). Beta-papillomavirus DNA loads in hair follicles of immunocompetent people and organ transplant recipients. *Med. Microbiol. Immunol.* 201, 117–125. doi: 10.1007/s00430-011-0212-3

Weissenborn, S. J., Nindl, I., Purdie, K., Harwood, C., Proby, C., Breuer, J., et al. (2005). Human papillomavirus-DNA loads in actinic keratoses exceed those in non-melanoma skin cancers. *J. Invest. Dermatol.* 125, 93–97. doi: 10.1111/j.0022-202X.2005.23733.x

Welsh, M. M., Karagas, M. R., Kuriger, J. K., Houseman, A., Spencer, S. K., Perry, A. E., et al. (2011). Genetic determinants of UV-susceptibility in non-melanoma skin cancer. *PLoS One* 6:e20019. doi: 10.1371/journal.pone.0020019

Wendel, S. O., and Wallace, N. A. (2017). Loss of genome fidelity: beta HPVs and the DNA damage response. *Front. Microbiol.* 8:2250. doi: 10.3389/fmicb.2017.02250

White, E. A., Walther, J., Javanbakht, H., and Howley, P. M. (2014). Genus beta human papillomavirus E6 proteins vary in their effects on the transactivation of p53 target genes. *J. Virol.* 88, 8201–8212. doi: 10.1128/JVI.01197-14

Wu, X., Nguyen, B. C., Dziunycz, P., Chang, S., Brooks, Y., Lefort, K., et al. (2010). Opposing roles for calcineurin and ATF3 in squamous skin cancer. *Nature* 465, 368–372. doi: 10.1038/nature08996

Xue, X. Y., Majerciak, V., Uberoi, A., Kim, B. H., Gotte, D., Chen, X., et al. (2017). The full transcription map of mouse papillomavirus type 1 (MmuPV1) in mouse wart tissues. *PLoS Pathog.* 13:e1006715. doi: 10.1371/journal.ppat.1006715

Yanofsky, V. R., Mercer, S. E., and Phelps, R. G. (2011). Histopathological variants of cutaneous squamous cell carcinoma: a review. *J. Skin Cancer* 2011, 210813. doi: 10.1155/2011/210813

Zhang, T., Liu, H., Chen, X., Wang, Z., Wang, S., Qu, C., et al. (2016). Lipidated L2 epitope repeats fused with a single-chain antibody fragment targeting human FcgammaRI elicited cross-neutralizing antibodies against a broad spectrum of human papillomavirus types. *Vaccine* 34, 5531–5539. doi: 10.1016/j.vaccine.2016.10.009

Zuckerman, V., Wolyniec, K., Sionov, R. V., Haupt, S., and Haupt, Y. (2009). Tumour suppression by p53: the importance of apoptosis and cellular senescence. *J. Pathol.* 219, 3–15. doi: 10.1002/path.2584

zur Hausen, H. (2002). Papillomaviruses and cancer: from basic studies to clinical application. *Nat. Rev. Cancer* 2, 342–350. doi: 10.1038/nrc798

4

HPV-Induced Field Cancerisation: Transformation of Adult Tissue Stem Cell Into Cancer Stem Cell

*Carlotta Olivero[1,2], Simone Lanfredini[2], Cinzia Borgogna[1], Marisa Gariglio[1] and Girish K. Patel[2]**

[1] *Virology Unit, Department of Translational Medicine, Novara Medical School, University of Eastern Piedmont, Novara, Italy,*
[2] *European Cancer Stem Cell Research Institute, Cardiff School of Biosciences, Cardiff University, Cardiff, United Kingdom*

Correspondence:
Girish K. Patel
patelgk@cardiff.ac.uk

Field cancerisation was originally described as a basis for multiple head and neck squamous cell carcinoma (HNSCC) and is a pre-malignant phenomenon that is frequently attributable to oncogenic human papillomavirus (HPV) infection. Our work on β-HPV-induced cutaneous squamous cell carcinomas identified a novel Lrig1+ hair follicle junctional zone keratinocyte stem cell population as the basis for field cancerisation. Herein, we describe the ability for HPV to infect adult tissue stem cells in order to establish persistent infection and induce their proliferation and displacement resulting in field cancerisation. By review of the HPV literature, we reveal how this mechanism is conserved as the basis of field cancerisation across many tissues. New insights have identified the capacity for HPV early region genes to dysregulate adult tissue stem cell self-renewal pathways ensuring that the expanded population preserve its stem cell characteristics beyond the stem cell niche. HPV-infected cells acquire additional transforming mutations that can give rise to intraepithelial neoplasia (IEN), from environmental factors such as sunlight or tobacco induced mutations in skin and oral cavity, respectively. With establishment of IEN, HPV viral replication is sacrificed with loss of the episome, and the tissue is predisposed to multiple cancer stem cell-driven carcinomas.

Keywords: HPV, field cancerization, adult tissue stem cells, skin cancer stem cells, squamous cell carcinoma

INTRODUCTION

Human papillomavirus (HPV) infection is associated with oropharyngeal and anogenital cancers in both men and women. Approximately 90% of all cervical cancers are attributed to high-risk alpha-genus HPV (α-HPV) infections, also ~60% of squamous cell carcinomas (SCC) of the vulva, vagina, anus and penis are due to infection of α-HPV (Crow, 2012). HPV infection is considered to be responsible for the rise in head and neck squamous cell carcinoma (HNSCC), particularly in cancers of the oropharynx and base of tongue (Marur et al., 2010; Leemans et al., 2011). Cutaneous HPVs, which are clustered in the evolutionarily distinct β-genus, have been also associated with the development of cutaneous SCC, especially in the immunosuppressed setting (Howley and Pfister, 2015; Quint et al., 2015).

Sequential genetic and epigenetic changes occur over several years and provide the transformational basis for both intraepithelial neoplasia (IEN) and ensuing epithelial cancers (carcinoma). The proportion of transformed cells within IEN can be graded and used to define the risk of invasive disease (FIGO Committee on Gynecologic Oncology, 2014). Progression to invasive carcinoma from IEN can take many years and there is often evidence of IEN at the excised tumor margins (Mao et al., 1996; Scholes et al., 1998).

As an entity, carcinoma account for over 70% of all malignancies and over 70% of all cancer mortality (Cancer Research UK, 2017[1]), hence the American Association for Cancer Research Task Force on the treatment and prevention of IEN recognizes the importance of early treatment to prevent invasive disease (O'Shaughnessy et al., 2002). Intriguingly, IEN can spontaneously regress. Although more often, IEN will progress to invasive malignancies (Dakubo et al., 2007). In epithelia susceptible to HPV infection, HPV early genes can cause IEN, notably E6 and E7 expression, and is therefore a mechanistic link to cancer, as such it represents a target for cancer prevention and is therefore the basis of this review.

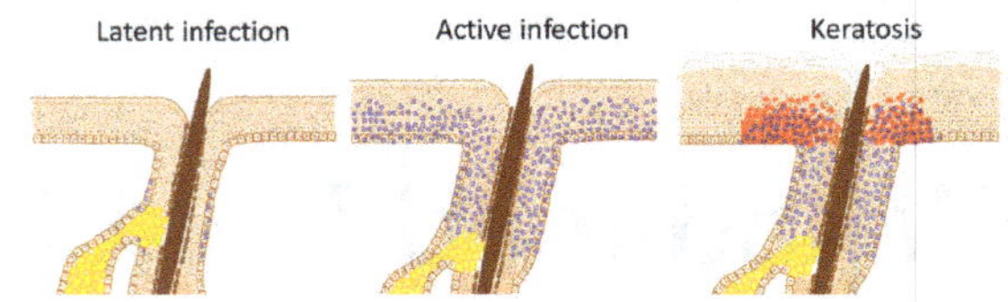

FIGURE 1 | HPV infection induced stem cell expansion. Latent HPV infection persists within epithelial stem cells and, in the case of β-HPV, within hair follicle keratinocyte stem cells; characterized herein by the presence of viral episomes (blue circles). Active replication, as occurs after immunosuppression or trauma, results in proliferation of stem cells beyond the niche; in the case of the skin into the interfollicular epidermis (IFE). Expansion and displacement of keratinocyte stem cells into the IFE renders them susceptible to UV induced transformation, resulting in field cancerisation. The archetypal initial lesion is clonal p53 mutation expression, within actinic keratoses (red cells).

FIELD CANCERISATION

Field cancerization, as a concept, was coined by Slaughter et al. (1953) to explain the occurrence of multiple foci of HNSCC. In all 783 HNSCC cases studied, the authors noted IEN at the peripheral margins of the resected primary malignancy. Where the tumor depth was less than 1 cm, they identified a second primary SCC focus in 43 of 88 cases. It is now clear that establishment of a premalignant epithelium, field cancerisation, is the basis for HNSCC, skin and cervical SCC.

Within field cancerisation, cells harbor a substantial number of mutations including those within known tumor suppressor genes, most frequently within the p53 gene (Bartkova et al., 1995; Ortiz et al., 2001; van Houten et al., 2002; Elgazzar et al., 2005; Merrick et al., 2006; Hu et al., 2012). In many tissues, the presence of mutant p53 clones is widely accepted as the hallmark of field cancerisation (**Figure 1**) (El-Naggar et al., 1995; Franklin et al., 1997). However, in cervical IEN, p53 is less frequently mutated (Akasofu and Oda, 1995). Within the early stage of field cancerisation there are multiple clones, but with increasing dysplasia severe field cancerisation becomes monoclonal (**Figure 2**) (Chung et al., 1995; Enomoto et al., 1997; Tate et al., 1997). Therefore, field cancerisation at its outset is polyclonal, implying that multiple cell lineages contribute to its occurrence as observed in active HPV infection.

Increasing mutational burden and greater dysplasia result in clonal selection, with a tendency toward mono-clonality (**Figure 2**). Clonal selection and expansion may result in a single clone in continuous epithelia (skin, oral and cervical tissues) or multiple clones in discontinuous epithelia (breast and lung) (Prevo et al., 1999; Simon et al., 2001; Larson et al., 2002; Tabor et al., 2002; Smeds et al., 2005). Within continuous epithelia, wherein HPV infection occurs, field cancerisation and ensuing cancers exhibit common epigenetic gene silencing, chromosomal anomalies, loss of heterozygosity, single nucleotide polymorphism, mutations, changes in mitochondrial genome, and altered gene expression (transcripts and proteins) (Ha et al., 2002; Tabor et al., 2004; Shen et al., 2005; Sui et al., 2006). Hence, severe IEN (part of the field cancerisation spectrum) that gives rise to multiple cancer, has limited numbers of clones.

The ensuing SCC that arise within continuous stratified squamous epithelia are clonal with respect to the underlying field cancerisation and severe IEN (**Figure 2**) (Sheu et al., 1995; Kim et al., 1996; Enomoto et al., 1997; Tate et al., 1997). However, the proliferative explosion of SCC cells results in multiple evolving clones, from acquisition of new mutations, which similarly undergo Darwinian evolutionary selection (McGranahan and Swanton, 2017). As a consequence, tumors arising from within IEN are genetically distinct (Nakashima et al., 1995; Shinmura et al., 1998). Hence, Darwinian evolutionary clonal selection determines the loss of clones in field cancerisation and determines the size of multiple clones within the emerging SCC.

HPV INFECTION AND STEM CELL EXPANSION

Human papillomavirus (HPV) binds epithelial cell heparan sulfate proteoglycans and cell specific receptors to gain entry by both clathrin-dependent and -independent endocytosis (McMillan et al., 1999; Day et al., 2003; Shafti-Keramat et al., 2003; Spoden et al., 2008; Schelhaas et al., 2012; Day and Schelhaas, 2014). Infection leads to the establishment of the HPV circular double-stranded genome as a stable episome within some cells of the basal layer (Dell et al., 2003). In the case of alpha-HPV, the viral genome can integrate into the host genome, whereas for beta-HPV, the viral genome remains episomal (Quint et al., 2015). Viral replication proteins E1 and E2 are required for the maintenance of the viral genome in the basal layer (Frattini et al., 1996; Stubenrauch et al., 1998; McBride, 2013). HPV infection of epithelial basal cells may be non-selective and by chance may involve adult tissue stem cells that reside in this layer.

[1] http://www.cancerresearchuk.org/health-professional/cancer-statistics/incidence/common-cancers-compared

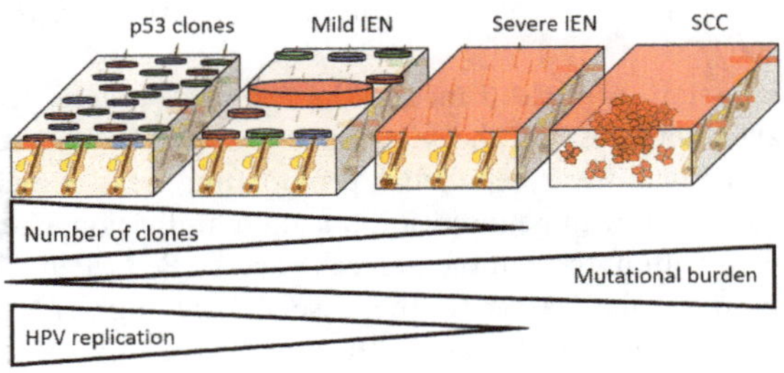

FIGURE 2 | Field cancerisation in the setting of HPV infection. The progression from IEN to SCC formation is characterized by the clonal selection, acquisition of mutations, and loss of HPV replication. Skin is used here as a HPV susceptible tissue, as we have previously shown that clonal expansion occurs from the hair follicle junctional zone. In mild IEN there are many clones, which in the case of p53 mutation susceptible tissues, may harbor individual distinct mutations as shown (circles with different colors). Progression of IEN is characterized by the selection and expansion of individual clones that have gained a proliferative advantage from additional mutations, culminating in severe IEN with full thickness epidermal dysplasia that is genetically uniform. With increasing mutational load, epidermal dysplasia increases and HPV episomes are lost. In the case of β-HPV types, the entire viral infection is lost, which accounts for the "hit and run" mechanism of transformation. From within the severe IEN, foci of SCC develop as shown, resulting in invasion into the underlying tissue.

Most HPV infections are spontaneously cleared. For example, the risk of α-HPV female genital infection over a lifetime is up to 80% (Syrjanen et al., 1990), but within 1–2 years most individuals clear the virus (Rodríguez et al., 2008). Although HPV may not specifically bind epithelial adult tissue stem cells for infection, as discussed earlier, persistent and or latent infection is presumed to involve epithelial adult tissue stem cells, but has not been determined for all tissues as stem cell markers are lacking (Schmitt et al., 1996; Boxman et al., 1997; Maglennon et al., 2011; Kranjec and Doorbar, 2016). Notably, the proposed reservoir for latent β-HPV infection has been the hair follicles (Boxman et al., 1997; De Koning et al., 2007; Galloway and Laimins, 2015; Quint et al., 2015; Hufbauer and Akgül, 2017; Tommasino, 2017). Animal models substantiated these clinical findings and moreover showed that the sub-populations of infected hair follicle cells have increased clonogenic potential, a hallmark of adult tissue stem cells (Schmitt et al., 1996; Lanfredini et al., 2017). In the oncogenic β-HPV8 transgenic mouse model we observed skin thickening (acanthosis), which was evident from birth and attributable to an expansion of the Lrig1 hair follicle adult tissue stem population (Lanfredini et al., 2017). In the absence of overt cutaneous lesions, such as papilloma or carcinoma, both unsorted and Lrig1+ keratinocytes demonstrated increased colony forming efficiency (increased clonogenicity) consistent with an expansion in keratinocyte stem cell numbers. Similarly, earlier studies on the cottontail rabbit model of HPV infection had also demonstrated the hair follicle to be the site of persistent HPV infection and, through similar colony forming assays, an expansion of the hair follicle junctional zone keratinocyte stem cells was reported (Schmitt et al., 1996). In these two studies, papilloma arose as a result of continued keratinocyte stem cell expansion into the adjacent overlying epidermis. For example, human benign cutaneous viral warts similarly result from keratinocyte stem cells expansion (Egawa, 2003). It is possible that the immune privilege provided by the stem cells niche prevents immune attack, thereby facilitating long term infection.

HPV-INDUCED EPIDERMAL PROLIFERATION

In cervical lesions caused by the α-HPVs, the viral oncogenes E6 and E7 increase proliferation of suprabasal epithelial cells. Along with E1 and E2, viral replication requires E6 and E7 for entry into S-phase. Upon leaving the basal layer, keratinocytes enter into a program of terminal differentiation in order to produce a protective barrier. However, in HPV infection, suprabasal cells continue to proliferate and are prevented from entering terminal differentiation (Sherman et al., 1997; Doorbar, 2006). Oncogenic viruses, including HPV, deregulate cell growth by disruption of pRb (retinoblastoma protein) binding to the E2F family of transcription factors though E7 binding pRb. Host p21 and p27 cyclin-dependent kinase inhibitors moderate the ability of E7 to drive cell proliferation in some cells (Doorbar, 2006; Tomaić, 2016). Inactive complexes with E7 and cyclin E occur within differentiating keratinocytes that express high levels of p21 and p27 (Noya et al., 2001; Akgül et al., 2006). In synchrony, high-risk α-HPV E6 prevent growth arrest or apoptosis by binding to p53, thus leading to p53 ubiquitination and degradation. In benign infections, proliferating cells remain in the epithelial basal layer, including within the hair follicle. As the infected cell enters the suprabasal cell layers of the epidermis, virus production is switched on resulting in viron assembly (Peh et al., 2002).

HPV INFECTION INDUCES STEM CELL EXPANSION AND SELF-RENEWAL PATHWAYS

Fluorescent labeling studies in mice using lineage tracing have concluded that stem cell division is prominently (~90%) asymmetric; in which there is renewal of the stem cell and a daughter cell that is committed to terminal differentiation (Clayton et al., 2007; Doupé et al., 2012). Stochastic cell division in basal cells, including stem cells, can lead to HPV infection clearance. Mathematical modeling together with epidemiological data suggests that natural stem cell dynamics contributes >80% toward viral clearance rather than rejection by the immune system (Ryser et al., 2015). Thus, factors that promote adult tissue stem cell symmetrical cell division resulting in an increase in stem cell numbers may perpetuate infection accounting for the correlation between the increased risk of persistent infections associated cervical cancer and long-term use of combined oral contraceptives (Muñoz et al., 2006). This may also explain the basis for why trauma, ultraviolet light and repetitive exposure to the virus are essential in maintaining site-specific HPV infection (Kranjec and Doorbar, 2016).

Adult tissue stem cell expansion, as proposed for the mechanism of HPV-induced field cancerisation, is dependent on symmetrical division of existing stem cells. As discussed, HPV viral oncogenes will drive proliferation of infected adult tissue stem cells by targeting p53 or pRb. Importantly, the binding of E7 to pRb releases repression of both sex determining region Y-box 2 (Sox2) and octamer-binding transcription factor 4 (Oct4) (Kareta et al., 2015). Similarly, α-HPV E6 mediated degradation of p53 results increased Nanog expression, which is normally transcriptionally repressed by p53 (Lin et al., 2005). Thus, HPV early region genes promote self-renewal pathways.

In addition, high-risk α-HPV E7 induces expression of the key transcription factor Oct4 and also directly to enhance activation of its target genes (Brehm et al., 1997, 1999; Organista-Nava et al., 2016). Another key transcription factor, Kruppel-like factor 4 (Klf4), is also upregulated and hypoSUMOylated by high risk α-HPV E6 (Gunasekharan et al., 2016). Simultaneously, β-HPV E6 blocks differentiation by inhibition of C/EBPα, Notch signaling and Hes1 upregulation (Tyagi et al., 2016; Kranjec et al., 2017; Marthaler et al., 2017; Meyers et al., 2017). β-HPV E6 specifically binds to a cellular target MAML1, resulting in the inhibition of Notch-mediated transcription, which is important to keep infected keratinocytes in a proliferative state (Meyers et al., 2017). α-HPV E7 also prevents histone3 Lysine27 (H3K27) trimethylation and therefore maintains adult tissue stem cells in a permissive epigenetic state (McLaughlin-Drubin et al., 2011). Thus, HPV causes proliferation of adult tissue stem cells and maintains stemness of these cells as they egress from the stem cell niche, consistent with expression of stem cell proteins and observations *in vitro* of increased colony forming efficiency (Hufbauer et al., 2013; Lindquist et al., 2014).

TRANSITION FROM HPV-INDUCED STEM CELL EXPANSION TO IEN

The earliest evolution of HPV-induced stem cell expansion into visible lesions is the presence of dysregulated stratification within the epidermis, resulting in benign keratoses (the archetypal lesion in epidermodysplasia verruciformis) or cutaneous warts. Similarly, mucosal HPV lesions include condyloma or leukoplakia within the genitalia and oral mucosa (Cubie, 2013). In addition, persistent infections with high-risk HPV types simultaneously trigger neoplastic change (Rodríguez et al., 2010).

The transition from benign to premalignant lesion has been characterized by TP53 immunostaining, resulting from mutation acquisition, and manifesting as a small micro-clonal expansion comprising of 60–3000 cells presenting clinically as an actinic (solar) keratosis or leukoplakia (Jonasson et al., 1996; Ren et al., 1966; Ponten et al., 1997; Waridel et al., 1997; Garcia et al., 1999; van Houten et al., 2002). In the skin, these p53 micro-clonal patches were larger and more frequent in sun-exposed than sun-shielded areas, suggesting that mutations arise from UV. In addition, HPV is able to inhibit DNA repair through E6 protein expression, facilitating acquisition of p53 mutations (Wallace et al., 2012; Hufbauer et al., 2015; McKinney et al., 2015). Gain-of-function p53 mutation acquisition results in persistence of the protein within cells to promote transformation (Caulin et al., 2007).

Progression of field cancerisation toward severe IEN is associated with loss of the viral episome. In HPV infection, such as benign warts, epithelial proliferating cells remain in the basal layers, with genome amplification and virion assembly occurring within the suprabasal cell layers (Peh et al., 2002; Middleton et al., 2003). In the case of the high-risk HPV types the relative thickness of the basal layers is increased, presumably due to expansion in the number of adult tissue stem cells. Progression to IEN is characterized by a loss of terminal differentiation and therefore the expression of viral coat proteins is retarded (**Figure 2**) (Middleton et al., 2003). For example in cervical IEN, increasing dysplasia is associated with reduced virion production and loss of viral episomes. This phenomenon is even more evident in the case of skin infection by β-HPV types, which do not integrate into the host genome, and do not maintain viral DNA in the late stages of skin cancer progression. For example, SCC that develop within HPV associated Organ Transplant Recipient (OTR) field cancerisation no longer express β-HPV proteins (Borgogna et al., 2014) Similarly, HPV expression was lost during actinic keratosis transformation to SCC in a nude mouse xenograft model (Borgogna et al., 2018). Hence, the progression to cancer from IEN occurs independent of virus production, and for the beta genotypes in the skin, this is referred to as the "hit and run" mechanism of carcinogenesis (Howley and Pfister, 2015; Quint et al., 2015).

Field cancerisation emerging from HPV induced amplification of adult tissue stem cells results from additional environmental induced mutations. The area of IEN can be large, in the oral cavity it can be over 7 cm in diameter and is predisposed to multiple primary HNSCC and therefore poor prognosis (Tabor et al., 2002, 2004; Baxi et al., 2014). Intriguingly, HPV associated HNSCC demonstrate a favorable response to chemotherapy (Hayes et al., 2015; Vokes et al., 2015). Likewise, HPV and non-HPV vulvar SCC have distinct mutational profiles and moreover multiple primaries developing from within HPV IEN demonstrate separate clonal basis (Rosenthal et al., 2002; Hampl et al., 2007). Hence, HPV-induced adult tissue stem cell expansion risks the generation of IEN that in turn is predisposed to further transformation resulting in multiple primary tumors.

HPV INFECTION DRIVEN CANCER STEM CELLS

Many cancers exhibit hierarchical growth with evidence of differentiation consistent with the cancer stem cell model (Colmont et al., 2012). Wherein a subset of cancer cells, called "cancer stem cells", which continue to exhibit stem cell characteristic, serve to promote tumor growth through self-renewal with symmetric and asymmetric cell division (Patel et al., 2012; Colmont et al., 2013). There is evidence of active self-renewal in HPV-induced female genital tract cancers, cervical and vulval cancers, which characteristically express the stem cell transcription factors Sox 2, Oct4, and Hes1

(Brustmann and Brunner, 2013; Kim et al., 2015; Napoletano et al., 2016; Gut et al., 2018). In cervical cancer, HPV gene E6 can enhance self-renewal associated hedgehog transcription factor Gli1 expression and therefore increase cancer stem cell numbers (Vishnoi et al., 2016).

Head and neck squamous cell carcinoma (HNSCC) identification and characterisation of cancer stem cells has been supported by *in vitro* and *in vivo* assays (Prince et al., 2007). Similar to HPV-induced female genital tract cancers, the self-renewal associated transcription factor Sox2 was found expressed in HPV associated HNSCC, resulting from HPV E6/7 associated PI3K-AKT pathway activation (Keysar et al., 2016; Xi et al., 2016). The ensuing HPV-associated HNSCC retain cancer stem cell markers, CD44, CD24, ALHD1, and functional side population characteristics (Tang et al., 2013; Lindquist et al., 2014; Pullos et al., 2015). Overall, HPV associated HNSCC has favorable outcome compared to non-HPV associated HNSCC, and intriguingly this has been attributed to reduced cancer stem cell frequency in HPV HNSCC (Rietbergen et al., 2014; Vlashi et al., 2016). High numbers of cancer stem cells in HNSCC, irrespective of HPV status, is associated with poor outcome and lack of response to both radiotherapy and chemotherapy (Linge et al., 2016; Modur et al., 2016). Hence, the role of HPV to cause both normal stem cell and cancer stem cell expansion, may establish the basis for cancer stem cell driven tumor growth and influence cancer outcome.

CONCLUSION

This review has focused on HPV infection, notably oncogenic genotypes from both the alpha and beta genus. Within the tropic tissue that was breached to allow viral entry, persistent infection requires that resident adult tissue stem cells are infected. HPV-infected adult tissue stem cells, similar to other HPV-infected cells are forced to proliferate, leading to their expansion as adult tissue stem cells beyond their native niche. This expansion renders them susceptible to environmental carcinogens. In the case of skin, β-HPV genotypes induce hair follicle junctional zone keratinocyte stem cells to proliferate and expand into the overlying epidermis, whereupon they are susceptible to UV-induced mutations. Transformational mutations result in field cancerisation, with additional driver mutations, causing clonal selection as IEN progresses from mild to severe. Additional mutations then can give rise to multiple cancers. Hence, HPV-induced stem cell expansion predisposes to and, through viral oncogene expression, induces the generation of cancer stem cells, which in turn can define the fate of tumor and patient prognosis. Hence, we propose that the ability of oncogenic HPV infection to manipulate adult tissue stem cells underpin its ability to drive cancer growth through promotion of cancer stem cells.

AUTHOR CONTRIBUTIONS

CO, SL, and GP conceived the idea. CO, SL, CB, MG, and GP drafted the manuscript with inputs from all authors. All authors have made final approval for the final version to be submitted.

FUNDING

GP was supported by British Skin Foundation (003/SG/17), Leo Foundation (LF17070), and Hywel Dda University Health Board. CO was funded by FCRT and Fondazione Goria-Bando Talenti della Società Civile 2016. MG was supported by Associazione Italiana per la Ricerca sul Cancro – AIRC grant IG2016. CB was supported by Compagnia di San Paolo (CSP2014) and the Italian Ministry for University and Research – MIUR (PRIN 2015).

REFERENCES

Akasofu, M., and Oda, Y. (1995). Immunohistochemical detection of p53 in cervical epithelial lesions with or without infection of human papillomavirus types 16 and 18. *Virchows Arch.* 425, 593–602. doi: 10.1007/BF00199349

Akgül, B., Cooke, J. C., and Storey, A. (2006). HPV-associated skin disease. *J. Pathol.* 208, 165–175. doi: 10.1002/path.1893

Bartkova, J., Lukas, J., Müller, H., Strauss, M., Gusterson, B., and Bartek, J. (1995). Abnormal patterns of D-type cyclin expression and G1 regulation in human head and neck cancer. *Cancer Res.* 55, 949–956.

Baxi, S. S., Pinheiro, L. C., Patil, S. M., Pfister, D. G., Oeffinger, K. C., and Elkin, E. B. (2014). Causes of death in long-term survivors of head and neck cancer. *Cancer* 120, 1507–1513. doi: 10.1002/cncr.28588

Borgogna, C., Lanfredini, S., Peretti, A., De Andrea, M., Zavattaro, E., Colombo, E., et al. (2014). Improved detection reveals β-papillomavirus infection in skin lesions from kidney transplant recipients. *Mod. Pathol.* 27, 1101–1115. doi: 10.1038/modpathol.2013.240

Borgogna, C., Olivero, C., Lanfredini, S., Calati, F., De Andrea, M., Zavattaro, E., et al. (2018). β-HPV infection correlates with early stages of carcinogenesis in skin tumors and patient-derived xenografts from a single center kidney transplant recipient cohort. *Front. Microbiol.* 9:117. doi: 10.3389/fmicb.2018.00117

Boxman, I. L., Berkhout, R. J., Mulder, L. H., Wolkers, M. C., Bouwes Bavinck, J. N., Vermeer, B. J., et al. (1997). Detection of human papillomavirus DNA in plucked hairs from renal transplant recipients and healthy volunteers. *J. Investig. Dermatol.* 108, 712–715. doi: 10.1111/1523-1747.ep12292090

Brehm, A., Ohbo, K., and Scholer, H. (1997). The carboxy-terminal transactivation domain of Oct-4 acquires cell specificity through the POU domain. *Mol. Cell. Biol.* 17, 154–162. doi: 10.1128/MCB.17.1.154

Brehm, A., Ohbo, K., Zwerschke, W., Botquin, V., Jansen-Durr, P., and Scholer, H. R. (1999). Synergism with germ line transcription factor Oct-4: viral oncoproteins share the ability to mimic a stem cell-specific activity. *Mol. Cell. Biol.* 19, 2635–2643. doi: 10.1128/MCB.19.4.2635

Brustmann, H., and Brunner, A. (2013). Immunohistochemical expression of SOX2 in vulvar intraepithelial neoplasia and squamous cell carcinoma. *Int. J. Gynecol. Pathol.* 32, 323–328. doi: 10.1097/PGP.0b013e31825d820e

Caulin, C., Nguyen, T., Lang, G. A., Goepfert, T. M., Brinkley, B. R., Cai, W. W., et al. (2007). An inducible mouse model for skin cancer reveals distinct roles for gain- and loss-of-function p53 mutations. *J. Clin. Invest.* 117, 1893–1901. doi: 10.1172/JCI31721

Chung, G. T., Sunderasan, V., Hasleton, P., Rudd, R., Taylor, R., and Rabbitts, P. (1995). Sequential molecular changes in lung cancer development. *Oncogene* 11, 2591–2598.

Clayton, E., Doupé, D., Klein, A., Winton, D., Simons, B., and Jones, P. H. (2007). A single type of progenitor cell maintains normal epidermis. *Nature* 446, 185–189. doi: 10.1038/nature05574

Colmont, C. S., Benketah, A., Reed, S. H., Hawk, N. V., Telford, W. G., Ohyama, M., et al. (2013). CD200-expressing human basal cell carcinoma cells initiate tumor growth. *Proc. Natl. Acad. Sci. U.S.A.* 110, 1434–1439. doi: 10.1073/pnas.1211655110

Colmont, C. S., Harding, K. G., Piguet, V., and Patel, G. K. (2012). Human skin cancer stem cells: a tale of mice and men. *Exp. Dermatol.* 21, 576–580. doi: 10.1111/j.1600-0625.2012.01533.x

Crow, J. M. (2012). HPV: the global burden. *Nature* 488, S2–S3. doi: 10.1038/488S2a

Cubie, H. A. (2013). Diseases associated with human papillomavirus infection. *Virology* 445, 21–34. doi: 10.1016/j.virol.2013.06.007

Dakubo, G., Jakupciak, J., Birch-Machin, M., and Parr, R. L. (2007). Clinical implications and utility of field cancerization. *Cancer Cell Int.* 7:2. doi: 10.1186/1475-2867-7-2

Day, P. M., Lowy, D. R., and Schiller, J. T. (2003). Papillomaviruses infect cells via a clathrin-dependent pathway. *Virology* 307, 1–11. doi: 10.1016/S0042-6822(02)00143-5

Day, P. M., and Schelhaas, M. (2014). Concepts of papillomavirus entry into host cells. *Curr. Opin. Virol.* 4, 24–31. doi: 10.1016/j.coviro.2013.11.002

De Koning, M. N., Struijk, L., Bavinck, J. N., Kleter, B., Ter Schegget, J., and Quint, W. G. (2007). Betapapillomaviruses frequently persist in the skin of healthy individuals. *J. Gen. Virol.* 88, 1489–1495. doi: 10.1099/vir.0.82732-0

Dell, G., Wilkinson, K. W., Tranter, R., Parish, J., Leo Brady, R., and Gaston, K. (2003). Comparison of the structure and DNA-binding properties of the E2 proteins from an oncogenic and a non-oncogenic human papillomavirus. *J. Mol. Biol.* 334, 979–991. doi: 10.1016/j.jmb.2003.10.009

Doorbar, J. (2006). Molecular biology of human papillomavirus infection and cervical cancer. *Clin. Sci.* 110, 525–541. doi: 10.1042/CS20050369

Doupé, D. P., Alcolea, M. P., Roshan, A., Zhang, G., Klein, A. M., Simons, B. D., et al. (2012). A single progenitor population switches behavior to maintain and repair esophageal epithelium. *Science* 337, 1091–1093. doi: 10.1126/science.1218835

Egawa, K. (2003). Do human papillomaviruses target epidermal stem cells? *Dermatology* 207, 251–254. doi: 10.1159/000073085

Elgazzar, R. F., Ali, A., Eldreeny, E., and Moustafa, K. (2005). Over expression of P53 and P21 in normal oral mucosa adjacent to resected squamous cell carcinomas may be an evidence of field cancerization. *Int. J. Cancer Prev.* 2, 1–8.

El-Naggar, A. K., Lai, S., Luna, M. A., Zhou, X. D., Weber, R. S., Goepfert, H., et al. (1995). Sequential p53 mutation analysis of the preinvasive and invasive head and squamous carcinoma. *Int. J. Cancer* 64, 196–201. doi: 10.1002/ijc.2910640309

Enomoto, T., Haba, T., Fujita, M., Hamada, T., Yoshino, K., Nakashima, R., et al. (1997). Clonal analysis of high-grade squamous intraepithelial lesions of the uterine cervix. *Int. J. Cancer* 73, 339–344. doi: 10.1002/(SICI)1097-0215(19971104)73:3<339::AID-IJC6>3.0.CO;2-0

FIGO Committee on Gynecologic Oncology (2014). FIGO staging for carcinoma of the vulva, cervix, and corpus uteri. *Int. J. Gynaecol. Obstet.* 125, 97–98. doi: 10.1016/j.ijgo.2014.02.003

Franklin, W. A., Gazdar, A. F., Haney, J., Wistuba, I. I., La Rosa, F. G., Kennedy, T., et al. (1997). Widely dispersed p53 mutation in respiratory epithelium. A novel mechanism for field carcinogenesis. *J. Clin. Invest.* 100, 2133–2137. doi: 10.1172/JCI119748

Frattini, M. G., Lim, H. B., and Laimins, L. A. (1996). In-vitro synthesis of oncogenic human papillomaviruses requires episomal genomes for differentiation-dependent late gene expression. *Proc. Natl. Acad. Sci. U.S.A.* 93, 3062–3067. doi: 10.1073/pnas.93.7.3062

Galloway, D. A., and Laimins, L. A. (2015). Human papillomaviruses: shared and distinct pathways for pathogenesis. *Curr. Opin. Virol.* 14, 87–92. doi: 10.1016/j.coviro.2015.09.001

Garcia, S. B., Park, H. S., Novelli, M., and Wright, N. A. (1999). Field cancerization, clonality, and epithelial stem cells: the spread of mutated clones in epithelial sheets. *J. Pathol.* 187, 61–81. doi: 10.1002/(SICI)1096-9896(199901)187:1<61::AID-PATH247>3.0.CO;2-I

Gunasekharan, V. K., Li, Y., Andrade, J., and Laimins, L. A. (2016). Post-transcriptional regulation of Klf4 by high-risk human papillomaviruses is necessary for the differentiation-dependent viral life cycle. *PLoS Pathog.* 12:e1005747. doi: 10.1371/journal.ppat.1005747

Gut, A., Moch, H., and Choschzick, M. (2018). SOX2 gene amplification and overexpression is linked to HPV-positive Vulvar Carcinomas. *Int. J. Gynecol. Pathol.* 37, 68–73. doi: 10.1097/PGP.0000000000000388

Ha, P. K., Tong, B. C., Westra, W. H., Sanchez-Cespedes, M., Parrella, P., and Zahurak, M. (2002). Mitochondrial C-tract alteration in premalignant lesions of the head and neck: a marker for progression and clonal proliferation. *Clin. Cancer Res.* 8, 2260–2265.

Hampl, M., Wentzensen, N., Vinokurova, S., von Knebel-Doeberitz, M., Poremba, C., Bender, H. G., et al. (2007). Comprehensive analysis of 130 multicentric intraepithelial female lower genital tract lesions by HPV typing and p16 expression profile. *J. Cancer Res. Clin. Oncol.* 133, 235–245. doi: 10.1007/s00432-006-0162-0

Hayes, D. N., Van Waes, C., and Seiwert, T. Y. (2015). Genetic landscape of human papillomavirus-associated head and neck cancer and comparison to tobacco-related tumors. *J. Clin. Oncol.* 33, 3227–3234. doi: 10.1200/JCO.2015.62.1086

Howley, P. M., and Pfister, H. J. (2015). Beta genus papillomaviruses and skin cancer. *Virology* 479–480, 290–296. doi: 10.1016/j.virol.2015.02.004

Hu, B., Castillo, E., Harewood, L., Ostano, P., Reymond, A., Dummer, R., et al. (2012). Multifocal epithelial tumors and field cancerization from loss of mesenchymal CSL signaling. *Cell* 149, 1207–1220. doi: 10.1016/j.cell.2012.03.048

Hufbauer, M., and Akgül, B. (2017). Molecular mechanisms of human papillomavirus induced skin carcinogenesis. *Viruses* 9:E187. doi: 10.3390/v9070187

Hufbauer, M., Biddle, A., Borgogna, C., Gariglio, M., Doorbar, J., Storey, A., et al. (2013). Expression of β-papillomavirus oncogenes increases the number of keratinocytes with stem cell-like properties. *J. Virol.* 87, 12158–12165. doi: 10.1128/JVI.01510-13

Hufbauer, M., Cooke, J., van der Horst, G. T., Pfister, H., Storey, A., and Akgül, B. (2015). Human papillomavirus mediated inhibition of DNA damage sensing and repair drives skin carcinogenesis. *Mol. Cancer.* 14:183. doi: 10.1186/s12943-015-0453-7

Jonasson, A. S., Kunala, S., Price, G. J., Restifo, R. J., Spinelli, H. M., Persing, J. A., et al. (1996). Frequent clones of p53-mutated keratinocytes in normal skin. *Proc. Natl. Acad. Sci. U.S.A.* 93, 14025–14029. doi: 10.1073/pnas.93.24.14025

Kareta, M. S., Gorges, L. L., Hafeez, S., Benayoun, B. A., Marro, S., Zmoos, A. F., et al. (2015). Inhibition of pluripotency networks by the Rb tumor suppressor restricts reprogramming and tumorigenesis. *Cell Stem Cell* 16, 39–50. doi: 10.1016/j.stem.2014.10.019

Keysar, S. B., Le, P. N., Miller, B., Jackson, B. C., Eagles, J. R., Nieto, C., et al. (2016). Regulation of head and neck squamous cancer stem cells by PI3K and SOX2. *J. Natl. Cancer Inst* 109:djw189. doi: 10.1093/jnci/djw189

Kim, B. W., Cho, H., Choi, C. H., Ylaya, K., Chung, J. Y., Kim, J. H., et al. (2015). Clinical significance of Oct4 and Sox2 protein expression in cervical cancer. *BMC Cancer* 15:1015. doi: 10.1186/s12885-015-2015-1

Kim, Y. T., Thomas, N. F., Kessis, T. D., Wilkinson, E. J., Hedrick, L., and Cho, K. R. (1996). p53 mutations and clonality in vulvar carcinoma and squamous hyperplasias; evidence suggesting that squamous hyperplasias do not serve as direct precursors of human papillomavirus-negative vulvar carcinomas. *Hum. Pathol.* 27, 389–395. doi: 10.1016/S0046-8177(96)90113-6

Kranjec, C., and Doorbar, J. (2016). Human papillomavirus infection and induction of neoplasia: a matter of fitness. *Curr. Opin. Virol.* 20, 129–136. doi: 10.1016/j.coviro.2016.08.011

Kranjec, C., Holleywood, C., Libert, D., Griffin, H., Mahmood, R., Isaacson, E., et al. (2017). Modulation of basal cell fate during productive and transforming HPV16 infection is mediated by progressive E6-driven depletion of Notch. *J. Pathol.* 242, 448–462. doi: 10.1002/path.4917

Lanfredini, S., Olivero, C., Borgogna, C., Calati, F., Powell, K., Davies, K. J., et al. (2017). HPV8 field cancerization in a transgenic mouse model is due to Lrig1+ keratinocyte stem cell expansion. *J. Invest. Dermatol.* 137, 2208–2216. doi: 10.1016/j.jid.2017.04.039

Larson, P. S., de las Morenas, A., Bennett, S. R., Cupples, L. A., and Rosenberg, C. L. (2002). Loss of heterozygosity or allele imbalance in histologically normal breast epithelium is distinct from loss of heterozygosity or allele imbalance in co-existing carcinomas. *Am. J. Pathol.* 161, 283–290. doi: 10.1016/S0002-9440(10)64180-6

Leemans, C. R., Braakhuis, B. J., and Brakenhoff, R. H. (2011). The molecular biology of head and neck cancer. *Nat. Rev. Cancer* 11, 9–22. doi: 10.1038/nrc2982

Lin, T., Chao, C., Saito, S., Mazur, S. J., Murphy, M. E., Appella, E., et al. (2005). p53 induces differentiation of mouse embryonic stem cells by suppressing nanog expression. *Nat. Cell. Biol.* 7, 165–171. doi: 10.1038/ncb1211

Lindquist, D., Näsman, A., Tarján, M., Henriksson, R., Tot, T., Dalianis, T., et al. (2014). Expression of LRIG1 is associated with good prognosis and human papillomavirus status in oropharyngeal cancer. *Br. J. Cancer* 110, 1793–1800. doi: 10.1038/bjc.2014.87

Linge, A., Lohaus, F., Löck, S., Nowak, A., Gudziol, V., Valentini, C., et al. (2016). HPV status, cancer stem cell marker expression, hypoxia gene signatures and tumour volume identify good prognosis subgroups in patients with HNSCC after primary radiochemotherapy: a multicentre retrospective study of the German Cancer Consortium Radiation Oncology Group (DKTK-ROG). *Radiother. Oncol.* 121, 364–373. doi: 10.1016/j.radonc.2016.11.008

Maglennon, G. A., McIntosh, P., and Doorbar, J. (2011). Persistence of viral DNA in the epithelial basal layer suggests a model for papillomavirus latency following immune regression. *Virology* 414, 153–163. doi: 10.1016/j.virol.2011.03.019

Mao, L., Lee, J. S., Fan, Y. H., Ro, J. Y., Batsakis, J. G., Lippman, S., et al. (1996). Frequent microsatellite alterations at chromosomes 9p21 and 3p14 in oral premalignant lesions and their value in cancer risk assessment. *Nat. Med.* 2, 682–685. doi: 10.1038/nm0696-682

Marthaler, A. M., Podgorska, M., Feld, P., Fingerle, A., Knerr-Rupp, K., Grässer, F., et al. (2017). Identification of C/EBPα as a novel target of the HPV8 E6 protein regulating miR-203 in human keratinocytes. *PLoS Pathog.* 13:e1006406. doi: 10.1371/journal.ppat.1006406

Marur, S., D'Souza, G., Westra, W. H., and Forastiere, A. A. (2010). HPV-associated head and neck cancer: a virus-related cancer epidemic. *Lancet Oncol.* 11, 781–789. doi: 10.1016/S1470-2045(10)70017-6

McBride, A. A. (2013). The papillomavirus E2 proteins. *Virology* 445, 57–79. doi: 10.1016/j.virol.2013.06.006

McGranahan, N., and Swanton, C. (2017). Clonal heterogeneity and tumor evolution: past, present, and the future. *Cell* 168, 613–628. doi: 10.1016/j.cell.2017.01.018

McKinney, C. C., Hussmann, K. L., and McBride, A. A. (2015). The role of the DNA damage response throughout the papillomavirus life cycle. *Viruses* 7, 2450–2469. doi: 10.3390/v7052450

McLaughlin-Drubin, M. E., Crum, C. P., and Münger, K. (2011). Human papillomavirus E7 oncoprotein induces KDM6A and KDM6B histone demethylase expression and causes epigenetic reprogramming. *Proc. Natl. Acad. Sci. U.S.A.* 108, 2130–2135. doi: 10.1073/pnas.1009933108

McMillan, N. A., Payne, E., Frazer, I. H., and Evander, M. (1999). Expression of the α6 integrin confers papillomavirus binding upon receptor-negative B-cells. *Virology* 261, 271–279. doi: 10.1006/viro.1999.9825

Merrick, D. T., Kittelson, J., Winterhalder, R., Kotantoulas, G., Ingeberg, S., Keith, R. L., et al. (2006). Analysis of c-ErbB1/epidermal growth factor receptor and c-ErbB2/HER-2 expression in bronchial dysplasia: evaluation of potential targets for chemoprevention of lung cancer. *Clin. Cancer Res.* 12, 2281–2288. doi: 10.1158/1078-0432.CCR-05-2291

Meyers, J. M., Uberoi, A., Grace, M., Lambert, P. F., and Munger, K. (2017). Cutaneous HPV8 and MmuPV1 E6 proteins target the NOTCH and TGF-β tumor suppressors to inhibit differentiation and sustain keratinocyte proliferation. *PLoS Pathog.* 13:e1006171. doi: 10.1371/journal.ppat.1006171

Middleton, K., Peh, W., Southern, S. A., Griffin, H., Sotlar, K., Nakahara, T., et al. (2003). Organization of the human papillomavirus productive cycle during neoplastic progression provides a basis for the selection of diagnostic markers. *J. Virol.* 77, 10186–10201. doi: 10.1128/JVI.77.19.10186-10201.2003

Modur, V., Joshi, P., Nie, D., Robbins, K. T., Khan, A. U., and Rao, K. (2016). CD24 expression may play a role as a predictive indicator and a modulator of cisplatin treatment response in head and neck squamous cellular carcinoma. *PLoS One* 11:e0156651. doi: 10.1371/journal.pone.0156651

Muñoz, N., Castellsagué, X., de González, A. B., and Gissmann, L. (2006). Chapter 1: HPV in the etiology of human cancer. *Vaccine* 24, S1–S10. doi: 10.1016/j.vaccine.2006.05.115

Nakashima, H., Honda, M., Inoue, H., Shibuta, K., Arinaga, S., Era, S., et al. (1995). Microsatellite instability in multiple gastric cancers. *Int. J. Pathol.* 64, 239–242. doi: 10.1002/ijc.2910640405

Napoletano, C., Bellati, F., Ruscito, I., Pernice, M., Zizzari, I. G., Caponnetto, S., et al. (2016). Immunological and clinical impact of cancer stem cells in vulvar cancer: role of CD133/CD24/ABCG2-expressing cells. *Anticancer Res.* 36, 5109–5116. doi: 10.21873/anticanres.11080

Noya, F., Chien, W. M., Broker, T. R., and Chow, L. T. (2001). p21cip1 degradation in differentiated keratinocytes is abrogated by costabilization with cyclin E induced by human papillomavirus E7. *J. Virol.* 75, 6121–6134. doi: 10.1128/JVI.75.13.6121-6134.2001

Organista-Nava, J., Gómez-Gómez, Y., Ocadiz-Delgado, R., García-Villa, E., Bonilla-Delgado, J., and Lagunas-Martínez, A. (2016). The HPV16 E7 oncoprotein increases the expression of Oct3/4 and stemness-related genes and augments cell self-renewal. *Virology* 499, 230–242. doi: 10.1016/j.virol.2016.09.020

Ortiz, B. H., Ailawadi, M., Colitti, C., Muto, M. G., Deavers, M., Silva, E. G., et al. (2001). Second primary or recurrence? Comparative patterns of p53 and K-ras mutations suggest that serous borderline ovarian tumors and subsequent serous carcinomas are unrelated tumors. *Cancer Res.* 61, 7264–7267.

O'Shaughnessy, J. A., Kelloff, G. J., Gordon, G. B., Dannenberg, A. J., Hong, W. K., Fabian, C. J., et al. (2002). Treatment and prevention of intraepithelial neoplasia: an important target for accelerated new agent development. *Clin. Cancer Res.* 8, 314–346.

Patel, G. K., Yee, C. L., Terunuma, A., Telford, W. G., Voong, N., Yuspa, S. H., et al. (2012). Identification and characterization of tumor-initiating cells in human primary cutaneous squamous cell carcinoma. *J. Invest. Dermatol.* 132, 401–409. doi: 10.1038/jid.2011.317

Peh, W. L., Middleton, K., Christensen, N., Nicholls, P., Egawa, K., Sotlar, K., et al. (2002). Life cycle heterogeneity in animal models of human papillomavirus-associated disease. *J. Virol.* 76, 10401–10416. doi: 10.1128/JVI.76.20.10401-10416.2002

Ponten, F., Berg, C., Ahmadian, A., Ren, Z. P., Nister, M., Lundeberg, J., et al. (1997). Molecular pathology in basal cell cancer with p53 as a genetic marker. *Oncogene* 15, 1059–1067. doi: 10.1038/sj.onc.1201435

Prevo, L. J., Sanchez, C. A., Galipeau, P. C., and Reid, B. J. (1999). p53-mutant clones and field effects in Barrett's esophagus. *Cancer Res.* 59, 4784–4787.

Prince, M. E., Sivanandan, R., Kaczorowski, A., Wolf, G. T., Kaplan, M. J., Dalerba, P., et al. (2007). Identification of a subpopulation of cells with cancer stem cell properties in head and neck squamous cell carcinoma. *Proc. Natl. Acad. Sci. U.S.A.* 104, 973–978. doi: 10.1073/pnas.0610117104

Pullos, A. N., Castilho, R. M., and Squarize, C. H. (2015). HPV infection of the head and neck region and its stem cells. *J. Dent. Res.* 94, 1532–1543. doi: 10.1177/0022034515605456

Quint, K. D., Genders, R. E., de Koning, M. N., Borgogna, C., Gariglio, M., Bouwes Bavinck, J. N., et al. (2015). Human Beta-papillomavirus infection and keratinocyte carcinomas. *J. Pathol.* 235, 342–354. doi: 10.1002/path.4425

Ren, Z. P., Ponten, F., Nister M., and Ponten, J. (1966). Two distinct p53 immunohistochemical patterns in human squamous skin cancer, precursors and normal epidermis. *Int. J. Cancer* 69, 174–179. doi: 10.1002/(SICI)1097-0215(19960621)69:3<174::AID-IJC4>3.0.CO;2-X

Rietbergen, M. M., Martens-de Kemp, S. R., Bloemena, E., Witte, B. I., Brink, A., Baatenburg de Jong, R. J., et al. (2014). Cancer stem cell enrichment marker CD98: a prognostic factor for survival in patients with human papillomavirus-positive oropharyngeal cancer. *Eur. J. Cancer* 50, 765–773. doi: 10.1016/j.ejca.2013.11.010

Rodríguez, A. C., Schiffman, M., Herrero, R., Hildesheim, A., Bratti, C., Sherman, M. E., et al. (2010). Longitudinal study of human papillomavirus persistence and cervical intraepithelial neoplasia grade 2/3: critical role of duration of infection. *J. Natl. Cancer Inst.* 102, 315–324. doi: 10.1093/jnci/djq001

Rodríguez, A. C., Schiffman, M., Herrero, R., Wacholder, S., Hildesheim, A., Castle, P. E., et al. (2008). Rapid clearance of human papillomavirus and implications for clinical focus on persistent infections. *J. Natl. Cancer Inst.* 100, 513–517. doi: 10.1093/jnci/djn044

Rosenthal, A. N., Ryan, A., Hopster, D., and Jacobs, I. J. (2002). Molecular evidence of a common clonal origin and subsequent divergent clonal evolution in vulval intraepithelial neoplasia, vulval squamous cell carcinoma and lymph node metastases. *Int. J. Cancer* 99, 549–554. doi: 10.1002/ijc.10362

Ryser, M. D., Myers, E. R., and Durrett, R. (2015). HPV clearance and the neglected role of stochasticity. *PLoS Comput. Biol.* 11:e1004113. doi: 10.1371/journal.pcbi.1004113

Schelhaas, M., Shah, B., Holzer, M., Blattmann, P., Kühling, L., Day, P. M., et al. (2012). Entry of human papillomavirus type 16 by actin-dependent, clathrin- and lipid raft-independent endocytosis. *PLoS Pathog.* 8:e1002657. doi: 10.1371/journal.ppat.1002657

Schmitt, A., Rochat, A., Zeltner, R., Borenstein, L., Barrandon, Y., Wettstein, F. O., et al. (1996). The primary target cells of the high-risk cottontail rabbit papillomavirus colocalize with hair follicle stem cells. *J. Virol.* 70, 1912–1922.

Scholes, A. G., Woolgar, J. A., Boyle, M. A., Brown, J. S., Vaughan, E. D., Hart, C. A., et al. (1998). Synchronous oral carcinomas: independent or common clonal origin? *Cancer Res.* 58, 2003–2006.

Shafti-Keramat, S., Handisurya, A., Kriehuber, E., Meneguzzi, G., Slupetzky, K., and Kirnbauer, R. (2003). Different heparan sulfate proteoglycans serve as cellular receptors for human papillomaviruses. *J. Virol.* 77, 13125–13135. doi: 10.1128/JVI.77.24.13125-13135.2003

Shen, L., Kondo, Y., Rosner, G. L., Xiao, L., Hernandez, N. S., and Vilaythong, J. (2005). MGMT promoter methylation and field defect in sporadic colorectal cancer. *J. Natl. Cancer Inst.* 97, 1330–1338. doi: 10.1093/jnci/dji275

Sherman, L., Jackman, A., Itzhaki, H., Stoppler, M. C., Koval, D., and Schlegel, R. (1997). Inhibition of serum- and calcium-induced differentiation of human keratinocytes by HPV16 E6 oncoprotein: role of p53 inactivation. *Virology* 237, 296–306. doi: 10.1006/viro.1997.8778

Sheu, L. F., Chen, A., Tseng, H. H., Leu, F. J., Lin, J. K., Ho, K. C., et al. (1995). The assessment of p53 expression in nasopharyngeal carcinoma. *Hum. Pathol.* 26, 380–386. doi: 10.1016/0046-8177(95)90137-X

Shinmura, K., Tani, M., Isogaki, J., Wang, Y., Sugimara, H., and Yokota, J. (1998). RER phenotype and its associated mutations in familial gastric cancer. *Carcinogenesis* 19, 247–251. doi: 10.1093/carcin/19.2.247

Simon, R., Eltze, E., Schafer, K. L., Burger, H., Semjonow, A., and Hertle, L. (2001). Cytogenetic analysis of multifocal bladder cancer supports a monoclonal origin and intraepithelial spread of tumor cells. *Cancer Res.* 61, 355–362.

Slaughter, D. P., Southwick, H. W., and Smejkal, W. (1953). Field cancerization in oral stratified squamous epithelium; clinical implications of multicentric origin. *Cancer* 6, 963–968. doi: 10.1002/1097-0142(195309)6:5<963::AID-CNCR2820060515>3.0.CO;2-Q

Smeds, J., Warnberg, F., Norberg, T., Nordgren, H., Holmberg, L., and Bergh, J. (2005). Ductal carcinoma in situ of the breast with different histopathological grades and corresponding new breast tumour events: analysis of loss of heterozygosity. *Acta Oncol.* 44, 41–49. doi: 10.1080/02841860410002842

Spoden, G., Freitag, K., Husmann, M., Boller, K., Sapp, M., Lambert, C., et al. (2008). Clathrin- and caveolin-independent entry of human papillomavirus type 16–involvement of tetraspanin-enriched microdomains (TEMs). *PLoS One* 3:e3313. doi: 10.1371/journal.pone.0003313

Stubenrauch, F., Lim, H. B., and Laimins, L. A. (1998). Differential requirements for conserved E2 binding sites in the life cycle of oncogenic human papillomavirus type 31. *J. Virol.* 72, 1071–1077.

Sui, G., Zhou, S., Wang, J., Canto, M., Lee, E. E., and Eshleman, J. R. (2006). Mitochondrial DNA mutations in preneoplastic lesions of the gastrointestinal tract: a biomarker for the early detection of cancer. *Mol. Cancer* 5:73.

Syrjanen, K., Hakama, M., Saarikoski, S., Väyrynen, M., Yliskoski, M., Syrjänen, S., et al. (1990). Prevalence, incidence, and estimated life-time risk of cervical human papillomavirus infections in a nonselected Finnish female population. *J. Sex. Transm. Dis.* 17, 15–19. doi: 10.1097/00007435-199017010-00004

Tabor, M. P., Brakenhoff, R. H., Ruijter-Schippers, H. J., Kummer, J. A., Leemans, C. R., and Braakhuis, B. J. (2004). Genetically altered fields as origin of locally recurrent head and neck cancer: a retrospective study. *Clin. Cancer Res.* 10, 3607–3613. doi: 10.1158/1078-0432.CCR-03-0632

Tabor, M. P., Brakenhoff, R. H., Ruijter-Schippers, H. J., Van Der Wal, J. E., Snow, G. B., and Leemans, C. R. (2002). Multiple head and neck tumors frequently originate from a single preneoplastic lesion. *Am. J. Pathol.* 161, 1051–1060. doi: 10.1016/S0002-9440(10)64266-6

Tang, A. L., Owen, J. H., Hauff, S. J., Park, J. J., Papagerakis, S., Bradford, C. R., et al. (2013). Head and neck cancer stem cells: the effect of HPV–an in vitro and mouse study. *Otolaryngol. Head Neck Surg.* 149, 252–260. doi: 10.1177/0194599813486599

Tate, J. E., Mutter, G. L., Boynton, K. A., and Crum, C. P. (1997). Monoclonal origin of vulvar intraepithelial neoplasia and some vulvar hyperplasias. *Am. J. Pathol.* 150, 315–322.

Tomaić, V. (2016). Functional roles of E6 and E7 oncoproteins in HPV-induced malignancies at diverse anatomical sites. *Cancers* 8:E95. doi: 10.3390/cancers8100095

Tommasino, M. (2017). The biology of beta human papillomaviruses. *Virus Res.* 231, 128–138. doi: 10.1016/j.virusres.2016.11.013

Tyagi, A., Vishnoi, K., Mahata, S., Verma, G., Srivastava, Y., Masaldan, S., et al. (2016). Cervical cancer stem cells selectively overexpress HPV oncoprotein E6 that controls stemness and self-renewal through upregulation of HES1. *Clin. Cancer Res.* 22, 4170–4184. doi: 10.1158/1078-0432.CCR-15-2574

van Houten, V. M., Tabor, M. P., van den Brekel, M. W., Kummer, J. A., Denkers, F., Dijkstra, J., et al. (2002). Mutated P53 as molecular marker for the diagnosis of head and neck cancer. *J. Pathol.* 198, 476–486. doi: 10.1002/path.1242

Vishnoi, K., Mahata, S., Tyagi, A., Pandey, A., Verma, G., Jadli, M., et al. (2016). Cross-talk between human papillomavirus oncoproteins and hedgehog signaling synergistically promotes stemness in cervical cancer cells. *Sci. Rep.* 28:34377. doi: 10.1038/srep34377

Vlashi, E., Chen, A. M., Boyrie, S., Yu, G., Nguyen, A., Brower, P. A., et al. (2016). Radiation-induced dedifferentiation of head and neck cancer cells into cancer stem cells depends on human papillomavirus status. *Int. J. Radiat. Oncol. Biol. Phys.* 94, 1198–1206. doi: 10.1016/j.ijrobp.2016.01.005

Vokes, E. E., Agrawal, N., and Seiwert, T. Y. (2015). HPV-associated head and neck cancer. *J. Natl. Cancer Inst.* 107:djv344. doi: 10.1093/jnci/djv344

Wallace, N. A., Robinson, K., Howie, H. L., and Galloway, D. A. (2012). HPV 5 and 8 E6 abrogate ATR activity resulting in increased persistence of UVB induced DNA damage. *PLoS Pathog.* 8:e1002807. doi: 10.1371/journal.ppat.1002807

Waridel, F., Estreicher, A., Bron, L., Flaman, J. M., Fontolliet, C., Monnier, P., et al. (1997). Field cancerisation and polyclonal p53 mutation in the upper aerodigestive tract. *Oncogene* 14, 163–169. doi: 10.1038/sj.onc.1200812

Xi, R., Pan, S., Chen, X., Hui, B., Zhang, L., Fu, S., et al. (2016). HPV16 E6-E7 induces cancer stem-like cells phenotypes in esophageal squamous cell carcinoma through the activation of PI3K/Akt signaling pathway in vitro and in vivo. *Oncotarget* 7, 57050–57065. doi: 10.18632/oncotarget.10959

5

β-HPV Infection Correlates with Early Stages of Carcinogenesis in Skin Tumors and Patient-Derived Xenografts from a Kidney Transplant Recipient Cohort

Cinzia Borgogna[1†], Carlotta Olivero[1,2†], Simone Lanfredini[2], Federica Calati[1], Marco De Andrea[1,3], Elisa Zavattaro[4], Paola Savoia[4], Elena Trisolini[5], Renzo Boldorini[5], Girish K. Patel[2] and Marisa Gariglio[1]*

[1] Virology Unit, Department of Translational Medicine, Novara Medical School, University of Eastern Piedmont, Novara Italy, [2] School of Biosciences, European Cancer Stem Cell Research Institute, Cardiff University, Cardiff, United Kingdom, [3] Virology Unit, Department of Public Health and Pediatric Sciences, Turin Medical School, University of Turin, Turin, Italy, [4] Dermatology Unit, Department of Health Sciences, Novara Medical School, Novara, Italy, [5] Pathology Unit, Department of Health Sciences, Novara Medical School, Novara, Italy

***Correspondence:**
Marisa Gariglio
marisa.gariglio@med.uniupo.it

† These authors have contributed equally to this work.

Many malignancies that occur in high excess in kidney transplant recipients (KTRs) are due to viruses that thrive in the setting of immunosuppression. Keratinocyte carcinoma (KC), the most frequently occurring cancer type in KTR, has been associated with skin infection by human papillomavirus (HPV) from the beta genus. In this report, we extend our previous investigation aimed at identifying the presence of active β-HPV infection in skin tumors from KTRs through detection of viral protein expression. Using a combination of antibodies raised against the E4 and L1 proteins of the β-genotypes, we were able to visualize infection in five tumors [one keratoacanthoma (KA), three actinic keratoses (AKs), and one seborrheic keratoses (SKs)] that were all removed from two patients who had been both transplanted twice, had developed multiple KCs, and presented with a long history of immunosuppression (>30 years). These infected tissues displayed intraepidermal hyperplasia and increased expression of the ΔNp63 protein, which extended into the upper epithelial layers. In addition, using a xenograft model system in nude mice displaying a humanized stromal bed in the site of grafting, we successfully engrafted three AKs, two of which were derived from the aforementioned KTRs and displayed β-HPV infection in the original tumor. Of note, one AK-derived xenograft, along with its ensuing lymph node metastasis, was diagnosed as squamous cell carcinoma (SCC). In the latter, both β-HPV infection and ΔNp63 expression were no longer detectable. Although the overall success rate of engrafting was very low, the results of this study show for the first time that β-HPV^{+} and ΔNp63^{+} intraepidermal hyperplasia can indeed progress to an aggressive SCC able to metastasize. Consistent with a series of reports attributing a causative role of β-HPV at early stages of skin carcinogenesis through ΔNp63 induction and increased keratinocytes stemness, here we provide *in vivo* evidence that these events are also occurring in the affected skin of KTRs. Due to these β-HPV-driven molecular pathways, the nascent tumor cell is able to acquire a high enough number of carcinogenic insults that its proliferation and survival will eventually become independent of viral gene expression.

Keywords: β-HPV, skin cancer, xenograft, carcinogenesis, organ transplant recipients

INTRODUCTION

The prolonged use of immunosuppressive drugs in kidney transplant recipients (KTRs) is a recognized risk factor for infectious diseases and ensuing complications, including infection-related malignancies (Vajdic and van Leeuwen, 2009; Krynitz et al., 2013; Geissler, 2015). Keratinocyte carcinoma (KC), which includes basal cell carcinoma (BCC) and squamous cell carcinoma (SCC), is the most frequent cancer type in KTRs, with an incidence rate ranging from 10 to 30% at 10 years post-transplantation (Kovach and Stasko, 2009; Madeleine et al., 2012).

Cutaneous human papillomaviruses (HPVs) from the β-genus, such as HPV5 and HPV8, have long been associated with KC in patients with a specific genetic background and in long-term immunosuppressed individuals (Genders et al., 2015; Howley and Pfister, 2015; Quint et al., 2015). Currently, more than 200 different HPV types have been described, which can be clustered into five genera (i.e., alpha-, beta-, gamma-, mu- and nu-papillomavirus) based on their taxonomy (http://pave.niaid.nih.gov/#home) (Bernard, 2013; Hufbauer and Akgül, 2017; Tommasino, 2017). Among them, mucosal α-genus HPV types are able to infect both oral and genital mucosa epithelia and are generally ranked as low-risk and high-risk types according to the tendency of the resulting neoplasm to undergo malignant progression (Kranjec and Doorbar, 2016). On the other hand, cutaneous HPVs, which are clustered in the evolutionarily distinct β-genus, can cause widespread unapparent or asymptomatic infections in the general population (Howley and Pfister, 2015; Quint et al., 2015). However, in immunosuppressed patients and in individuals suffering from the rare inherited disease epidermodysplasia verruciformis (EV), these viruses can spread unchecked and promote the development of KC. For example, β-HPV-associated wart-like lesions in EV patients are at high risk for progression to KC (Borgogna et al., 2012; Landini et al., 2014), and the ensuing tumors are positive for β-HPV DNA and protein expression (Dell'Oste et al., 2009).

Unlike cancers associated with mucosal HPV infections, cutaneous HPV-associated KC arises mainly in sun-exposed body areas, and hence these viruses are thought to cooperate with UV to induce cancer (Bouwes Bavinck et al., 2010, 2017; Quint et al., 2015). A series of reports have indeed demonstrated that expression of either β-HPV5 or 8 E6 substantially increases the mutagenic potential of UVB exposure (Wallace et al., 2012). For example, HPV8 E2, E6, and E7 each have oncogenic activities when expressed in basal epithelial cells of transgenic mice (Schaper et al., 2005; Pfefferle et al., 2008; Marcuzzi et al., 2009; Heuser et al., 2016). Furthermore, β-HPV E6s can alter Notch-mediated keratinocyte differentiation, thereby fostering a cellular environment conducive to viral replication (Meyers et al., 2013; Wallace and Galloway, 2014).

Although recent publications have, for the most part, characterized *in vitro* the effects of β-HPV oncogenes on host signaling pathways, it has become increasingly apparent that the dissection of the mechanisms underlying viral pathogenesis and oncogenesis in the affected skin areas during long-term HPV persistence would further our understanding of how such tissues are primed for cancer progression. Unfortunately, the exquisite host specificity of HPVs, which prevents experimental infections of heterologous hosts, has so far hindered the development of tractable animal models of infection. Moreover, it appears that β-HPV sequences are not essential for the maintenance of the transformed state as they are apparently lost from cancer cells, especially in non-EV tumors, at later stages of disease (Weissenborn et al., 2005).

In an effort to correlate β-HPV infection with disease pathology during progression of premalignant lesions to KC, we have set up an immunofluorescence protocol that allows both visualization of productive HPV infection in affected skin areas and evaluation of skin homeostasis through detection of the minichromosome maintenance complex component 7 (MCM7), a cellular proliferation marker (Borgogna et al., 2012, 2014). Using this protocol, in a previous study of a single center KTR cohort (Borgogna et al., 2014), we could observe active β-HPV infection in hyperplastic edges of skin SCC and BCC as well as in premalignant lesions, such as actinic keratoses (AK). Of note, while the $E4^+$ areas were mainly found within the disorganized epithelium of AK lesions, in more advanced tumors, such as skin SCC and BCC, they were always localized in the adjacent pathological epithelium. Furthermore, we detected MCM7 expression extending into the upper epithelial layers of E4 expressing areas ($E4^+$), indicating that epithelial cells were actively proliferating in areas of productive viral infection. Thus, based on these findings, we hypothesized that β-HPV-induced basal cell proliferation in the immunosuppressed setting alongside other transforming agents, such as UVB irradiation, might play a causative role at early stages of neoplastic transformation, while it may not be necessarily involved at later stages of the disease (Quint et al., 2015).

Emerging evidence also indicates that β-HPV can perturb p63 expression, a master regulator of development and maintenance of multilayered epithelia, including the epidermis (Meyers et al., 2013; Marthaler et al., 2017). p63, predominantly the ΔNp63 isoform, is selectively distributed in basal cells of stratified epithelia where it is required for the replenishment of stem cells (Senoo et al., 2007; Romano et al., 2009; Koster, 2010; Melino et al., 2015). In this regard, we have recently shown that HPV8-induced field cancerization in a transgenic mouse model is due to Lrig1$^+$ keratinocyte stem cell expansion, which is accompanied by aberrant nuclear p63 expression in the expanded infundibulum and adjoining interfollicular epidermis. EV and non-EV keratoses displayed similar histology associated with β-HPV reactivation and nuclear p63 expression (Lanfredini et al., 2017).

In this study, we have further extended our previous analysis of a single center cohort of KTRs by (i) analyzing 128 additional skin lesions excised from 29 KTRs; (ii) correlating ΔNp63 expression levels with those of E4 and MCM7 in skin areas of productive HPV infection; and (iii) establishing and characterizing patient-derived xenografts as models to study skin cancer progression of β-HPV-infected skin lesions. In particular, we provide evidence of two KTRs with multiple β-HPV$^+$ skin tumors and demonstrate progression of a β-HPV$^+$ AK lesion into SCC in a patient-derived xenograft.

MATERIALS AND METHODS

Sample Collection

Tissue sections were obtained from 171 formalin-fixed and paraffin-embedded blocks (FFPE) corresponding to either the core or the edges of the tumor, collected from 128 skin lesions excised from 29 KTRs attending the dermatology unit in the University Hospital-Novara. Thirty-two tumors were derived from KTRs already described in our previous work (patients 1M, 3M, 9M, 14M, 15M, and 17M respectively; Borgogna et al., 2014).

The study was approved by the local ethic committee: Comitato Etico Interaziendale Novara (Prot. CE 168/15) and written informed consent was obtained by all subjects according to the Declaration of Helsinki.

Transplantation of Human Skin Tumors

The immunodeficient mice used for xenograft development were male athymic Nude-Foxn1nu (Envigo, Huntingdon, UK). Mice were housed under pathogen-free conditions in our animal facilities in accordance with The Guide for the Care and Use of Laboratory Animals and the experimentation was approved by the CESAPO (Comitato Etico Sperimentazione Animale Piemonte Orientale, Prot. 20093). Mice were anesthetized with an Ohmeda TEC4 Vaporizer using Isoflurane Vet (Merial, Ingelheim am Rhein, Germany) and Gelfoam dressing (Johnson & Johnson, New Brunswick, NJ) was implanted into the dorsal sub-cutaneous space together with primary human fibroblasts suspended in 100 μl Matrigel (BD Biosciences, Milano, Italia), and wounds were closed with surgical stitches (Ethicon, Johnson & Johnson, New Brunswick, NJ). After 14 days, mice were anesthetized and human skin tumors (~0.5 cm^3) were xenografted into the stromal bed together with 10^6 primary human fibroblasts suspended in 100 μl Matrigel (Patel et al., 2012). Xenograft growth was weekly monitored by measuring the longer diameter of the tumor mass by caliper. After 3 or 6 months, mice were sacrified *via* CO_2 inhalation and tumors were removed: half of them was fixed in 10% neutral-buffered formalin and embedded in paraffin blocks, while the other half was snap frozen and stored at −80°C. Five-μm sections were cut from the FFPE blocks and stained with hematoxylin and eosin (H&E) as performed for human skin biopsies.

HPV Genotyping

Total DNA was extracted from the frozen xenograft or plucked hair bulbs from eyebrows using QIAamp DNA Mini Kit following the manufacturer's instructions (Qiagen, Milan, Italy). β-HPV DNA analysis was carried out using broad spectrum PCR (PM-PCR) in combination with a reverse hybridization system [RHA Kit Skin (beta) HPV (Diassay, Rijswijk, the Netherlands)] as previously described (de Koning et al., 2006).

Immunofluorescence Labeling

DNA-FISH and immunofluorescence detection of β-HPV E4, MCM7, β-HPV L1 were performed on formalin-fixed and paraffin-embedded skin biopsies or xenografts using standard techniques as previously described (Borgogna et al., 2012, 2014). Briefly, DNA-FISH was performed using as probe the complete biotin-labeled (Biotin-nick translation kit, Roche Diagnostics GmbH, Mannheim, Germany) genomic HPV plasmid DNA (100 ng/ml). For the other markers analyzed (β-HPV E4, MCM7, β-HPV L1, and ΔNp63), antigen unmasking was performed by heating the slides in a conventional decloaking chamber for 10 min at 121°C in 10 mM citrate buffer at pH 6.0 (Vector Laboratories, Burlingame, CA, USA). Immunofluorescence was carried out using the following antibodies: rabbit anti-β-HPV E4 (kindly provided by John Doorbar, 1:1,000), mouse anti-MCM7 (1:200, Neomarkers Fremont, Fremont, CA), rabbit anti-ΔNp63 antibody (clone Poly6190) (BioLegend, San Diego, CA, USA) (1:500) and rabbit anti-β-HPV L1 (1:1,000). Images were acquired using a digital scanner (Pannoramic MIDI; 3D Histech Kft., Budapest, Hungary). For the assessment of histological features, the slides analyzed by immunofluorescence were disassembled and stained with H&E. The production of polyclonal antibodies to β-HPV E4 (HPV5E4) and β-HPV L1 has been previously described (Borgogna et al., 2012, 2014). Briefly, the broad spectrum anti-L1 antibodies were raised against the highly conserved region between amino acid 200 and 300 of the L1 protein, while those against the HPV5E4 crossreact with many genotypes from species 1 only, including HPV8, 14, 20, 24, 25, and 36.

RESULTS

Visualization of β-HPV Viral Protein Expression in Skin Tumors from the KTR Cohort

In our previous work, we had already analyzed 111 FFPE blocks obtained from 79 skin lesions of 17 patients from a cohort of KTRs for the presence of active β-HPV infection by immunostaining with anti-E4 and anti-L1 antibodies. Among those specimens, we could find E4$^+$ areas in six FFPE blocks from four patients corresponding to four AK lesions and the adjacent pathological area of one SCC and one BCC (**Table 1**). In this study, we have analyzed 171 additional FFPE blocks from 128 skin lesions excised from 29 KTRs following the same procedure. Within this second group, two patients, who were not included

TABLE 1 | Overview of the skin biopsy blocks from the KTR cohort study examined by immunohistochemistry for the presence of β-HPV infection and grouped according to pathology diagnosis.

	Seborrheic keratoses, n = 18	***Keratoacanthoma, n = 16***	***Bowen's disease, n = 3***	***Actinic keratoses, n = 54***	***Basal cell carcinoma, n = 77***	***Squamous cell carcinoma, n = 39***	***Total Lesions, n = 207***
	FFPE blocks n = 20	***FFPE blocks n = 21***	***FFPE blocks n = 3***	***FFPE blocks n = 71***	***FFPE blocks n = 107***	***FFPE blocks n = 60***	***Total FFPE blocks n = 282***
β-HPV-positive lesions	1	1		7	1	1	11
Previous study (Borgogna et al., 2014)				4	1	1	6
This study	1	1		3			5

The skin biopsies found positive for β-HPV E4 expression in our previous study (Borgogna et al., 2014) and this current one are indicated separately.

in the previous survey, presented with multiple skin lesions some of which displayed areas of β-HPV infection.

The first case was a female KTR who underwent a second kidney transplant (KTx) in 2016 due to the failure of her first one after 25 years. She displayed many flat, reddish papular lesions widespread in the total body skin as shown by the representative picture of the forehead (**Figure 1A**) that were very much resembled the EV keratoses, and her clinical history reported the development of many proliferative skin lesions (>15) in different body sites starting approximately 10 years after her first kidney transplant, which was carried out in 1980. A total of 22 FFPE blocks corresponding to the 13 tumors excised from this patient from 2014 in our hospital, each diagnosed as SCC (n = 5), BCC (n = 3), AK (n = 2), or keratoacanthoma (KA) (n = 3), were made available for immunofluorescence analysis. β-HPV$^+$ areas were found in one KA located on the leg, and in two AKs located on the hand and the leg (**Table 1**). As shown in representative (**Figures 1C,D**), E4$^+$ cells were clearly evident in the areas of an AK lesion presenting with hyperkeratosis and parakeratosis; some of them were trapped in the keratin layers where L1$^+$ nuclei were also observed (data not shown). The cellular proliferation marker MCM7, a subunit of DNA helicase, was more evident in the E4$^+$ area compared with the adjacent epithelium, and extended to suprabasal layers, indicating that cells were primed to enter the cell cycle. In the AK found on the hand, E4 expression was not detected, while nuclei stained with the β-HPV late capsidic protein (L1) were well evident in the upper layers of the epithelium where some differentiation was still occurring, indicating the presence of productive viral infection (data not shown).

The second case was a male KTR born in 1960 who underwent kidney transplant twice, with the first one taking place in 1996. From 2012 onwards, the patient developed five skin cancers in different body sites diagnosed as BCC (n = 2), AK (n = 2) and seborrheic keratoses (SK; n = 1). Positivity for β-HPV markers was found in one AK and in the SK removed from the back and the left forearm, respectively. The virus-positive AK displayed highly keratotic epithelium with clear signs of β-HPV-related cytopathic effects (**Figures 2A,B**). Immunofluorescence analysis showed large areas of β-HPV E4 expression in the most superficial layers of the epithelium and increased MCM7 expression in the basal and suprabasal layers (**Figure 2C**). Likewise, in the SK we found a large number of E4$^+$ cells spread throughout the entire lesion as shown in **Figures 2E–G**. Consistent with the benign nature of this skin tumor, MCM7 expression in the basal layer was less evident, while it was highly expressed in the suprabasal cells overexpressing cytoplasmic E4. These cells located in the mid to upper epithelial layers had likely re-entered the cell cycle to support viral genome amplification as E4 expression usually occurs in cells where viral DNA is replicating.

ΔNp63 Expression in Skin Tumors

To ascertain whether p63 induction could also be visualized in virus-positive skin cancers from the KTR cohort, tissue sections from all the skin lesions excised from the two aforementioned patients (n = 18) were co-labeled with antibodies against ΔNp63 and MCM7. In addition, six skin lesions (SCC n = 1, BCC n = 1 and AK n = 4) with areas positive for E4 expression from our previous survey were similarly analyzed. As depicted in the representative **Figure 3** showing a KTR-derived BCC identified in the first round of screening (patient 5M, Borgogna et al., 2014), the ΔNp63 protein was highly expressed in the neoplastic area in comparison with the non-pathological adjoining epithelium (**Figure 3D** vs. **Figure 3J**), and its expression generally overlapped with that of MCM7 (**Figures 3C,I** respectively). This staining pattern was reproducibly observed in the high-grade lesions, including SCC (n = 6) and BCC (n = 6). Of note, in the adjacent β-HPV-infected hyperplastic epithelium as determined by E4 staining (**Figure 3F**), ΔNp63 expression extended in the middle-superficial layers, higher than those expressing MCM7, indicating that ΔNp63 was expressed in cells either proliferating or with a great potential of proliferation although not yet transformed. A similar pattern of ΔNp63 expression was also observed in the benign SK shown in **Figure 2**, where it spread across the entire epithelium despite the fact that MCM7 was restricted to some cells in the basal layer and some cells in the intermediate layers (**Figures 2G,H**). Also in the case of AK (n = 8) and KA (n = 3), ΔNp63 expression exceeded that of MCM7 as it was still detectable in the more superficial nucleated cells. Quantification of ΔNp63 and MCM7 positive cells confirmed the increase

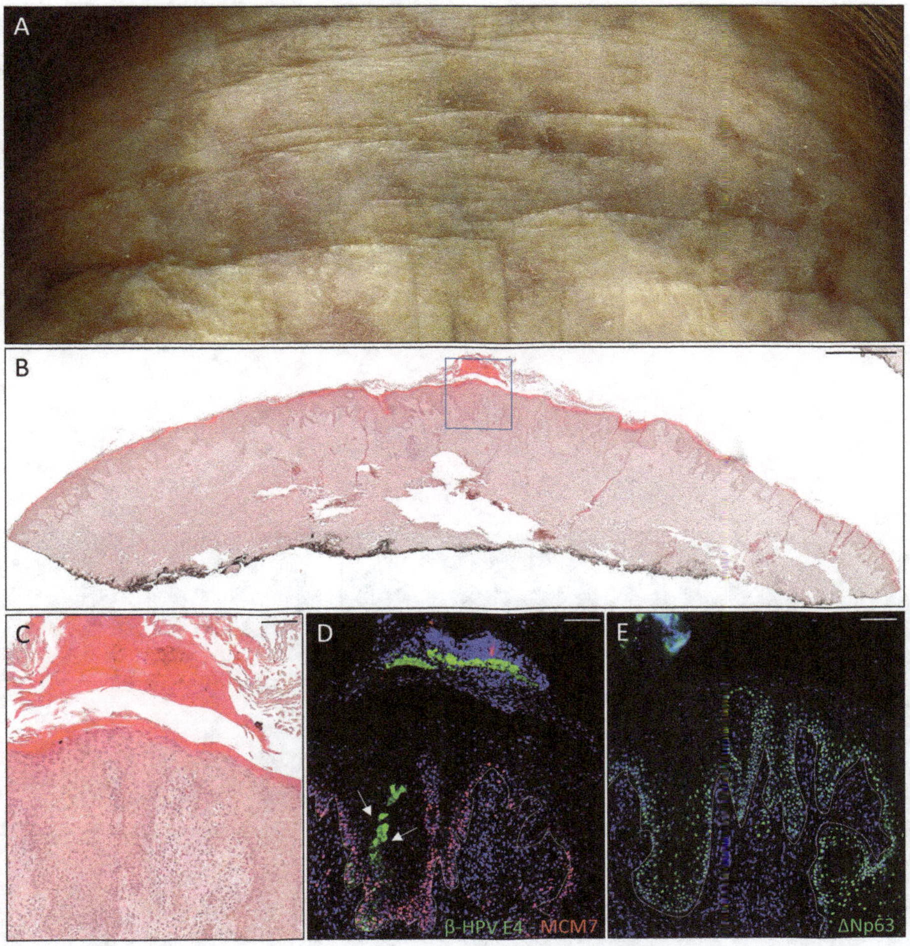

FIGURE 1 | Histopathological analysis of an actinic keratoses (AK) from a female kidney transplant recipient (KTR). **(A)** Flat whitish and reddish papular lesions on her forehead. **(B)** Hematoxylin and eosin (H&E) staining of a representative tissue section (scale bar: 1,000 μm) from one AK lesion on the leg of the patient. **(C)** Magnification of the region highlighted by the blue box shown in panel B (scale bar: 100 μm). **(D)** Immunofluorescence staining for beta human papillomavirus (β-HPV) E4 and minichromosome maintenance complex component 7 (MCM7) (β-HPV E4 in green; MCM7 in red) of the same tissue section shown in **(B,C)**. The white arrows indicate E4 staining. **(E)** Immunofluorescence staining for ΔNp63 (green) of a serial section. The white dotted line indicates the basal layer. Sections in **(D,E)** were counterstained with 4′,6-diamidino-2-phenylindole (DAPI) (blue) to visualize cell nuclei.

in $\Delta Np63^+$ cells in both β-HPV-infected cells and tumors vs. non-pathological epithelium (Supplementary Figure 1). In the case of β-HPV-infected cells, the number of $\Delta Np63^+$ cells was significantly higher than that of $MCM7^+$ cells.

Development of Xenografts in Athymic Nude Mice

A well-established model to study tumor progression and clinical outcome is represented by patient-derived xenograft (PDX) models. PDXs are developed by implanting tumor samples obtained directly from patients in immunodeficient mice. In this regard, we have previously shown that the creation of a humanized stromal bed, by first implanting Gelfoam dressing along with HDF, facilitates primary human skin SCC xenograft growth in nude mice (Patel et al., 2012).

Thus, we asked whether premalignant skin lesions could be similarly engrafted so that we could monitor progression or regression of a lesion that otherwise would be surgically removed from the patient. For this purpose, we engrafted all skin lesions available from the cohort study in the period of observation (3 years), including those that clinically appeared as benign and/or premalignant. From a total of 42 lesions engrafted following this procedure, we were able to collect 38 xenografts—in four cases no tumor growth was detected. The main characteristics of the KTRs whose skin tumors were grafted into nude mice are shown in Supplementary Table 1, and the histological features of the tumors are listed in **Table 2**. At the beginning, tumors were removed 6 months after the graft (15 out of 38). Following this timeline, growth was obtained for two BCCs whose xenograft histology closely mirrored that found in the original tumor. The human origin of the xenograft tumors was confirmed by staining

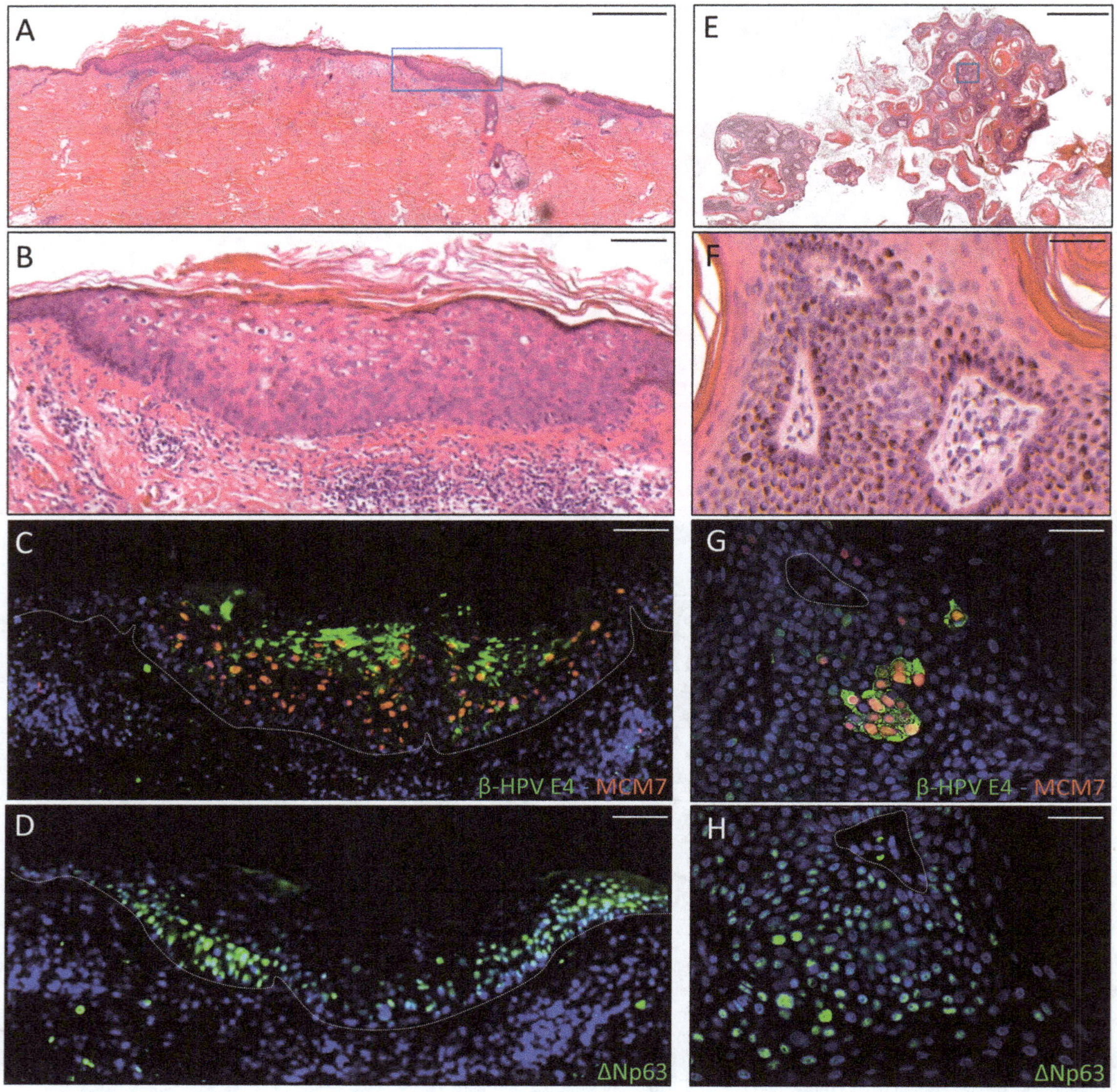

FIGURE 2 | Immunohistochemical staining for β-HPV E4, MCM7, and ΔNp63 in one AK lesion **(A–D)** and one seborrheic keratoses (SK) lesions **(E–H)** derived from a male KTR. **(A)** H&E staining of a representative tissue section (scale bar: 1,000 μm) from one AK lesion on the back of the patient. **(B)** Magnification of the region highlighted by the blue box shown in **A** (scale bar: 100 μm). **(C)** Immunofluorescence staining for β-HPV E4 (green) and MCM7 (red) of the same tissue section shown in **(A,B)**. **(D)** Immunofluorescence staining for ΔNp63 (green) of a serial section. The white dotted line indicates the basal layer. **(E)** H&E staining of a representative tissue section (scale bar: 1,000 μm) from one SK lesion on the forearm of the patient. **(F)** Magnification of the region highlighted by the blue box shown in **E** (scale bar: 50 μm). **(G)** Immunofluorescence staining for β-HPV E4 (green) and MCM7 (red) of the same tissue section shown in **(E,F)**. **(H)** Immunofluorescence staining for ΔNp63 (green) of a serial section. Sections **(C,D,G,H)** were counterstained with DAPI (blue) to visualize cell nuclei.

with human cytokeratin (data not shown). Unfortunately, all other cases ($n = 13$) turned out to be epidermal cysts filled with cornified material and surrounded by dying epithelial cells. This pitfall prompted us to shorten the length of the growing period in nude mice to 3 months. Using this modified timeline, three out of the 23 skin tumors engrafted gave rise to a tumor mass with well-defined histological features. Three AKs successfully grew in nude mice; two of them displayed a growth curve similar to that of the two BCCs, while one grew faster, especially after week 8 (Supplementary Figure 2). While the formers xenografts retained the original histological features, the latter, which was derived from the aforementioned male KTR, was diagnosed as SCC along with its ensuing lymph node metastasis (**Figure 4**). Although β-HPV markers were well evident in multiple areas of the original AK (**Figures 2A–D**), they were no longer detectable in the SCC, not even by PCR amplification of xenograft total DNA using broad spectrum primers for beta genotypes (data not shown, de Koning et al., 2006). This SCC turned out to be

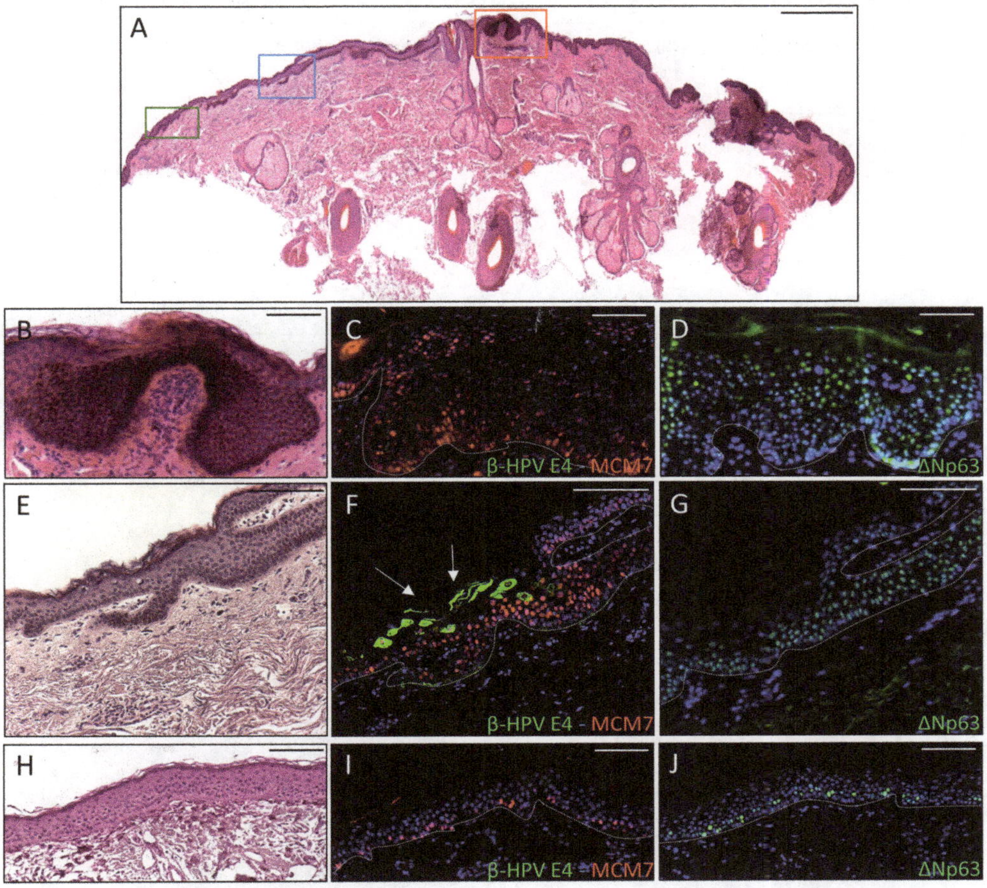

FIGURE 3 | Immunohistochemical staining for β-HPV E4, MCM7, and ΔNp63 in one basal cell carcinoma (BCC) from a KTR (patient 5M, Borgogna et al., 2014). **(A)** H&E staining of a representative tissue section (scale bar: 1,000 μm). The red square highlights the BCC, the blue square indicates the HPV-infected area in the adjacent epithelium, and the green square shows non-pathological epithelium. **(B,E,H)** Magnification of the regions highlighted by the boxes shown in **A** (**B**: red square; **E**: blue square; **H**: green square). Scale bar: 100 μm. **(C,F,I)** Serial sections obtained from the same specimens depicted in panels B, E, and H, respectively, were subject to double staining using antibodies against β-HPV E4 (green) and MCM7 (red). The white arrows indicate E4 staining. **(D,G,J)** Serial sections obtained from the same specimens depicted in **(B,E,H)**, respectively, were stained with antibodies against ΔNp63 (green). The white dotted line indicates the basal layer. All sections were counterstained with DAPI (blue) to visualize cell nuclei.

negative for ΔNp63 expression by immunohistochemistry (data not shown), while it was strongly positive for MCM7. From the same patient, we also implanted the β-HPV$^+$ SK shown in **Figures 2E–H**, which failed to grow in nude mice probably due to its benign nature. One of the two other AKs was from a patient transplanted in 1995 who had developed three AKs and one SCC after 20 years of transplantation. In this case, we failed to detect any viral protein expression in both xenograft and original tumor as it was the case in all the other skin lesions excised from this KTR (data not shown). The second AK was from the KTR female described above (**Figure 1**). Consistent with the fact that a documented β-HPV reactivation was reported in the female patient as well as in her original skin lesion, in this latter xenograft, we were able to detect in some cells both viral protein E4 expression and the presence of the HPV5 genome by FISH (**Figure 5**). The HPV5 probe was used because this genotype was detected in plucked hair bulbs from the eyebrows (data not shown), which are regarded as representative samples of the virus carriage on a person's skin. Furthermore, one SCC and one BCC were engrafted from the same patient, but they failed to grow in nude mice.

DISCUSSION

In this study, we extend our previous investigation aimed at identifying the presence of active β-HPV infection in skin tumors from KTRs through the detection of viral protein expression, such as E4 and L1 (Borgogna et al., 2014). In this new round of screening, we found positive staining in five tumors that were all removed from two patients who had been both transplanted twice and presented with a long history of immunosuppression (>30 years). The female patient had developed many skin cancers (>15) accompanied by the development of a clinical picture highly resembling that of an EV patient. Consistent with

TABLE 2 | Histological features of the skin tumors grafted into nude mice, timeline of excision and outcome of xenograft establishment.

	No. of tumors (tot: 42)	Xenograft excision after		Xenograft establishment	
		3 months	6 months	Failure	Growth
Squamous cell carcinoma	6	6	0	6	
Basal cell carcinoma	16	9	7	14	2 (BCC)
Keratoacanthoma	1	0	1	1	
Actinic keratoses	14	6	8	11	- 2 (AK) - 1 (SCC+ metastasis)
Seborrheic keratoses	5	3	2	5	

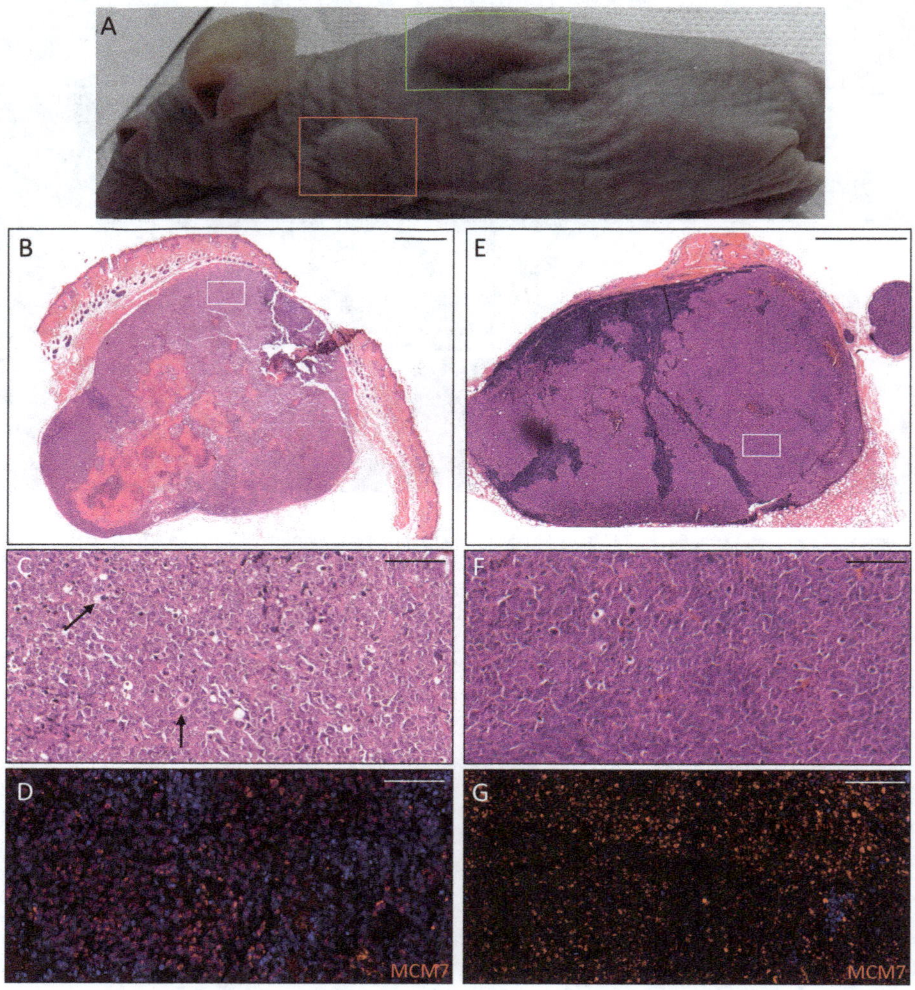

FIGURE 4 | Histopathological analysis of an AK xenograft derived from the male KTR. **(A)** Nude mouse in which the xenograft was diagnosed as SCC (green box) giving rise to a lymph node metastasis (red box). **(B,E)** Histopathological features (H&E staining) of the lesions corresponding to the boxes highlighted in **A** (**B**: SCC; **E**: lymph node metastasis). Scale bars: 1,000 μm. **(C,F)** Magnification of the areas highlighted by the white boxes depicted in **(B,E)**. Scale bar 100 μm. The black arrows indicate cells in mitotic phase. **(D,G)** Immunofluorescence staining for MCM7 (red) of the same tissue section shown in the **(C,F)** respectively. Sections **(D,G)** were counterstained with DAPI (blue) to visualize cell nuclei.

her clinical manifestations revealing diffuse actinic damage on her forehead and dorsum of the hands, β-HPV viral protein expression was observed in three skin tumors, corresponding to two AKs and one KA. Likewise, among the five skin tumors removed from the other male patient, one AK and one SK showed extensive E4 expression.

According to our previous findings, E4 expression was mostly detected at early stages of disease, confirming that virus expansion was taking place in the skin under condition of prolonged immunosuppression, albeit no longer detectable in more advanced stages of disease (Borgogna et al., 2012, 2014; Landini et al., 2014). These infected tissues displayed intraepidermal hyperplasia as demonstrated by histology, enhanced expression of the MCM7 proliferation marker in the suprabasal layers, and ΔNp63 expression. Intriguingly, ΔNp63 protein expression levels were also high in both benign and premalignant lesions as well as in cells that did not express MCM7 and, therefore, were not regarded as actively proliferating.

Overall, given the important role of p63 in the proliferation and maintenance of epidermal stem cells, and a number of *in vitro* and *in vivo* data linking β-HPV infection to ΔNp63 upregulation (Lanfredini et al., 2017; Marthaler et al., 2017), our findings further strengthen the proposed model of β-HPV-induced skin carcinogenesis in an immunosuppressed setting through p63 activation and increased keratinocyte stemness. Consistently, using a novel bitransgenic mouse model where ΔNp63 is overexpressed moderately in the basal layer of stratified epithelia, Devos et al. have recently demonstrated that overexpression of ΔNp63 favors early steps of skin tumorigenesis (Devos et al., 2017). Development of benign lesions, such as papilloma, was indeed accelerated following ΔNp63 overexpression in a dose-dependent manner in a classical two-stage chemical carcinogenesis protocol where an increased number of papilloma was observed.

Emerging evidence clearly indicates that β-HPVs contribute to skin cancer development at early stages and through molecular mechanisms that are different from those reported for high-risk α-types, such as HPV16 and 18 (Howley and Pfister, 2015; Quint et al., 2015). Our group and others have reported that β-HPV can increase stemness properties of keratinocytes in both monolayer cultures of keratinocytes transduced with HPV8 E6 and E7 viral proteins and an HPV8 transgenic mouse model where the skin-specific transcription of the early region of HPV8 is driven by the K14 promoter (Hufbauer et al., 2013; Lanfredini et al., 2017). In all these experimental models, as well as in β-HPV-infected human skin, this increased stemness is always accompanied by ΔNp63 overexpression (Marthaler et al., 2017). Thus, together with previous reports pointing to a possible cooperation between E6 expression and UVB exposure in skin carcinogenesis, our findings provide *in vivo* evidence that β-HPV infection might be a co-factor of early stages of skin cancer progression. This hypothesis is fully compatible with the "hit-and-run" mechanisms of carcinogenesis, with cutaneous β-HPV playing an important role for tumor initiation and progression, but not required for tumor maintenance. Assuming that viral replication is more active at very early stages of carcinogenesis, or when lesions are not yet even clinically evident and rarely removed, it seems reasonable to propose that at later stages of disease, when lesions require surgical excision, β-HPV infection is no longer detectable or otherwise restricted to some residual areas at the edges of the lesion. These assumptions can explain the low percentage of positivity found in our study. However, the observed reactivation of β-HPV infection occurring in the skin of KTRs alongside the demonstration that these viruses can increase keratinocyte stemness and interfere with the DNA damage response argues in favor of a model whereby the cooperation between β-HPV and UVB, which triggers skin carcinogenesis, is no longer required to maintain the malignant state at later stages of neoplastic development (Hufbauer and Akgül, 2017; Lanfredini et al., 2017; Wendel and Wallace, 2017).

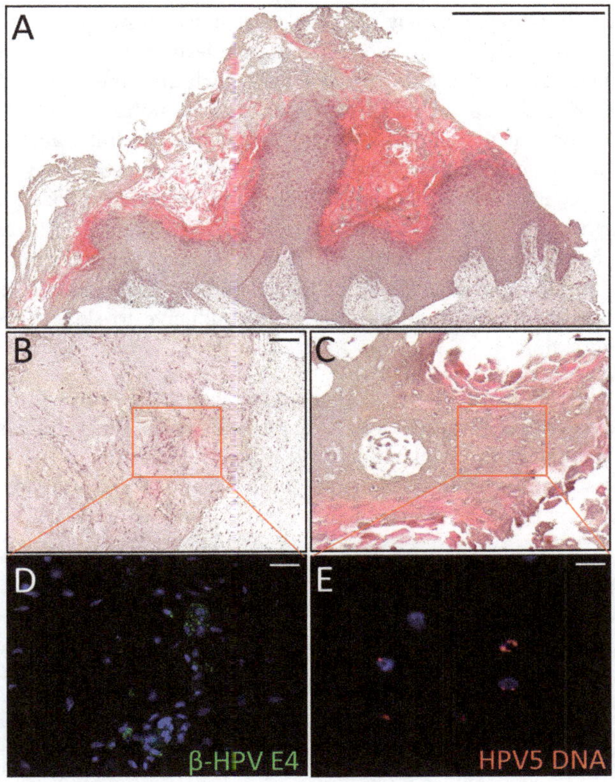

FIGURE 5 | Histopathological analysis of an AK xenograft derived from the female KTR. **(A)** H&E staining of a representative sections of the xenograft. Scale bar 1,000 μm. **(B,C)** H&E staining of two representative areas positive for the viral markers. Scale bars: 100 μm. **(D,E)** Magnification of the areas corresponding to the red squares highlighted in the top pictures and immunostained for β-HPV E4 protein (green, **D**) and HPV5 DNA (red, **E**). Sections **(D,E)** were counterstained with DAPI (blue) to visualize cell nuclei. Scale bars: 10 μm.

Another important aspect of the current study is the optimization and implementation of a unique xenograft model system in nude mice (Patel et al., 2012). Thanks to the creation of a humanized stromal bed in the site of grafting, here we show that it is possible to obtain xenograft growth also from small biopsy samples from relatively benign skin lesions such as AKs. However, the overall success rate of this procedure was very low as only three out of 14 engrafted AKs grew as PDXs. Furthermore, we failed to grow any SCCs while two out of the 16 engrafted BCCs gave rise to a tumor mass with the same histological features of the original tumor. This low rate of success may be due to the low proliferating index of the tumor, especially for the AK, or the size of the engrafted tumor, which in some cases was small and very likely did not include enough cells with high proliferating capacity. Despite these limitations, the results of this study are extremely exciting because we show for the first time that β-HPV$^+$ and ΔNp63$^+$ intraepidermal hyperplasia can indeed progress to an aggressive SCC, including metastasis. As this SCC developed in 12 weeks in a nude mouse, we cannot rule out that the engrafted AK already harbored small amount of SCC. Nevertheless, cancer cells were originated from the infected epithelium that clinically appeared as field cancerization. Furthermore, the observation that both ΔNp63 and β-HPV are no longer detectable in the SCC suggests that their roles might be more important at premalignant stages where they likely cooperate to create an environment conducive to skin cancer progression.

Overall, the xenografts obtained following our protocol may prove useful not only in following the fate of each lesion but also in increasing the availability of biological samples for molecular investigations, which is generally limited due to surgical removal of premalignant lesions. In this regard, every effort should be made by clinicians involved in the daily management of KTRs to identify patients with clinically evident virus reactivation in the skin, and as such at increased risk of developing cancer.

AUTHOR CONTRIBUTIONS

MG, MD and GP conceived the project. CB and CO designed experiments. CB, CO, SL, FC, RB, and ET performed experiments and collected, analysed data. EZ and PS enrolled patients and collected clinical samples. MG drafted the manuscript with inputs from all authors. CB and MG handled funding, supervision, and coordination. All authors have made final approval for the final version to be submitted.

ACKNOWLEDGMENTS

We would like to thank John Doorbar, Cambridge University-UK, for providing us the anti-β-HPV-E4 antibodies and Marcello Arsura for critically reviewing the manuscript.

REFERENCES

Bernard, H. U. (2013). Taxonomy and phylogeny of papillomaviruses: an overview and recent developments. *Infect. Genet. Evol.* 18, 357–361. doi: 10.1016/j.meegid.2013.03.011

Borgogna, C., Lanfredini, S., Peretti, A., De Andrea, M., Zavattaro, E., Colombo, E., et al. (2014). Improved detection reveals active β-papillomavirus infection in skin lesions from kidney transplant recipients. *Mod. Pathol.* 27, 1101–1115. doi: 10.1038/modpathol.2013.240

Borgogna, C., Zavattaro, E., De Andrea, M., Griffin, H. M., Dell'Oste, V., Azzimonti, B., et al. (2012). Characterization of beta papillomavirus E4 expression in tumours from Epidermodysplasia Verruciformis patients and in experimental models. *Virology.* 423, 195–204. doi: 10.1016/j.virol.2011.11.029

Bouwes Bavinck, J. N., Feltkamp, M. C. W., Green, A. C., Fiocco, M., Euvrard, S., Harwood, C. A., et al. (2017). Human papillomavirus and post-transplant cutaneous squamous-cell carcinoma: a multicenter, prospective cohort study. *Am. J. Transplant.* doi: 10.1111/ajt.14537. [Epub ahead of print].

Bouwes Bavinck, J. N., Neale, R. E., Abeni, D., Euvrard, S., Green, A. C., Harwood, C. A., et al. (2010). Multicenter study of the association between betapapillomavirus infection and cutaneous squamous cell carcinoma. *Cancer. Res.* 70, 9777–9786. doi: 10.1158/0008-5472.CAN-10-0352

de Koning, M., Quint, W., and Struijk, L. (2006). Evaluation of a novel highly sensitive, broad-spectrum PCR-reverse hybridization assay for detection and identification of beta-papillomavirus DNA. *J. Clin. Microbiol.* 44, 1792–1800. doi: 10.1128/JCM.44.5.1792-1800.2006

Dell'Oste, V., Azzimonti, B., De Andrea, M., Mondini, M., Zavattaro, E., Leigheb, G., et al. (2009). High β-HPV DNA loads and strong seroreactivity are present in Epidermodysplasia Verruciformis. *J. Invest. Dermatol.* 129, 1026–1034. doi: 10.1038/jid.2008.317

Devos, M., Gilbert, B., Denecker, G., Leurs, K., Mc Guire, C., Lemeire, K., et al. (2017). Elevated ΔNp63α levels facilitate epidermal and biliary oncogenic transformation. *J. Invest. Dermatol.* 137, 494–505. doi: 10.1016/j.jid.2016.09.026

Geissler, E. K. (2015). Post-transplantation malignancies: here today, gone tomorrow? *Nat. Rev. Clin. Oncol.* 12, 705–717. doi: 10.1038/nrclinonc.2015.186

Genders, R. E., Mazlom, H., Michel, A., Plasmeijer, E. I., Quint, K. D., Pawlita, M., et al. (2015). The presence of betapapillomavirus antibodies around transplantation predicts the development of Keratinocyte Carcinoma in Organ transplant recipients: a cohort study. *J. Invest. Dermatol.* 135, 1275–1282. doi: 10.1038/jid.2014.456

Heuser, S., Hufbauer, M., Steiger, J., Marshall, J., Sterner-Kock, A., Mauch, C., et al. (2016). The fibronectin/α3β1 integrin axis serves as molecular basis for keratinocyte invasion induced by βHPV. *Oncogene* 35, 4529–4539. doi: 10.1038/onc.2015.512

Howley, P. M., and Pfister, H. J. (2015). Beta genus papillomaviruses and skin cancer. *Virology* 479-480, 290–296. doi: 10.1016/j.virol.2015.02.004

Hufbauer, M., and Akgül, B. (2017). Molecular mechanisms of human Papillomavirus induced skin carcinogenesis. *Viruses* 9:187. doi: 10.3390/v9070187

Hufbauer, M., Biddle, A., Borgogna, C., Gariglio, M., Doorbar, J., Storey, A., et al. (2013). Expression of betapapillomavirus oncogenes increases the number of keratinocytes with stem cell-like properties. *J. Virol.* 87, 12158–12165. doi: 10.1128/JVI.01510-13

Koster, M. (2010). p63 in skin development and ectodermal dysplasias. *J. Invest. Dermatol.* 130, e2352–e2358. doi: 10.1038/jid.2010.119

Kovach, B. T., and Stasko, T. (2009). Skin cancer after transplantation. *Transplant. Rev.* 23, 178–189. doi: 10.1016/j.trre.2009.02.004

Kranjec, C., and Doorbar, J. (2016). Human papillomavirus infection and induction of neoplasia: a matter of fitness. *Curr. Opin. Virol.* 20, 129–136. doi: 10.1016/j.coviro.2016.08.011

Krynitz, B., Edgren, G., Lindelöf, B., Baecklund, E., Brattström, C., Wilczek, H., et al. (2013). Risk of skin cancer and other malignancies in kidney, liver, heart and lung transplant recipients 1970 to 2008–a Swedish population-based study. *Int. J. Cancer.* 132, 1429–1438. doi: 10.1002/ijc.27765

Landini, M. M., Borgogna, C., Peretti, A., Colombo, E., Zavattaro, E., Boldorini, R., et al. (2014). α- and β-Papillomavirus infection in a young patient with an unclassified primary T-cell immunodeficiency and multiple mucosal and cutaneous lesions. *J. Am. Acad. Dermatol.* 71, 108–115.e1. doi: 10.1016/j.jaad.2014.01.859

Lanfredini, S., Olivero, C., Borgogna, C., Calati, F., Powell, K., Davies, K. J., et al. (2017). HPV8 field cancerization in a transgenic mouse model is due to Lrig1+ Keratinocyte stem cell expansion. *J. Invest. Dermatol.* 137, 2208–2216. doi: 10.1016/j.jid.2017.04.039

Madeleine, M. M., Johnson, L. G., Daling, J. R., Schwartz, S. M., Carter, J. J., Berg, D., et al. (2012). Cohort profile: the skin cancer after organ transplant study. *Int. J. Epidemiol.* 42, 1669–1677. doi: 10.1093/ije/dys179

Marcuzzi, G. P., Hufbauer, M., Kasper, H. U., Weissenborn, S. J., Smola, S., and Pfister, H. (2009). Spontaneous tumour development in human papillomavirus type 8 E6 transgenic mice and rapid induction by UV-light exposure and wounding. *J. Gen. Virol.* 90(Pt 12), 2855–2864. doi: 10.1099/vir.0.012872-0

Marthaler, A. M., Podgorska, M., Feld, P., Fingerle, A., Knerr-Rupp, K., Grässer, F., et al. (2017). Identification of C/EBPα as a novel target of the HPV8 E6 protein regulating miR-203 in human keratinocytes. *PLoS. Pathog.* 13:e1006406. doi: 10.1371/journal.ppat.1006406

Melino, G., Memmi, E. M., Pelicci, P. G., and Bernassola, F. (2015). Maintaining epithelial stemness with p63. *Sci. Signal.* 8:re9. doi: 10.1126/scisignal.aaa1033

Meyers, J. M., Spangle, J. M., and Munger, K. (2013). The human Papillomavirus Type 8 E6 during Keratinocyte Differentiation Protein Interferes with NOTCH Activation. *J. Virol.* 87:4762. doi: 10.1128/JVI.02527-12

Patel, G. K., Yee, C. L., Yuspa, S. H., and Vogel, J. C. (2012). A humanized stromal bed is required for engraftment of isolated human primary squamous cell carcinoma cells in immunocompromised mice. *J. Invest. Dermatol.* 132, 284–290. doi: 10.1038/jid.2011.284

Pfefferle, R., Marcuzzi, G. P., Akgül, B., Kasper, H. U., Schulze, F., Haase, I., et al. (2008). The human papillomavirus type 8 E2 protein induces skin tumors in transgenic mice. *J. Invest. Dermatol.* 128, 2310–2315. doi: 10.1038/jid.2008.73

Quint, K. D., Genders, R. E., de Koning, M. N., Borgogna, C., Gariglio, M., Bouwes Bavinck, J. N., et al. (2015). Human Beta-papillomavirus infection and keratinocyte carcinomas. *J. Pathol.* 235, 342–354. doi: 10.1002/path.4425.

Romano, R. A., Ortt, K., Birkaya, B., Smalley, K., and Sinha, S. (2009). An active role of the DeltaN isoform of p63 in regulating basal keratin genes K5 and K14 and directing epidermal cell fate. *PLoS ONE* 4:e5623. doi: 10.1371/journal.pone.0005623

Schaper, I. D., Marcuzzi, G. P., Weissenborn, S. J., Kasper, H. U., Dries, V., Smyth, N., et al. (2005). Development of skin tumors in mice transgenic for early genes of human papillomavirus type 8. *Cancer Res.* 65, 1394–1400. doi: 10.1158/0008-5472

Senoo, M., Pinto, F., Crum, C. P., and McKeon, F. (2007). p63 is essential for the proliferative potential of stem cells in stratified epithelia. *Cell.* 129, 523–536. doi: 10.1016/j.cell.2007.02.045

Tommasino, M. (2017). The biology of beta human papillomaviruses. *Virus. Res.* 231, 128–138. doi: 10.1016/j.virusres.2016.11.013

Vajdic, C. M., and van Leeuwen, M. T. (2009). Cancer incidence and risk factors after solid organ transplantation. *Int. J. Cancer* 125, 1747–1754. doi: 10.1002/ijc.24439

Wallace, N. A., and Galloway, D. A. (2014). Manipulation of cellular DNA damage repair machinery facilitates propagation of human papillomaviruses. *Semin. Cancer Biol.* 26, 30–42. doi: 10.1016/j.semcancer.2013.12.003

Wallace, N. A., Robinson, K., Howie, H. L., and Galloway, D. A. (2012). HPV 5 and 8 E6 abrogate ATR activity resulting in increased persistence of UVB induced DNA damage. *PLoS. Pathog.* 8:e1002807. doi: 10.1371/journal.ppat.1002807

Weissenborn, S. J., Nindl, I., Purdie, K., Harwood, C., Proby, C., Breuer, J., et al. (2005). Human papillomavirus-DNA loads in actinic keratoses exceed those in non-melanoma skin cancers. *J. Invest. Dermatol.* 125, 93–97. doi: 10.1111/j.0022-202X.2005.23733.x

Wendel, S. O., and Wallace, N. A. (2017). Loss of genome fidelity: beta HPVs and the DNA damage response. *Front. Microbiol.* 15:2250. doi: 10.3389/fmicb.2017.02250

6

Novel Insights Into Cellular Changes in HPV8-E7 Positive Keratinocytes: A Transcriptomic and Proteomic Analysis

*Matthias Kirschberg[1], Adnan Shahzad Syed[1], Hanife Güler Dönmez[1,2], Sandra Heuser[1], Astrid Wilbrand-Hennes[3], Angel Alonso[4], Martin Hufbauer[1] and Baki Akgül[1]**

[1] Medical Faculty and University Hospital Cologne, Institute of Virology, University of Cologne, Cologne, Germany, [2] Department of Biology, Hacettepe University, Ankara, Turkey, [3] Cologne Excellence Cluster on Cellular Stress Responses in Aging-Associated Diseases (CECAD) and Center for Molecular Medicine (CMMC), University of Cologne, Cologne, Germany, [4] German Cancer Research Center (DKFZ), Heidelberg, Germany

Correspondence:
Baki Akgül
baki.akguel@uk-koeln.de
orcid.org/0000-0002-6564-9412

Human papillomavirus type 8 (HPV8) is associated with the development of non-melanoma skin cancer. In the past we already delved into the mechanisms involved in keratinocyte invasion, showing that the viral E7 oncoprotein is a key player that drives invasion of basal keratinocytes controlled by the extracellular protein fibronectin. To unravel further downstream effects in E7 expressing keratinocytes we now aimed at characterizing gene and protein/phosphoprotein alterations to narrow down on key cellular targets of HPV8-E7. We now show that gene expression of GADD34 and GDF15 are strongly activated in the presence of E7 in primary human keratinocytes. Further analyses of fibronectin-associated factors led to the identification of the Src kinase family members Fyn and Lyn being aberrantly activated in the presence of HPV8-E7. Phospho-proteomics further revealed that E7 not only targets cell polarity and cytoskeletal organization, but also deregulates the phosphorylation status of nuclear proteins involved in DNA damage repair and replication. Many of these differentially phosphorylated proteins turned out to be targets of Fyn and Lyn. Taken together, by using unbiased experimental approaches we have now arrived at a deeper understanding on how fibronectin may affect the signaling cascades in HPV8 positive keratinocytes, which may be key for skin tumorigenesis and that may also aid in the development of novel therapeutic approaches for betaHPV-mediated cancers.

Keywords: betapapillomavirus, skin cancer, E7 oncoprotein, keratinocyte invasion, fibronectin

INTRODUCTION

Cutaneous squamous cell carcinoma (SCC) is the most common metastatic skin cancer, and its incidence is increasing worldwide. DNA damage, as a consequence of excessive UV light exposure, is known to be the main causative factor for the development of cutaneous SCC which arises from a precancerous lesion termed actinic keratosis (Fania et al., 2021). Recent epidemiological

Abbreviations: ECM, extracellular matrix; PHAK, primary human adult keratinocyte; PHFK, primary human foreskin keratinocyte; DED, de-epidermalized human dermis.

data strongly implicate that human papillomavirus (HPV) of genus betapapillomavirus (betaHPV) has a co-factorial role in this process (Hasche et al., 2017, 2018; Hufbauer and Akgül, 2017). The oncogenic potential of betaHPV in skin carcinogenesis was originally identified in patients suffering from the rare inherited disease Epidermodysplasia verruciformis (EV), who have an increased susceptibility to betaHPV infections (Howley and Pfister, 2015). However, betaHPV can also be found in skin cancers of non-EV patients. Particularly, immunosuppressed patients, such as organ-transplant-recipients, also have a higher susceptibility to betaHPV infections of the skin as well as an increased risk of developing SCC compared with healthy individuals (Bouwes Bavinck et al., 2018; Rollison et al., 2019; Smola, 2020).

Despite the more detailed analyses of the viral E6 oncoprotein in keratinocyte transformation, the precise molecular mechanisms by which the E7 oncoprotein may interact with the host cells are still being investigated. We have previously described already that the E7 protein of the oncogenic betaHPV type 8 (HPV8) plays a pivotal role in inducing keratinocyte hyperproliferation and invasion when expressed in primary human adult keratinocytes (PHAK) differentiating in de-epidermalized human dermis (DED)-based organotypic skin cultures (Akgül et al., 2005; Heuser et al., 2016). These keratinocytes display hyperproliferation in the regenerated epithelium and are positive for both cyclin E and p16INK4a, indicating that E7 is able to overcome p16INK4a induced cell cycle arrest (Westphal et al., 2009). In addition, HPV8-E7 positive keratinocytes lose their physiological polarity and invade the underlying dermis (Akgül et al., 2005). Here, downward migration of keratinocytes is facilitated by the degradation of basement membrane components such as collagen VII, collagen IV and laminin V, a process that is paralleled by increased expression of the matrix metalloproteinases (MMP)-1, MMP-8, and membrane-type (MT)1-MMP (Akgül et al., 2005; Smola-Hess et al., 2005). In light of the fact that E7 positive keratinocytes do not exhibit invasive behavior on a collagen type I matrix (Boxman et al., 2001), but do so when cultivated as DED-based organotypic skin cultures, we hypothesized that components of the extracellular matrix (ECM) may be critical in eliciting the invasive behavior of HPV8-E7 positive cells. To address the mechanism by which E7 mediates invasion we tested for a possible cadherin-switch which is commonly seen in invasion-related epithelial-mesenchymal transition. To this end, we examined the E-cadherin and N-cadherin mRNA expression in cells cultured on collagen type IV, laminin V, or fibronectin. Only when HPV8-E7 positive keratinocytes were grown on fibronectin, a reduction in E-cadherin and an increase in N-cadherin levels were detected. These data identified fibronectin as an inducer of the observed cadherin-switch in the presence of HPV8-E7. In subsequent experiments we could detect increased fibronectin levels in peritumoral areas in betaHPV positive SCC as opposed to betaHPV negative tissues. In addition, we showed that E7 positive keratinocytes have elevated levels of integrin α3β1 on their cell surface. Silencing of the α3 chain and the usage of the invasion deficient E7 mutant L23A led to a drastic reduction in the invasive potential of HPV8-E7 cells, thus providing evidence for a direct role of the fibronectin/α3β1 integrin axis in invasion of HPV8-E7 expressing keratinocytes (Heuser et al., 2016). The overall goal of the present follow-up project therefore was to identify further gene expression and protein/phospho-protein alterations using unbiased global transcriptomic and proteomic approaches in order to further pinpoint key downstream cellular targets of HPV8-E7 which may extend our knowledge on the mechanisms underlying betaHPV associated skin carcinogenesis.

MATERIALS AND METHODS

Cell Culture

N/TERT keratinocytes (Dickson et al., 2000) and the spontaneously immortalized human skin keratinocyte cell line PM1 (Proby et al., 2000) were cultivated either in KGM-Gold (0.05 mM Calcium, Lonza, Cologne, Germany) or in RM+ medium (consisting of a 3:1 ratio of Dulbecco's modified Eagle's medium (DMEM) and DMEM-F12, supplemented with 10% fetal calf serum (FCS), 1% glutamine, 0.4 μg hydrocortisone, 10^{-10} M cholera toxin, 5 μg/mL transferrin, 2 × 10^{-11} M liothyronine, 5 μg/mL insulin, 10 ng/mL epidermal growth factor, 1 × penicillin–streptomycin mixture) (Hufbauer et al., 2013). The PT67 cell line was maintained in DMEM with 10% FCS and penicillin-streptomycin mixture. All cell lines were cultivated at 37°C and 6% CO_2.

Retroviral Expression Vectors and Infection of Keratinocytes

The generation of the pLXSN-based retroviral vectors coding for HPV8 E1, E2, E6, E7, or E6E7 has been previously described (Akgül et al., 2005, 2007; Leverrier et al., 2007). Production of retroviruses and retroviral transduction of N/TERT and PM1 keratinocytes were performed as previously described (Hufbauer et al., 2013). Briefly, keratinocytes were seeded out in 6 cm dishes. Next day, retroviral supernatants were mixed with an equal volume of DMEM in the presence of 5 μg/mL of hexadimethrine bromide (polybrene) and added to the keratinocytes. Spin infection was made by centrifugation for 1 h at 300 × g. Cells were then washed with PBS and cultured further for 2 days. Then, cells were selected against G418 (500 μg/mL) until only infected keratinocytes had survived. In subsequent experiments we used pooled stable cell populations to minimize possible variations due to the randomness of the viral integration site in the cellular chromosomes.

RTqPCR and PrimePCR

To quantify mRNA levels of cellular genes, quantitative reverse transcription-PCR (RTqPCR) using the LightCycler system (Roche, Mannheim, Germany) was performed as previously described (Hufbauer et al., 2015). The primers used for this study were:

ATF3-fw: TTTGCCATCCAGAACAAGC;
ATF3-rev: CATCTTCTTCAGGGGCTACCT;
GADD34-fw: GCTTCTGGCAGACCGAAC;

GADD34-rev: GTAGCCTGATGGGGTGCTT;
GDF15-fw: CCCGGGACCCTCAGAGTT;
GDF15-rev: CCGCAGCCTGGTTAGCA;
HPRT1-fw: TGACACTGGCAAAACAATGCA;
HPRT1-rev: GGTCCTTTTCACCAGCAAGCT.

The RTqPCR based PrimePCR (Fibronectin-Binding Integrin in Cell Motility H96, BIORAD, Feldkirchen, Germany) was performed in quadruplicate using 96-well plates with pre-spotted primers in each well of the plate. The plates were designed to be analyzed using a Roche LC 480 light cycler, using the SsoAdvanced™ Universal SYBR® Green Supermix. Analyses of these plates were carried out following manufacturer's instructions.

DNA Microarrays

The cDNA microarray analyses performed in the Akgül group used total RNA extracted from monolayer cultures of PHAKs in total passage 3 (passage 2 after transduction). The RNA was analyzed in biological triplicates from cells containing either the empty vector control pLXSN or pLXSN-HPV8-E7. Changes in gene expression were measured using the Human Genome U133A arrays according to Affymetrix protocols. Microarray data were analyzed using Transcriptome Analysis Console software (Thermo Fisher Scientific, v4.0.1.36). For analysis of differential gene expression, we applied the following conditions to determine statistically relevant genes: (a) ANOVA test: ebayes, (b) a fold change cut-off of < -2 or > 2, and (c) determination of statistical significance with $p < 0.05$. Gene ontology analysis was carried out using the PANTHER (Protein ANalysis THrough Evolutionary Relationships) database (v14.1). These microarray data files have been uploaded to the Gene Expression Omnibus (GEO) database (GSE133813) (Kirschberg et al., 2019).

The cDNA microarray analyses performed in the Alonso group at the DKFZ were performed with RNA isolated from primary keratinocytes also transduced with pLXSN or pLXSN-HPV8-E7 coding retroviruses. The Affymetrix chip-based experiments and data analyses were performed at the core facility of the German Cancer Center (DKFZ) (**Supplementary Table 1**). Differentially expressed genes (DEG) from both independent studies were overlapped to minimize bias of the data in respect to genetic variations among keratinocyte donors, cell culture media effects, thus making the results more robust.

ELISA

The Human GDF15 Quantikine ELISA Kit (RnD systems) was used to measure GDF15 in cell culture supernatants. For this N/TERT-8E7 were cultured on fibronectin and cell culture supernatants were harvested after 4 days. Collected supernatants were treated with protease/phosphatase inhibitors (Protease/Phosphatase Inhibitor Cocktail, Cell Signaling). The ELISA was performed according to the manufacturer's protocol.

Western Blotting and Phospho-Kinase Array Analysis

Western blotting was performed as previously described (Marx et al., 2018). Briefly, cell pellets were resuspended in radioimmunoprecipitation assay (RIPA) buffer containing protease inhibitors, incubated on ice for 30 min, sonicated and then centrifuged at 15,000 × g at 4°C for 15 min. Protein concentrations were measured with the Pierce™ BCA Protein Assay Kit (Thermo Fisher Scientific, Dreieich, Germany). SDS gels were transferred upon completion to nitrocellulose membranes, which were then blocked with either 5% bovine serum albumin or 5% dry milk in TBST [10 mM Tris/HCl (pH 8.0), 150 mM NaCl, 0.05% Tween 20]. The primary antibodies used targeted 14-3-3β (sc-59419, clone 60C10, Santa Cruz), ERK1/2 (#4695, clone 137F5, Cell Signaling), Fyn (#4023, Cell Signaling), p-Tyr^{530}-Fyn (#PA5-36644, Invitrogen), Lyn (#4576, clone 5G2, Cell Signaling), p-Tyr^{397}-Lyn (#orb6340, Biobyrt, Cambridge, United Kingdom), GAPDH-Alexa680 (sc-365062, cloneG9, Santa Cruz). HuT78 whole cell lysates (sc-2208, Santa Cruz) were used as positive controls. Antibodies were incubated for 2 h at RT or overnight at 4°C. Following washing, membranes were incubated with corresponding secondary antibodies (IRDye, LI-COR, Lincoln, Nebraska, United States). Western blots were visualized by employing the LI-COR ODYSSEY FC Imaging system with the Image Studio Ver 5.2. software.

The Human Phospho-Kinase Array Kit (RnD Systems, Minneapolis, United States), spotted with antibodies targeting phospho-sites in kinases associated with malignant processes, was used to identify potentially deregulated kinases in HPV8-E7 expressing keratinocytes grown for 96 h on fibronectin coated tissue culture plates. Cells were rinsed with PBS and then lysed using the provided buffer supplemented with 10 μg/mL Aprotinin, 10 μg/mL Leupeptin, and 10 μg/mL Pepstatin. The lysates were gently incubated at 4°C for 30 min and then centrifuged at 14,000×g for 5 min, before transferring the supernatants into a clean test tube. Samples were then further processed according to the manufacturer's protocol. Visualization of the membranes and evaluation of individual spot densities were carried out employing the LI-COR ODYSSEY FC Imaging system with the Image Studio Ver 5.2. software.

Proteomics

Proteomic and phospho-proteomic analyses were performed with total cell extracts from HPV8-E7 expressing N/TERT keratinocytes (N/TERT-8E7) grown for 96 h on fibronectin coated tissue culture plates which were lysed using 8M urea supplemented with protease and phosphatase inhibitors. The whole cell lysates were prepared in triplicates in two separate experiments ($n = 6$) were analyzed at the proteomics core facility of the Cologne Excellence Cluster on Cellular Stress Responses in Aging-Associated Diseases (CECAD) by means of "stable isotope labeling with amino acids in cell culture" (SILAC)-based mass-spectrometry. The protein profile was submitted to the Proteomics Identifications Database (PRIDE) and is available via ProteomeXchange with the identifier PXD026099. Briefly, samples were reduced with DTT (100 mM) and alkylated with 550 mM Iodoacetic acid (IAA) prior to digestion with trypsin and Lys-C overnight at 37°C. Generated peptides were extracted by incubation with increasing amount of acetonitrile, concentrated in a speed-vac and primed prior to LC-MS/MS analysis by the STAGE tip technique (Rappsilber et al., 2003). For liquid chromatography and tandem mass spectrometry (LC-MS/MS), an easy nLC 1,000 (Thermo Fisher Scientific) was coupled to the quadrupole-based Q Exactive Plus (Thermo Fisher Scientific) instrument by a nano-spray ionization source. Peptides were separated on a 50 cm in-house-packed column by a two-solvent buffer system: buffer A (0.1% formic acid) and B (0.1% formic acid in acetonitrile). The content of buffer B was increased from 7 to 23% within 40 min and followed by an increase to 45% in 5 min and a washing and re-equilibration step before continuing with the injection of the next sample. Proteins were considered differentially expressed or phosphorylated under the following criteria: (a) $\log_2$fold change < -2.5 or > 2.5, (b) p-value of $p < 0.05$, and (c) same phosphorylation status in all data sets. Data analysis was performed using the Perseus software suite, KinasePhos2.0 and ShinyGO (v0.61). The differentially phosphorylated protein targets of E7 were imported into the STRING database (Szklarczyk et al., 2019) to identify relevant protein-protein interactions and functional enrichment networks. STRING holds physical as well as functional interaction information derived from high-throughput experimental data, published literature, and computationally predicted co-expression studies.

For secretomic analyses the supernatants of N/TERT-8E7^{wt}, N/TERT-8E7^{L23A} as well as empty vector control grown for 96 h on fibronectin coated tissue culture plates ($n = 6$) were harvested and treated with protease/phosphatase inhibitors (Protease/Phosphatase Inhibitor Cocktail, Cell Signaling). Afterward, the supernatants were concentrated using Amicon ultra-15 centrifugation 3K tubes (Merck Millipore, Darmstadt, Germany). Concentrated supernatants as well as a media-only control were then further processed at the CECAD proteomics facility and subjected to mass-spectrometric analysis. The profile of secreted proteins was submitted to the PRIDE Database and is available via ProteomeXchange with the identifier PXD026100.

Statistical Analysis

Microarray data analyses were analyzed using ANOVA test, setting a $\log_2$fold change < -2.5 or > 2.5 with a p-value of $p < 0.01$. Gene ontology analysis was carried out using PANTHER (v14.1) and ShinyGO (v0.61). RTqPCRs were repeated at least three times in duplicate, and the results are presented as mean ± standard deviation (SD). Statistical significance was determined with an unpaired 2-tailed Student's t-test calculated with GraphPad Prism (Version 9.0). Asterisks shown in the figures indicate significant differences of experimental groups in comparison with the corresponding control conditions ($^*p < 0.05$; $^{**}p < 0.01$; $^{***}p < 0.001$). Images from immunoblots are from a representative experiment and were qualitatively similar in $n = 3$ experiments. The ANOVA two sample t-test was performed to identify statistically significant ($p < 0.05$) peptides in proteomics and the phospho-proteomic data sets.

RESULTS

Identification of HPV8-E7 Gene Targets

We previously published a cDNA oligonucleotide microarray (Affymetrix) data set based on HPV8-E7 expressing PHAK which had been grown in KGM-Gold (Kirschberg et al., 2019). In parallel to our own works similar experiments had been carried out by the Alonso group at the DKFZ in Heidelberg using primary human foreskin keratinocytes (PHFK) (**Supplementary Table 1**). Both experiments were carried out with cells grown on uncoated cell culture dishes. In an effort to identify similarities in gene expression profiles in these HPV8-E7 positive keratinocytes we created an overlap of both sets. After filtering and normalization ($\log_2$fold-change < -2.5 or > 2.5 and $p < 0.01$) we identified a total of 81 and 73 genes, respectively, in the Cologne and Heidelberg data sets. Interestingly, using these highly stringent cut-off values we still found an overlap of 4 genes (**Figure 1A**). Three of these genes, namely ATF3 (activating transcription factor 3), GADD34 (growth arrest and DNA damage-inducible protein), and GDF15 (growth differentiation factor–15) were found to be upregulated in both data sets and may therefore be the most relevant target genes of HPV8-E7. In contrast, the THBS1 (Thrombospondin 1) gene showed an opposite regulation which is why this gene was occluded from further analysis (**Figure 1B**).

In order to further validate our results in cutaneous keratinocytes, the PM1 cell line (Proby et al., 2000) was used which is one of very few keratinocyte lines that can be cultivated in different cell culture growth media. This enabled us to grow keratinocytes under both undifferentiating (KGM-Gold, low-calcium) as well as differentiating (RM+, high-calcium) conditions using the same cell line. Furthermore, in order to underpin the importance of the interaction of E7 with cellular genes the PM1 cells were not only retrovirally transduced with vectors harboring the E7 gene, but also in parallel with constructs expressing E1, E2, or E6.

In the PM1 cell line our experiments showed that E1 and E2 do not have an influence on GDF15 expression. We could, however, confirm a significant effect of HPV8-E7 on GDF15 under non-differentiating conditions, unveiling a fivefold upregulation in gene expression. Most intriguingly, we observed a cumulative effect of E6 and E7 on GDF15 with an up to 15-fold increase in gene expression. Curiously E6 expression alone had appeared to have a slight suppressive effect on GDF15 expression (**Figure 1C**). Somewhat unexpectedly, these effects on gene expression were greatly diminished, yet still significant under differentiating growth conditions (**Figure 1D**). Since GDF15 is a member of the transforming growth factor beta superfamily (TGFβ) and therefore a secretory protein we next tested via ELISA whether the elevated GDF15 gene expression may also result in higher protein contents in cell culture supernatants. As shown in **Figure 1E**, an increase in GDF15 protein levels could also be confirmed in cell culture supernatants of cells grown under non-differentiating conditions. Despite the fact that an upregulation of ATF3 had been predicted in the microarray analyses we could not confirm this by means of RTqPCR.

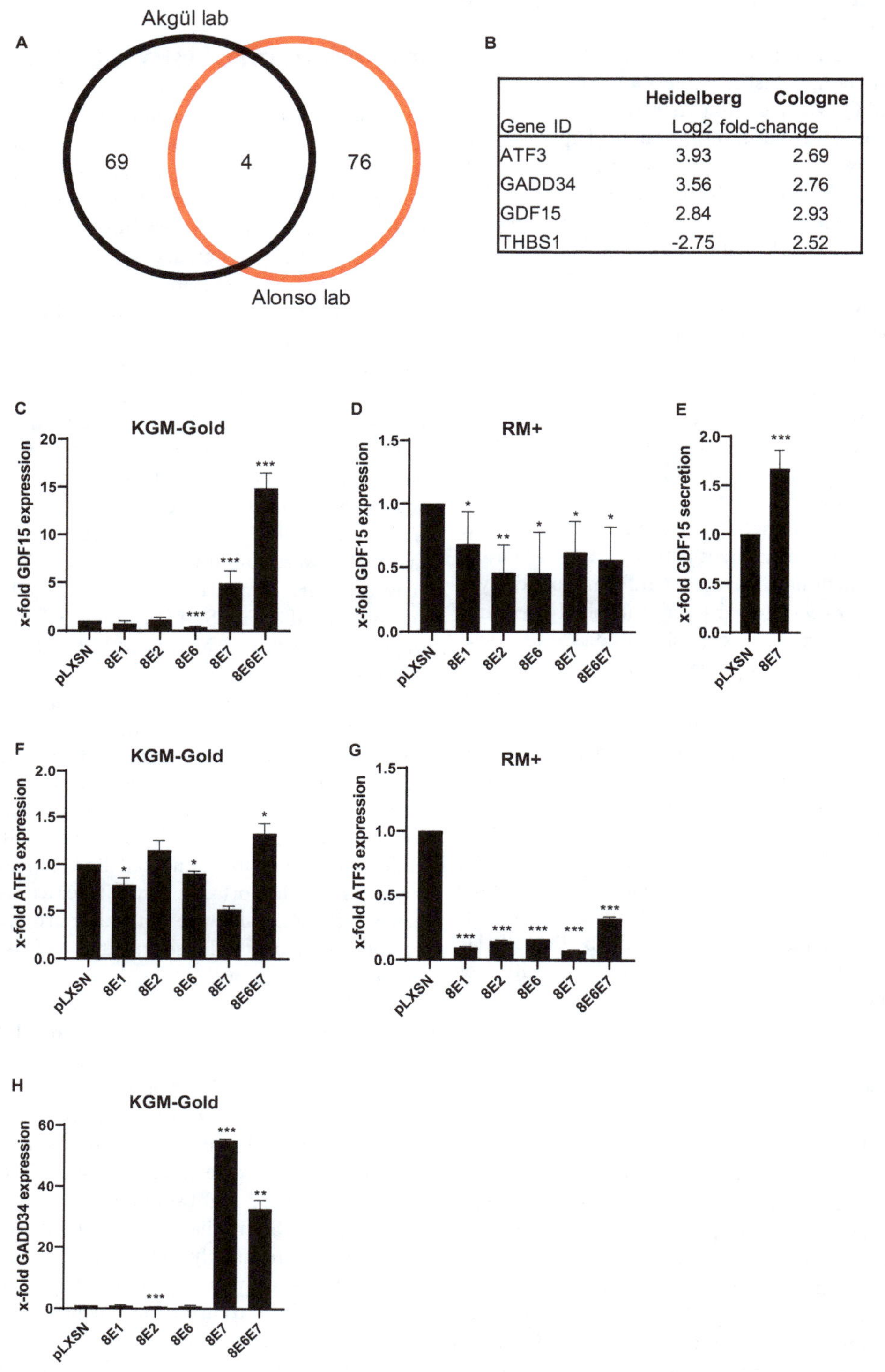

FIGURE 1 | Transcriptional changes in HPV8-E7 positive keratinocytes. **(A)** Venn Diagram comparison of two independent cDNA microarray analyses carried out with PHAK expressing HPV8-E7 in the Akgül lab in Cologne and with PHFK expressing HPV8-E7 in the Alonso lab at the DKFZ in Heidelberg. **(B)** Gene IDs of 4 genes differentially expressed in both array studies. **(C,D)** GDF15 mRNA expression in isogenic PM1 keratinocytes cultured either in KGM-Gold or RM+, respectively. **(E)** GDF15 ELISA performed with cell culture supernatants of HPV8-E7 expressing keratinocytes grown in KGM-Gold medium. **(F,G)** ATF3 mRNA expression in isogenic PM1 keratinocytes cultured either in KGM-Gold or RM+, respectively. **(H)** GADD34 mRNA expression in PM1 keratinocytes cultured in KGM-Gold. RTqPCRs were normalized to HPRT1 mRNA levels (n = 3 independent experiments performed in duplicate). Error bars represent standard deviations. Asterisks shown in the figures indicate significant differences of experimental groups in comparison with the corresponding control conditions (*$p < 0.05$; **$p < 0.01$; ***$p < 0.001$).

All viral proteins seem to only exert neglible control over ATF3 under undifferentiating conditions (**Figure 1F**). Under differentiating conditions, however, all virus genes have a strong and highly statistically significant suppressive effect on ATF3 gene expression (**Figure 1G**). The most profound effect of E7 on gene expression was measured for GADD34 and to a lesser degree for E6E7 positive cells under undifferentiating conditions. The presence of E1, E2, and E6 did not have any effect (**Figure 1H**). GADD34 gene expression could not be detected at all in isogenic keratinocytes grown in RM+ medium, implying that GADD34 may only play a vital role in undifferentiated basal keratinocytes (data not shown).

HPV8-E7 Mediated Alterations in Fibronectin Associated Signaling Pathways

Since we already knew that the ECM protein fibronectin is key in the regulation of cell fate and also has an important effect on invasive behavior of HPV8-E7 positive keratinocytes (Heuser et al., 2016), we first investigated how HPV8-E7 may alter the secretome of keratinocytes relevant for a crosstalk between epidermal keratinocytes and the ECM. Here, we cultivated both the N/TERT-8E7wt, N/TERT-8E7^{L23A} (which codes for the invasion deficient mutant) as well as the empty vector control on a fibronectin matrix and collected the cell culture supernatants after 96 h. In the mass-spectrometric analysis we unveiled 11 proteins that were exclusively differentially secreted in N/TERT-8E7 cells compared to control and N/TERT-8E7^{L23A} (**Figures 2A,B** and **Supplementary Table 2**). A further GO enrichment analysis pointed toward most of the identified proteins (except for GALNT2 and UGP2) to be involved in processes associated with cell growth and proliferation (**Figure 2C**). Interestingly, 14-3-3 family members, which are known to be scaffolds that facilitate a multitude of protein-protein interactions, were present in these pathways and may therefore represent an important regulatory axis. In order to check if the reduced quantity of 14-3-3 in the secretome was the result of decreased protein expression we next performed Western blots with cell extracts of the same cells. Here, we could again show that the presence of HPV8-E7 had a suppressive effect on 14-3-3 β expression (**Figure 2D**).

To narrow down on gene expression changes of known fibronectin-associated genes in HPV8-E7 positive keratinocytes we next performed PrimePCRs using the Fibronectin-Binding Integrin in Cell Motility H96 assay. These RTqPCRs were performed in quadruplicate, with RNA derived from both control as well as HPV8-E7 positive N/TERT grown on fibronectin coated cell culture dishes for 96 h. The PrimePCR revealed four genes that were more than 15-fold up- or down regulated, namely PIK3R2 (phosphoinositide-3-kinase regulatory subunit 2), Fyn as well as RhoA (ras homolog family member A) and Cfl1 (cofilin 1), respectively (**Figure 3A**). Since Src kinase family members, like Fyn, are known to be key modulators of cancer cell invasion and metastasis including the skin (Serrels et al., 2009), we next performed Western blots and could confirm higher protein levels and observed four major splice variants. Interestingly, Fyn phosphorylation at pTyr530, which is a negative regulatory tyrosine residue for this kinase (Qayyum et al., 2012) was weaker in E7 cells compared to the empty vector control (**Figure 3B**).

This observation sparked the idea to have a deeper look at differentially phosphorylated kinases in HPV8-E7 positive keratinocytes. We therefore used a phosphokinase array kit (Proteome Profiler^{TM} Array) with total cell extracts from N/TERT-8E7 grown on fibronectin-coated tissue culture plates for 96 h. Based on the obtained experimental data we discovered that now particularly the Src kinase family member Lyn seemed to be strongly hyperphosphorylated in HPV8-E7 positive cells (**Figure 3C**). Subsequent Western blot analyses proved that Lyn was indeed hyperphosphorylated at residue Tyr397 in HPV8-E7 positive keratinocytes whilst total protein levels remained unchanged (**Figure 3D**). Taken together, our findings show that Src-kinases are deregulated in HPV8-E7 positive keratinocytes grown on fibronectin.

Identification of Differentially Phosphorylated Proteins in HPV8-E7 Positive Cells

Considering that protein kinases appear to play an important role in downstream signaling from fibronectin in HPV8-E7 positive cells we next expanded our studies to investigate the phospho-proteome of these cells. We first performed total proteome and phospho-proteome analyses of HPV8-E7 positive cells compared to control cells using the Perseus software suite. After subtracting the total proteins from the phopho-proteins we report 40 statistically significant phospho-proteins in HPV8-E7 expressing keratinocytes. Out of these 40 proteins, 16 were hyperphosphorylated and 24 proteins hypophosphorylated (**Figure 4**). The Perseus output table, showing the kinase target motif enrichments, excluding the results for Fyn and Lyn kinases, additionally predicts 14-3-3 binding motifs for several hypo- and hyperphosphorylated proteins as presented in **Supplementary Table 3**.

To pinpoint potential Fyn and Lyn targets, we performed an additional kinase motif enrichment analysis using the online tool KinasePhos2.0 (Wong et al., 2007). This analysis revealed that a great number of the identified differentially phosphorylated proteins are targets of the Src kinase family members Fyn and Lyn which may point toward HPV8-E7 hijacking these kinases to enact post-translational modifications in HPV8 infected cells (**Figures 4A,C**).

These aberrantly phosphorylated proteins could be grouped into two enriched pathway clusters, namely "cytoskeletal organization and cell polarity" and "DNA replication and repair" (**Figures 4B,D**). STRING database analyses further revealed that a majority of the identified proteins form protein-protein interaction networks (**Supplementary Figure 1**).

DISCUSSION

HPV8-E7 is the main viral oncoprotein exerting control over both proliferation and invasive behavior of keratinocytes

A

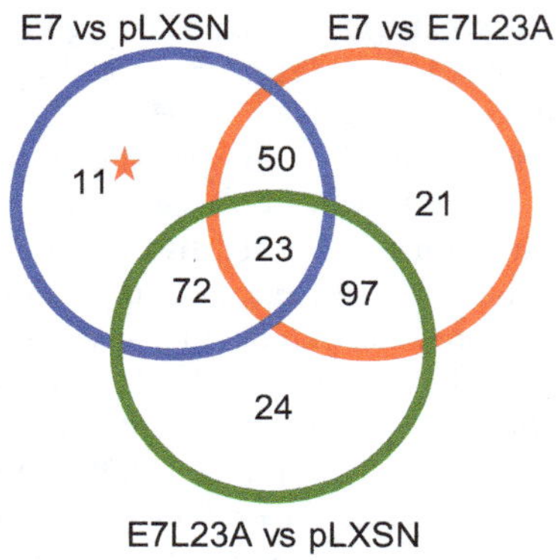

B

Gene ID	Description	fold-change in secretion levels
PITPNB	Phosphatidylinositol transfer protein beta isoform	8.8
GALNT2	Polypeptide N-acetylgalactosaminyltransferase 2	7.2
IGFBP7	Insulin-like growth factor-binding protein 7	6.7
UGP2	UTP--glucose-1-phosphate uridylyltransferase	5.7
PRDX6	Peroxiredoxin-6	4.5
SFN	14-3-3 protein sigma	-4.8
YWHAB	14-3-3 protein beta/alpha	-4.9
LGMN	Legumain	-4.9
CTSC	Cathepsin C	-5.5
PRDX1	Peroxiredoxin-1	-5.6
CNPY2	Protein canopy homolog 2	-7.9

C

N	GO category	Genes
6	Response to stress	CTSC IGFBP7 LGMN PRDX1 PRDX6 SFN
5	Catabolic process	CTSC LGMN PRDX1 PRDX6 YWHAB
5	Regulation of signaling in response to stimulus	CTSC LGMN PRDX1 SFN YWHAB
5	Regulation of biological quality	LGMN PRDX1 PRDX6 SFN YWHAB
4	Cell proliferation	IGFBP7 LGMN PRDX1 SFN
4	Regulation of multicellular organismal process	CNPY2 CTSC LGMN SFN
3	Regulation of localization and molecular function	LGMN SFN YWHAB
3	Macromolecule localization	PITPNB SFN YWHAB
3	Regulation of growth	LGMN IGFBP7 SFN
3	Regulation of developmental process	CTSC LGMN SFN

D

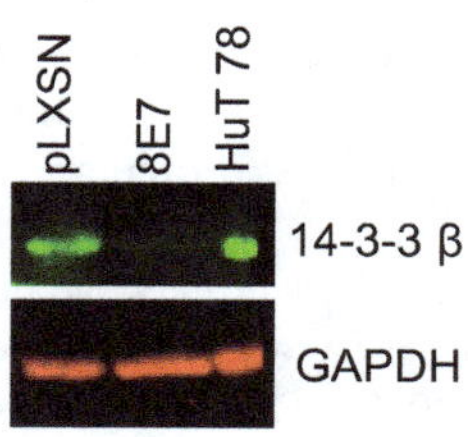

FIGURE 2 | Secretome analysis of N/TERT-8E7^{wt} or N/TERT-8E7^{L23A} grown on fibronectin. **(A)** Venn diagram depicting a three set comparison of differentially secreted proteins taken from N/TERT-pLXSN, N/TERT8-E7^{wt}, or N/TERT8-E7^{L23A}. The starred number indicates proteins targeted only by HPV8-E7^{wt}. **(B)** Description of differentially proteins exclusively secreted by HPV8-E7^{wt} positive keratinocytes as depicted in subfigure A The log2-fold changes of the secretome results from N/TERT-8E7 and N/TERT-pLXSN were compared to calculate the difference. **(C)** Gene ontology analysis of differentially secreted proteins using ShinyGO v0.61. **(D)** Representative immunoblots of RIPA extracts from N/TERTs expressing HPV8-E7 tested for 14-3-3β protein expression (n = 3). HuT78 whole cell lysate served as a positive control. Equal loading was confirmed by immunoblotting for GAPDH.

(Akgül et al., 2005, 2007; Heuser et al., 2016; Hufbauer and Akgül, 2017). More detailed molecular insights on the mechanisms involved would therefore be invaluable to further expand our understanding of how these invasive processes are initiated and propagated. In order to shed more light on these issues this comprehensive study employed several different unbiased experimental angles, including transcriptomic, secretomic and proteomic/phospho-proteomic approaches.

From previous studies we already knew that a broad range of genes deregulated in HPV8-E7 positive primary keratinocytes are controlled upstream through Sp1/Sp3 binding sites in the promoter region (Kirschberg et al., 2019). Here, we now compared our data with a data set generated in the Alonso laboratory, with both data sets having been generated with either PHAK or PHFK, both grown on plastic. We thus identified three genes, namely ATF3, GADD34, and GDF15, as they showed the

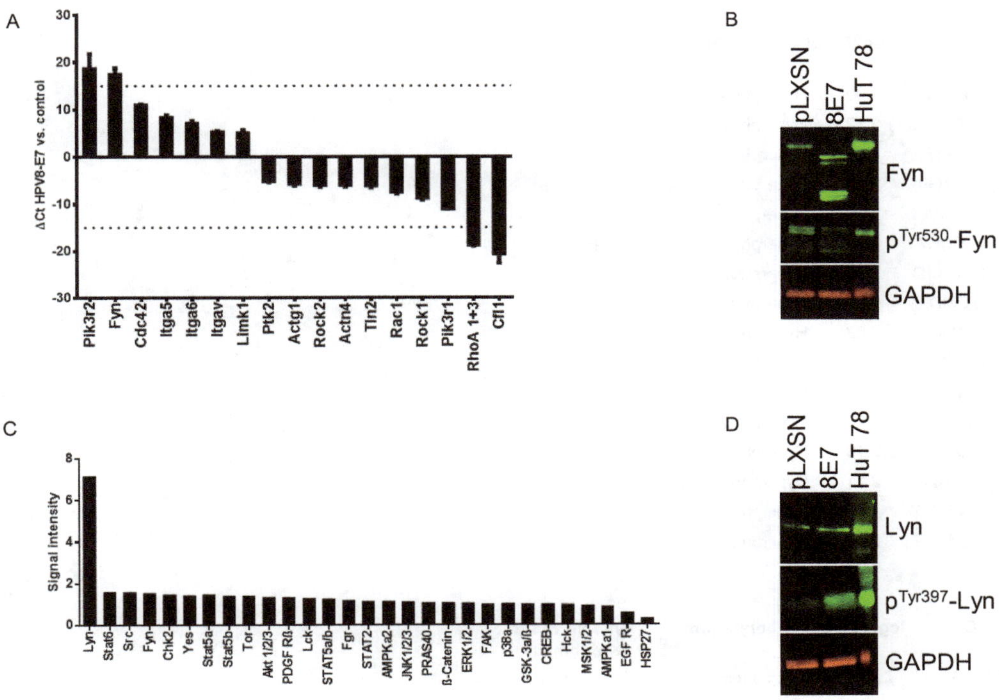

FIGURE 3 | Analysis of fibronectin associated gene expression and protein kinase phosphorylation changes in HPV8-E7 positive keratinocytes. **(A)** PrimePCR results for N/TERT-8E7 grown on fibronectin for 96 h (*n* = 4). **(B)** Representative immunoblots of RIPA extracts from N/TERT-8E7 tested for total Fyn and p^{Tyr530}-Fyn (*n* = 3). HuT78 whole cell lysates served as a positive control. Equal loading was confirmed by immunoblotting for GAPDH. **(C)** Protein kinase phosphorylation patterns in N/TERT-8E7 cells cultured on fibronectin for 96 h were analyzed using the Proteome Profiler Human Phospho- Kinase Array Kit (RnD Systems). The cut-off value for up- and down-regulated genes was set to fivefold. The dashed line indicates the 15-fold change. **(D)** Representative immunoblots of RIPA extracts of N/TERT-8E7 tested for total Lyn and p^{Tyr397}-Lyn (*n* = 3). HuT78 whole cell lysates served as a positive control. Equal loading was confirmed by immunoblotting for GAPDH.

same expression pattern in the cDNA data sets of both studies. By means of RTqPCR we could validate both GADD34 and GDF15 as novel gene targets of E7 but not ATF3. One possible reason for this discrepancy could be that ATF3 might only be specifically targeted in primary keratinocytes but not in a cell line. Interestingly, the upregulation of GADD34 and GDF15 could only be detected in keratinocytes grown under undifferentiating conditions (grown in KGM-Gold), thus confirming these genes as novel gene targets of HPV8-E7. Despite the fact that both genes are known to be regulated by Sp1/Sp3 the exact mechanism by which this upregulation is achieved in HPV8-E7 positive cells should be further researched in future studies.

E7 co-expression with E6 even had a synergistic effect on GDF15 over-expression under undifferentiating conditions. In contrast, co-expression had a repressive effect on GADD34, whose expression was, however, still highly elevated compared to the control. When isogenic keratinocytes were grown under differentiating conditions the activating effect of E7 on GDF15 expression was abolished. Under these conditions, the GADD34 transcripts could not be detected at all pointing toward an exclusive role in undifferentiated keratinocytes. GDF15 is a member of the TGF-β superfamily. However, its role in keratinocyte biology has thus far not been extensively studied. It is known that GDF15 overexpression in melanoma cells is associated with tumor invasion and metastasis (Unal et al., 2015). In line with our data, it is reasonable to speculate that the E7 mediated upregulation and secretion of GDF15 may disturb the physiological keratinocyte differentiation program. This may also have an influence on epidermal-dermal crosstalk, which may ultimately result in aberrant cell growth. GADD34, on the other hand, belongs to a family of genes which are induced by DNA damage and apoptotic cell death, and which are also known to enhance the apoptotic response to DNA damage (Grishin et al., 2001). In later studies, GADD34 was shown to dephosphorylate several kinases that function in various important signaling cascades (Collier et al., 2017). Our observation that GADD34 is only detectable and thus seemingly targeted by E7 in undifferentiated keratinocytes with a basal cell phenotype points toward a role of this regulation axis in manipulating the growth of undifferentiated basal keratinocytes.

Since previous results of our group had shown the importance of fibronectin in modulating the phenotype of HPV8-E7 expressing keratinocytes we now aimed at identifying signaling molecules and cascades that are altered under these conditions.

Our secretomic and proteomic data both hint at a possible involvement of 14-3-3 family members in HPV8-E7 mediated

A

ID	log2fc	phosphorylation	Fyn/Lyn motif enrichment
SRRM2	4.00	Hyperphos.	Lyn
CEP170B	3.72	Hyperphos.	-
CEP170	3.06	Hyperphos.	-
SPAG9	2.40	Hyperphos.	-
RBMX	2.37	Hyperphos.	Fyn
DOCK7	2.35	Hyperphos.	Fyn
CSNK1D	2.35	Hyperphos.	-
EMD	2.34	Hyperphos.	Fyn, Lyn
TANC2	2.32	Hyperphos.	Fyn, Lyn
RANBP2	2.30	Hyperphos.	-
NFIA	2.26	Hyperphos.	Fyn
TMPO	2.20	Hyperphos.	-
CLASP2	2.16	Hyperphos.	-
LMNA	2.11	Hyperphos.	-
ZNF687	2.06	Hyperphos.	Fyn, Lyn
CDC42EP1	2.02	Hyperphos.	-

B

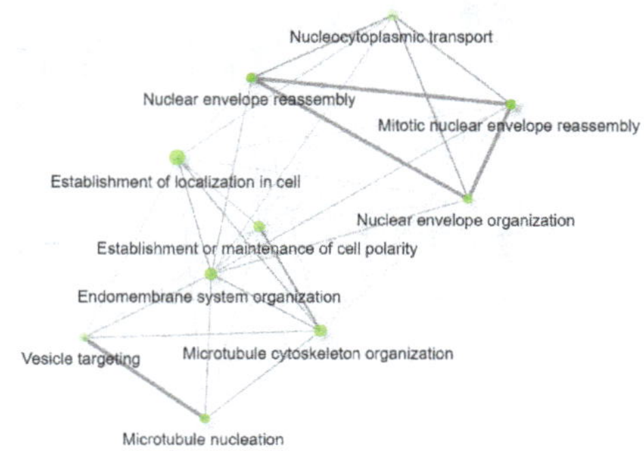

C

ID	log2fc	phosphorylation	Fyn/Lyn motif enrichment
NDRG1	-2.00	Hypophos.	Fyn, Lyn
MYO1E	-2.04	Hypophos.	Fyn, Lyn
AHNAK	-2.05	Hypophos.	Fyn, Lyn
BRIP1	-2.07	Hypophos.	-
SIPA1L1	-2.08	Hypophos.	Fyn
MAGI3	-2.12	Hypophos.	-
PLEKHG3	-2.17	Hypophos.	Lyn
ZNF281	-2.22	Hypophos.	-
MCM4	-2.24	Hypophos.	-
U2SURP	-2.24	Hypophos.	-
PPIP5K2	-2.25	Hypophos.	-
PSIP1	-2.28	Hypophos.	Fyn, Lyn
PHRF1	-2.35	Hypophos.	Fyn, Lyn
PTRF	-2.38	Hypophos.	-
LEMD3	-2.40	Hypophos.	-
INCENP	-2.40	Hypophos.	Fyn
PRRC2C	-2.47	Hypophos.	-
RAP1GAP2	-2.56	Hypophos.	-
MDC1	-2.72	Hypophos.	Fyn, Lyn
ANLN	-2.74	Hypophos.	-
SF3B1	-2.82	Hypophos.	Fyn, Lyn
EPN3	-3.09	Hypophos.	-
COL17A1	-3.20	Hypophos.	Lyn
RPS6	-4.42	Hypophos.	-

D

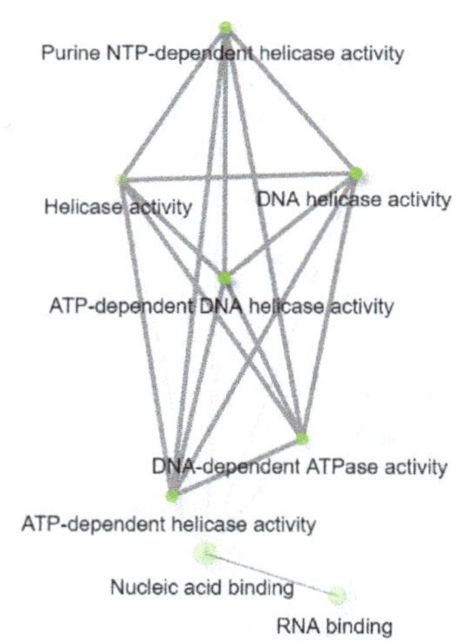

FIGURE 4 | Phospho-proteome analysis of N/TERT-8E7 cultured on fibronectin. **(A)** List of proteins found to be hyper-phosphorylated in between HPV8-E7 positive keratinocytes. **(B)** Gene Ontology Enrichment Analysis of hyper-phosphorylated proteins. **(C)** List of proteins found to be hypo-phosphorylated in between HPV8-E7 positive keratinocytes. **(D)** Gene Ontology Enrichment Analysis of hypo-phosphorylated proteins. Fyn and Lyn kinase substrates identified using KinasePhos2.0 were highlighted in **(A,C)**.

cellular changes. The 14-3-3 family is comprised of a number of scaffolding proteins that serve as platforms for several protein-protein interactions. The 14-3-3 protein family fulfills various regulatory functions involved in signaling pathways, cell proliferation, DNA damage response, apoptosis, differentiation and cell survival. By altering key regulatory proteins 14-3-3 family members play pivotal roles in cancer initiation and progression (Khorrami et al., 2017; Liu et al., 2021). It is therefore not unreasonable to assume that the observed E7-mediated changes in 14-3-3 protein levels as well as changes in global protein phosphorylation patterns may also lead to changes in 14-3-3 binding motif availabilities as well. Considering that we found a downregulation of 14-3-3 protein levels both in cell culture supernatants as well as in full cell lysates our experimental results may thus have unveiled a modulatory axis hijacked by the HPV8-E7 oncoprotein which may contribute to disturbing physiological keratinocyte functions.

Using different experimental approaches and bioinformatical tools we identified the Src kinase family members Fyn and Lyn, among others (**Figures 3,4** and **Supplementary Table 3**), as novel crucial kinases deregulated by E7 that may play a vital role in altering the phosphorylation profile of cellular proteins involved in cytoskeletal organization and cell polarity as well as proteins associated with DNA replication and repair, which may ultimately contribute HPV8-E7 mediated keratinocyte transformation.

In that light, Src kinases are comprised of a family of 11 non-receptor tyrosine kinases and interestingly only Fyn and Lyn seem to become over-abundantly activated in HPV8-E7 positive keratinocytes grown on fibronectin. Here, Lyn expression has also been implicated to be activated in response to DNA damage. Also, Lyn—but not other Src kinases—is activated following genotoxic stress, where Lyn is associated with cell cycle arrest and apoptotic processes (Yoshida et al., 2000). Furthermore, Lyn is known to act as a negative regulator of GADD34 in DNA damage-induced cell death (Grishin et al., 2001). As in HPV8-E7 positive cells Lyn is overly activated one would expect now that GADD34 expression would also be repressed (as described above). Surprisingly, this does not seem to be the case, which points toward an uncoupling of this regulatory circuit in the presence of E7 and E6E7, respectively. Moving on to Fyn, this kinase has three known splice variants, namely FynT, FynB, and FynC, which arise from alternative splicing of exon 7 of the Fyn gene (Brignatz et al., 2009; Uddin et al., 2020). The observation of a fourth Fyn signal in Western blots of HPV8-E7 positive cells grown on fibronectin may potentially have unveiled a fourth unknown Fyn splice variant, which may be associated with E7 expression and contribute to the complexity of Src kinase regulation in betaHPV positive skin. Interestingly, in a previous study on HPV16-E7 the authors also described phosphorylation of Src family kinases Yes and Fyn in the presence of HPV16-E7 (Szalmas et al., 2013).

In addition to the already known HPV8-E7 binding partners (Enzenauer et al., 1998; Rozenblatt-Rosen et al., 2012; Sperling et al., 2012; White et al., 2012; White and Howley, 2013; Grace and Munger, 2017; Oswald et al., 2017, 2019) we now identified novel cellular targets which are differentially regulated in HPV8-E7 positive keratinocytes. The finding that the Src kinases Fyn and Lyn are significantly over-activated and likely change the phosphorylation status of several proteins when cells are grown on fibronectin may possibly represent the most profound results of our study. As Src kinase inhibitors already exist our results may therefore pave the way for novel therapeutic approaches in which these inhibitors could be used for treatment of skin SCCs in which betaHPV involvement has been demonstrated.

AUTHOR CONTRIBUTIONS

MK, ASS, HGD, SH, AW-H, AA, and MH performed the experiments. MK, ASS, HGD, SH, AW-H, AA, MH, and BA analyzed the data. MK and BA designed the experiments and wrote the manuscript. All authors contributed to the article and approved the submitted version.

ACKNOWLEDGMENTS

N/TERT keratinocytes were kindly provided by the James Rheinwald, Harvard Medical School, Boston, MA, United States.

REFERENCES

Akgül, B., Garcia-Escudero, R., Ghali, L., Pfister, H. J., Fuchs, P. G., Navsaria, H., et al. (2005). The E7 protein of cutaneous human papillomavirus type 8 causes invasion of human keratinocytes into the dermis in organotypic cultures of skin. *Cancer Res.* 65, 2216–2223. doi: 10.1158/0008-5472.can-04-1952

Akgül, B., Ghali, L., Davies, D. Pfister, H., Leigh, I. M., and Storey, A. (2007). HPV8 early genes modulate differentiation and cell cycle of primary human adult keratinocytes. *Exp. Dermatol.* 16, 590–599. doi: 10.1111/j.1600-0625.2007.00569.x

Bouwes Bavinck, J. N., Feltkamp, M. C. W., Green, A. C., Fiocco, M., Euvrard, S., Harwood, C. A., et al. (2018). Human papillomavirus and posttransplantation cutaneous squamous cell carcinoma: a multicenter, prospective cohort study. *Am. J.Transplant.* 18, 1220–1230. doi: 10.1111/ajt.14537

Boxman, I. L., Mulder, L. H., Noya, F., De Waard, V., Gibbs, S., Broker, T. R., et al. (2001). Transduction of the E6 and E7 genes of epidermodysplasia-verruciformis-associated human papillomaviruses alters human keratinocyte growth and differentiation in organotypic cultures. *J. Invest. Dermatol.* 117, 1397–1404. doi: 10.1046/j.0022-202x.2001.01602.x

Brignatz, C., Paronetto, M. P., Opi, S., Cappellari, M., Audebert, S., Feuillet, V., et al. (2009). Alternative splicing modulates autoinhibition and SH3 accessibility in the Src kinase Fyn. *Mol. Cell Biol.* 29, 6438–6448. doi: 10.1128/mcb.00398-09

Collier, A. E., Wek, R. C., and Spandau, D. F. (2017). Human keratinocyte differentiation requires translational control by the eIF2alpha kinase GCN2. *J. Invest. Dermatol.* 137, 1924–1934. doi: 10.1016/j.jid.2017.04.029

Dickson, M. A., Hahn, W. C., Ino, Y., Ronfard, V., Wu, J. Y., Weinberg, R. A., et al. (2000). Human keratinocytes that express hTERT and also bypass a p16(INK4a)-enforced mechanism that limits life span become immortal yet retain normal growth and differentiation characteristics. *Mol. Cell Biol.* 20, 1436–1447. doi: 10.1128/mcb.20.4.1436-1447.2000

Enzenauer, C., Mengus, G., Lavigne, A., Davidson, I., Pfister, H., and May, M. (1998). Interaction of human papillomavirus 8 regulatory proteins E2, E6 and E7 with components of the TFIID complex. *Intervirology* 41, 80–90. doi: 10.1159/000024918

Fania, L., Didona, D., Di Pietro, F. R., Verkhovskaia, S., Morese, R., Paolino, G., et al. (2021). Cutaneous squamous cell carcinoma: from pathophysiology to novel therapeutic approaches. *Biomedicines* 9:171. doi: 10.3390/biomedicines9020171

Grace, M., and Munger, K. (2017). Proteomic analysis of the gamma human papillomavirus type 197 E6 and E7 associated cellular proteins. *Virology* 500, 71–81. doi: 10.1016/j.virol.2016.10.010

Grishin, A. V., Azhipa, O., Semenov, I., and Corey, S. J. (2001). Interaction between growth arrest-DNA damage protein 34 and Src kinase Lyn negatively regulates genotoxic apoptosis. *Proc. Natl. Acad. Sci. U S A* 98, 10172–10177. doi: 10.1073/pnas.191130798

Hasche, D., Stephan, S., Braspenning-Wesch, I., Mikulec, J., Niebler, M., Grone,

H. J., et al. (2017). The interplay of UV and cutaneous papillomavirus infection in skin cancer development. *PLoS Pathog.* 13:e1006723. doi: 10.1371/journal.ppat.1006723

Hasche, D., Vinzon, S. E., and Rosl, F. (2018). Cutaneous papillomaviruses and

Heuser, S., Hufbauer, M., Steiger, J., Marshall, J., Sterner-Kock, A., Mauch, C., et al. (2016). The fibronectin/alpha3beta1 integrin axis serves as molecular basis for keratinocyte invasion induced by betaHPV. *Oncogene* 35, 4529–4539. doi: 10.1038/onc.2015.512

Howley, P. M., and Pfister, H. J. (2015). Beta genus papillomaviruses and skin cancer. *Virology* 47, 290–296. doi: 10.1016/j.virol.2015.02.004

Hufbauer, M., and Akgül, B. (2017). Molecular mechanisms of human papillomavirus induced skin carcinogenesis. *Viruses* 9:187. doi: 10.3390/v9070187

Hufbauer, M., Biddle, A., Borgogna, C., Gariglio, M., Doorbar, J., Storey, A., et al. (2013). Expression of betapapillomavirus oncogenes increases the number of keratinocytes with stem cell-like properties. *J. Virol.* 87, 12158–12165. doi: 10.1128/jvi.01510-13

Hufbauer, M., Cooke, J., Van Der Horst, G. T., Pfister, H., Storey, A., and Akgül, B. (2015). Human papillomavirus mediated inhibition of DNA damage sensing and repair drives skin carcinogenesis. *Mol. Cancer* 14:183. doi: 10.1186/s12943-015-0453-7

Khorrami, A., Sharif Bagheri, M., Tavallaei, M., and Gharechahi, J. (2017). The functional significance of 14-3-3 proteins in cancer: focus on lung cancer. *Horm. Mol. Biol. Clin. Investig.* 32. doi: 10.1515/hmbci-2017-0032

Kirschberg, M., Heuser, S., Syed, A. S., Steger, G., Majewski, S., Hufbauer, M., et al. (2019). HPV8 activates cellular gene expression mainly through Sp1/3 binding sites. *Virology* 535, 136–143. doi: 10.1016/j.virol.2019.06.019

Leverrier, S., Bergamaschi, D., Ghali, L., Ola, A., Warnes, G., Akgül, B., et al. (2007). Role of HPV E6 proteins in preventing UVB-induced release of pro-apoptotic factors from the mitochondria. *Apoptosis* 12, 549–560. doi: 10.1007/s10495-006-0004-1

Liu, J., Cao, S., Ding, G., Wang, B., Li, Y., Zhao, Y., et al. (2021). The role of 14-3-3 proteins in cell signalling pathways and virus infection. *J. Cell. Mol. Med.* 25, 4173–4182. doi: 10.1111/jcmm.16490

Marx, B., Hufbauer, M., Zigrino, P., Majewski, S., Markiefka, B., Sachsenheimer, T., et al. (2018). Phospholipidation of nuclear proteins by the human papillomavirus E6 oncoprotein: implication in carcinogenesis. *Oncotarget* 9, 34142–34158. doi: 10.18632/oncotarget.26140

Oswald, E., Kirschberg, M., Aubin, F., Alonso, A., Hufbauer, M., Akgül, B., et al. (2019). BetaHPV E6 and E7 colocalize with NuMa in dividing keratinocytes. *Virus Genes* 55, 600–609. doi: 10.1007/s11262-019-01685-9

Oswald, E., Reinz, E., Voit, R., Aubin, F., Alonso, A., and Auvinen, E. (2017). Human papillomavirus type 8 E7 protein binds nuclear myosin 1c and downregulates the expression of pre-rRNA. *Virus Genes* 53, 807–813. doi: 10.1007/s11262-017-1491-6

Proby, C. M., Purdie, K. J., Sexton, C. J., Purkis, P., Navsaria, H. A., Stables, J. N., et al. (2000). Spontaneous keratinocyte cell lines representing early and advanced stages of malignant transformation of the epidermis. *Exp. Dermatol.* 9, 104–117. doi: 10.1034/j.1600-0625.2000.009002104.x

Qayyum, T., Mcardle, P. A., Lamb, G. W., Jordan, F., Orange, C., Seywright, M., et al. (2012). Expression and prognostic significance of Src family members in renal clear cell carcinoma. *Br. J. Cancer* 107, 856–863. doi: 10.1038/bjc.2012.314

Rappsilber, J., Ishihama, Y., and Mann, M. (2003). Stop and go extraction tips for matrix-assisted laser desorption/ionization, nanoelectrospray, and LC/MS sample pretreatment in proteomics. *Anal. Chem.* 75, 663–670. doi: 10.1021/ac026117i

Rollison, D. E., Viarisio, D., Amorrortu, R. P., Gheit, T., and Tommasino, M. (2019). An emerging issue in oncogenic virology: the role of beta HPV types in development of cutaneous squamous cell carcinoma. *J. Virol.* 93, e01003–18 doi: 10.1128/JVI.01003-18

Rozenblatt-Rosen, O., Deo, R. C., Padi, M., Adelmant, G., Calderwood, M. A., Rolland, T., et al. (2012). Interpreting cancer genomes using systematic host network perturbations by tumour virus proteins. *Nature* 487, 491–495. doi: 10.1038/nature11288

Serrels, B., Serrels, A., Mason, S. M., Baldeschi, C., Ashton, G. H., Canel, M., et al. (2009). A novel Src kinase inhibitor reduces tumour formation in a skin carcinogenesis model. *Carcinogenesis* 30, 249–257. doi: 10.1093/carcin/bgn278

Smola, S. (2020). Human papillomaviruses and skin cancer. *Adv. Exp. Med. Biol.* 1268, 195–209. doi: 10.1007/978-3-030-46227-7_10

Smola-Hess, S., Pahne, J., Mauch, C., Zigrino, P., Smola, H., and Pfister, H. J. (2005). Expression of membrane type 1 matrix metalloproteinase in papillomavirus-positive cells: role of the human papillomavirus (HPV) 16 and HPV8 E7 gene products. *J. Gen. Virol.* 86, 1291–1296. doi: 10.1099/vir.0.80551-0

Sperling, T., Oldak, M., Walch-Ruckheim, B., Wickenhauser, C., Doorbar, J., Pfister, H., et al. (2012). Human papillomavirus type 8 interferes with a novel C/EBPbeta-mediated mechanism of keratinocyte CCL20 chemokine expression and Langerhans cell migration. *PLoS Pathog.* 8:e1002833. doi: 10.1371/journal.ppat.1002833

Szalmas, A., Gyongyosi, E., Ferenczi, A., Laszlo, B., Karosi, T., Csomor, P., et al. (2013). Activation of Src. Fyn and Yes non-receptor tyrosine kinases in keratinocytes expressing human papillomavirus (HPV) type 16 E7 oncoprotein. *Virol. J.* 10:79. doi: 10.1186/1743-422x-10-79

Szklarczyk, D., Gable, A. L., Lyon, D., Junge, A., Wyder, S., Huerta-Cepas, J., et al. (2019). STRING v11: protein-protein association networks with increased coverage, supporting functional discovery in genome-wide experimental datasets. *Nucleic Acids Res.* 47, D607–D613. doi: 10.1093/nar/gky1131

Uddin, M. J., Dorotea, D., Pak, E. S., and Ha, H. (2020). Fyn kinase: a potential therapeutic target in acute kidney injury. *Biomol. Ther. (Seoul)* 28, 213–221. doi: 10.4062/biomolther.2019.214

Unal, B., Alan, S., Bassorgun, C. I., Karakas, A. A., Elpek, G. O., and Ciftcioglu, M. A. (2015). The divergent roles of growth differentiation factor-15 (GDF-15) in benign and malignant skin pathologies. *Arch. Dermatol. Res.* 307, 551–557. doi: 10.1007/s00403-015-1546-2

Westphal, K., Akgül, B., Storey, A., and Nindl, I. (2009). Cutaneous human papillomavirus E7 type-specific effects on differentiation and proliferation of organotypic skin cultures. *Cell Oncol.* 31, 213–226. doi: 10.1155/2009/584185

White, E. A., and Howley, P. M. (2013). Proteomic approaches to the study of papillomavirus-host interactions. *Virology* 435, 57–69. doi: 10.1016/j.virol.2012.09.046

White, E. A., Sowa, M. E., Tan, M. J., Jeudy, S., Hayes, S. D., Santha, S., et al. (2012). Systematic identification of interactions between host cell proteins and E7 oncoproteins from diverse human papillomaviruses. *Proc. Natl. Acad. Sci. U.S.A.* 109, E260–E267. doi: 10.1073/pnas.1116776109

Wong, Y. H., Lee, T. Y., Liang, H. K., Huang, C. M., Wang, T. Y., Yang, Y. H., et al. (2007). KinasePhos 2.0: a web server for identifying protein kinase-specific phosphorylation sites based on sequences and coupling patterns. *Nucleic Acids Res.* 35, W588–W594. doi: 10.1093/nar/gkm322

Yoshida, K., Weichselbaum, R., Kharbanda, S., and Kufe, D. (2000). Role for Lyn tyrosine kinase as a regulator of stress-activated protein kinase activity in response to DNA damage. *Mol. Cell Biol.* 20, 5370–5380. doi: 10.1128/mcb.20.15.5370-5380.2000

7

Loss of Genome Fidelity: Beta HPVs and the DNA Damage Response

Sebastian O. Wendel and Nicholas A. Wallace*

Division of Biology, Kansas State University, Manhattan, KS, United States

***Correspondence:**
Nicholas A. Wallace
nwallac@ksu.edu

While the role of genus alpha human papillomaviruses in the tumorigenesis and tumor maintenance of anogenital and oropharyngeal cancers is well-established, the role of genus beta human papilloviruses (β-HPVs) in non-melanoma skin cancers (NMSCs) is less certain. Persistent β-HPV infections cause NMSCs in sun-exposed skin of people with a rare genetic disorder, epidermodysplasia verruciformis. However, β-HPV infections in people without epidermodysplasia verruciformis are typically transient. Further, β-HPV gene expression is not necessary for tumor maintenance in the general population as on average there is fewer than one copy of the β-HPV genome per cell in NMSC tumor biopsies. Cell culture, epidemiological, and mouse model experiments support a role for β-HPV infections in the initiation of NMSCs through a "hit and run" mechanism. The virus is hypothesized to act as a cofactor, augmenting the genome destabilizing effects of UV. Supporting this idea, two β-HPV proteins (β-HPV E6 and E7) disrupt the cellular response to UV exposure and other genome destabilizing events by abrogating DNA repair and deregulating cell cycle progression. The aberrant damage response increases the likelihood of oncogenic mutations capable of driving tumorigenesis independent of a sustained β-HPV infection or continued viral protein expression. This review summarizes what is currently known about the deleterious effects of β-HPV on genome maintenance in the context of the virus's putative role in NMSC initiation.

Keywords: beta HPV, DNA-damage response, skin cancer, genomic fidelity, tumorigenesis, epidermodysplasia verruciformis, viral oncogenesis, p300

INTRODUCTION

Human papillomavirus (HPV) is a family of small, non-enveloped double-stranded DNA viruses that infect mucosal and cutaneous epithelia. This family is comprised of five genera (alpha, beta, gamma, nu, and mu) spanning across over 396 different HPV types potentially inhabiting human skin (Bzhalava et al., 2014). Classification of the HPV family is based on the sequence of the L1 capsid protein (Bernard et al., 2010; de Villiers, 2013). The alpha and beta genera are most widely studied because of the pathogenesis associated with some members of these genera. α-HPV causes genital warts (low risk types, HPV 6, and 11 for example) and genital cancer (high risk types, HPV 16, 18, 31, and 45 for example) (Tommasino, 2014; Doorbar et al., 2015). While β-HPV is known to cause flat warts and non-melanoma skin cancer in individuals with compromised immune systems (Cubie, 2013), there is a growing interest in determining if these viruses can cause tumors in the general population. Further, while so called "high risk" α-HPVs have been identified, the relative oncogenic potential among the beta genus of HPV is still being discussed. Moreover, despite already consisting of ~50 types of HPV that are sub-classified in five species (Van Doorslaer, 2013), it is likely that a large portion of β-HPV types have yet to be discovered (Ekström et al., 2013;

Bzhalava et al., 2014, 2015). Because the first β-HPV types isolated were HPV 5 and HPV 8 from cutaneous squamous cell carcinomas (cSCC) of patients with the rare disorder Epidermodysplasia Verruciformis (EV) (Pfister et al., 1981; Kremsdorf et al., 1982, 1983), these two β-HPVs have been the most extensively examined.

Because β-HPVs do not generally persist in tumors, they are hypothesized to act through a "hit and run" mechanism (Pfister, 2003; Hufbauer and Akgül, 2017). Specifically, β-HPVs are believed to hinder the repair of DNA damage caused by UV radiation making mutations more likely. For a virus that infects an area frequently exposed to UV radiation and yet requires proliferating cells to complete its lifecycle, it is reasonable that β-HPVs have developed mechanisms to prevent the cell cycle arrest that accompanies repair of UV damaged DNA. However, this could have severe consequences for the host cell as the UV-induced mutations will remain after the viral infection is cleared and could drive the development of non-melanoma skin cancers (NMSCs) without continued expression of β-HPV genes. In this review, we will begin by providing a brief synapsis of the evidence that β-HPV infections cause NMSCs as well as the cellular signaling pathways that respond to UV insults. We will provide a concise discussion of α-HPV associated tumorigenesis, as these more clearly defined mechanisms of transformation provide a useful and relevant comparison for β-HPV associated oncogenesis. Then, we will move on to the *in vitro* and *in vivo* data that demonstrate the ability of β-HPV genes to disrupt the repair of DNA, destabilizing the host genome in a manner consistent with a "hit and run" mechanism of tumorigenesis.

Transformation by Alpha Genus HPV Oncogenes

Extensive evidence has established α-HPV as the causative agent in cervical cancers and in many other malignancies in the oropharynx and throughout the anogenital tract (Hobbs et al., 2006; Moody and Laimins, 2010; Carter et al., 2011; D'Souza and Dempsey, 2011; Tommasino, 2014). Infections with high risk α-HPVs can begin a multi-decade process where cells are immortalized, accumulate destabilized genomes, and are ultimately transformed into deadly malignant tumors. Two oncogenes, α-HPV E6 and E7 proteins drive this progression by activating telomerase and degrading two tumor suppressor, p53 and pRB (Dyson et al., 1989; Münger et al., 1989; Scheffner et al., 1990; Werness et al., 1990; Huibregtse et al., 1991; Boyer et al., 1996; Klingelhutz et al., 1996; Kiyono et al., 1998; Oh et al., 2001). These oncogenes also induce aberrant activation of the DNA damage response (DDR) and in some case, impair the cells ability to repair DNA damage (Patel et al., 1999; Zimmermann et al., 1999; Moody and Laimins, 2009; Sakakibara et al., 2011; Gillespie et al., 2012; Reinson et al., 2013; Hong et al., 2015; Wallace et al., 2017). In notable contrast to β-HPV associated malignancies, tumors caused by α-HPV are dependent on the continued expression of α-HPV E6 and E7 (Hwang et al., 1993; Goodwin and DiMaio, 2000; Goodwin et al., 2000). Because the β-HPV homologs of these α-HPV oncogenes are believed to be the primary contributors to NMSC, β-HPV E6, and E7 are frequently compared to α-HPV E6 and E7. When informative, we will make similar comparisons.

Beta-HPV in Epidermodysplasia Verruciformis Patients and Organ Transplant Recipients

The oncogenic potential of β-HPV is most firmly established in people with compromised immune systems. β-HPV associated cSCCs occur in 30–60% of people with the rare genetic disorder epidermodysplasia verruciformis (EV) and presented the first link between β-HPV infections and skin carcinogenesis (Orth, 1986). β-HPV+ tumors found in people with EV generally contain a high copy number (~300 copies/cell) of viral DNA (Dell'Oste et al., 2009). In contrast, β-HPV+ tumors of non-EV patients show a very low viral DNA copy number <1 per cell (Weissenborn et al., 2005; Arron et al., 2011). The most frequently β-HPV types associated with EV are β-HPV 5 and 8 (also less often β-HPV 14 and 20) (de Oliveira et al., 2004; Dell'Oste et al., 2009). Tumors in individuals with EV occur predominantly in parts of the body frequently exposed to the sun, suggesting a role for UV in β-HPV associated tumorigenesis (Pfister, 2003). Another group at risk for β-HPV associated cSCCs are people receiving immunosuppressive therapy following organ transplant. Organ transplant recipients (OTRs) (Bouwes Bavinck et al., 2001) show an increased susceptibility to β-HPV infections, a higher prevalence of viral DNA and a greater risk of developing non-melanoma skin cancer (Boyle et al., 1984; Kiviat, 1999). This increased risk is particularly notable if they are seropositive for β-HPV, with a hazard ratio of 2.8 (Genders et al., 2015). Both, EV-patients and OTRs display a significantly elevated viral load than the immunocompetent population (Dell'Oste et al., 2009; Weissenborn et al., 2012). Further, OTRs that have similar β-HPV viral loads to patients with EV show a 100-fold increase of cSCC incidence (Weissenborn et al., 2012). Investigations in to NMSCs in EV and OTR patient groups provide strong evidence that β-HPV infections have oncogenic potential. Additionally, the OTR patient group shows that β-HPV associated cSCCs are not limited to patients with the rare EV disorder (Howley and Pfister, 2015; Tommasino, 2017). These "special" scenarios provide the proof of context specific β-HPV induced oncogenesis, but defining the breath of β-HPV's contribution to NMSC development is a critical area of research as millions of people are diagnosed with these malignancies each year.

Beta-HPV in the General Population

β-HPVs inhabit the cutaneous epithelium and are found in abundance throughout the population (Casabonne et al., 2009; de Koning et al., 2009; Weissenborn et al., 2012; Farzan et al., 2013). A particularly frequent site of infection is the hair follicles of eyebrows (Weissenborn et al., 2012; Neale et al., 2013; Iannacone et al., 2014). Unlike α-HPV infections, which are usually sexually transmitted and occur later in life, β-HPV infections often occur during early childhood through skin to skin contact (Antonsson et al., 2003; Weissenborn et al., 2009). The persistence of α- and β-HPVs is a further differentiating factor, although the exact mechanisms driving this difference are not fully appreciated. Median β-HPV infection duration is 8.6 months in eyebrow hairs, while infections of the skin are less common but have a median persistence of 11.3 months (Hampras et al., 2014). In contrast α-HPV infections persist longer (18.3 months on average), and upon accidental genome-integration are present for decades (Richardson et al., 2003). Suggesting reinfections, β-HPV infections can persist within a family for several years without manifestation of clinical symptoms (Hsu et al., 2009). While infections first occur in infants, advanced age is a risk-factor for a β-HPV infection (Hazard et al., 2007; Weissenborn et al., 2009). Sunburn is another risk factor, potentially due to local immune suppression (Hampras et al., 2014). The evidence of β-HPV's involvement in cSCCs of EV patients led to the classification of HPV 5 and HPV 8 as possibly carcinogenic by a WHO-IARC 2009 work group (Bouvard et al., 2009).

Epidemiology

Epidemiologically, β-HPV antibody positivity is associated with an increased risk for cSCCs, especially for infections by β-HPV 38 (Bzhalava et al., 2013; Chahoud et al., 2016). There is also a difference of β-HPV prevalence by anatomical site (Hampras et al., 2017). The most common site of infection was genital skin (81.6%), followed by forearm skin (64.4%), eyebrow hairs (60.9%), oral mucosa (35.6%), and anal mucosa (33.3%). The most common type on the sunlight exposed and therefore risk associated sites eyebrows and forearm are β-HPV 38 and β-HPV 12 respectively. High loads of β-HPV DNA are statistically associated with increased cutaneous SCC incidences at an odds ratio of ~3 in immunocompetent Australians and immunosuppressed OTRs (Bouwes et al., 2010; Neale et al., 2013). People with cSCCs more frequently test positive for viral DNA in skin as well as anti β-HPV L1 antibodies than the general population (Forslund et al., 2007; Waterboer et al., 2008; Karagas et al., 2010; Iannacone et al., 2012; Farzan et al., 2013). The involvement of β-HPV in cSCC carcinogenesis is somewhat challenged by the low relative incidence rate of β-HPV+ cSCCs considering the high prevalence of 80% for β-HPV infections. Furthermore, unlike α-HPV+ cancers, the expression of β-HPV viral proteins is not required for tumor maintenance and the viral DNA copy-number is <1 per cell in β-HPV associated cSCCs (Meyer et al., 2001; Nindl et al., 2006). Since cSCC tumors typically occur in parts of the body exposed mutagenic UV radiation from the sun, the role of β-HPV is thought to be in the initiation and acceleration of genomic destabilization.

The phrase "hit and run" was coined to describe the hypothesize contribution of β-HPV infections to NMSCs, where the virus acts as a cofactor along with UV during tumor initiation (Bavinck et al., 2008). The destabilization of the host genome caused by sun exposure is augmented by β-HPV's ability to attenuate the cellular response to UV damage and thus increase the risk of oncogenic mutations capable of driving tumor development independent of continued β-HPV gene expression. Epidemiological studies support this hypothesis (Forslund et al., 2007; Iannacone et al., 2012) as there is increased prevalence and frequency of β-HPV in precancerous, actinic keratinosis lesions (AK). AK, otherwise known as solar keratinosis, is an abnormal growth of the skin, induced by UV exposure (Moy, 2000). Consistent with a role in tumor initiation, despite being found at very low copy numbers in cSCCs, the β-HPV viral load in AK is >50 copies/cell (Weissenborn et al., 2005). Together these data form the foundation that supports the "hit and run" model of β-HPV associated skin cancer, but this hypothesis is dependent on the ability of β-HPV infections to make UV more mutagenic.

DNA Damage Response-Pathways

The most likely way that β-HPV could amplify the destabilization of the host genome induced by UV is through the aberration of the cellular DDR. The primary type of DNA damage caused by UV are DNA intrastrand crosslinks, most often cyclobutane purimidine dimers or CPDs (Yang, 2011). Failure to properly repair these lesions can result in point mutations (Brash et al., 1991; Keohavong et al., 1991). Crosslinked DNA can also cause a replication fork collapse and subsequent double strand break in DNA (DSB) (Jeggo and Löbrich, 2007). If DSBs are not repaired, the damage becomes much more deleterious, including chromosome rearrangement or loss of entire chromosome arms (Pankotai and Soutoglou, 2013). In this section, we will introduce the biochemical pathways that coordinate the cellular response to UV-damage to preserve the integrity of the human genome. A graphical representation of the cellular response to UV induced DNA damage in S-phase can be found in **Figure 1**. During S-phase, translesion synthesis (TLS) prevents UV-induced DNA crosslinks from causing replication fork collapse by facilitating the bypass of the damaged bases (Lerner et al., 2017). Depending on the position in the cell cycle, nucleotide excision repair (NER), and the Fanconi Anemia (FA) pathways repair these crosslinks (Moldovan and D'Andrea, 2009; Marteijn et al., 2014). While FA requires sister chromosomes to complete repair and is thus limited to cells that have undergone replication, NER is not bound by cell cycle position. UV-induced DSBs are the result of replication fork collapse and therefore must occur during S-phase. Although DSB repair occurs through two major pathways, non-homologous end joining (NHEJ) and homologous recombination (HR), DSBs occurring during S-phase are repaired predominantly by HR (Mao et al., 2008). Repairing DNA lesions usually requires pausing the cell cycle to avoid escalating the damage during replication (Willis and Rhind, 2009). Finally, should the cell receive more damage than can be repaired, the intrinsic apoptosis pathway will initiate program cell death (Offer et al., 2002).

Although recognized as distinct pathways, the individual proteins that make up these repair mechanisms are often shared. This is particularly true for repair kinases (Yang et al., 2003; Yan et al., 2014). For instance, ATR controls the rate limiting step of NER (through phosphorylation mediated stabilization of XPA) and facilitates translesion synthesis by phosphorylating the TLS-specific polymerase, Polη (Chen et al., 2008; Göhler et al., 2011; Lee et al., 2014). ATR's kinase activity is similarly necessary for the repair of crosslinked DNA by the FA pathway and plays a role in DSB repair via the homologous recombination pathway (Jazayeri et al., 2006; Shiotani and Zou, 2009; Shigechi et al., 2012;

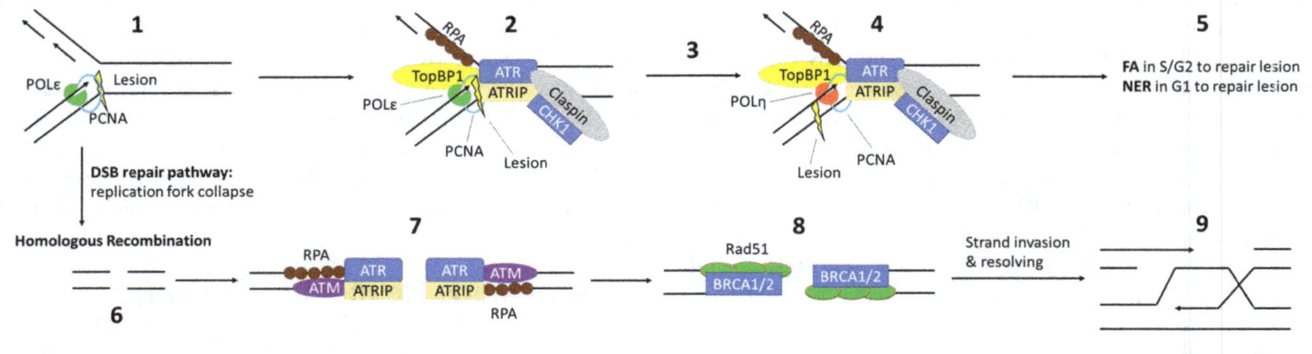

FIGURE 1 | Critical DDR Pathways for UV induced DNA Damage: (1) UV induces an intrastrand lesion, causing the replication fork to stall in S-pase. (2) Exposed ssDNA is coated with RPA, followed by recruitment of TopBP1 and ATR/ATRIP. TopBP1 accelerates autophosphorylation of ATR. Claspin and CHK1 are recruited and phosphorylated, promoting fork stabilization. (3) This leads to Rad6/Rad18 recruitment and mono-ubiquitination of PCNA (not shown), triggering the switch from high fidelity replication DNA-polymerases to y-family polymerase Polη. (4) Then, Polη replicates past the lesion and normal replication can continue after a repeated polymerase switch back to the high-fidelity replication polymerase. (5) The lesion itself is repaired by either the FA or NER pathway. (6) Prolonged stalling leads to replication fork collapse into a DSB. The MRE11, Rad50 and Nbs1 complex (not shown) is recruited to this DSB, initiating strand resection and recruitment/activation of ATM. (7) After strand resection, the exposed ssDNA is coated by RPA and ATR/ATRIP is recruited. (8) RPA is then replaced by RAD51, with the assistance of BRCA1 and BRCA2. (9) This facilitates homology-dependent single strand invasion and resolution of the lesion.

Maréchal and Zou, 2013). A similar situation exists for the related kinase, ATM. ATM phosphorylates proteins critical for the FA, NER, and HR repair pathways (Ray et al., 2013, 2016; Shiloh and Ziv, 2013). It may also play a role in translesion synthesis. Further, both ATM and ATR can stabilize p53 in response to DNA damage, causing p53-dependent DNA repair or apoptosis (Kruse and Gu, 2009; Cheng and Chen, 2010). ATM and ATR are both classically involved in DNA damage induced cell cycle arrest (Reinhardt and Yaffe, 2009). Both of these kinases also help pause the cell cycle progression by phosphorylating/activating cell cycle regulatory proteins (CHK1 and CHK2) (Branzei and Foiani, 2008). Finally, ATM and ATR also facilitate programed cell death or apoptosis should the cell's DNA be too extensively damaged. Specifically, their phosphorylation of p53 stabilizes the tumor suppressor and can result in p53-dependent apoptosis (Banin et al., 1998; Tibbetts et al., 1999; Shiloh and Ziv, 2013).

The RPA complex (RPA14, RPA32, and RPA70), BRCA1 and BRCA2 are similarly important for a myriad of DDRs (Yoshida and Miki, 2004; Maréchal and Zou, 2015). The RPA heterotrimer binds single stranded DNA (ssDNA) protecting it from degradation. Because ssDNA intermediates occur during both homologous recombination and translesion synthesis, RPA proteins are essential for these repair mechanisms. Both the FA and HR pathways require BRCA1 and BRCA2. FA pathway proteins contain the prefix "FANC" in their names indicating that many of these proteins were named after loss of the gene was shown to result in the clinical manifestation (Fanconi Anemia) from which the repair pathway derives its name, for example, FANCA, FANCB, FANC. Indicative of its requirement for FA repair an alternative name for BRCA2 is FANCD1. Moreover, BRCA1 was recently shown to be a critical component of the FA pathway (Domchek et al., 2013; Sawyer et al., 2015) and even described as the pathway's "missing link" (D'Andrea, 2013). The requirement of BRCA1 and BRCA2 in repair of DSBs by homologous recombination has been established for over a decade. Further indicative of how intertwined the cellular DNA response is, ATR and ATM both play regulatory roles in repair by phosphorylating the RPA complex, BRCA1 as well as BRCA2.

EFFECTS OF β-HPV E6 ON DNA DAMAGE RESPONSE

Inhibition of Apoptosis

The E6 protein of β-HPV can hinder both DNA repair machinery and apoptotic pathways in response to DNA damage. Unlike high risk α-HPVs, it does not commonly degrade the "guardian of the genome," p53, one of the most prominent high-risk E6 targets, directly (Scheffner et al., 1990; White et al., 2014). The tumor-suppressor, p53, is an important signaling protein that regulates two large subsets of target proteins: negative regulators of cell cycle progression (p21, 14-3-3, GADD45α) and pro-apoptotic proteins (PUMA, BAX, BAK). In normal cells, p53 has to balance on a fine line between sufficient activity to ensure genome fidelity and tumor suppression as well as avoiding hyperactivity that would induce abnormal aging by depleting stem-cell populations (Vogelstein et al., 2000; Reinhardt and Schumacher, 2012). Compared to high risk α-HPV E6s, β-HPV E6, apart from β-HPV 49, have a lower affinity for a cellular E3 ubiquitin ligase, known as E6AP or UBE3A, and are therefore not able to form the E6-E6AP complex required for proteasomal degradation of p53 (Huibregtse et al., 1991; Cornet et al., 2012). Instead, β-HPV types 17, 38, and 92 have been shown to bind to p53 directly and stabilize it (White et al., 2012), while β-HPV 23 has been shown to interfere with the phosphorylation-dependent activation of p53 by inhibiting HIPK2 (Muschik et al., 2011). β-HPV 5 and β-HPV 8 delay the stabilization and phosphorylation after UV irradiation (Wallace et al., 2014). HIPK2 is a protein kinase that can phosphorylate p53 at Ser 46, which subsequently leads to the acetylation of p53 at Lys 382 and a promotion of p53 target gene expression. More specifically, HIPK2's activity is UV-induced and UV exposure leads to HIPK2 mediated growth arrest or apoptosis via p53. β-HPV 38 E6 induces the accumulation of ΔNp73, altering p53 functions (Accardi et al., 2006). These effects cause the alteration or loss of p53's activity as a transcriptional co-factor and impact both apoptosis- (Fas, BAX) and cell cycle checkpoint pathway (p21) gene expression (White et al., 2014). p53 is also a known transcription factor for the TLS polymerase Polη, implying the TLS DDR pathway as a suitable target for investigation (Lerner et al., 2017).

The selection between a p53-mediated checkpoint activation and p53-mediated apoptosis depends on a cell type specific threshold of p53 expression and activation (Kracikova et al., 2013). Mild DNA damage triggers p53-dependent checkpoint activation and subsequent DNA repair while moderate DNA damage causes p53-mediated senescence. Excessive DNA damage or failed cytokinesis induce apoptosis (Chen et al., 1996). β-HPV E6 can also inhibit apoptosis downstream of p53. The interaction of E6 with a pro-apoptotic protein, Bcl2 homologous antagonist killer (BAK), is a highly conserved function across HPV types and genera (Thomas and Banks, 1999; Simmonds and Storey, 2008; Underbrink et al., 2008; Jackson and Bartek, 2009; Holloway et al., 2015; Tomaić, 2016). Increases in BAK abundance are an essential step in the intrinsic apoptotic pathway (Chittenden et al., 1995). β-HPV E6 prevents the accumulation of Bak following UV-irradiation inducing DNA damage. An overview of the different pathways for β-HPV E6 mediated inhibition of apoptosis and the β-HPV types involved can be found in the upper right panel of **Figure 2**.

Interference with Checkpoint Signaling & DNA Damage Repair

Upstream of the inhibition of apoptosis, β-HPV E6 can attenuate G1 to S-phase cell cycle checkpoint induction in response to DNA damage (Wallace et al., 2012; Hufbauer et al., 2015) and continue cellular proliferation while DNA damage repair is attenuated (Giampieri and Storey, 2004). These effects arise from the interaction of β-HPV E6 with the acetyltransferase p300 (Muench et al., 2010; Howie et al., 2011). As an important coactivator of DDR gene transcription, the loss of p300 activity has far reaching consequences. β-HPV 5 and 8 have been shown to facilitate the destabilization of p300 (Howie et al., 2011; Wallace et al., 2012, 2013), while β-HPV 38 has been shown to inhibit p300 acetyltransferase activity (Muench et al., 2010). The steady state levels of the DDR kinases ATM and ATR as well as BRCA1 and BRCA2 are reduced because of the lack of p300 in β-HPV 5 and β-HPV 8 E6 expressing cells (Wallace et al., 2012, 2013, 2015). This attenuates the repair of UV induced cyclobutane pyrimidine dimer (CPD), increases the UV-induced frequency of DSBs and attenuates LINE-1 retrotransposition. Double strand breaks can be a secondary effect of UV-induced DNA damage, occurring when a replication fork collapses at an unrepaired CPD. Both the repair of CPDs (ATR dependent) as well as the repair of DSBs (ATM, BRCA1 and BRCA2 dependent) are significantly delayed by β-HPV 5 and β-HPV 8 E6 (Giampieri and Storey, 2004; Wallace et al., 2012, 2015). γH2AX is a known marker for DSBs and its foci kinetics can be utilized as indicators for DSB-repair. The (β-HPV 5 E6 and 8 E6) p300 degradation-dependent attenuation of BRCA1/BRCA2 expression and foci formation led

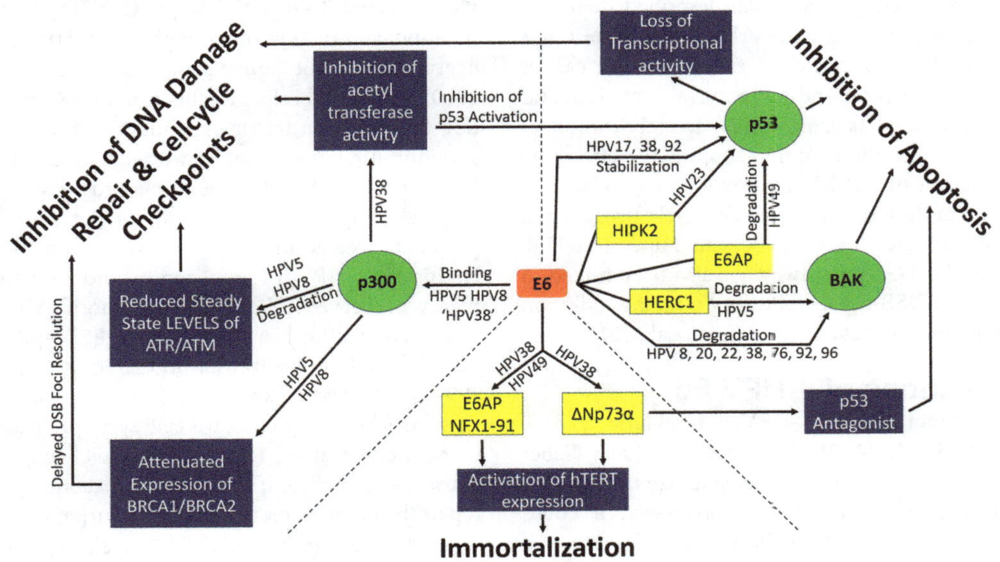

FIGURE 2 | β-HPV E6 and its effects on genome stability. Interactions among β-HPV E6s and proteins involved in DNA repair and cell cycle check points (upper left third), apoptotic signaling (upper right third), and immortalization (bottom third) are depicted. Green circles denote cellular proteins that are central to β-HPV E6's ability to alter the cellular response to DNA damage. Blue boxes depict the diversity of cellular processes altered through the manipulation of the green circular proteins. Yellow boxes represent proteins that cooperate in the manipulation of the green circular proteins or facilitate immortalization. 'HPV 38' refers to the fact that while β-HPV 38 E6 can bind p300, it does not bind it strong enough to destabilize the histone acetyltransferase.

to delayed γH2AX foci resolution after DSBs were induced by ionizing radiation (Wallace et al., 2015).

ATR and ATM activate cell cycle checkpoints by phosphorylating checkpoint kinases Chk1 and Chk2 respectively. Activation of Chk1/Chk2 induces cell cycle arrest and DDR (Reinhardt and Yaffe, 2009). β-HPV 5 and 8 E6 reduce steady state levels of ATM and ATR *in vitro* as well as reduced pATM and pATR levels *in vitro* and *in vivo* (Hufbauer et al., 2015). This leads to an attenuated Chk1 phosphorylation and impaired G1 to S-phase checkpoint activation, presenting a bypass to an important tumor-suppressing barrier. Furthermore, p300 is an important transcriptional cofactor for BRCA1, BRCA2 (Both essential proteins for HR) (Goodman and Smolik, 2000; Pao et al., 2000; Yoshida and Miki, 2004) and has been shown to be essential for proper cytokinesis and the faithful resolution of mitotic figures (Turnell et al., 2005; Xia et al., 2012). Attenuation of proper checkpoint signaling and the consequent possible unscheduled cell cycle progression leaves pre-existing DNA damage unaddressed. This allows less severe types of damage (for example, UV-induced intrastrand crosslinks) to evolve into more deleterious types of DNA damage like DSBs. β-HPV E6 expressing cells have been shown to contain a significantly larger portion of multinucleated cells *in vitro* (Wallace et al., 2014), pointing to a possible attenuation of the Hippo pathway. The Hippo pathway stabilizes p53, inactivates the oncogene YAP and induces apoptosis in the event of failed cytokinesis (Harvey et al., 2013; Ganem et al., 2014). The mechanisms through which β-HPV E6 disrupts the DDR are depicted in the upper left panel of **Figure 2**.

In addition to p300-dependent checkpoint inhibition, β-HPV 5E6 and 8E6 can bind the transcription factor SMAD3, thereby inhibiting the transforming growth factor-beta (TGF-β) pathway (Mendoza et al., 2006). TGF-β has a well-described dual role in carcinogenesis. In normal cells and early carcinomas, it acts as tumor suppressor through cytostatic effects. As the cancer progresses, the TGF-β aids proliferation, survival, invasion, and angiogenesis of tumor cells (Lebrun, 2012). Destabilization of the SMAD3 may attenuate these tumor suppressive effects by inhibiting the expression of CDK inhibitors p16, p17, p21, and p27 and possibly promoting unscheduled cell cycle progression from G1- into S-phase (Itoh et al., 2000; ten Dijke and Hill, 2004). Disruption of the TGF-β pathway has also been linked to an impaired function of DSB-repair following ionizing radiation (Kirshner et al., 2006; Bouquet et al., 2011; Kim et al., 2015).

Additional Functions of β-HPV E6

Additional notable functions of β-HPV E6 include hTERT stabilization (β-HPV 5, 20, 22, 38; Bedard et al., 2008; Gabet et al., 2008; Cornet et al., 2012), which may stabilize the genome by preventing unstably short telomers. Conversely, it could decrease genome fidelity by aborting the role of telomers as a "cellular clock" that prevent proliferation of older cells that are more likely to contain mutations (Sharma et al., 2003). Another target of β-HPV 5 and 8 E6 is the Notch signaling pathway. The Notch signaling pathway has been shown to have tumor suppressive functions in epithelial cells (Reichrath and Reichrath, 2012) and can decide cell fate (Lai, 2004). It can also act as a negative regulator of the ATM-dependent DDR (Vermezovic et al., 2015). β-HPV 5 and 8 interfere with the Notch signaling pathway through interaction with MAML1. The β-HPV E6-mediated repression of Notch signaling delays S-phase cell cycle exit and differentiation (Brimer et al., 2012; Meyers et al., 2013). Prolonged or perpetual existence in S-phase in combination with impaired DNA-damage signaling and attenuated DDR could lead to cross-amplification of these individual effects.

Summary

β-HPV E6 attenuates UV-induced apoptosis and DDR through interaction with multiple targets. BAK degradation and prevention of apoptosis is highly conserved throughout the β-HPV genus. Less common is the inhibition of apoptosis through direct interaction with and degradation of p53 (β-HPV 49, E6AP mediated) or the inhibition of p53 activation (β-HPV 23 through HIPK2 interaction). β-HPV 17, 38, and 92 E6 interact with p53 directly, leading to its stabilization but altering or restricting p53's transcriptional activity. β-HPV 5, 8, and 38 E6 interfere with DDR and checkpoint signaling through interaction with p300. A combination of inhibited apoptosis, impaired DNA damage signaling and attenuated DSB response bears a potential to destabilize the genome over time or cause carcinogenesis in combination with DNA-damaging agents that is consistent with β-HPV's proposed contribution to skin cancer. Notably, although through markedly different mechanisms, high risk α-HPV oncogenes similarly contribute to tumorigenesis by impairing the cellular response to genome destabilizing events.

E7 AND ITS INFLUENCE ON CELL CYCLE PROGRESSION AND DDR

Promotion of Cell Cycle Progression

A canonical function of the high risk α-HPV E7 oncogene is the degradation of the tumor suppressor pRb (Moody and Laimins, 2010). In normal cells, the function of pRb is the suppression of E2F transcription factor dependent genes through binding E2F and inhibiting its association with promoters (Dyson, 1998). E2F-family proteins facilitate cell cycle progression and proliferation by promoting the expression of a variety of genes encoding for proteins involved in G1/S-phase transition (Bertoli et al., 2013). High risk α-HPV E7 oncogenes bind directly to pRb via the highly conserved LXCXE binding motif (Münger et al., 1989). This leads to the disruption of the E2F—pRb complex, allows E2F to bind to its transcriptional targets (Chellappan et al., 1992). E2F target expression (for example cyclin A or cyclin E) then facilitate premature cell cycle progression and S-phase entry (Zerfass et al., 1995). Cell cycle checkpoints are meant to pause the cell cycle in case of DNA damage and allow time to repair the damage, or, if the damage surpasses a threshold, induce senescence or apoptosis. Cell cycle checkpoints are an integral part of a cells quest to maintain genome integrity. Consequently, attenuated checkpoint activation leads to a destabilization of the genome through accumulating DNA damage (Malumbres and Barbacid, 2009). α-HPV E7 allows keratinocytes with damaged DNA to progress through cell cycle check points, even when p53 is induced (Demers et al., 1994). Much like these α-HPV

E7s, several of the β-HPV E7s (β-HPV 5, 8, 38, 49) can interact with Rb (Yamashita et al., 1993; Caldeira et al., 2003; Cornet et al., 2012). However, the β-HPV E7 interactions tend to cause a hyperphosphorylation of Rb in Keratinocytes, rather than its destabilization (Caldeira et al., 2003; Cornet et al., 2012). Hyperphosphorylation of Rb inhibits its ability to bind and inactivate E2F, allowing E2F to promote transcription of its target genes (Bertoli et al., 2013). Additionally, β-HPV 24, 38, and 49 E7 severely attenuate pRb half-life in rodent fibroblasts, while β-HPV 14, 22, 23, and 36 do not affect pRb's half-life (Cornet et al., 2012). Cornet et al. also found that in the context of E6 and E7 expressing cells, β-HPV 14 and 22 can degrade pRb, but do not induce the expression of cyclin A or Cdk1. Cdk1 is essential for cell cycle progression(Santamaria et al., 2007).

Alteration of the p53-Transcriptional Network

The tumor suppressor p53 is an essential factor in the avoidance of inappropriate cell proliferation in the presence of genotoxic stress. It has transcriptional targets in several pathways, including DNA damage tolerance and apoptosis (Espinosa et al., 2003; Yu and Zhang, 2005; Beckerman and Prives, 2010). While the mechanisms of how high Risk α-HPV E7 disrupts p53 activity remain a poorly defined, significantly more is known about how some β-HPV E7 proteins disrupt this essential tumor suppressor. ΔNp73 is an important antagonist of the p53 gene family and participating in a negative feedback loop with p53 (Bailey et al., 2011). β-HPV-38 E7 promotes the accumulation and stability of ΔNp73α through both transcriptional and post-translational mechanisms (Accardi et al., 2006, p.73; Saidj et al., 2013). β-HPV 38 E7 promotes the accumulation of double monophosphorylated p53 (serine 15 and 392) in the nucleus. These dual p53 phosphorylation events increase ΔNp73α expression. β-HPV 38 E7 also mediates the nuclear translocation of the IκB kinase (IKKβ) that increases the stability of ΔNp73α by phosphorylating it at serine 422 (Accardi et al., 2011). Furthermore, IKKβ, ΔNp73α, DNMT1, and EZH2 form a transcription regulatory complex. This complex is able to bind to a subset of p53 regulated promoters and interferes with the expression of DDR pathway- and apoptosis-related genes, but not with pro-survival genes like Survivin. This implies a role of β-HPV-38 E7 in the inhibition of p53 dependent apoptosis and allows for speculation on the influence of β-HPV E7 over DDR-proteins that depend on p53 activity as a transcriptional factor (for example Polη of the TLS pathway and XPC of the NER pathway) (Fischer, 2017).

Other Functions Related to DDR

A systematic screening of E7 interacting protein has shown that E7 from β-HPVs 8, 25, and 92 can interact with the tyrosine phosphatase and tumor suppressor PTPN14. While several high- and low-risk α-HPV types have been shown to degrade PTPN14 (White et al., 2016; Szalmás et al., 2017), the role of the β-HPV E7—PTPN14 interaction is yet to be investigated. PTPN14 is a required regulator of the Hippo signaling pathway, as it is necessary for the translocation of the Hippo transcription factor, YAP1, from the nucleus to the cytoplasm (Wang et al., 2012). This indicates that β-HPV E7 may attenuate the Hippo pathway, if β-HPV E7 proves to also be capable of PTPN14 destabilization. The Hippo pathway plays a crucial role in the control of proliferation and induces apoptosis in the event of cytokinesis (Ganem et al., 2014). Phosphorylation of Yap1, a part of the hippo pathway, is a critical step in the induction of apoptosis in response to DNA damage (Levy et al., 2008). β-HPV infections occur in the skin and thus in an environment where UV-induced cell cycle arrest and apoptosis occur with some frequency. As a result, it would not be surprising if there yet undiscovered abilities of β-HPV E7 to disconnect the cellular response to UV in manners that promote the β-HPV lifecycle.

MOUSE MODELS: EVIDENCE FOR A ROLE OF β-HPV IN CARCINOGENESIS VIA A HIT AND RUN MECHANISM

Mouse models can be an effective tool for elucidating the oncogenic potential of β-HPVs. The most common of these is the transgenic (tg) mouse model that expresses can individual and groups of β-HPV genes (E2, E6, E7, E6/E7) or the entire early region of the virus under a keratin promoter. Placing the expression under a keratin promoter restricts expression to keratinocytes, the cell type infected by β-HPV. The result is that genes are only expressed at anatomical sites relevant in the context of β-HPV infections. Our review of the literature shows that β-HPV 8 is the most frequently investigated β-HPV type, followed by β-HPV 38, β-HPV 49, and β-HPV 20. Additionally, one study has investigated β-HPV 5 E7 in a nude mouse/artificial skin graft model (Buitrago-Pérez et al., 2012).

β-HPV 8 Transgenic-Mouse Models

Schaper et al. established the first β-HPV tg-model using the Keratin 14 (K14) promoter to express the entire early gene region of β-HPV 8. Transgene expression was the highest for E2, followed by E6 and E7 (Schaper et al., 2005). While the tg-negative littermates did not develop lesions on the skin or other organs, 91% of the β-HPV 8 tg-positive mice developed single- or multifocal benign tumors. Of this population, 25% showed varying degrees of dysplasia and finally 6% developed SCCs spontaneously. The SCCs developed without additional DNA-damaging events. This established an *in vivo* link between β-HPV 8 and carcinogenesis. A caveat, however, is the stable oncogene expression in tg-mice. β-HPV infections, and therefore expression of β-HPV genes in the immunocompetent population, are transient.

In a follow up study, a possible role of β-HPV 8 E2 in skin tumor induction was revealed when 60% of the E2 positive population, but none of the E2 negative population developed spontaneous ulcerous lesions of the skin (Pfefferle et al., 2008). Moreover, 3 weeks after UV irradiation, 87% of a tg-mouse line with high E2 expression levels and 36% of a tg-mouse line with lower E2 expression levels developed skin tumors. On the other hand, irradiation of tg-negative mice did not lead to tumor formation. This could point toward a potential synergy between β-HPV 8 E2, E6, and E7 for their role in carcinogenesis.

Later, by expressing E6 individually under the K14 promoter, it was shown that β-HPV 8 E6 is the major driving force behind both spontaneous tumor development in tg-mice and that tumor formation could be prevented via DNA vaccination (Marcuzzi et al., 2009, 2014). Rapid tumor development by induction, either through UV irradiation or wounding, was demonstrated. This observation that persistent β-HPV 8 infections combined with UV exposure and wound healing processes pose a significant risk factor for skin cancer is consistent with observations in individuals with persistent β-HPV 8 infections due to EV. A potential role of the signal transducer and activator of transcription 3 (Stat3) was demonstrated in tg mice expressing the early region of β-HPV 8 that additionally had an epidermis restricted ablation of Stat3 (Andrea et al., 2010, p.3). The Stat3 heterozygous line was significantly less prone to spontaneous tumor development and these tumors did not progress to malignancy. Hufbauer et al. showed that β-HPV 8 E6 expressing tg-mice dysregulate mi-RNA expression (Hufbauer et al., 2011). Following UV induced inflammation and wound healing, the levels of mi-RNA for regulatory targets including cell-cycle (Rb) and apoptosis (PTEN, PDCD4) remained dysregulated, while dysregulation in wt-mice was transient. Hufbauer et al. also demonstrated that β-HPV 8 E6 expression leads to an impaired DNA-damage response in tg-mice following UV irradiation (Hufbauer et al., 2015). β-HPV 8 E6 expressing mice were shown to be thymine-dimer positive for an extended period while wt-mice efficiently repaired the UV induced DNA damage within 48 h. More importantly, probing for the DSB marker, γH2AX, revealed that the persistence of UV induced lesions in β-HPV 8 E6 expressing cells ultimately led to the formation of highly mutagenic and more dangerous DSBs. Immunohistochemical analysis of tg-mouse skin biopsies showed an increased signal for γH2AX at both, early (3d, 5d) and later (13d, 24d) timepoints. This not only demonstrates β-HPV 8 E6's attenuation of DDR, but also its ability to enhance the cells tolerance of persistent and increasingly severe DNA-damage. UV radiation typically causes intrastrand lesions that are tolerated by TLS- and repaired by NER-pathway. If this type of damage persists it will lead to increased rates of DSBs. The emergence and persistence of DSBs could point toward a broad influence of β-HPV 8 E6 on the DNA-damage response machinery, stretching from pathways meant to handle minor DNA damage (TLS, NER) to pathways that control and repair highly mutagenic DSBs (NHEJ, HR).

The role of β-HPV 8 E7 has also been investigated in tg-mice (Sperling et al., 2012; Heuser et al., 2016). It was shown that β-HPV 8 E7, but not β-HPV 8 E6 enables an escape from the immune response of β-HPV 8^+ lesions. β-HPV 8 E7 achieved this by inhibiting chemotactic signaling. β-HPV 8 E7 binds to C/EBPβ and inhibits its interaction with the CCL20 promoter, leading to decreased levels of CCL20, a chemoattractant for Langerhans cells. β-HPV 8 E7 is also critical for the invasiveness of hyperproliferating keratinocytes by dysregulating cell-cell interactions.

β-HPV 38 Transgenic-Mouse Models

While β-HPV 8 tg-mice demonstrated spontaneous tumor formation, tg-models of other β-HPV types do not exhibit the same behavior. Dong et al. showed that a mouse model for β-HPV 38 E6/E7 expressing mice under the Keratin 10 promoter exhibit hyperproliferation of the skin, but require external stimuli for carcinogenesis (Dong et al., 2005). Furthermore, ΔNp73α has been identified as integral to the attenuation of cell cycle arrest after UV exposure (Dong et al., 2007). Loss of p53 attenuated ΔNp73α expression and partially restored cell cycle arrest while loss of p73 lead to loss of ΔNp73α and consequently to high levels of p21 expression and cell cycle arrest after UV exposure. Differential susceptibility to chemically induced (DMBA/TPA) carcinogenesis correlates with differential oncogene expression levels and indicates a dose-dependency for risk of carcinogenesis. Irradiation of wt-mice with a single UV-dose led to accumulation of p21 and cell cycle arrest in the epidermis, while β-HPV 38 E6/E7 expressing mice inhibited cell cycle arrest through attenuation of p21 accumulation. Chronic irradiation of tg-mice with UV led to the formation of AK-like lesions that are considered precursors to SCCs in humans, while wt-mice did not develop lesions. Some of the AK-like lesions progressed to SCCs after 22 weeks (Viarisio et al., 2011). This provides evidence for the carcinogenesis-risk amplifying potential of the β-HPV 38 oncogenes E6 and E7.

Other β-HPV Transgenic-Mouse Models

The K14 tg-model for β-HPV 49 E6/E7 does neither show spontaneous tumor development nor tumor development after UV-irradiation (Viarisio et al., 2016). However, the β-HPV 49 tg-mice lines where susceptible to chemically induced carcinogenesis of the upper digestive tract. When exposed to 4 nitroquinoline 1-oxide (4NQO), 87% of the β-HPV 49 tg-mice developed tumors in the upper digestive tract while 4NQO treatment had little effect on β-HPV 38 tg-mice, which are susceptible to UV-triggered skin carcinogenesis.

A model for β-HPV 20 E6/E7 showed enhanced proliferation and papilloma formation in the evaluated transgenic lines, when compared to non-transgenic controls (Michel et al., 2006). Chronic exposure to UV radiation led to the development of SCCs and proliferation was enhanced for several weeks after UV treatment. The tg-lines also showed a reduced expression of differentiation markers (involucrin & loricrin and irregular patterns of p53 expression post UV, while controls showed a continued expression of proliferation markers and even expression of p53.

Summary

Mouse models provide a valuable *in vivo* tool to dissect the relative ability of β-HPV genes to induce tumorigenesis. They also allow a distinction between different carcinogenic potentials exhibited by E2, E6, or E7 to be accessed. The mouse models make it evident that β-HPV E6 carries a particularly high potential due to its effects on both apoptotic pathways and the DDR. The tg-mouse models also support the "hit and run" hypothesis regarding β-HPV induced malignancies, since most models require external stimuli to induce malignant tumors. β-HPV 8 has the potential for spontaneous transformation in tg-models, but it remains unclear whether the potential persists when β-HPV 8 early gene expression is transient, as it is the case in most humans. It also should be pointed out that the average daily UV dose of an American is ~94 J/m^2 (Godar et al., 2001), while the dosages used in the β-HPV tg-model studies discussed here reach 45-fold great levels. Although constrains in experimental design may require doses of this magnitude, it is a necessary caveat to considered when evaluating tg models of β-HPV induced skin cancer.

CONCLUSIONS

The impact of genus β-HPV on the DNA damage as well as the ability of these viruses to induce carcinogenesis is diverse and manifest in both *in vitro* and *in vivo* investigations. Generally, β-HPV viruses effect on DDR may be explained by their interest of uninterrupted proliferation, despite the presence of DNA damage. While most β-HPV E6 inhibit apoptosis by degrading the pro-apoptotic protein BAK, only a subset (β-HPV 5 and 8 E6) bind p300 strongly enough to destabilize the histone acetyltransferase, causing delayed repair of thymine dimers and double strand breaks (Giampieri and Storey, 2004; Muench et al., 2010; Howie et al., 2011; Hufbauer et al., 2011; Wallace et al., 2012, 2013, 2015). A larger subset of β-HPV E6 proteins (β-HPV 5, 8, 17, 23, 38, 49, and 92) interfere with p53 activity, but they do so through different mechanisms. Continuing the theme of diversity among β-HPVs, β-HPV 38 E6 immortalizes cells through a ΔNp73α-dependent mechanism, while β-HPV 49 E6 acts more similarly to high risk α-HPV E6, immortalizing cells through interactions with E6AP and NFX1-91 (Caldeira et al., 2003; Gabet et al., 2008; Muench et al., 2010). **Figure 2** depicts these diverse effects of β-HPV E6.

There are notable differences between β-HPV E7 proteins as well. A large cohort of these viral proteins (β-HPV 5, 8, 24, 38, and 49 E7) impair pRB function. The sole mechanism of pRB interference by β-HPV 5 and 8 E7 is through binding and induction of hyperphosphorylation of pRB. In addition to promoting the phosphorylation of pRB, β-HPV 38 and 49 E7 also decrease the half-life of pRB. β-HPV 24 E7 is only known to reduce pRB's half-life. Further, β-HPV 38 E7 has the ability to interfere with p53 activity by stabilizing the p53 antagonist, ΔNp73α, and increase inhibitory post-translational modifications of p53.

Not surprisingly, *in vivo* transgenic mouse models of β-HPV associated tumorigenesis reflect the varied ability of β-HPV to degrade the fidelity of host cells (Dong et al., 2005; Michel et al., 2006; Viarisio et al., 2011). The tg-mouse models of β-HPV 8 show spontaneous tumor formation (Schaper et al., 2005; Pfefferle et al., 2008; Marcuzzi et al., 2009). While carcinogenesis is augmented by UV exposure in β-HPV 8 mouse models, similar models of other β-HPV induced cancers (β-HPV 20, 38, and 49) require external stimulants to develop tumors. The required stimulants vary as well. Expression of β-HPV 20 and 38 proteins cause cancer in mice exposed to UV, but only β-HPV 49 proteins cause upper digestive tract tumors after exposure to 4NQO. Notably, the transient nature of β-HPV infections in immunocompetent individuals is not reflected in the mouse models discussed above and the ability of persistent β-HPV infection to cause cancer is generally accepted. Further, the amount of UV exposure necessary to cause tumors in β-HPV tg mice is often well above what humans typically receive. Thus, new *in vivo* models will be quintessential to drive the field forward and may include mice infected with the murine papillomavirus (MmuPV1) that recapitulates some but not all of the characteristics of β-HPV (Meyers et al., 2017).

The bulk of evidence for β-HPV infections playing a role in NMSCs suggests that β-HPV 5, 8, and 38 are the most tumorigenic, with a particular and unsurprising emphasis on

TABLE 1 | Characteristics and differences of several β-HPV strands and high risk α-HPVs.

	HPV5	HPV8	HPV38	HPV49	high risk αHPVs
Impact on DDR	•Delay UV repair •Destabilize p300 •ATM, ATR, BRCA1/2 ↓	•Delay UV repair •Destabilize p300 •ATM, ATR, BRCA1/2 ↓	•Delayed UV repair •ΔNp73α ↑ •Inhibit p300	•Unknown	•Attenuate and repurpose several DDR proteins
Prevention of Apoptosis	•Degrade BAK	•Degrade BAK	•Stabilize p53 •Alter p53 activity •Degrade BAK	•Degrade p53	•Degrade p53
Proliferation	•Hyperphosphorylate pRb	•Hyperphosphorylate pRb	•Attenuate p21 accumulation •Phosphorylate pRB	•Hyperphosphorylate pRb	•Degrade pRb
Immortalization	•No	•No	•Yes	•Yes	•Yes
Tumor maintenance	•Not required	•Not required	•Not required	•Not required	•Required
E6 motif	•No PDZ domain	•No PDZ domain	•No PDZ domain	•No PDZ domain	•PDZ domain present
Animal Models	•Artificial skin graft model •UV-induced lesion formation	•Spontaneous tumor formation	•UV DNA damage induced tumor formation	•No cSCC formation •Chemically-induced carcinogenesis in digestive tract	•Spontaneous tumor formation

This table compares the impact of several β-HPVs and high risk α-HPVs on DDR and other pathways relevant to carcinogenesis. ↑ and ↓ indicate increased or decreased abundance, respectively.

the homologous of high risk α-HPV oncogenes (E6 and E7). These viruses are expected to promote carcinogenesis via the "hit and run" model that is dependent on their amplification of UV's genome destabilizing effects and otherwise decreasing genome fidelity. Since the mechanisms of abrogating genome stability vary among β-HPVs, it is reasonable to expect that the carcinogenic potential of individual β-HPVs depends on their cellular environment during infection. As a result, not only is the clear delineation of pathways and proteins impacted by β-HPV necessary to understand their oncogenic potential, but also the relative ability among β-HPVs to disrupt these pathways. A major knowledge gap regarding β-HPV induced oncogenesis is the extent that the reduced availability of ATM, ATR, BRCA1, and BRCA2 affects the activity of these proteins in each of the repair pathways that they participate in. This could expand the known ability of β-HPV proteins to disrupt DNA repair to include nearly every cellular response to damaged DNA. Alternatively, if the impairment of these repair proteins was context specific, it could highlight particularly deleterious situations for a β-HPV infection to occur. Further, there is a diversity of genome destabilizing events beyond DNA damage (failed cytokinesis, centrosome duplication errors, etc.) that if disrupted would fit the ascribed "hit and run" model of tumorigenesis. Defining the mutagenic potential of β-HPV infections is essential to take next steps in preventing disease associated with these viruses. **Table 1** compares β-HPV 5, 8, 38, and 49 as well as high-risk α-HPV oncogenes regarding their oncogenic potential. A possible intervention is the development of β-HPV specific vaccines. While β-HPV infection occurs in early childhood, a vaccine against specific "high-risk" types may prevent re-infection. Additionally, immunity acquired through vaccination may be more effective than immunity through infection. The FDA-approved technology to make the current vaccine could be readily adapted to prevent β-HPV infections or specific inhibitors of β-HPVs could be developed and added to sunscreens to precisely target the intersection of UV and viral infection. A commonly stated challenge to the development of a vaccine against β-HPV is the fact that these infections are initially acquired soon after birth and that β-HPV infections do not illicit a protective immune response. Although true, vaccination could mitigate disease by preventing reinfection and potential initial infection with particularly oncogenic β-HPVs not necessarily acquired at birth. Further, vaccination is effective against members of the alpha HPV genus despite poor natural adaptive immune responses to those infections. Ultimately, these ambitious goals are dependent on advancements in the dissection of β-HPV biology and its ability to hinder the cellular DDR.

AUTHOR CONTRIBUTIONS

Wrote the manuscript: SW and NW. Reviewed and edited the manuscript: SW and NW.

ACKNOWLEDGMENTS

The authors would like to thank Dr. Zhilong Yang for providing his valuable insight and feedback on the manuscript.

REFERENCES

Accardi, R., Dong, W., Smet, A., Cui, R., Hautefeuille, A., Gabet, A. S., et al. (2006). Skin human papillomavirus type 38 alters p53 functions by accumulation of deltaNp73. *EMBO Rep.* 7, 334–340. doi: 10.1038/sj.embor.7400615

Accardi, R., Scalise, M., Gheit, T., Hussain, I., Yue, J., Carreira, C., et al. (2011). IkappaB kinase beta promotes cell survival by antagonizing p53 functions through DeltaNp73alpha phosphorylation and stabilization. *Mol. Cell. Biol.* 31, 2210–2226. doi: 10.1128/MCB.00964-10

Andrea, M. D., Rittà, M., Landini, M. M., Borgogna, C., Mondini, M., Kern, F., et al. (2010). Keratinocyte-specific stat3 heterozygosity impairs development of skin tumors in human papillomavirus 8 transgenic mice. *Cancer Res.* 70, 7938–7948. doi: 10.1158/0008-5472.CAN-10-1128

Antonsson, A., Karanfilovska, S., Lindqvist, P. G., and Hansson, B. G. (2003). General acquisition of human papillomavirus infections of skin occurs in early infancy. *J. Clin. Microbiol.* 41, 2509–2514. doi: 10.1128/JCM.41.6.2509-2514.2003

Arron, S. T., Ruby, J. G., Dybbro, E., Ganem, D., and DeRisi, J. L. (2011). Transcriptome sequencing demonstrates that human papillomavirus is not active in cutaneous squamous cell carcinoma. *J. Invest. Dermatol.* 131, 1745–1753. doi: 10.1038/jid.2011.91

Bailey, S. G., Cragg, M. S., and Townsend, P. A. (2011). Family friction as ΔNp73 antagonises p73 and p53. *Int. J. Biochem. Cell Biol.* 43, 482–486. doi: 10.1016/j.biocel.2010.12.022

Banin, S., Moyal, L., Shieh, S., Taya, Y., Anderson, C. W., Chessa, L., et al. (1998). Enhanced phosphorylation of p53 by ATM in response to DNA damage. *Science* 281, 1674–1677. doi: 10.1126/science.281.5383.1674

Bavinck, J. N. B., Plasmeijer, E. I., and Feltkamp, M. C. W. (2008). β-Papillomavirus infection and skin cancer. *J. Invest. Dermatol.* 128, 1355–1358. doi: 10.1038/jid.2008.123

Beckerman, R., and Prives, C. (2010). Transcriptional Regulation by P53. *Cold Spring Harb. Perspect. Biol.* 2:a000935. doi: 10.1101/cshperspect.a000935

Bedard, K. M., Underbrink, M. P., Howie, H. L., and Galloway, D. A. (2008). The E6 oncoproteins from human betapapillomaviruses differentially activate telomerase through an E6AP-dependent mechanism and prolong the lifespan of primary keratinocytes. *J. Virol.* 82, 3894–3902. doi: 10.1128/JVI.01818-07

Bernard, H. U., Burk, R. D., Chen, Z., van Doorslaer, K., zur Hausen, H., and de Villiers, E. M. (2010). Classification of papillomaviruses (PVs) based on 189 PV types and proposal of taxonomic amendments. *Virology* 401, 70–79. doi: 10.1016/j.virol.2010.02.002

Bertoli, C., Skotheim, J. M., and de Bruin, R. A. M. (2013). Control of cell cycle transcription during G1 and S phases. *Nat. Rev. Mol. Cell Biol.* 14, 518–528. doi: 10.1038/nrm3629

Bouquet, F., Pal, A., Pilones, K. A., Demaria, S., Hann, B., Akhurst, R. J., et al. (2011). TGFβ1 inhibition increases the radiosensitivity of breast cancer cells *in vitro* and promotes tumor control by radiation *in vivo*. *Clin. Cancer Res. Off. J. Am. Assoc. Cancer Res.* 17, 6754–6765. doi: 10.1158/1078-0432.CCR-11-0544

Bouvard, V., Baan, R., Straif, K., Grosse, Y., Secretan, B., Ghissassi, F. E., et al. (2009). A review of human carcinogens—Part B: biological agents. *Lancet Oncol.* 10, 321–322. doi: 10.1016/S1470-2045(09)70096-8

Bouwes, B., Neale, R. E., Abeni, D., Euvrard, S., Green, A. C., Harwood, C. A., et al. (2010). Multicenter study of the association between betapapillomavirus infection and cutaneous squamous cell carcinoma. *Cancer Res.* 70, 9777–9786. doi: 10.1158/0008-5472.CAN-10-0352

Bouwes Bavinck, J. N., Feltkamp, M., Struijk, L., and ter Schegget, J. (2001). Human papillomavirus infection and skin cancer risk in organ transplant recipients. *J. Investig. Dermatol. Symp. Proc.* 6, 207–211. doi: 10.1046/j.0022-202x.2001.00048.x

Boyer, S. N., Wazer, D. E., and Band, V. (1996). E7 protein of human papilloma virus-16 induces degradation of retinoblastoma protein through the ubiquitin-proteasome pathway. *Cancer Res.* 56, 4620–4624.

Boyle, J., Briggs, J. D., Mackie, R., Junor, B. J. R., and Aitchison, T. C. (1984). Cancer, warts, and sunshine in renal transplant patients. *Lancet* 323, 702–705. doi: 10.1016/S0140-6736(84)92221-9

Branzei, D., and Foiani, M. (2008). Regulation of DNA repair throughout the cell cycle. *Nat. Rev. Mol. Cell Biol.* 9, 297–308. doi: 10.1038/nrm2351

Brash, D. E., Rudolph, J. A., Simon, J. A., Lin, A., McKenna, G. J., Baden, H. P., et al. (1991). A role for sunlight in skin cancer: UV-induced p53 mutations in squamous cell carcinoma. *Proc. Natl. Acad. Sci. U.S.A.* 88, 10124–10128. doi: 10.1073/pnas.88.22.10124

Brimer, N., Lyons, C., Wallberg, A. E., and Vande Pol, S. B. (2012). Cutaneous papillomavirus E6 oncoproteins associate with MAML1 to repress transactivation and NOTCH signaling. *Oncogene* 31, 4639–4646. doi: 10.1038/onc.2011.589

Buitrago-Pérez, Á., Hachimi, M., Dueñas, M., Lloveras, B., Santos, A., Holguín, A., et al. (2012). A humanized mouse model of HPV-associated pathology driven by E7 expression. *PLoS ONE* 7:e41743. doi: 10.1371/journal.pone.0041743

Bzhalava, D., Eklund, C., and Dillner, J. (2015). International standardization and classification of human papillomavirus types. *Virology* 476, 341–344. doi: 10.1016/j.virol.2014.12.028

Bzhalava, D., Guan, P., Franceschi, S., Dillner, J., and Clifford, G. (2013). A systematic review of the prevalence of mucosal and cutaneous human papillomavirus types. *Virology* 445, 224–231. doi: 10.1016/j.virol.2013.07.015

Bzhalava, D., Mühr, L. S. A., Lagheden, C., Ekström, J., Forslund, O., Dillner, J., et al. (2014). Deep sequencing extends the diversity of human papillomaviruses in human skin. *Sci. Rep.* 4:5807. doi: 10.1038/srep05807

Caldeira, S., Zehbe, I., Accardi, R., Malanchi, I., Dong, W., Giarrè, M., et al. (2003). The E6 and E7 proteins of the cutaneous human papillomavirus type 38 display transforming properties. *J. Virol.* 77, 2195–2206. doi: 10.1128/JVI.77.3.2195-2206.2003

Carter, J. R., Ding, Z., and Rose, B. R. (2011). HPV infection and cervical disease: a review. *Aust. N. Z. J. Obstet. Gynaecol.* 51, 103–108. doi: 10.1111/j.1479-828X.2010.01269.x

Casabonne, D., Waterboer, T., Michael, K. M., Pawlita, M., Mitchell, L., Newton, R., et al. (2009). The seroprevalence of human papillomavirus by immune status and by ethnicity in London. *Infect. Agent. Cancer* 4:14. doi: 10.1186/1750-9378-4-14

Chahoud, J., Semaan, A., Chen, Y., Cao, M., Rieber, A. G., Rady, P., et al. (2016). Association between β-genus human papillomavirus and cutaneous squamous cell carcinoma in immunocompetent individuals—a meta-analysis. *JAMA Dermatol.* 152, 1354–1364. doi: 10.1001/jamadermatol.2015.4530

Chellappan, S., Kraus, V. B., Kroger, B., Munger, K., Howley, P. M., Phelps, W. C., et al. (1992). Adenovirus E1A, simian virus 40 tumor antigen, and human papillomavirus E7 protein share the capacity to disrupt the interaction between transcription factor E2F and the retinoblastoma gene product. *Proc. Natl. Acad. Sci. U.S.A.* 89, 4549–4553. doi: 10.1073/pnas.89.10.4549

Chen, X., Ko, L. J., Jayaraman, L., and Prives, C. (1996). p53 levels, functional domains, and DNA damage determine the extent of the apoptotic response of tumor cells. *Genes Dev.* 10, 2438–2451. doi: 10.1101/gad.10.19.2438

Chen, Y.-W., Cleaver, J. E., Hatahet, Z., Honkanen, R. E., Chang, J.-Y., Yen, Y., et al. (2008). Human DNA polymerase eta activity and translocation is regulated by phosphorylation. *Proc. Natl. Acad. Sci. U.S.A.* 105, 16578–16583. doi: 10.1073/pnas.0808589105

Cheng, Q., and Chen, J. (2010). Mechanism of p53 stabilization by ATM after DNA damage. *Cell Cycle Georget. Tex* 9, 472–478. doi: 10.4161/cc.9.3.10556

Chittenden, T., Harrington, E. A. O., Connor, R., Flemington, C., Lutz, R. J., Evan, G. I., et al. (1995). Induction of apoptosis by the Bcl-2 homologue Bak. *Nature* 374, 733–736. doi: 10.1038/374733a0

Cornet, I., Bouvard, V., Campo, M. S., Thomas, M., Banks, L., Gissmann, L., et al. (2012). Comparative analysis of transforming properties of E6 and E7 from different beta human papillomavirus types. *J. Virol.* 86, 2366–2370. doi: 10.1128/JVI.06579-11

Cubie, H. A. (2013). Diseases associated with human papillomavirus infection. *Virology* 445, 21–34. doi: 10.1016/j.virol.2013.06.007

D'Andrea, A. D. (2013). BRCA1: a missing link in the Fanconi anemia/BRCA pathway. *Cancer Discov.* 3, 376–378. doi: 10.1158/2159-8290.CD-13-0044

D'Souza, G., and Dempsey, A. (2011). The role of HPV in head and neck cancer and review of the HPV vaccine. *Prev. Med.* 53, S5–S11. doi: 10.1016/j.ypmed.2011.08.001

de Koning, M. N. C., Weissenborn, S. J., Abeni, D., Bouwes Bavinck, J. N., Euvrard, S., Green, A. C., et al. (2009). Prevalence and associated factors of betapapillomavirus infections in individuals without cutaneous squamous cell carcinoma. *J. Gen. Virol.* 90, 1611–1621. doi: 10.1099/vir.0.010017-0

Dell'Oste, V., Azzimonti, B., De Andrea, M., Mondini, M., Zavattaro, E., Leigheb, G., et al. (2009). High β-HPV DNA loads and strong seroreactivity are present in epidermodysplasia verruciformis. *J. Invest. Dermatol.* 129, 1026–1034. doi: 10.1038/jid.2008.317

Demers, G. W., Foster, S. A., Halbert, C. L., and Galloway, D. A. (1994). Growth arrest by induction of p53 in DNA damaged keratinocytes is bypassed by human papillomavirus 16 E7. *Proc. Natl. Acad. Sci. U.S.A.* 91, 4382–4386. doi: 10.1073/pnas.91.10.4382

de Oliveira, W. R. P., He, Q., Rady, P. L., Hughes, T. K., Neto, C. F., Rivitti, E. A., et al. (2004). HPV typing in Brazilian patients with epidermodysplasia verruciformis: high prevalence of EV-HPV 25. *J. Cutan. Med. Surg.* 8, 110–115. doi: 10.1177/120347540400800206

de Villiers, E.-M. (2013). Cross-roads in the classification of papillomaviruses. *Virology* 445, 2–10. doi: 10.1016/j.virol.2013.04.023

Domchek, S. M., Tang, J., Stopfer, J., Lilli, D. R., Hamel, N., Tischkowitz, M., et al. (2013). Biallelic deleterious BRCA1 mutations in a woman with early-onset ovarian cancer. *Cancer Discov.* 3, 399–405. doi: 10.1158/2159-8290.CD-12-0421

Dong, W., Arpin, C., Accardi, R., Gissmann, L., Sylla, B. S., Marvel, J., et al. (2007). Loss of p53 or p73 in human papillomavirus type 38 E6 and E7 transgenic mice partially restores the UV-activated cell cycle checkpoints. *Oncogene* 27, 2923–2928. doi: 10.1038/sj.onc.1210944

Dong, W., Kloz, U., Accardi, R., Caldeira, S., Tong, W.-M., Wang, Z.-Q., et al. (2005). Skin hyperproliferation and susceptibility to chemical carcinogenesis in transgenic mice expressing e6 and e7 of human papillomavirus type 38. *J. Virol.* 79, 14899–14908. doi: 10.1128/JVI.79.23.14899-14908.2005

Doorbar, J., Egawa, N., Griffin, H., Kranjec, C., and Murakami, I. (2015). Human papillomavirus molecular biology and disease association. *Rev. Med. Virol.* 25, 2–23. doi: 10.1002/rmv.1822

Dyson, N. (1998). The regulation of E2F by pRB-family proteins. *Genes Dev.* 12, 2245–2262. doi: 10.1101/gad.12.15.2245

Dyson, N., Howley, P. M., Munger, K., and Harlow, E. (1989). The human papilloma virus-16 E7 oncoprotein is able to bind to the retinoblastoma gene product. *Science* 243, 934–937. doi: 10.1126/science.2537532

Ekström, J., Mühr, L. S. A., Bzhalava, D., Söderlund-Strand, A., Hultin, E., Nordin, P., et al. (2013). Diversity of human papillomaviruses in skin lesions. *Virology* 447, 300–311. doi: 10.1016/j.virol.2013.09.010

Espinosa, J. M., Verdun, R. E., and Emerson, B. M. (2003). p53 functions through stress- and promoter-specific recruitment of transcription initiation components before and after DNA damage. *Mol. Cell* 12, 1015–1027. doi: 10.1016/S1097-2765(03)00359-9

Farzan, S. F., Waterboer, T., Gui, J., Nelson, H. H., Li, Z., Michael, K. M., et al. (2013). Cutaneous alpha, beta and gamma human papillomaviruses in relation to squamous cell carcinoma of the skin: a population-based study. *J. Int. Cancer* 133, 1713–1720. doi: 10.1002/ijc.28176

Fischer, M. (2017). Census and evaluation of p53 target genes. *Oncogene* 36, 3943–3956. doi: 10.1038/onc.2016.502

Forslund, O., Iftner, T., Andersson, K., Lindelof, B., Hradil, E., Nordin, P., et al. (2007). Cutaneous human papillomaviruses found in sun-exposed skin: beta-papillomavirus species 2 predominates in squamous cell carcinoma. *J. Infect. Dis.* 196, 876–883. doi: 10.1086/521031

Gabet, A.-S., Accardi, R., Bellopede, A., Popp, S., Boukamp, P., Sylla, B. S., et al. (2008). Impairment of the telomere/telomerase system and genomic instability are associated with keratinocyte immortalization induced by the skin human papillomavirus type 38. *FASEB J.* 22, 622–632. doi: 10.1096/fj.07-8389com

Ganem, N. J., Cornils, H., Chiu, S. Y., O'Rourke, K. P., Arnaud, J., Yimlamai, D., et al. (2014). Cytokinesis failure triggers hippo tumor suppressor pathway activation. *Cell* 158, 833–848. doi: 10.1016/j.cell.2014.06.029

Genders, R. E., Mazlom, H., Michel, A., Plasmeijer, E. I., Quint, K. D., Pawlita, M., et al. (2015). The presence of betapapillomavirus antibodies around transplantation predicts the development of keratinocyte carcinoma in organ transplant recipients: a cohort study. *J. Invest. Dermatol.* 135, 1275–1282. doi: 10.1038/jid.2014.456

Giampieri, S., and Storey, A. (2004). Repair of UV-induced thymine dimers is compromised in cells expressing the E6 protein from human papillomaviruses types 5 and 18. *Br. J. Cancer* 90, 2203–2209. doi: 10.1038/sj.bjc.6601829

Gillespie, K. A., Mehta, K. P., Laimins, L. A., and Moody, C. A. (2012). Human papillomaviruses recruit cellular DNA repair and homologous recombination factors to viral replication centers. *J. Virol.* 86, 9520–9526. doi: 10.1128/JVI.00247-12

Godar, D. E., Wengraitis, S. P., Shreffler, J., and Sliney, D. H. (2001). UV doses of americans. *Photochem. Photobiol.* 73, 621–629. doi: 10.1562/0031-8655(2001)074<0787:udoaca>2.0.co;2

Göhler, T., Sabbioneda, S., Green, C. M., and Lehmann, A. R. (2011). ATR-mediated phosphorylation of DNA polymerase η is needed for efficient recovery from UV damage. *J. Cell Biol.* 192, 219–227. doi: 10.1083/jcb.201008076

Goodman, R. H., and Smolik, S. (2000). CBP/p300 in cell growth, transformation, and development. *Genes Dev.* 14, 1553–1577. doi: 10.1101/gad.14.13.1553

Goodwin, E. C., and DiMaio, D. (2000). Repression of human papillomavirus oncogenes in HeLa cervical carcinoma cells causes the orderly reactivation of dormant tumor suppressor pathways. *Proc. Natl. Acad. Sci. U.S.A.* 97, 12513–12518. doi: 10.1073/pnas.97.23.12513

Goodwin, E. C., Yang, E., Lee, C.-J., Lee, H.-W., DiMaio, D., and Hwang, E.-S. (2000). Rapid induction of senescence in human cervical carcinoma cells. *Proc. Natl. Acad. Sci. U.S.A.* 97, 10978–10983. doi: 10.1073/pnas.97.20.10978

Hampras, S. S., Giuliano, A. R., Lin, H.-Y., Fisher, K. J., Abrahamsen, M. E., Sirak, B. A., et al. (2014). Natural history of Cutaneous Human Papillomavirus (HPV) infection in men: the HIM study. *PLoS ONE* 9:e104843. doi: 10.1371/journal.pone.0104843

Hampras, S. S., Rollison, D. E., Giuliano, A. R., McKay-Chopin, S., Minoni, L., Sereday, K., et al. (2017). Prevalence and concordance of cutaneous beta human papillomavirus infection at mucosal and cutaneous sites. *J. Infect. Dis.* 216, 92–96. doi: 10.1093/infdis/jix245

Harvey, K. F., Zhang, X., and Thomas, D. M. (2013). The Hippo pathway and human cancer. *Nat. Rev. Cancer* 13, 246–257. doi: 10.1038/nrc3458

Hazard, K., Karlsson, A., Andersson, K., Ekberg, H., Dillner, J., and Forslund, O. (2007). Cutaneous human papillomaviruses persist on healthy skin. *J. Invest. Dermatol.* 127, 116–119. doi: 10.1038/sj.jid.5700570

Heuser, S., Hufbauer, M., Marx, B., Tok, A., Majewski, S., Pfister, H., et al. (2016). The levels of epithelial anchor proteins β-catenin and zona occludens-1 are altered by E7 of human papillomaviruses 5 and 8. *J. Gen. Virol.* 97, 463–472. doi: 10.1099/jgv.0.000363

Hobbs, C. G., Sterne, J. A. C., Bailey, M., Heyderman, R. S., Birchall, M. A., and Thomas, S. J. (2006). Human papillomavirus and head and neck cancer: a systematic review and meta-analysis. *Clin. Otolaryngol.* 31, 259–266. doi: 10.1111/j.1749-4486.2006.01246.x

Holloway, A., Simmonds, M., Azad, A., Fox, J. L., and Storey, A. (2015). Resistance to UV-induced apoptosis by β-HPV5 E6 involves targeting of activated BAK for proteolysis by recruitment of the HERC1 ubiquitin ligase. *Int. J. Cancer* 136, 2831–2843. doi: 10.1002/ijc.29350

Hong, S., Cheng, S., Iovane, A., and Laimins, L. A. (2015). STAT-5 regulates transcription of the topoisomerase IIβ-binding protein 1 (TopBP1) gene to activate the ATR pathway and promote human papillomavirus replication. *mBio* 6, e02006–e02015. doi: 10.1128/mBio.02006-15

Howie, H. L., Koop, J. I., Weese, J., Robinson, K., Wipf, G., Kim, L., et al. (2011). Beta-HPV 5 and 8 E6 promote p300 degradation by blocking AKT/p300 association. *PLOS Pathog.* 7:e1002211. doi: 10.1371/journal.ppat.1002211

Howley, P. M., and Pfister, H. J. (2015). Beta genus papillomaviruses and skin cancer. *Virology* 479, 290–296. doi: 10.1016/j.virol.2015.02.004

Hsu, J. Y.-C., Chen, A. C. H., Keleher, A., McMillan, N. A. J., and Antonsson, A. (2009). Shared and persistent asymptomatic cutaneous human papillomavirus infections in healthy skin. *J. Med. Virol.* 81, 1444–1449. doi: 10.1002/jmv.21529

Hufbauer, M., and Akgül, B. (2017). Molecular mechanisms of human papillomavirus induced skin carcinogenesis. *Viruses* 9:187. doi: 10.3390/v9070187

Hufbauer, M., Cooke, J., van der, H., Pfister, H., Storey, A., and Akgül, B. (2015). Human papillomavirus mediated inhibition of DNA damage sensing and repair drives skin carcinogenesis. *Mol. Cancer* 14:183. doi: 10.1186/s12943-015-0453-7

Hufbauer, M., Lazic, D., Reinartz, M., Akgül, B., Pfister, H., and Weissenborn, S. J. (2011). Skin tumor formation in human papillomavirus 8 transgenic mice is associated with a deregulation of oncogenic miRNAs and their tumor suppressive targets. *J. Dermatol. Sci.* 64, 7–15. doi: 10.1016/j.jdermsci.2011.06.008

Huibregtse, J. M., Scheffner, M., and Howley, P. M. (1991). A cellular protein mediates association of p53 with the E6 oncoprotein of human papillomavirus types 16 or 18. *EMBO J.* 10, 4129–4135.

Hwang, E. S., Riese, D. J., Settleman, J., Nilson, L. A., Honig, J., Flynn, S., et al. (1993). Inhibition of cervical carcinoma cell line proliferation by the introduction of a bovine papillomavirus regulatory gene. *J. Virol.* 67, 3720–3729.

Iannacone, M. R., Gheit, T., Pfister, H., Giuliano, A. R., Messina, J. L., Fenske, N. A., et al. (2014). Case-control study of genus-beta human papillomaviruses in plucked eyebrow hairs and cutaneous squamous cell carcinoma. *J. Int. Cancer* 134, 2231–2244. doi: 10.1002/ijc.28552

Iannacone, M. R., Gheit, T., Waterboer, T., Giuliano, A. R., Messina, J. L., Fenske, N. A., et al. (2012). Case-control study of cutaneous human papillomaviruses in squamous cell carcinoma of the skin. *Cancer Epidemiol. Biomark. Prev.* 21, 1303–1313. doi: 10.1158/1055-9965.EPI-12-0032

Itoh, S., Itoh, F., Goumans, M. J., and Ten Dijke, P. (2000). Signaling of transforming growth factor-beta family members through Smad proteins. *Eur. J. Biochem.* 267, 6954–6967. doi: 10.1046/j.1432-1327.2000.01828.x

Jackson, S. P., and Bartek, J. (2009). The DNA-damage response in human biology and disease. *Nature* 461, 1071–1078. doi: 10.1038/nature08467

Jazayeri, A., Falck, J., Lukas, C., Bartek, J., Smith, G. C. M., Lukas, J., et al. (2006). ATM- and cell cycle-dependent regulation of ATR in response to DNA double-strand breaks. *Nat. Cell Biol.* 8, 37–45. doi: 10.1038/ncb1337

Jeggo, P. A., and Löbrich, M. (2007). DNA double-strand breaks: their cellular and clinical impact? *Oncogene* 26, 7717–7719. doi: 10.1038/sj.onc.1210868

Karagas, M. R., Waterboer, T., Li, Z., Nelson, H. H., Michael, K. M., Bavinck, J. N. B., et al. (2010). Genus β human papillomaviruses and incidence of basal cell and squamous cell carcinomas of skin: population based case-control study. *BMJ* 341:c2986. doi: 10.1136/bmj.c2986

Keohavong, P., Liu, V. F., and Thilly, W. G. (1991). Analysis of point mutations induced by ultraviolet light in human cells. *Mutat. Res.* 249, 147–159. doi: 10.1016/0027-5107(91)90141-A

Kim, M.-R., Lee, J., An, Y. S., Jin, Y. B., Park, I.-C., Chung, E., et al. (2015). TGFβ1 protects cells from γ-IR by enhancing the activity of the NHEJ repair pathway. *Mol. Cancer Res.* 13, 319–329. doi: 10.1158/1541-7786.MCR-14-0098-T

Kirshner, J., Jobling, M. F., Pajares, M. J., Ravani, S. A., Glick, A. B., Lavin, M. J., et al. (2006). Inhibition of transforming growth factor-β1 signaling attenuates ataxia telangiectasia mutated activity in response to genotoxic stress. *Cancer Res.* 66, 10861–10869. doi: 10.1158/0008-5472.CAN-06-2565

Kiviat, N. B. (1999). Papillomaviruses in non-melanoma skin cancer: epidemiological aspects. *Semin. Cancer Biol.* 9, 397–403. doi: 10.1006/scbi.1999.0143

Kiyono, T., Foster, S. A., Koop, J. I., McDougall, J. K., Galloway, D. A., and Klingelhutz, A. J. (1998). Both Rb/p16INK4a inactivation and telomerase activity are required to immortalize human epithelial cells. *Nature* 396, 84–88. doi: 10.1038/23962

Klingelhutz, A. J., Foster, S. A., and McDougall, J. K. (1996). Telomerase activation by the E6 gene product of human papillomavirus type 16. *Nature* 380, 79–82. doi: 10.1038/380079a0

Kracikova, M., Akiri, G., George, A., Sachidanandam, R., and Aaronson, S. A. (2013). A threshold mechanism mediates p53 cell fate decision between growth arrest and apoptosis. *Cell Death Differ.* 20, 576–588. doi: 10.1038/cdd.2012.155

Kremsdorf, D., Jablonska, S., Favre, M., and Orth, G. (1982). Biochemical characterization of two types of human papillomaviruses associated with epidermodysplasia verruciformis. *J. Virol.* 43, 436–447.

Kremsdorf, D., Jablonska, S., Favre, M., and Orth, G. (1983). Human papillomaviruses associated with epidermodysplasia verruciformis. II. Molecular cloning and biochemical characterization of human papillomavirus 3a, 8, 10, and 12 genomes. *J. Virol.* 48, 340–351.

Kruse, J. P., and Gu, W. (2009). Modes of p53 Regulation. *Cell* 137, 609–622. doi: 10.1016/j.cell.2009.04.050

Lai, E. C. (2004). Notch signaling: control of cell communication and cell fate. *Development* 131, 965–973. doi: 10.1242/dev.01074

Lebrun, J.-J. (2012). The dual role of TGF in human cancer: from tumor suppression to cancer metastasis. *Int. Sch. Res. Not.* 2012:381428. doi: 10.5402/2012/381428

Lee, T. H., Park, J. M., Leem, S. H., and Kang, T. H. (2014). Coordinated regulation of XPA stability by ATR and HERC2 during nucleotide excision repair. *Oncogene* 33, 19–25. doi: 10.1038/onc.2012.539

Lerner, L. K., Francisco, G., Soltys, D. T., Rocha, C. R. R., Quinet, A., Vessoni, A. T., et al. (2017). Predominant role of DNA polymerase eta and p53-dependent translesion synthesis in the survival of ultraviolet-irradiated human cells. *Nucleic Acids Res.* 45, 1270–1280. doi: 10.1093/nar/gkw1196

Levy, D., Adamovich, Y., Reuven, N., and Shaul, Y. (2008). Yap1 phosphorylation by c-Abl Is a critical step in selective activation of proapoptotic genes in response to DNA damage. *Mol. Cell* 29, 350–361. doi: 10.1016/j.molcel.2007.12.022

Malumbres, M., and Barbacid, M. (2009). Cell cycle, CDKs and cancer: a changing paradigm. *Nat. Rev. Cancer* 9, 153–166. doi: 10.1038/nrc2602

Mao, Z., Bozzella, M., Seluanov, A., and Gorbunova, V. (2008). DNA repair by nonhomologous end joining and homologous recombination during cell cycle in human cells. *Cell Cycle Georget. Tex* 7, 2902–2906. doi: 10.4161/cc.7.18.6679

Marcuzzi, G. P., Awerkiew, S., Hufbauer, M., Schädlich, L., Gissmann, L., Eming, S., et al. (2014). Tumor prevention in HPV8 transgenic mice by HPV8-E6 DNA vaccination. *Med. Microbiol. Immunol.* 203, 155–163. doi: 10.1007/s00430-014-0327-4

Marcuzzi, G. P., Hufbauer, M., Kasper, H. U., Weißenborn, S. J., Smola, S., and Pfister, H. (2009). Spontaneous tumour development in human papillomavirus type 8 E6 transgenic mice and rapid induction by UV-light exposure and wounding. *J. Gen. Virol.* 90, 2855–2864. doi: 10.1099/vir.0.012872-0

Maréchal, A., and Zou, L. (2013). DNA damage Sensing by the ATM and ATR kinases. *Cold Spring Harb. Perspect. Biol.* 5:a012716. doi: 10.1101/cshperspect.a012716

Maréchal, A., and Zou, L. (2015). RPA-coated single-stranded DNA as a platform for post-translational modifications in the DNA damage response. *Cell Res.* 25, 9–23. doi: 10.1038/cr.2014.147

Marteijn, J. A., Lans, H., Vermeulen, W., and Hoeijmakers, J. H. J. (2014). Understanding nucleotide excision repair and its roles in cancer and ageing. *Nat Rev. Mol. Cell Biol.* 15, 465–481. doi: 10.1038/nrm3822

Mendoza, J.-A., Jacob, Y., Cassonnet, P., and Favre, M. (2006). Human papillomavirus type 5 E6 oncoprotein represses the transforming growth factor β signaling pathway by binding to SMAD3. *J. Virol.* 80, 12420–12424. doi: 10.1128/JVI.02576-05

Meyer, T., Arndt, R., Christophers, E., Nindl, I., and Stockfleth, E. (2001). Importance of human papillomaviruses for the development of skin cancer. *Cancer Detect. Prev.* 25, 533–547.

Meyers, J. M., Spangle, J. M., and Munger, K. (2013). The human papillomavirus type 8 E6 protein interferes with NOTCH activation during keratinocyte differentiation. *J. Virol.* 87, 4762–4767. doi: 10.1128/JVI.02527-12

Meyers, J. M., Uberoi, A., Grace, M., Lambert, P. F., and Munger, K. (2017). Cutaneous HPV8 and MmuPV1 E6 proteins target the NOTCH and TGF-β tumor suppressors to inhibit differentiation and sustain keratinocyte proliferation. *PLOS Pathog.* 13:e1006171. doi: 10.1371/journal.ppat.1006171

Michel, A., Kopp-Schneider, A., Zentgraf, H., Gruber, A. D., and de Villiers, E.-M. (2006). E6/E7 expression of human papillomavirus type 20 (HPV-20) and HPV-27 influences proliferation and differentiation of the skin in UV-irradiated SKH-hr1 transgenic mice. *J. Virol.* 80, 11153–11164. doi: 10.1128/JVI.00954-06

Moldovan, G. L., and D'Andrea, A. D. (2009). How the Fanconi Anemia pathway guards the genome. *Annu. Rev. Genet.* 43, 223–249. doi: 10.1146/annurev-genet-102108-134222

Moody, C. A., and Laimins, L. A. (2009). Human papillomaviruses activate the ATM DNA damage pathway for viral genome amplification upon differentiation. *PLOS Pathog.* 5:e1000605. doi: 10.1371/journal.ppat.1000605

Moody, C. A., and Laimins, L. A. (2010). Human papillomavirus oncoproteins: pathways to transformation. *Nat. Rev. Cancer* 10, 550–560. doi: 10.1038/nrc2886

Moy, R. L. (2000). Clinical presentation of actinic keratoses and squamous cell carcinoma. *J. Am. Acad. Dermatol.* 42, S8–S10. doi: 10.1067/mjd.2000.103343

Muench, P., Probst, S., Schuetz, J., Leiprecht, N., Busch, M., Wesselborg, S., et al. (2010). Cutaneous papillomavirus E6 proteins must interact with p300 and block p53-mediated apoptosis for cellular immortalization and tumorigenesis. *Cancer Res.* 70, 6913–6924. doi: 10.1158/0008-5472.CAN-10-1307

Münger, K., Werness, B. A., Dyson, N., Phelps, W. C., Harlow, E., and Howley, P. M. (1989). Complex formation of human papillomavirus E7 proteins with the retinoblastoma tumor suppressor gene product. *EMBO J.* 8, 4099–4105.

Muschik, D., Braspenning-Wesch, I., Stockfleth, E., Rösl, F., Hofmann, T. G., and Nindl, I. (2011). Cutaneous HPV23 E6 prevents p53 phosphorylation through interaction with HIPK2. *PLoS ONE* 6:e27655. doi: 10.1371/journal.pone.0027655

Neale, R. E., Weissenborn, S., Abeni, D., Bavinck, J. N. B., Euvrard, S., Feltkamp, M. C. W., et al. (2013). Human papillomavirus load in eyebrow hair follicles and risk of cutaneous squamous cell carcinoma. *Cancer Epidemiol. Prev. Biomark.* 22, 719–727. doi: 10.1158/1055-9965.EPI-12-0917-T

Nindl, I., Koehler, A., Meyer, T., Forschner, T., Meijer, C. J. L. M., Snijders, P. J. F., et al. (2006). Detection of human papillomavirus DNA in primary squamous cell carcinoma and metastases. *Br. J. Dermatol.* 154, 797–799. doi: 10.1111/j.1365-2133.2006.07173.x

Offer, H., Erez, N., Zurer, I., Tang, X., Milyavsky, M., Goldfinger, N., et al. (2002). The onset of p53-dependent DNA repair or apoptosis is determined by the level of accumulated damaged DNA. *Carcinogenesis* 23, 1025–1032. doi: 10.1093/carcin/23.6.1025

Oh, S. T., Kyo, S., and Laimins, L. A. (2001). Telomerase activation by human papillomavirus type 16 E6 protein: induction of human telomerase reverse transcriptase expression through Myc and GC-Rich Sp1 binding sites. *J. Virol.* 75, 5559–5566. doi: 10.1128/JVI.75.12.5559-5566.2001

Orth, G. (1986). Epidermodysplasia verruciformis: a model for understanding the oncogenicity of human papillomaviruses. *Ciba Found. Symp.* 120, 157–174.

Pankotai, T., and Soutoglou, E. (2013). Double strand breaks. *Transcription* 4, 34–38. doi: 10.4161/trns.22879

Pao, G. M., Janknecht, R., Ruffner, H., Hunter, T., and Verma, I. M. (2000). CBP/p300 interact with and function as transcriptional coactivators of BRCA1. *Proc. Natl. Acad. Sci. U.S.A.* 97, 1020–1025. doi: 10.1073/pnas.97.3.1020

Patel, D., Huang, S. M., Baglia, L. A., and McCance, D. J. (1999). The E6 protein of human papillomavirus type 16 binds to and inhibits co-activation by CBP and p300. *EMBO J.* 18, 5061–5072. doi: 10.1093/emboj/18.18.5061

Pfefferle, R., Marcuzzi, G. P., Akgül, B., Kasper, H. U., Schulze, F., Haase, I., et al. (2008). The Human papillomavirus type 8 E2 protein induces skin tumors in transgenic mice. *J. Invest. Dermatol.* 128, 2310–2315. doi: 10.1038/jid.2008.73

Pfister, H. (2003). Chapter 8: human papillomavirus and skin cancer. *J. Natl. Cancer Inst. Monogr.* 52–56. doi: 10.1093/oxfordjournals.jncimonographs.a003483

Pfister, H., Nürnberger, F., Gissmann, L., and zur Hausen, H. (1981). Characterization of a human papillomavirus from epidermodysplasia verruciformis lesions of a patient from upper-volta. *Int. J. Cancer* 27, 645–650. doi: 10.1002/ijc.2910270511

Ray, A., Blevins, C., Wani, G., and Wani, A. A. (2016). ATR- and ATM-mediated DNA damage response is dependent on excision repair assembly during G1 but not in S phase of cell cycle. *PLoS ONE* 11:e0159344. doi: 10.1371/journal.pone.0159344

Ray, A., Milum, K., Battu, A., Wani, G., and Wani, A. A. (2013). NER initiation factors, DDB2 and XPC, regulate UV radiation response by recruiting ATR and ATM kinases to DNA damage sites. *DNA Repair* 12, 273–283. doi: 10.1016/j.dnarep.2013.01.003

Reichrath, J., and Reichrath, S. (2012). Notch-signaling and nonmelanoma skin cancer: an ancient friend, revisited. *Adv. Exp. Med. Biol.* 727, 265–271. doi: 10.1007/978-1-4614-0899-4_20

Reinhardt, H. C., and Schumacher, B. (2012). The p53 network: cellular and systemic DNA damage responses in aging and cancer. *Trends Genet.* 28, 128–136. doi: 10.1016/j.tig.2011.12.002

Reinhardt, H. C., and Yaffe, M. B. (2009). Kinases that control the cell cycle in response to DNA damage: Chk1, Chk2, and MK2. *Curr. Opin. Cell Biol.* 21, 245–255. doi: 10.1016/j.ceb.2009.01.018

Reinson, T., Toots, M., Kadaja, M., Pipitch, R., Allik, M., Ustav, E., et al. (2013). Engagement of the ATR-dependent DNA damage response at the human papillomavirus 18 replication centers during the initial amplification. *J. Virol.* 87, 951–964. doi: 10.1128/JVI.01943-12

Richardson, H., Kelsall, G., Tellier, P., Voyer, H., Abrahamowicz, M., Ferenczy, A., et al. (2003). The natural history of type-specific human papillomavirus infections in female university students. *Cancer Epidemiol. Prev. Biomark* 12, 485–490.

Saidj, D., Cros, M. P., Hernandez-Vargas, H., Guarino, F., Sylla, B. S., Tommasino, M., et al. (2013). Oncoprotein E7 from beta human papillomavirus 38 induces formation of an inhibitory complex for a subset of p53-regulated promoters. *J. Virol.* 87, 12139–12150. doi: 10.1128/JVI.01047-13

Sakakibara, N., Mitra, R., and McBride, A. A. (2011). The papillomavirus E1 helicase activates a cellular DNA damage response in viral replication foci?. *J. Virol.* 85, 8981–8995. doi: 10.1128/JVI.00541-11

Santamaria, D., Barrière, C., Cerqueira, A., Hunt, S., Tardy, C., Newton, K., et al. (2007). Cdk1 is sufficient to drive the mammalian cell cycle. *Nature* 448, 811–815. doi: 10.1038/nature06046

Sawyer, S. L., Tian, L., Kähkönen, M., Schwartzentruber, J., Kircher, M., and University of Washington Centre for Mendelian Gnomics (2015). Biallelic mutations in BRCA1 cause a new Fanconi anemia subtype. *Cancer Discov.* 5, 135–142. doi: 10.1158/2159-8290.CD-14-1156

Schaper, I. D., Marcuzzi, G. P., Weissenborn, S. J., Kasper, H. U., Dries, V., Smyth, N., et al. (2005). Development of skin tumors in mice transgenic for early genes of human papillomavirus type 8. *Cancer Res.* 65, 1394–1400. doi: 10.1158/0008-5472.CAN-04-3263

Scheffner, M., Werness, B. A., Huibregtse, J. M., Levine, A. J., and Howley, P. M. (1990). The E6 oncoprotein encoded by human papillomavirus types 16 and 18 promotes the degradation of p53. *Cell* 63, 1129–1136. doi: 10.1016/0092-8674(90)90409-8

Sharma, G. G., Gupta, A., Wang, H., Scherthan, H., Dhar, S., Gandhi, V., et al. (2003). hTERT associates with human telomeres and enhances genomic stability and DNA repair. *Oncogene* 22, 131–146. doi: 10.1038/sj.onc.1206063

Shigechi, T., Tomida, J., Sato, K., Kobayashi, M., Eykelenboom, J. K., Pessina, F., et al. (2012). ATR-ATRIP kinase complex triggers activation of the Fanconi anemia DNA repair pathway. *Cancer Res.* 72, 1149–1156. doi: 10.1158/0008-5472.CAN-11-2904

Shiloh, Y., and Ziv, Y. (2013). The ATM protein kinase: regulating the cellular response to genotoxic stress, and more. *Nat. Rev. Mol. Cell Biol.* 14, 197–210. doi: 10.1038/nrm3546

Shiotani, B., and Zou, L. (2009). Single-stranded DNA orchestrates an ATM-to-ATR switch at DNA breaks. *Mol. Cell* 33, 547–558. doi: 10.1016/j.molcel.2009.01.024

Simmonds, M., and Storey, A. (2008). Identification of the regions of the HPV 5 E6 protein involved in Bak degradation and inhibition of apoptosis. *Int. J. Cancer* 123, 2260–2266. doi: 10.1002/ijc.23815

Sperling, T., Ołdak, M., Walch-Ruckheim, B., Wickenhauser, C., Doorbar, J., Pfister, H., et al. (2012). Human papillomavirus type 8 interferes with a novel C/EBPβ-mediated mechanism of keratinocyte CCL20 chemokine expression and langerhans cell migration. *PLoS Pathog.* 8:e1002833. doi: 10.1371/journal.ppat.1002833

Szalmás, A., Tomaić, V., Basukala, O., Massimi, P., Mittal, S., Kónya, J., et al. (2017). The PTPN14 tumor suppressor is a degradation target of human papillomavirus E7. *J. Virol.* 91:e00057-17. doi: 10.1128/JVI.00057-17

ten Dijke , P., and Hill, C. S. (2004). New insights into TGF-β-Smad signalling. *Trends Biochem. Sci.* 29, 265–273. doi: 10.1016/j.tibs.2004.03.008

Thomas, M., and Banks, L. (1999). Human papillomavirus (HPV) E6 interactions with Bak are conserved amongst E6 proteins from high and low risk HPV types. *J. Gen. Virol.* 80(Pt 6), 1513–1517. doi: 10.1099/0022-1317-80-6-1513

Tibbetts, R. S., Brumbaugh, K. M., Williams, J. M., Sarkaria, J. N., Cliby, W. A., Shieh, S. Y., et al. (1999). A role for ATR in the DNA damage-induced phosphorylation of p53. *Genes Dev.* 13, 152–157. doi: 10.1101/gad.13.2.152

Tomaić, V. (2016). Functional roles of E6 and E7 oncoproteins in HPV-induced malignancies at diverse anatomical sites. *Cancers* 8:95. doi: 10.3390/cancers8100095

Tommasino, M. (2014). The human papillomavirus family and its role in carcinogenesis. *Semin. Cancer Biol.* 26, 13–21. doi: 10.1016/j.semcancer.2013.11.002

Tommasino, M. (2017). The biology of beta human papillomaviruses. *Virus Res.* 231, 128–138. doi: 10.1016/j.virusres.2016.11.013

Turnell, A. S., Stewart, G. S., Grand, R. J. A., Rookes, S. M., Martin, A., Yamano, H., et al. (2005). The APC/C and CBP/p300 cooperate to regulate transcription and cell-cycle progression. *Nature* 438, 690–695. doi: 10.1038/nature04151

Underbrink, M. P., Howie, H. L., Bedard, K. M., Koop, J. I., and Galloway, D. A. (2008). E6 Proteins from multiple human betapapillomavirus types degrade Bak and protect keratinocytes from apoptosis after UVB irradiation. *J. Virol.* 82, 10408–10417. doi: 10.1128/JVI.00902-08

Van Doorslaer, K. (2013). Evolution of the papillomaviridae. *Virology* 445, 11–20. doi: 10.1016/j.virol.2013.05.012

Vermezovic, J., Adamowicz, M., Santarpia, L., Rustighi, A., Forcato, M., Lucano, C., et al. (2015). Notch is a direct negative regulator of the DNA-damage response. *Nat. Struct. Mol. Biol.* 22, 417–424. doi: 10.1038/nsmb.3013

Viarisio, D., Mueller-Decker, K., Kloz, U., Aengeneyndt, B., Kopp-Schneider, A., Gröne, H. J., et al. (2011). E6 and E7 from Beta Hpv38 cooperate with ultraviolet light in the development of actinic keratosis-like lesions and squamous cell carcinoma in mice. *PLOS Pathog.* 7:e1002125. doi: 10.1371/journal.ppat.1002125

Viarisio, D., Müller-Decker, K., Zanna, P., Kloz, U., Aengeneyndt, B., Accardi, R., et al. (2016). Novel ß-HPV49 transgenic mouse model of upper digestive tract cancer. *Cancer Res.* 76, 4216–4225. doi: 10.1158/0008-5472.CAN-16-0370

Vogelstein, B., Lane, D., and Levine, A. J. (2000). Surfing the p53 network. *Nature* 408, 307–310. doi: 10.1038/35042675

Wallace, N. A., Gasior, S. L., Faber, Z. J., Howie, H. L., Deininger, P. L., and Galloway, D. A. (2013). HPV 5 and 8 E6 expression reduces ATM protein levels and attenuates LINE-1 retrotransposition. *Virology* 443, 69–79. doi: 10.1016/j.virol.2013.04.022

Wallace, N. A., Khanal, S., Robinson, K. L., Wendel, S. O., Messer, J. J., and Galloway, D. A. (2017). High-risk *alphapapillomavirus* oncogenes impair the homologous recombination pathway. *J. Virol.* 91:e01084-17. doi: 10.1128/JVI.01084-17

Wallace, N. A., Robinson, K., and Galloway, D. A. (2014). Beta human papillomavirus E6 expression inhibits stabilization of p53 and increases tolerance of genomic instability. *J. Virol.* 88, 6112–6127. doi: 10.1128/JVI.03808-13

Wallace, N. A., Robinson, K., Howie, H. L., and Galloway, D. A. (2012). HPV 5 and 8 E6 abrogate ATR activity resulting in increased persistence of UVB induced DNA damage. *PLoS Pathog.* 8:e1002807. doi: 10.1371/journal.ppat.1002807

Wallace, N. A., Robinson, K., Howie, H. L., and Galloway, D. A. (2015). β-HPV 5 and 8 E6 disrupt homology dependent double strand break repair by attenuating BRCA1 and BRCA2 expression and foci formation. *PLoS Pathog.* 11:e1004687. doi: 10.1371/journal.ppat.1004687

Wang, W., Huang, J., Wang, X., Yuan, J., Li, X., Feng, L., et al. (2012). PTPN14 is required for the density-dependent control of YAP1. *Genes Dev.* 26, 1959–1971. doi: 10.1101/gad.192955.112

Waterboer, T., Abeni, D., Sampogna, F., Rother, A., Masini, C., Sehr, P., et al. (2008). Serological association of beta and gamma human papillomaviruses with squamous cell carcinoma of the skin. *Br. J. Dermatol.* 159, 457–459. doi: 10.1111/j.1365-2133.2008.08621.x

Weissenborn, S. J., De Koning, M. N. C., Wieland, U., Quint, W. G. V., and Pfister, H. J. (2009). Intrafamilial transmission and family-specific spectra of cutaneous betapapillomaviruses. *J. Virol.* 83, 811–816. doi: 10.1128/JVI.01338-08

Weissenborn, S. J., Nindl, I., Purdie, K., Harwood, C., Proby, C., Breuer, J., et al. (2005). Human Papillomavirus-DNA loads in actinic keratoses exceed those in non-melanoma skin cancers. *J. Invest. Dermatol.* 125, 93–97. doi: 10.1111/j.0022-202X.2005.23733.x

Weissenborn, S., Neale, R. E., Waterboer, T., Abeni, D., Bavinck, J. N. B., Green, A. C., et al. (2012). Beta-papillomavirus DNA loads in hair follicles of immunocompetent people and organ transplant recipients. *Med. Microbiol. Immunol.* 201, 117–125. doi: 10.1007/s00430-011-0212-3

Werness, B. A., Levine, A. J., and Howley, P. M. (1990). Association of human papillomavirus types 16 and 18 E6 proteins with p53. *Science* 248, 76–79. doi: 10.1126/science.2157286

White, E. A., Kramer, R. E., Tan, M. J. A., Hayes, S. D., Harper, J. W., and Howley, P. M. (2012). Comprehensive analysis of host cellular interactions with human papillomavirus E6 proteins identifies new E6 binding partners and reflects viral diversity. *J. Virol.* 86, 13174–13186. doi: 10.1128/JVI.02172-12

White, E. A., Münger, K., and Howley, P. M. (2016). high-risk human papillomavirus E7 proteins target PTPN14 for degradation. *mBio* 7:e01530-16. doi: 10.1128/mBio.01530-16

White, E. A., Walther, J., Javanbakht, H., and Howley, P. M. (2014). Genus beta human papillomavirus E6 proteins vary in their effects on the transactivation of p53 target genes. *J. Virol.* 88, 8201–8212. doi: 10.1128/JVI.01197-14

Willis, N., and Rhind, N. (2009). Regulation of DNA replication by the S-phase DNA damage checkpoint. *Cell Div.* 4:13. doi: 10.1186/1747-1028-4-13

Xia, P., Wang, Z., Liu, X., Wu, B., Wang, J., Ward, T., et al. (2012). EB1 acetylation by P300/CBP-associated factor (PCAF) ensures accurate kinetochore-microtubule interactions in mitosis. *Proc. Natl. Acad. Sci. U.S A.*109, 16564–16569. doi: 10.1073/pnas.1202639109

Yamashita, T., Segawa, K., Fujinaga, Y., Nishikawa, T., and Fujinaga, K. (1993). Biological and biochemical activity of E7 genes of the cutaneous human papillomavirus type 5 and 8. *Oncogene* 8, 2433–2441.

Yan, S., Sorrell, M., and Berman, Z. (2014). Functional interplay between ATM/ATR-mediated DNA damage response and DNA repair pathways in oxidative stress. *Cell. Mol. Life Sci. CMLS* 71, 3951–3967. doi: 10.1007/s00018-014-1666-4

Yang, J., Yu, Y., Hamrick, H. E., and Duerksen-Hughes, P. J. (2003). ATM, ATR and DNA-PK: initiators of the cellular genotoxic stress responses. *Carcinogenesis* 24, 1571–1580. doi: 10.1093/carcin/bgg137

Yang, W. (2011). Surviving the sun: repair and bypass of DNA UV lesions. *Protein Sci. Publ. Protein Soc.* 20, 1781–1789. doi: 10.1002/pro.723

Yoshida, K., and Miki, Y. (2004). Role of BRCA1 and BRCA2 as regulators of DNA repair, transcription, and cell cycle in response to DNA damage. *Cancer Sci.* 95, 866–871. doi: 10.1111/j.1349-7006.2004.tb02195.x

Yu, J., and Zhang, L. (2005). The transcriptional targets of p53 in apoptosis control. *Biochem. Biophys. Res. Commun.* 331, 851–858. doi: 10.1016/j.bbrc.2005.03.189

Zerfass, K., Schulze, A., Spitkovsky, D., Friedman, V., Henglein, B., and Jansen-Dürr, P. (1995). Sequential activation of cyclin E and cyclin A gene expression by human papillomavirus type 16 E7 through sequences necessary for transformation. *J. Virol.* 69, 6389–6399.

Zimmermann, H., Degenkolbe R., Bernard, H.-U., and O'Connor, M. J. (1999). The human papillomavirus type 16 E6 oncoprotein can down-regulate p53 activity by targeting the transcriptional coactivator CBP/p300. *J. Virol.* 73, 6209–6219.

8

Chronic Inflammatory Microenvironment in Epidermodysplasia Verruciformis Skin Lesions: Role of the Synergism Between HPV8 E2 and C/EBPβ to Induce Pro-Inflammatory S100A8/A9 Proteins

*Marta Podgórska[1], Monika Ołdak[1,2], Anna Marthaler[1], Alina Fingerle[1], Barbara Walch-Rückheim[1], Stefan Lohse[1], Cornelia S. L. Müller[3], Thomas Vogt[3], Mart Ustav[4], Artur Wnorowski[1], Magdalena Malejczyk[5], Sławomir Majewski[6] and Sigrun Smola[1]**

[1] Institute of Virology, Saarland University Medical Center, Homburg, Germany, [2] Department of Histology and Embryology, Center of Biostructure Research, Medical University of Warsaw, Warsaw, Poland, [3] Department of Dermatology, Saarland University Medical Center, Homburg, Germany, [4] Icosagen Cell Factory OÜ, Institute of Technology, University of Tartu, Tartu, Estonia, [5] Diagnostic Laboratory of STDs, Department of Dermatology and Venereology, Medical University of Warsaw, Warsaw, Poland, [6] Department of Dermatology and Venereology, Medical University of Warsaw, Warsaw, Poland

Correspondence:
Sigrun Smola
sigrun.smola@uks.eu

Persistent genus β-HPV (human papillomavirus) infection is a major co-factor for non-melanoma skin cancer in patients suffering from the inherited skin disease epidermodysplasia verruciformis (EV). Malignant EV lesions are particularly associated with HPV type 5 or 8. There is clinical and molecular evidence that HPV8 actively suppresses epithelial immunosurveillance by interfering with the recruitment of Langerhans cells, which may favor viral persistence. Mechanisms how persistent HPV8 infection promotes the carcinogenic process are, however, less well understood. In various tumor types chronic inflammation has a central role in tumor progression. The calprotectin complex consisting of S100A8 and S100A9 proteins has recently been identified as key driver of chronic and tumor promoting inflammation in skin carcinogenesis. It induces chemotaxis of neutrophil granulocytes and modulates inflammatory as well as immune responses. In this study, we demonstrate that skin lesions of EV-patients are massively infiltrated by inflammatory cells, including CD15^{+} granulocytes. At the same time we observed a very strong expression of S100A8 and S100A9 proteins in lesional keratinocytes, which was mostly confined to the suprabasal layers of the epidermis. Both proteins were hardly detected in non-lesional skin. Further experiments revealed that the HPV8 oncoproteins E6 and E7 were not involved in S100A8/A9 up-regulation. They rather suppressed differentiation-induced S100A8/A9 expression. In contrast, the viral transcription factor E2 strongly enhanced PMA-mediated S100A8/A9 up-regulation in primary human keratinocytes. Similarly, a tremendous up-regulation of both S100 proteins was observed, when minute amounts of the PMA-inducible CCAAT/enhancer binding protein β (C/EBPβ), which is expressed at low levels in the suprabasal layers of the epidermis, were co-expressed together with HPV8 E2. This confirmed our previous observation that C/EBPβ interacts and functionally synergizes with the HPV8 E2 protein in differentiation-dependent gene expression. Potent synergistic up-regulation of S100A8/A9 was seen at transcriptional and protein levels. S100A8/A9 containing supernatants from keratinocytes co-expressing HPV8 E2 and C/EBPβ significantly induced chemotaxis of granulocytes in migration assays supporting the relevance of our finding. In conclusion, our data suggest that the HPV8 E2 protein actively contributes to the recruitment of myeloid cells into EV skin lesions, which may support chronic inflammation and progression to skin cancer.

Keywords: HPV, E2, epidermodysplasia verruciformis, inflammation, C/EBP, S100A8/A9

INTRODUCTION

Human papillomaviruses (HPVs) infect keratinocytes of mucosa and skin and cause a wide range of clinical outcomes from benign to malignant lesions. Mucosal HPV types have a well-established role in anogenital tumors, particularly in cervical carcinoma. Cutaneous HPVs of the genus beta (β-HPV) were first discovered in patients with epidermodysplasia verruciformis (EV) (Majewski and Jablonska, 2006). This rare genetic skin condition mostly results from recessive mutations in *EVER1* or *EVER2* genes, which confer predisposition to persistent β-HPV infection (Shamanin et al., 1994; Ramoz et al., 2002). EV begins early in childhood with widespread flat warts and macules, which can, later in life, evolve to cutaneous squamous cell carcinoma (SCC), mainly at sun-exposed sites. Multiple HPVs, e.g., HPV5, 8, 17, 20, 27, 38, or 47, can be found within the EV skin lesions but HPV5 or 8 are the most frequently detected in EV-associated skin carcinomas (Orth et al., 1978; Orth, 1986; Pfister, 2003).

Viral persistence is a major prerequisite for HPV-induced tumor development in cervix uteri and potentially in the skin and it requires an escape of the virus from host immune surveillance (zur Hausen, 2009; Smola, 2017; Smola et al., 2017). Recently, we have proposed a novel molecular mechanism how HPV8 might disrupt innate immunity in skin. We found reduced numbers of antigen-presenting Langerhans cells in EV lesions and showed that it is a consequence of HPV8-mediated suppression of CCL20, which is a chemokine attracting Langerhans cells (Sperling et al., 2012; Smola, 2014).

A set of *in vivo* data employing transgenic mouse models established a role of EV-associated HPVs in the development of skin tumors. HPV38, 20, and 27 transgenic mice expressing E6 and E7, the main viral oncoproteins, displayed increased susceptibility to carcinogenesis after UV or chemical treatment (Michel et al., 2006; Viarisio et al., 2011). In mice expressing the complete early region of HPV8 under the keratin 14 (K14) promoter even spontaneous development of skin cancers was observed. Transcript analysis in the affected tissue revealed high mRNA levels of the viral transcription factor E2, which prevailed over E7 and E6 and did not change during tumor progression (Schaper et al., 2005). Interestingly tumor development was also observed in transgenic mice expressing only the HPV8 E2 gene under the K14 promoter and this process was accompanied by a massive stromal infiltration of immune cells (Pfefferle et al., 2008). These findings emphasized the importance of the E2 protein in tumor formation and raised the hypothesis that E2 might augment tumor-promoting inflammatory responses in skin.

Recently, S100A8 (calgranulin A, MRP-8) and S100A9 (calgranulin B, MRP-14) have been identified as key drivers of skin carcinogenesis in a mouse model (Gebhardt et al., 2008). Both proteins belong to the S100 multigenic family of non-ubiquitous Ca^{2+}-binding low molecular weight proteins. They associate in a higher-ordered heteromeric complex called calprotectin, which is essential for their biological activity (Leukert et al., 2006). In skin their expression has been observed under inflammatory conditions, such as wound healing or psoriasis (Kerkhoff et al., 2012). Beside the intracellular activity of S100A8 and S100A9 proteins, they are also found in the extracellular milieu, where they function as damage-associated molecular pattern molecules (DAMPs) or alarmins and induce immune cell migration, particularly of granulocytes (Ryckman et al., 2003).

In this report, we demonstrate that S100A8/A9 proteins are potently up-regulated in HPV8-positive EV lesions and S100 expression was paralleled by a strong inflammatory response. Detailed molecular analysis revealed that not the HPV8 E6 or E7 oncoproteins, but the viral transcription factor E2 plays a major role in S100A8/A9 induction.

MATERIALS AND METHODS

Ethics Statement

This study was carried out in accordance with the recommendations of the Declaration of Helsinki with written informed consent from all subjects. All subjects gave written informed consent in accordance with the Declaration of Helsinki. The protocol was approved by the Bioethics Committee at the Medical University of Warsaw, Poland, and the Saarland University at the Saarland Ärztekammer.

Immunohistochemistry, Immunofluorescence, and HPV Genotyping

Formalin fixed paraffin-embedded (FFPE) skin specimens from EV-lesions were obtained from the Department of Dermatology, Medical University of Warsaw, Warsaw, Poland. The presence of HPV8 was confirmed by quantitative real-time PCR (qRT-PCR) as described in Weissenborn et al. (2010). Sections were stained with mouse monoclonal anti-CD15 antibody (clone Carb-3, Dako, Glostrup, Denmark), rabbit monoclonal anti-S100A8 antibody (clone EPR3554; Novus Biologicals, Cambridge, United Kingdom), rabbit polyclonal anti-S100A9 antibody (H-90, sc-20173, Santa Cruz Biotechnology, Heidelberg, Germany) or mouse anti-CD45 (Abcam, Cambridge, United Kingdom). Staining was performed using the Dako instrument Autostainer Plus (Dako) or Immpress AP Reagent kit (Vector, Burlingame, CA, United States). For immunofluorescence, cells were grown on cover slips, fixed with 2% buffered paraformaldehyde, permeabilized with 0.1% Triton X-100 and stained with rabbit anti-HPV8 E2 (from Mart Ustav, University of Tartu, Tartu, Estonia) and mouse monoclonal anti-pan-cytokeratin (clone C11; Sigma-Aldrich, Steinheim, Germany) and secondary goat anti-rabbit Alexa Fluor 546 goat and goat anti-mouse Alexa Fluor 488 (Life Technologies, Eugene, OR, United States), respectively.

Plasmid Constructs

Expression vectors of HPV8 E2 and E6/E7 cloned in pLXSN, HPV8 E2, E6, E7, HPV16 E2, C/EBPβ, cloned in pcDNA3.1+ and HPV8 E2ΔC in pXJ42 were reported previously (Hadaschik et al., 2003). S100A8 in pcDNA3.1/myc-His(-) and S100A9 in pcDNA3.1+ expression vectors were kind gifts from Peter Angel (German Cancer Research Centre, Heidelberg, Germany). The S100A8 luciferase reporter construct containing a fragment (−917 to +456 bp) of the murine S100A8 promoter region cloned upstream of the firefly luciferase gene in the pGL2-basic vector was a kind gift from Kenneth Hsu (Sydney, NSW, Australia). It comprises a functional C/EBPβ binding site, which is highly conserved in mammalian S100A8 promoters, particularly in human and murine promoters, and has been shown to bind to C/EBPβ by chromatin immunoprecipitation (Miao et al., 2012).

Cell Culture and Retroviral Infection

Normal human foreskin keratinocytes (NFKs) were cultured in KBM-Gold medium with supplements (Lonza, Basel, Switzerland). NFK stably expressing HPV8 E2 or E6/E7 were generated by retroviral gene transfer as previously described (Oldak et al., 2010). Viral gene expression was confirmed by HPV8 E2-, E6-, and E7-specific qRT-PCR. The HPV-negative skin SCC-derived RTS3b cell line (Purdie et al., 1993) was grown as previously reported (Hadaschik et al., 2003). Organotypic 3-dimensional cultures (OC) were generated as described in Smola et al. (1993) with minor modifications. Dermal equivalents were prepared by seeding 0.5×10^6 primary foreskin fibroblasts (usually between passage 3 and 6) in 4 mg/ml rat-tail collagen. Next day 0.5×10^6 RTS3b cells were seeded onto the fibroblast-collagen matrix. Twenty-four hours later OC were lifted on metal grids at the air-medium interphase, grown for 14 days, fixed with 4% buffered paraformaldehyde, embedded in paraffin and sectioned.

Granulocyte Isolation and Migration Assay

Granulocytes were obtained from whole blood of healthy volunteers by dextran-sedimentation of red blood cell pellets. The purity of granulocyte isolation was 93–99% as determined by CD15 and CD66 surface expression (mouse anti-human CD15-PE BD Biosciences, Heidelberg, Germany and mouse anti-human CD66abce-APC, Miltenyi Biotec, Bergisch Gladbach, Germany). Contaminating monocytes, T- and B-cells in granulocyte isolates were discriminated with CD14-FITC, CD3-FITC, and CD19-PE antibodies. Prior to the assessment of migration, granulocytes were cultured for 2 h under endotoxin-free conditions in RPMI 1640 supplemented with 5% FCS, 1% penicillin-streptomycin and 1% sodium pyruvate. 0.25×10^6 granulocytes were then seeded onto transwell chambers placed in 24-well plates (3 μm pore size, Corning Costar Corp., Corning, NY, United States). The migration capacity of granulocytes was assessed after 2 h. Background migration in culture medium only was subtracted.

Transient Transfection and Luciferase Assay

Normal human foreskin keratinocytes were transfected with TransFast reaching transfection efficiencies between 10 and 15% (Promega, Mannheim, Germany) and RTS3b cells with Lipofectamine 2000 reagent reaching transfection efficiencies between 50 and 70% (Invitrogen, Karlsruhe, Germany) according to the manufacturers' protocols. Twenty-four hours later NFKs were stimulated with PMA for another 24 h (Sigma-Aldrich, Taufkirchen, Germany). Afterward, the cells were lysed and assayed for luciferase activity as described previously (Marthaler et al., 2017). The values of luciferase activities were normalized to protein content of the respective lysates.

RNA Isolation and qRT-PCR

RNA was isolated using NucleoSpin RNA kit (Macherey-Nagel, Düren, Germany) and cDNA was generated from 0.5 to 1 μg of RNA with the Maxima Reverse Transcriptase (Thermo Fisher Scientific, Rockford, IL, United States). qRT-PCR was performed using gene-specific primers and the Universal Probe Library System (Roche, Mannheim, Germany) as follows: S100A8: 5′-CAAGTCCGTGGG CATCAT-3′, 5′-GACGTCGATGATAGAGTTCAAGG-3′, probe #78, S100A9: 5′-GTGCGAAAAGATCTGCAAAA-3′, 5′-CCA GCTGCTTGTCTGCATTT-3′, probe #85, RPL13A: 5′-AGCG GATGAACACCAACC-3′, 5′-TTTGTGGGGCAGCATACTC-3′, probe #28, HPV8 E2: 5′-GACGGCGATCAACCTCAA-3′, 5′-CTCCCCTTTGTGACCGTTT-3′, probe #22, HPV8 E6: 5′-CCGCAACGTTTGAATTTAATG-3′, 5′-ATTGAACGTCCT GTAGCTAATTCA-3′, probe #13 and HPV8 E7: 5′-AGG AATTACCAAACGAACAGGA-3′, 5′-CACGGTGCAACAATTT TGAATA-3′, probe #63. Expression levels were measured using

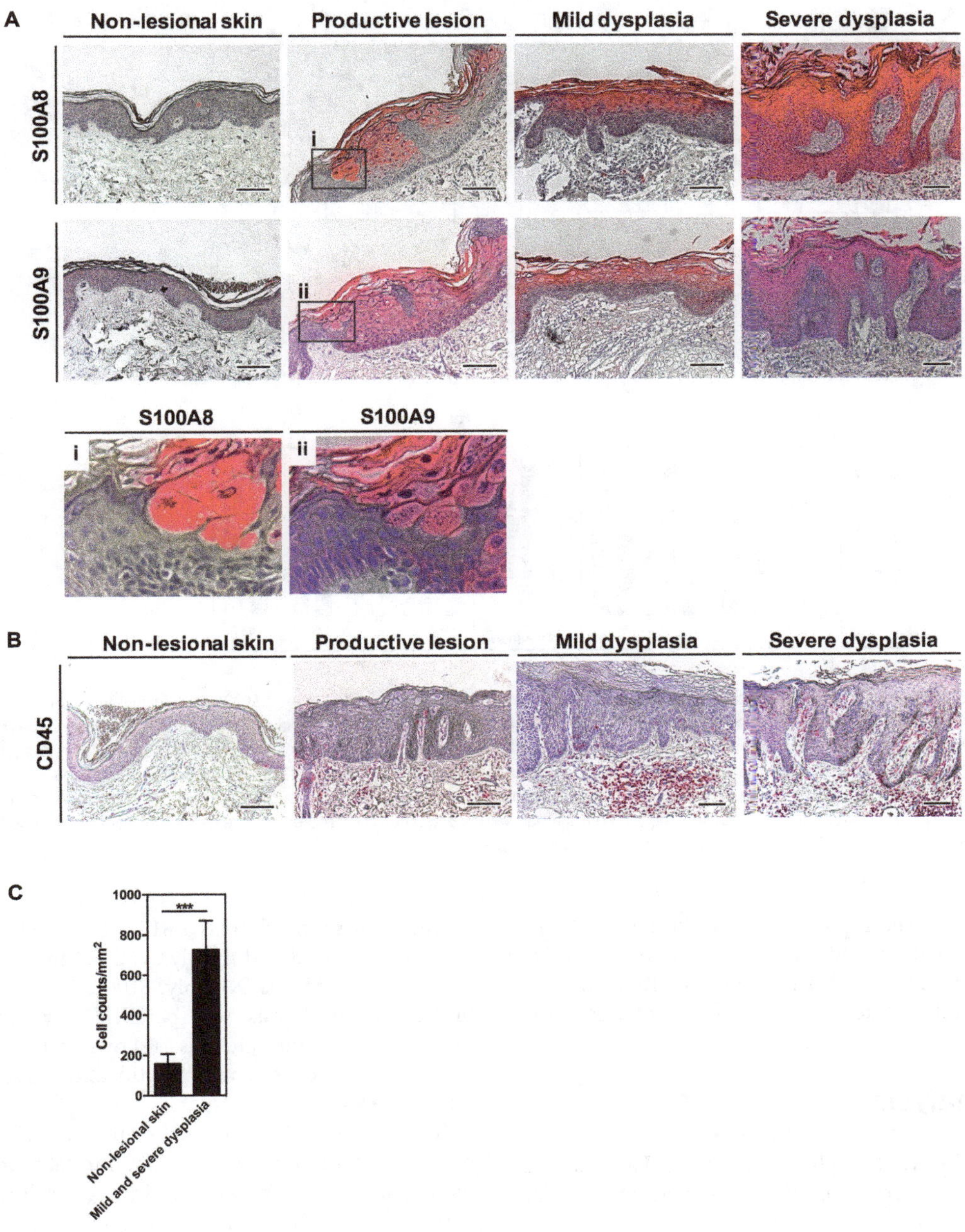

FIGURE 1 | Strong expression of S100A8/A9 in HPV8-positive EV-lesions corresponds to an inflammatory infiltrate. **(A)** Serial sections of HPV8-positive EV-lesions were analyzed by IHC for S100A8 and S100A9 (magnifications in **i** and **ii**) or **(B)** CD45 (all red) and counterstained with hematoxylin. Scale bars 100 μm. **(C)** Infiltrating immune cells were counted in the stroma of mild and severe dysplasia of EV-lesions versus non-lesional skin of EV-patients based on hematoxylin counterstaining and are given as cell counts per mm^2. Values represent counts ± SD from six different areas. ***$p < 0.001$, unpaired t-test.

LightCycler 480 II instrument (Roche) and normalized to RPL13A housekeeping gene expression (Marthaler et al., 2017).

Western Blot Analysis and ELISAs

The cells were lysed in buffer containing 62.5 mM Tris-Cl pH 6.8, 10% glycerol and 2% SDS. Thirty micrograms of the samples were separated by 9.5–20% gradient SDS-PAGE and subjected to Western blotting. Anti-S100A8, anti-S100A9, mouse monoclonal anti-actin (clone AC-15, Sigma-Aldrich, St. Louis, MO, United States) as well as horseradish peroxidase-labeled goat anti-rabbit and rabbit anti-mouse (both Sigma-Aldrich) antibodies were used followed by chemiluminescence detection (Thermo Fisher Scientific). ChemiDoc XRS$^+$ Molecular Imager and Quantity One analysis software (both Bio-Rad, Philadelphia, PA, United States) were used for quantification. Interleukin-8 (IL-8, CXCL8), Epithelial-derived Neutrophil-Activating peptide

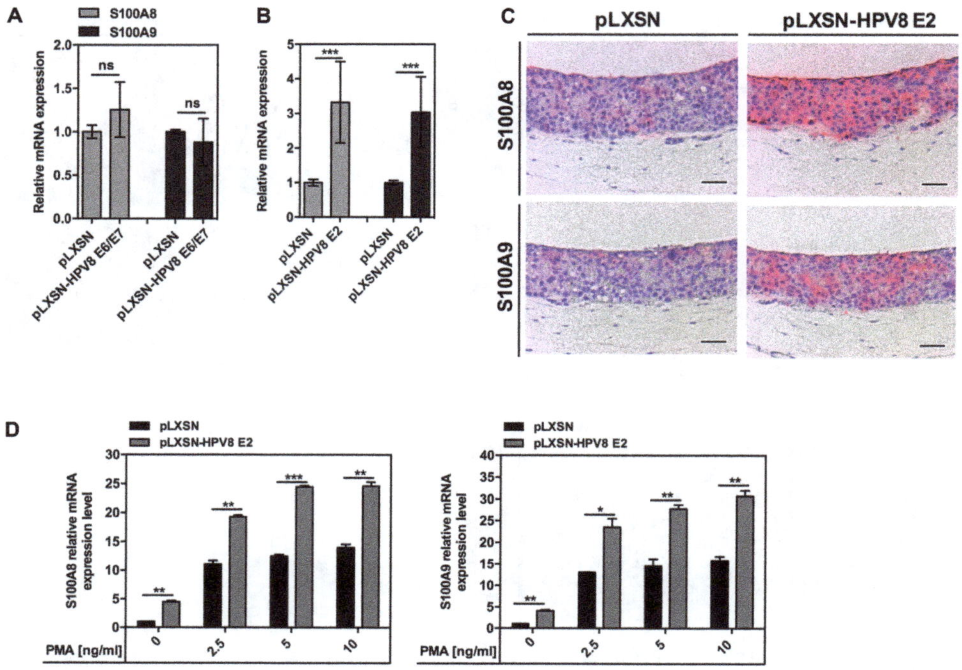

FIGURE 2 | Not HPV8 E6/E7 oncoproteins but the E2 transcription factor induces both S100A8 and S100A9. S100A8/A9 mRNA levels in NFK stably expressing **(A)** HPV8 E6/E7 or **(B)** HPV8 E2 and corresponding control pLXSN cells were measured by qRT-PCR in relation to RPL13A. The amount of S100A8 and S100A9 in pLXSN control cells was set at 1. Shown are the mean values ± SD from $n \geq 2$ independent experiments performed in duplicates. **(C)** Serial sections of OC of HPV8 E2-expressing or control pLXSN RTS3b cells were analyzed by IHC for S100A8 and S100A9 (both red) and counterstained with hematoxylin. Scale bars 100 μm. **(D)** NFK stably expressing HPV8 E2 or control pLXSN cells were stimulated with PMA or DMSO as a vehicle control and 24 h later S100A8 and S100A9 mRNA levels were measured by qRT-PCR in relation to RPL13A. Shown are the mean values ± SD from one representative experiment out of three performed in duplicates. ns, not significant, $^{*}p < 0.05$, $^{**}p < 0.01$, $^{***}p < 0.001$, unpaired t-test.

78 (ENA-78, CXCL5), Neutrophil Activating Protein-2 (NAP-2, CXCL7) and Growth-Regulated Oncogene-α (GRO-α, CXCL1) concentrations were measured with DuoSet (R&D Systems, South Beloit, IL, United States) according to the manufacturer's protocols.

Statistical Analysis

Statistical differences were determined with unpaired t-test using Prism 5 software (GraphPad Software, La Jolla, CA, United States). Significances are indicated by asterisks ($^{*}p < 0.05$, $^{**}p < 0.01$, $^{***}p < 0.001$, $^{****}p < 0.0001$).

RESULTS

In this study, we investigated S100A8 and S100A9 protein expression in the skin of EV-patients. In non-lesional skin both proteins were occasionally detectable in the keratinocytes of the granular layer or were completely lacking (**Figure 1A**). HPV8-positive lesional skin of EV-patients, however, revealed a dramatic induction of S100A8 and S100A9 proteins in keratinocytes of suprabasal spinous and granular layers. In productive EV-lesions staining of both proteins was particularly prominent in keratinocytes displaying viral cytopathic effects as demonstrated in higher magnifications (**Figures 1A i** and **ii**). Also in mild and severe dysplasia S100A8 and S100A9 staining was strongly enhanced and mostly confined to the suprabasal layers of infected epidermis. Notably, S100A8 and S100A9 expression in lesional epidermis was paralleled by significant stromal infiltration with immune cells as shown by CD45 staining, a pan-marker for leukocytes, and quantification of stromal infiltrating cells (**Figures 1B,C**).

To investigate the potential impact of HPV8 early proteins on S100A8 and S100A9 induction, normal human keratinocytes (NFKs) and the RTS3b skin keratinocyte cell line were engineered to stably express HPV8 E2 or combined E6/E7 genes by retroviral gene transfer. Expression of HPV8 E2, E6, and E7 genes was confirmed by qRT-PCR and E2 additionally on protein level by double immunofluorescence (Supplementary Figure S1). Presence of HPV8 E6/E7 in NFK did not influence S100A8 and S100A9 expression (**Figure 2A**). However, a significant increase in S100A8/A9 mRNA levels was observed in HPV8 E2-expressing NFK (**Figure 2B**). This was further validated at the protein level by strong S100A8 and S100A9 IHC staining in OC of HPV8 E2-expressing RTS3b keratinocytes compared to control cells with empty pLXSN vector only (**Figure 2C**).

Since in EV-lesions S100A8 and S100A9 staining was confined to the suprabasal more differentiated layers, we were interested whether HPV8 E2 might cooperate with differentiation-regulating factors to up-regulate the calgranulins. To test

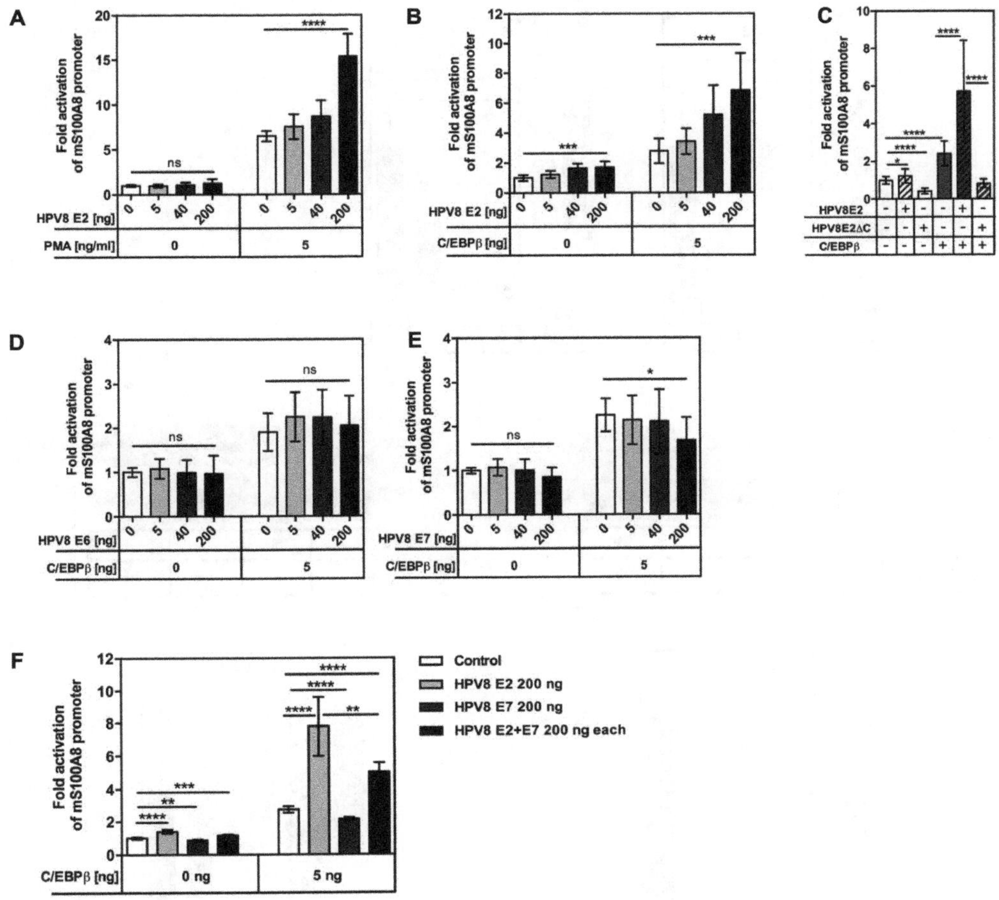

FIGURE 3 | HPV8 E2 enhances PMA- or C/EBPβ-induced activation of the S100A8 promoter in human keratinocytes. **(A)** 0.1 × 10^6 NFKs were seeded onto 12-well plates, next day co-transfected with 0.2 μg S100A8 reporter vector and 0.005, 0.04, or 0.2 μg HPV8 E2 expression vector and 6 h later stimulated with PMA or DMSO as a vehicle control. 0.61 × 10^5 RTS3b cells were seeded onto 12-well plates and next day co-transfected with 0.2 μg S100A8 reporter vector together with 0.005 μg C/EBPβ and in **(B)** 0.005, 0.04, or 0.2 μg HPV8 E2, **(C)** 0.2 μg HPV8 E2 or HPV8 E2ΔC, **(D)** 0.005, 0.04 or 0.2 μg HPV8 E6, **(E)** 0.005, 0.04, or 0.2 μg HPV8 E7 or **(F)** HPV8 E2 and E7 expression vectors (0.2 μg each). Total amount of DNA in all transfections was adjusted up to 0.8 μg with pcDNA3.1+ empty vector. 24 h post-transfection the luciferase activity was measured and normalized to protein concentration. Control transfection was set at 1. Shown are the mean values ± SD from $n \geq 3$ independent experiments performed in triplicates. ns, not significant, $*p < 0.05$, $**p < 0.01$, $***p < 0.001$, $****p < 0.0001$, unpaired *t*-test.

this hypothesis, HPV8 E2-expressing NFKs were stimulated with phorbol 12-myristate 13-acetate (PMA), a well-known activator of protein kinase C (PKC) and inducer of keratinocyte differentiation (Agarwal et al., 1999; Balasubramanian et al., 2000; Goethe et al., 2007). PMA significantly enhanced the effect of HPV8 E2 on S100A8 and S100A9 mRNA in NFK from two different donors (**Figure 2D** and Supplementary Figure S2).

To study whether regulation took place at the promoter level, the interplay of PMA activation and HPV8 E2 expression was examined in reporter gene assays. In NFK, transient expression of HPV8 E2 alone had only a minor effect, while PMA stimulation strongly synergized with HPV8 E2 in S100A8 promoter activation (**Figure 3A**). Others and we have previously demonstrated that PMA potently induces the transcription factor C/EBPβ in primary human keratinocytes (Park et al., 2008; Sperling et al., 2012). Furthermore, our previous data had shown that HPV8 E2 can bind to and synergize with C/EBPβ to transactivate the involucrin promoter (Hadaschik et al., 2003). Notably, a functional C/EBPβ binding site is also highly conserved in mammalian S100A8 promoters, particularly in human and murine promoters (Miao et al., 2012). Since C/EBPβ is expressed at low levels in suprabasal layers of the skin (Sperling et al., 2012), minute amounts of C/EBPβ (5 ng) were co-transfected together with the HPV8 E2 expression vector in RTS3b cells. In these cells transient transfection of HPV8 E2 alone significantly activated the murine S100A8 promoter up to 1.64-fold while co-expression of HPV8 E2 and C/EBPβ significantly increased promoter activity in a dose-dependent manner up to 7-fold, similar to the results obtained with the involucrin promoter (**Figure 3B**) (Hadaschik et al., 2003). HPV8 E2 interacts with C/EBPβ via its C-terminus. We therefore investigated the impact of the C-terminal E2 deletion mutant (HPV8 E2ΔC) on S100A8 promoter activity. While full length HPV8 E2 strongly synergized with C/EBPβ, this was not observed

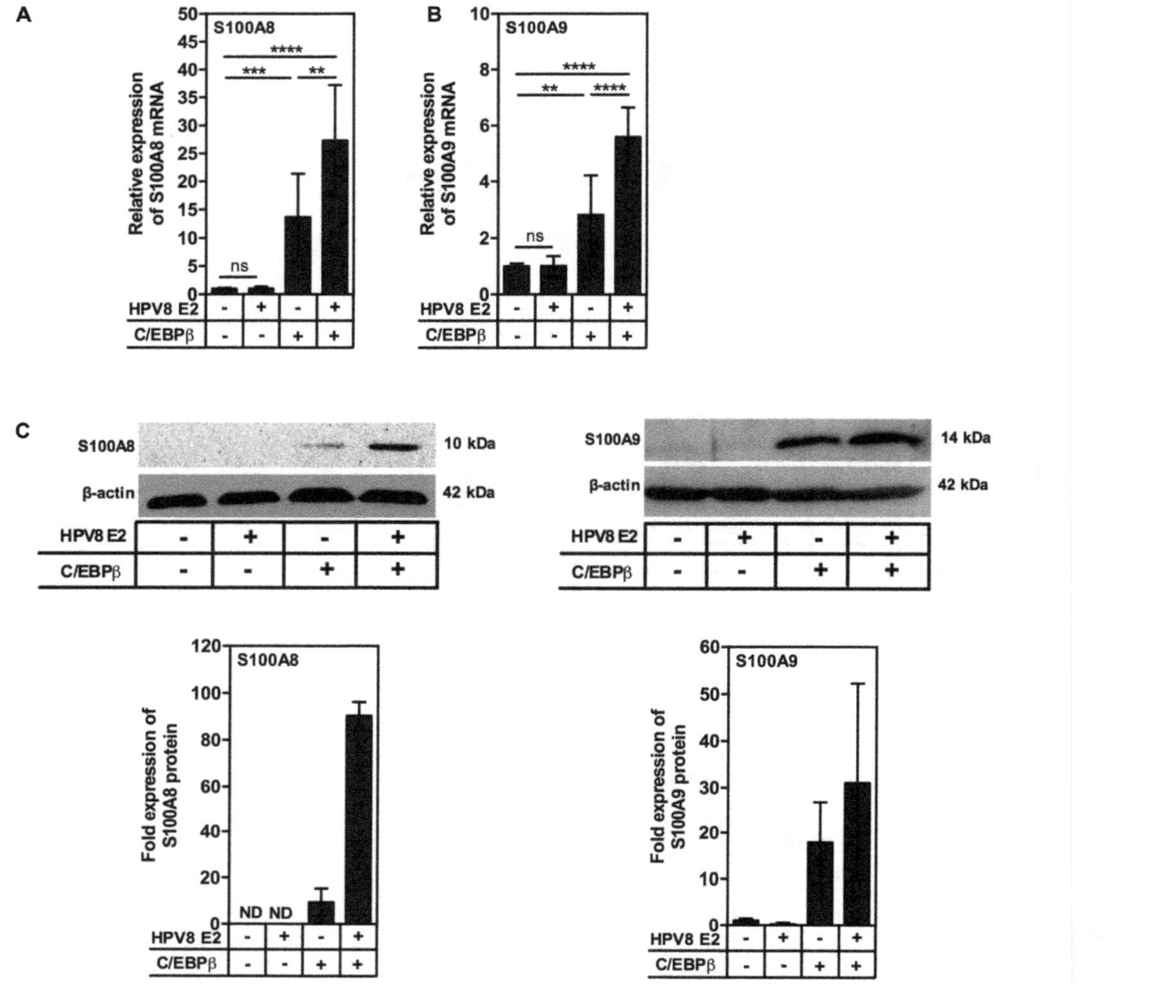

FIGURE 4 | HPV8 E2 synergizes with minute amounts of C/EBPβ to up-regulate S100A8 and S100A9 in human keratinocytes. RTS3b cells were seeded onto 6-cm dishes at a density of 0.4 × 10^6 cells per dish and transiently co-transfected with 2.64 μg HPV8 E2 and 0.1 μg C/EBPβ expression vectors and 24 h later were analyzed for **(A)** S100A8 and **(B)** S100A9 mRNA expression by qRT-PCR in relation to RPL13A. Shown are the mean values ± SD from n = 3 independent experiments performed in duplicates. **(C)** For Western blot analysis 1 × 10^6 RTS3b cells were seeded onto 10-cm dishes and next day co-transfected with 0.27 μg C/EBPβ and 7.2 μg HPV8 E2 expression vectors. Forty-eight hours later whole-cell extracts were analyzed for S100A8 (left) and S100A9 (right) protein expression. β-actin served as a loading control. Shown is one representative experiment out of n = 3. Diagrams summarize n = 3 experiments. ND, not detected; ns, not significant, $^{**}p < 0.01$, $^{***}p < 0.001$, $^{****}p < 0.0001$, unpaired t-test.

for the E2 mutant lacking the C-terminal C/EBPβ-interacting domain (**Figure 3C**). To investigate the influence of HPV8 E6 and E7 on C/EBPβ-induced S100A8 promoter activity, we performed co-transfection experiments in RTS3b cells. Neither E6 nor E7 alone increased C/EBPβ-induced promoter activity. HPV8 E7 even led to a suppression of C/EBPβ-induced promoter activity (**Figures 3D,E**). This corresponded well to our previous observation that HPV8 E7 can interfere with C/EBPβ-mediated induction of the Langerhans cell attracting chemokine CCL20 (Sperling et al., 2012). Since E7 is predominantly expressed in the granular layer of EV-lesions, we investigated its potential impact on the synergism between C/EBPβ and E2 on the S100A8 promoter. HPV8 E7 alone was able to reduce C/EBPβ-dependent promoter activity. When equal amounts of HPV8 E2 and E7 were co-transfected together with C/EBPβ, however, the positive E2 activity prevailed over the negative effect of HPV8 E7 (**Figure 3F**).

Next, we analyzed the impact of transient HPV8 E2 and C/EBPβ expression on the regulation of endogenous S100A8 and S100A9. Expression of HPV8 E2 led to a strong enhancement of C/EBPβ-mediated S100A8 induction (more than 25-fold, **Figure 4A**) and S100A9 (up to 6-fold, **Figure 4B**) at mRNA level. In parallel experiments the cells were subjected to Western blot analysis. While control cells expressed minimal levels of calgranulins, HPV8 E2 enhanced the impact of C/EBPβ on the levels of endogenous S100A8 and S100A9 proteins up to 90- and 31-fold, respectively, as shown by quantification (**Figure 4C**).

This effect was not seen for its mucosal counterpart HPV16 E2, which did not enhance but rather suppressed

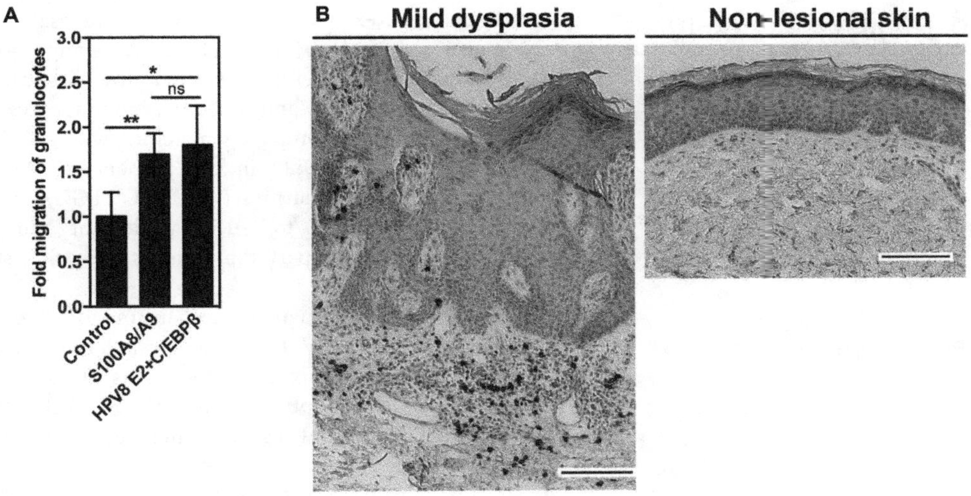

FIGURE 5 | Co-expression of HPV8 E2 and C/EBPβ induces migration of granulocytes *in vitro*. **(A)** Granulocyte migration toward conditioned media collected from RTS3b cells co-transfected with S100A8 and S100A9 or HPV8 E2 and C/EBPβ expression vectors or control vectors was measured by transwell chemotaxis assay. Number of migrated granulocytes toward control conditioned media was set at 1. Shown are the mean values ± SD from $n = 3$ independent experiments performed in duplicates. **(B)** Sections of EV-lesions were stained with anti-CD15 antibody by IHC (red). Counterstaining with hematoxylin reveals the segmented appearance of nuclei in CD15-positive cells indicating infiltration with granulocytes. Scale bars 100 μm. ns, not significant, $^{*}p < 0.05$, $^{**}p < 0.01$, unpaired *t*-test.

C/EBPβ-activated S100A8 promoter activity and S100A8/A9 mRNA levels (Supplementary Figure S3).

Since the S100A8/A9 complex is chemotactic for neutrophils, we set up an *in vitro* migration assay. Freshly prepared conditioned media from transiently transfected keratinocytes were applied onto transwells containing granulocytes. Keratinocytes ectopically expressing S100A8/A9 significantly induced the migration of granulocytes. Notably, conditioned media obtained from the keratinocytes co-transfected with HPV8 E2 and minute amounts of C/EBPβ induced migration of granulocytes at least as strong as overexpressed S100A8/A9 (**Figure 5A**).

To validate this finding *in vivo*, the EV-lesions were further investigated. We observed that the stroma of HPV8-positive EV-lesions was strongly infiltrated with CD15-positive granulocytes in comparison to non-lesional skin, where granulocytes were not detected (**Figure 5B**).

DISCUSSION

In this study, we demonstrate that HPV8-positive skin lesions of EV patients are characterized by a dramatic increase of suprabasal alarmin S100A8/A9 expression and stromal inflammation starting in productive lesions and still observed in mild and severe dysplasia. Analysis of the underlying molecular mechanism revealed that the viral transcription factor HPV8 E2 synergizes with the cellular differentiation-dependent transcription factor C/EBPβ to up-regulate S100A8/A9 expression and to enhance recruitment of granulocytes. Our data indicate that the HPV8 E2 protein hijacks a differentiation-associated pathway to create a chronic inflammatory microenvironment in EV-patients that may pave the way for carcinogenic progression (**Figure 6**).

Epidermodysplasia verruciformis patients are highly susceptible to β-HPV-associated skin carcinogenesis at sun-exposed sites (Smola, 2014). However, the HPV-mediated molecular mechanisms that support the carcinogenic process are poorly understood so far. Our study strongly indicates that the cutaneous β-HPV type 8 can actively trigger inflammation, a hallmark of cancer (Hanahan and Weinberg, 2011). In human organ transplant recipients as well as in mouse models of skin carcinogenesis, this involves the induction of the alarmins S100A8/A9 promoting a pro-tumorigenic inflammatory microenvironment (Gebhardt et al., 2008; Iotzova-Weiss et al., 2015). S100A8/A9 proteins gained a unique interest over the last decades with respect to their role in cancer progression since they can propel cancer cell proliferation, migration, and invasion (Bresnick et al., 2015). Despite the well-defined role of S100A8/A9 in carcinogenesis, however, little is known about factors altering their expression, particularly in HPV-associated carcinogenesis.

Our data clearly demonstrate that S100A8/A9 expression is accompanied by strong immune cell infiltration starting during the productive phase of viral infection in EV-lesions. Tumor-promoting inflammation was previously also observed in mucosal HPV-driven carcinogenesis (Schroer et al., 2011; Walch-Ruckheim et al., 2015, 2016; Smola, 2017; Smola et al., 2017). From published data it was unclear, whether β-HPV oncoproteins contribute to increased inflammatory cytokine production (De Andrea et al., 2007; Akgul et al., 2010). For HPV8 E7, it was rather shown that it interferes with Langerhans recruitment via repression of the chemokine CCL20 (Sperling et al., 2012). This is consistent with observations in anogenital

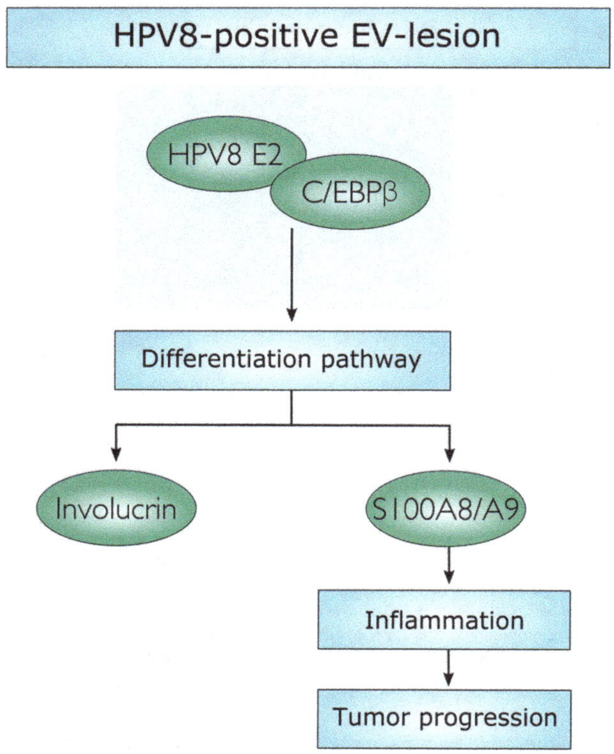

FIGURE 6 | Schematic presentation. Molecular mechanism, by which HPV8 E2 synergizes with C/EBPβ to induce keratinocyte differentiation and to up-regulate S100A8/A9 expression.

HPV infection, where mucosal high-risk HPV oncoproteins were shown to suppress inflammatory responses in keratinocytes (Guess and McCance, 2005; Smola-Hess and Pfister, 2006; Karim et al., 2011, 2013). Here, we demonstrate that neither expression of the HPV8 E6 nor the E7 protein in primary human keratinocytes resulted in higher levels of S100A8 and S100A9. Rather, our study provides evidence that the β-HPV type 8-encoded transcription factor E2 up-regulates S100A8 and S100A9 on mRNA and protein levels. The relevance of this finding was further supported by the observation that calgranulin expression converges spatially with HPV5 E2 mRNA (Haller et al., 1995) in EV-lesions that display characteristic cytopathic effects of β-HPV infection. Notably, this activity seemed to be a unique feature of cutaneous HPV E2, since mucosal high-risk HPV16 E2 was unable to induce S100A8/A9 mRNA expression.

The HPV E2 protein regulates viral transcription through direct binding via its C-terminal domain to the palindromic $ACCN_6GGT$ motif in the HPV non-coding regulatory region, which can result either in gene induction or repression (McBride, 2013), and HPV8 E2 was additionally shown to bind to a non-classical site $ATCGN_4CGAT$ (Akgul et al., 2003). We have previously demonstrated that HPV8 E2 can also modulate the expression of a cellular gene, β4-integrin, via E2-binding sites (Oldak et al., 2004, 2010). E2-expressing cells lose β4-integrin expression, which normally anchors keratinocytes to the basement membrane. This may push E2-expressing cells into suprabasal layers, where they are destined to differentiate. Applying bioinformatic tools, however, we neither detected any classical E2 binding site in the S100A8 and S100A9 promoter regions nor a non-canonical site completely matching with $ATCGN_4CGAT$ (Akgul et al., 2003). Only in the human S100A8 promoter, a site with some similarities (ATCTGGCTGGAT) was detectable at positions −168 to −156, while not being present in the murine counterpart that was used in this study for reporter assays.

As an alternative mechanism to regulate cellular gene expression, HPV E2 engages cellular transcription factors via direct protein-protein interactions. This was first shown for cellular transcription factors of the C/EBP family (Hadaschik et al., 2003) and also for other factors (McBride et al., 2004; McPhillips et al., 2006; Wu et al., 2016). It was shown that E2 can form a ternary complex with C/EBP factors in a DNA-bound state at a C/EBP-specific binding site within the human involucrin gene, a classical marker of keratinocyte differentiation. As a consequence of its interaction with C/EBP factors, E2 leads to potent activation of the involucrin promoter (Hadaschik et al., 2003). Notably, C/EBPβ also directly binds to the S100A8 promoter region as demonstrated by chromatin immunoprecipitation (Miao et al., 2012). In fact, in our transient transfection experiments in RTS3b cells, HPV8 E2 alone was able to activate the murine S100A8 promoter containing the C/EBP but no putative E2-binding site. Moreover, in both, primary human keratinocytes as well as RTS3b cells, HPV8 E2 significantly enhanced PMA- or C/EBPβ-induced promoter activation, respectively. This strongly supported the notion that the molecular mechanism underlying the synergism between HPV8 E2 and C/EBPβ does not necessarily depend on a classical or non-classical E2-binding site but rather resembles the situation previously described for the human involucrin promoter (Hadaschik et al., 2003). However, with respect to the human S100A8 promoter, we cannot exclude that the ATCTGGCTGGAT sequence might further contribute to the E2 effect. In addition, human and murine S100A8 promoter regions are very similar with respect to their C/EBPβ binding site (Miao et al., 2012) but they are not identical. Therefore, we cannot exclude that the promoter region of the murine gene, we used for the reporter assays, can also bind to other transcription factors than those involved in the regulation of the human gene.

S100A8/A9 are potent pro-inflammatory mediators. Our preliminary analysis indicates that calgranulins are not the only pro-inflammatory factors that are up-regulated in cells co-expressing E2 and C/EBPβ, since we could also detect several other neutrophil attracting chemokines in their supernatants. These included IL-8, ENA-78 and NAP-2. The chemokine GRO-α was expressed constitutively and only slightly but non-significantly up-regulated in the E2 and C/EBPβ expressing cells (Supplementary Figure S4). The exact mechanisms underlying the regulation of these chemokines remain to be determined in the future. In our preliminary analyses, recombinant S100A8/A9 did not lead to induction of these chemokines indicating that their up-regulation was parallel to and not via S100A8/A9. In contrast, it has been demonstrated that calgranulins are involved in the induction matrix-metalloproteinases, such as MMP-9, which are involved in tumor growth and angiogenesis (Moon et al., 2008; Saha et al., 2010; Kerkhoff et al., 2012; Lim et al., 2016). From this it can be speculated that the E2-C/EBPβ-S100A8/A9 axis might exert further pleiotropic effects during carcinogenesis.

Apart from this, S100A8/A9, loss of β4-integrin and the induction of involucrin are all involved in keratinocyte differentiation. A role for HPV8 E2 in keratinocyte differentiation was also supported by observations in transgenic mice expressing the HPV8 E2 protein under the K14-promoter (Pfefferle et al., 2008). Morphologically, their skin presented obvious ulcerations and thinning of the epidermis. This was discussed as a putative consequence of premature keratinocyte differentiation and a reduced pool of proliferative keratinocytes consistent with our previous observation of β4-integrin suppression and involucrin induction (Hadaschik et al., 2003; Oldak et al., 2004, 2010; Pfefferle et al., 2008). Importantly, the skin of HPV8 E2-transgenic mice was also characterized by chronic immune cell infiltration and it was associated with spontaneous tumorigenic progression in a significant proportion of the mice (Pfefferle et al., 2008).

Collectively, these data provided evidence for a role of the E2 protein not only in differentiation but also in inflammation and skin tumor formation. This raised the question, how HPV8 E2 might augment tumor-promoting inflammation in skin.

The data presented in this study may provide this missing link. We demonstrate that HPV8 E2 engages the differentiation-inducing C/EBPβ pathway to up-regulate S100A8/A9 factors, which are not only part of the epidermal differentiation complex (Kuruto-Niwa et al., 1998; Miao et al., 2012) but also part of an inflammatory response promoting tumorigenesis (**Figure 6**).

AUTHOR CONTRIBUTIONS

SS, MP, and MO: conceptualization. SS and SL: funding acquisition. SS, MP, MO, AM, SL, and AW: investigation. SS, MP, AM, MO, CM, and BW-R: methodology. SS, CM, TV, MU, MM, and SM: resources. SS: supervision. SS, MP, MO, SL, and BW-R: validation. MP: visualization. SS and MP: writing the original draft. SS, MP, and SL: reviewing and editing the manuscript.

ACKNOWLEDGMENTS

We thank B. Best, B. Glombitza, and A. Kerber for excellent technical assistance.

REFERENCES

Agarwal, C., Efimova, T., Welter, J. F., Crish, J. F., and Eckert, R. L. (1999). CCAAT/enhancer-binding proteins. A role in regulation of human involucrin promoter response to phorbol ester. *J. Biol. Chem.* 274, 6190–6194. doi: 10.1074/jbc.274.10.6190

Akgul, B., Bostanci, N., Westphal, K., Nindl, I., Navsaria, H., Storey, A., et al. (2010). Human papillomavirus 5 and 8 E6 downregulate interleukin-8 secretion in primary human keratinocytes. *J. Gen. Virol.* 91(Pt 4), 888–892. doi: 10.1099/vir.0.016527-0

Akgul, B., Karle, P., Adam, M., Fuchs, P. G., and Pfister, H. J. (2003). Dual role of tumor suppressor p53 in regulation of DNA replication and oncogene E6-promoter activity of *epidermodysplasia verruciformis*-associated human papillomavirus type 8. *Virology* 308, 279–290. doi: 10.1016/S0042-6822(02)00133-2

Balasubramanian, S., Agarwal, C., Efimova, T., Dubyak, G. R., Banks, E., Welter, J., et al. (2000). Thapsigargin suppresses phorbol ester-dependent human involucrin promoter activity by suppressing CCAAT-enhancer-binding protein alpha (C/EBPalpha) DNA binding. *Biochem. J.* 350(Pt 3), 791–796. doi: 10.1042/bj3500791

Bresnick, A. R., Weber, D. J., and Zimmer, D. B. (2015). S100 proteins in cancer. *Nat. Rev. Cancer* 15, 96–109. doi: 10.1038/nrc3893

De Andrea, M., Mondini, M., Azzimonti, B., Dell'Oste, V., Germano, S., Gaudino, G., et al. (2007). Alpha- and betapapillomavirus E6/E7 genes differentially modulate pro-inflammatory gene expression. *Virus Res.* 124, 220–225. doi: 10.1016/j.virusres.2006.09.010

Gebhardt, C., Riehl, A., Durchdewald, M., Nemeth, J., Furstenberger, G., Muller-Decker, K., et al. (2008). RAGE signaling sustains inflammation and promotes tumor development. *J. Exp. Med.* 205, 275–285. doi: 10.1084/jem.20070679

Goethe, R., Basler, T., and Phi-van, L. (2007). Regulation of C/EBPbeta mRNA expression and C/EBPbeta promoter activity by protein kinases A and C in a myelomonocytic cell line (HD11). *Inflamm. Res.* 56, 274–281. doi: 10.1007/s00011-007-6170-y

Guess, J. C., and McCance, D. J. (2005). Decreased migration of Langerhans precursor-like cells in response to human keratinocytes expressing human papillomavirus type 16 E6/E7 is related to reduced macrophage inflammatory protein-3alpha production. *J. Virol.* 79, 14852–14862. doi: 10.1128/JVI.79.23.14852-14862.2005

Hadaschik, D., Hinterkeuser, K., Oldak, M., Pfister, H. J., and Smola-Hess, S. (2003). The Papillomavirus E2 protein binds to and synergizes with C/EBP factors involved in keratinocyte differentiation. *J. Virol.* 77, 5253–5265. doi: 10.1128/JVI.77.9.5253-5265.2003

Haller, K., Stubenrauch, F., and Pfister, H. (1995). Differentiation-dependent transcription of the epidermodysplasia verruciformis-associated human papillomavirus type 5 in benign lesions. *Virology* 214, 245–255. doi: 10.1006/viro.1995.0028

Hanahan, D., and Weinberg, R. A. (2011). Hallmarks of cancer: the next generation. *Cell* 144, 646–674. doi: 10.1016/j.cell.2011.02.013

Iotzova-Weiss, G., Dziunycz, P. J., Freiberger, S. N., Lauchli, S., Hafner, J., Vogl, T., et al. (2015). S100A8/A9 stimulates keratinocyte proliferation in the development of squamous cell carcinoma of the skin via the receptor for advanced glycation-end products. *PLoS One* 10:e0120971. doi: 10.1371/journal.pone.0120971

Karim, R., Meyers, C., Backendorf, C., Ludigs, K., Offringa, R., van Ommen, G. J., et al. (2011). Human papillomavirus deregulates the response of a cellular network comprising of chemotactic and proinflammatory genes. *PLoS One* 6:e17848. doi: 10.1371/journal.pone.0017848

Karim, R., Tummers, B., Meyers, C., Biryukov, J. L., Alam, S., Backendorf, C., et al. (2013). Human papillomavirus (HPV) upregulates the cellular deubiquitinase UCHL1 to suppress the keratinocyte's innate immune response. *PLoS Pathog.* 9:e1003384. doi: 10.1371/journal.ppat.1003384

Kerkhoff, C., Voss, A., Scholzen, T. E., Averill, M. M., Zanker, K. S., and Bornfeldt, K. E. (2012). Novel insights into the role of S100A8/A9 in skin biology. *Exp. Dermatol.* 21, 822–826. doi: 10.1111/j.1600-0625.2012.01571.x

Kuruto-Niwa, R., Nakamura, M., Takeishi, K., and Nozawa, R. (1998). Transcriptional regulation by C/EBP alpha and -beta in the expression of the gene for the MRP14 myeloid calcium binding protein. *Cell Struct. Funct.* 23, 109–118. doi: 10.1247/csf.23.109

Leukert, N., Vogl, T., Strupat, K., Reichelt, R., Sorg, C., and Roth, J. (2006). Calcium-dependent tetramer formation of S100A8 and S100A9 is essential for biological activity. *J. Mol. Biol.* 359, 961–972. doi: 10.1016/j.jmb.2006.04.009

Lim, S. Y., Yuzhalin, A. E., Gordon-Weeks, A. N., and Muschel, R. J. (2016). Tumor-infiltrating monocytes/macrophages promote tumor invasion and migration by upregulating S100A8 and S100A9 expression in cancer cells. *Oncogene* 35, 5735–5745. doi: 10.1038/onc.2016.107

Majewski, S., and Jablonska, S. (2006). Current views on the role of human papillomaviruses in cutaneous oncogenesis. *Int. J. Dermatol.* 45, 192–196. doi: 10.1111/j.1365-4632.2006.02758.x

Marthaler, A. M., Podgorska, M., Feld, P., Fingerle, A., Knerr-Rupp, K., Grasser, F., et al. (2017). Identification of C/EBPalpha as a novel target of the HPV8 E6 protein regulating miR-203 in human keratinocytes. *PLoS Pathog.* 13:e1006406. doi: 10.1371/journal.ppat.1006406

McBride, A. A. (2013). The papillomavirus E2 proteins. *Virology* 445, 57–79. doi: 10.1016/j.virol.2013.06.006

McBride, A. A., McPhillips, M. G., and Oliveira, J. G. (2004). Brd4: tethering, segregation and beyond. *Trends Microbiol.* 12, 527–529. doi: 10.1016/j.tim.2004.10.002

McPhillips, M. G., Oliveira, J. G., Spindler, J. E., Mitra, R., and McBride, A. A. (2006). Brd4 is required for e2-mediated transcriptional activation but not genome partitioning of all papillomaviruses. *J. Virol.* 80, 9530–9543. doi: 10.1128/JVI.01105-06

Miao, L., Grebhardt, S., Shi, J., Peipe, I., Zhang, J., and Mayer, D. (2012). Prostaglandin E2 stimulates S100A8 expression by activating protein kinase A and CCAAT/enhancer-binding-protein-beta in prostate cancer cells. *Int. J. Biochem. Cell Biol.* 44, 1919–1928. doi: 10.1016/j.biocel.2012.06.015

Michel, A., Kopp-Schneider, A., Zentgraf, H., Gruber, A. D., and de Villiers, E. M. (2006). E6/E7 expression of human papillomavirus type 20 (HPV-20) and HPV-27 influences proliferation and differentiation of the skin in UV-irradiated SKH-hr1 transgenic mice. *J. Virol.* 80, 11153–11164. doi: 10.1128/JVI.00954-06

Moon, A., Yong, H. Y., Song, J. I., Cukovic, D., Salagrama, S., Kaplan, D., et al. (2008). Global gene expression profiling unveils S100A8/A9 as candidate markers in H-ras-mediated human breast epithelial cell invasion. *Mol. Cancer Res.* 6, 1544–1553. doi: 10.1158/1541-7786.MCR-08-0189

Oldak, M., Maksym, R. B., Sperling, T., Yaniv, M., Smola, H., Pfister, H. J., et al. (2010). Human papillomavirus type 8 E2 protein unravels JunB/Fra-1 as an activator of the beta4-integrin gene in human keratinocytes. *J. Virol.* 84, 1376–1386. doi: 10.1128/JVI.01220-09

Oldak, M., Smola, H., Aumailley, M., Rivero, F., Pfister, H., and Smola-Hess, S. (2004). The human papillomavirus type 8 E2 protein suppresses beta4-integrin expression in primary human keratinocytes. *J. Virol.* 78, 10738–10746. doi: 10.1128/JVI.78.19.10738-10746.2004

Orth, G. (1986). Epidermodysplasia verruciformis: a model for understanding the oncogenicity of human papillomaviruses. *Ciba Found. Symp.* 120, 157–174.

Orth, G., Jablonska, S., Favre, M., Croissant, O., Jarzabek-Chorzelska, M., and Rzesa, G. (1978). Characterization of two types of human papillomaviruses in lesions of epidermodysplasia verruciformis. *Proc. Natl. Acad. Sci. U.S.A.* 75, 1537–1541. doi: 10.1073/pnas.75.3.1537

Park, M. H., Park, S. Y., and Kim, Y. (2008). Induction of proline-rich tyrosine kinase2 (Pyk2) through C/EBPbeta is involved in PMA-induced monocyte differentiation. *FEBS Lett.* 582, 415–422. doi: 10.1016/j.febslet.2008.01.001

Pfefferle, R., Marcuzzi, G. P., Akgul, B., Kasper, H. U., Schulze, F., Haase, I., et al. (2008). The human papillomavirus type 8 E2 protein induces skin tumors in transgenic mice. *J. Invest. Dermatol.* 128, 2310–2315. doi: 10.1038/jid.2008.73

Pfister, H. (2003). Chapter 8: Human papillomavirus and skin cancer. *J. Natl. Cancer Inst. Monogr.* 31, 52–56. doi: 10.1093/oxfordjournals.jncimonographs.a003483

Purdie, K. J., Sexton, C. J., Proby, C. M., Glover, M. T., Williams, A. T., Stables, J. N., et al. (1993). Malignant transformation of cutaneous lesions in renal allograft patients: a role for human papillomavirus. *Cancer Res.* 53, 5328–5333.

Ramoz, N., Rueda, L. A., Bouadjar, B., Montoya, L. S., Orth, G., and Favre, M. (2002). Mutations in two adjacent novel genes are associated with epidermodysplasia verruciformis. *Nat. Genet.* 32, 579–581. doi: 10.1038/ng1044

Ryckman, C., Vandal, K., Rouleau, P., Talbot, M., and Tessier, P. A. (2003). Proinflammatory activities of S100: proteins S100A8, S100A9, and S100A8/A9 induce neutrophil chemotaxis and adhesion. *J. Immunol.* 170, 3233–3242. doi: 10.4049/jimmunol.170.6.3233

Saha, A., Lee, Y. C., Zhang, Z., Chandra, G., Su, S. B., and Mukherjee, A. B. (2010). Lack of an endogenous anti-inflammatory protein in mice enhances colonization of B16F10 melanoma cells in the lungs. *J. Biol. Chem.* 285, 10822–10831. doi: 10.1074/jbc.M109.083550

Schaper, I. D., Marcuzzi, G. P., Weissenborn, S. J., Kasper, H. U., Dries, V., Smyth, N., et al. (2005). Development of skin tumors in mice transgenic for early genes of human papillomavirus type 8. *Cancer Res.* 65, 1394–1400. doi: 10.1158/0008-5472.CAN-04-3263

Schroer, N., Pahne, J., Walch, B., Wickenhauser, C., and Smola, S. (2011). Molecular pathobiology of human cervical high-grade lesions: paracrine STAT3 activation in tumor-instructed myeloid cells drives local MMP-9 expression. *Cancer Res.* 71, 87–97. doi: 10.1158/0008-5472.CAN-10-2193

Shamanin, V., Glover, M., Rausch, C., Proby, C., Leigh, I. M., zur Hausen, H., et al. (1994). Specific types of human papillomavirus found in benign proliferations and carcinomas of the skin in immunosuppressed patients. *Cancer Res.* 54, 4610–4613.

Smola, H., Thiekotter, G., and Fusenig, N. E. (1993). Mutual induction of growth factor gene expression by epidermal-dermal cell interaction. *J. Cell Biol.* 122, 417–429. doi: 10.1083/jcb.122.2.417

Smola, S. (2014). Human papillomaviruses and skin cancer. *Adv. Exp. Med. Biol.* 810, 192–207.

Smola, S. (2017). Immunopathogenesis of HPV-associated cancers and prospects for immunotherapy. *Viruses* 9:E254. doi: 10.3390/v9090254

Smola, S., Trimble, C., and Stern, P. L. (2017). Human papillomavirus-driven immune deviation: challenge and novel opportunity for immunotherapy. *Ther. Adv. Vaccines* 5, 69–82. doi: 10.1177/2051013617717914

Smola-Hess, S., and Pfister, H. (2006). "Immune evasion in genital papillomavirus infection and cervical cancer: role of cytokines and chemokines," in *Papillomavirus Research: From Natural History to Vaccines and Beyond*, ed. M. S. Campo (Wymondham: Caister Academic), 423.

Sperling, T., Oldak, M., Walch-Ruckheim, B., Wickenhauser, C., Doorbar, J., Pfister, H., et al. (2012). Human papillomavirus type 8 interferes with a novel C/EBPbeta-mediated mechanism of keratinocyte CCL20 chemokine expression and Langerhans cell migration. *PLoS Pathog.* 8:e1002833. doi: 10.1371/journal.ppat.1002833

Viarisio, D., Mueller-Decker, K., Kloz, U., Aengeneyndt, B., Kopp-Schneider, A., Grone, H. J., et al. (2011). E6 and E7 from beta HPV38 cooperate with ultraviolet light in the development of actinic keratosis-like lesions and squamous cell carcinoma in mice. *PLoS Pathog.* 7:e1002125. doi: 10.1371/journal.ppat.1002125

Walch-Ruckheim, B., Mavrova, R., Henning, M., Vicinus, B., Kim, Y. J., Bohle, R. M., et al. (2015). Stromal fibroblasts induce CCL20 through IL6/C/EBPbeta to support the recruitment of Th17 cells during cervical cancer progression. *Cancer Res.* 75, 5248–5259. doi: 10.1158/0008-5472.CAN-15-0732

Walch-Ruckheim, B., Pahne-Zeppenfeld, J., Fischbach, J., Wickenhauser, C., Horn, L. C., Tharun, L., et al. (2016). STAT3/IRF1 pathway activation sensitizes cervical cancer cells to chemotherapeutic drugs. *Cancer Res.* 76, 3872–3883. doi: 10.1158/0008-5472.CAN-14-1306

Weissenborn, S. J., Wieland, U., Junk, M., and Pfister, H. (2010). Quantification of beta-human papillomavirus DNA by real-time PCR. *Nat. Protoc.* 5, 1–13. doi: 10.1038/nprot.2009.153

Wu, S. Y., Nin, D. S., Lee, A. Y., Simanski, S., Kodadek, T., and Chiang, C. M. (2016). BRD4 phosphorylation regulates HPV E2-mediated viral transcription, origin replication, and cellular MMP-9 expression. *Cell Rep.* 16, 1733–1748. doi: 10.1016/j.celrep.2016.07.001

zur Hausen, H. (2009). Papillomaviruses in the causation of human cancers - a brief historical account. *Virology* 384, 260–265. doi: 10.1016/j.virol.2008.11.046

9

From Merkel Cell Polyomavirus Infection to Merkel Cell Carcinoma Oncogenesis

Nathan A. Krump[†] and Jianxin You[*]

Department of Microbiology, Perelman School of Medicine, University of Pennsylvania, Philadelphia, PA, United States

***Correspondence:**
Jianxin You
jianyou@pennmedicine.upenn.edu

[†]Present address:
Nathan A. Krump,
Integral Molecular, Inc., Philadelphia, PA, United States

Merkel cell polyomavirus (MCPyV) infection causes near-ubiquitous, asymptomatic infection in the skin, but occasionally leads to an aggressive skin cancer called Merkel cell carcinoma (MCC). Epidemiological evidence suggests that poorly controlled MCPyV infection may be a precursor to MCPyV-associated MCC. Clearer understanding of host responses that normally control MCPyV infection could inform prophylactic measures in at-risk groups. Similarly, the presence of MCPyV in most MCCs could imbue them with vulnerabilities that-if better characterized-could yield targeted intervention solutions for metastatic MCC cases. In this review, we discuss recent developments in elucidating the interplay between host cells and MCPyV within the context of viral infection and MCC oncogenesis. We also propose a model in which insufficient restriction of MCPyV infection in aging and chronically UV-damaged skin causes unbridled viral replication that licenses MCC tumorigenesis.

Keywords: Merkel cell polyomavirus, Merkel cell carcinoma, persistence, innate immune response, integration, dysbiosis, oncogenesis

INTRODUCTION

Merkel cell polyomavirus (MCPyV) infection can be detected on the skin of most healthy adults (Tolstov et al., 2009; Schowalter et al., 2010), yet details of its virology and infectious cycle remain sparse. Evidence from serological studies suggests that MCPyV infects most people during early childhood with exposure to the virus increasing as populations age (Chen et al., 2011; Viscidi et al., 2011; Martel-Jantin et al., 2013). A vast majority of MCPyV infections are asymptomatic (Tolstov et al., 2011), but some result in an aggressive neuroendocrine skin cancer called Merkel cell carcinoma (MCC) (Feng et al., 2008; Gjoerup and Chang, 2010; Harms, 2017; Schadendorf et al., 2017). The etiology of over 80% of MCC tumors can be traced to MCPyV by the presence of integrated MCPyV genomic sequence in the cellular DNA (Feng et al., 2008; Santos-Juanes et al., 2015).

Though MCC cases are rare, the incidence of MCC has tripled over the last two decades and is projected to increase further in the future (Fitzgerald et al , 2015; Paulson et al., 2018a; Stang et al., 2018; Freeman et al., 2019; Jacobs et al., 2020). MCC has a high rate of mortality with 5-year overall survival around 51% for patients presenting with local disease at the time of diagnosis, and worse prognoses for those with more advanced stages of disease (Harms K. L. et al., 2016). Primary MCC malignancies are combatted by surgical resection, sentinel lymph node biopsy, and/or adjuvant radiation (Cassler et al., 2016). In metastatic MCC, chemotherapies have thus far failed to produce durable responses (Iyer et al., 2016; Cowey et al., 2017). Promisingly, a recent bourgeoning of anti-PD1 and anti-PDL1 treatments for MCC has yielded prolonged responses in patients with advanced disease, though a significant proportion of patients do not respond and the durability of responses varies (Iyer et al., 2016; Becker et al., 2017; D'angelo et al., 2018; Nghiem et al., 2019). The pursuit of more targeted and effective MCC therapies necessitates a better understanding of the oncogenic underpinnings of MCC and the role of MCPyV in tumorigenesis.

Despite the status of MCPyV as a member of the human skin virome and its relevance to human disease, much is unknown about its biology. For instance, while it is clear that MCPyV integration and oncogene expression enable MCC cell growth, the conditions that lead to MCPyV integration are not known. Neither has a consensus been reached regarding the MCC cell of origin. Most pressingly, methods of limiting MCPyV infection and thereby preventing MCC onset have yet to be discovered. In recent years, however, efforts have been aimed at exploiting the presence of MCPyV oncoproteins in MCCs to develop targeted therapies for virus-positive MCC tumors (Chapuis et al., 2014; Gavvovidis et al., 2018; Longino et al., 2019; Sarma et al., 2020). The potential for expanding on these opportunities to provide prophylactic or therapeutic interventions for a highly lethal skin cancer should not be overlooked.

Merkel Cell Carcinoma

MCC was first described in 1972 by Cyril Toker, MD (Toker, 1972). He and his colleagues discovered that the tumors arose in the dermis or lower subcutis layers of the skin and that they metastasized readily via the lymphatic system. Because the malignancies shared neuroendocrine markers with Merkel cells, such as cytokeratin-20 (CK20) and neuron-specific enolase (NSE), the disease was named Merkel cell carcinoma (De Wolff-Peeters et al., 1980; Gu et al., 1983; Moll et al., 1992).

The next breakthrough in characterizing MCC came in 2008 when the Chang and Moore group identified a novel polyomavirus genome monoclonally integrated in the DNA of MCC tumor cells (Feng et al., 2008). Previously, they had correctly predicted the viral etiology of AIDS-associated Kaposi's sarcoma (KS) (Chang et al., 1994), hypothesizing that the altered immune status of these individuals engendered dysbiosis between the host and virus to trigger oncogenesis. Following the same principle, they suspected viral involvement in MCCs given the knowledge that MCCs were far more likely to occur in HIV-positive individuals (Engels et al., 2002). Probing MCC primary tumors and metastases by digital transcriptome subtraction and viral genome walking revealed the presence and sequence of the MCPyV genome, respectively (Feng et al., 2008).

As a result of their discovery, assays to determine the status of MCPyV have provided definitive markers and more assured diagnosis for a subset of MCCs (Buck and Lowy, 2009; Decaprio, 2009; Duncavage et al., 2009; Haugg et al., 2014; Starrett et al., 2020). Moreover, it is now widely acknowledged that immunocompromised individuals are more likely to develop virus-driven cancers (Ellerbrock et al., 2000; Weber et al., 2006; Chadburn et al., 2013; Ponce et al., 2014; Schadendorf et al., 2017). The discovery of MCPyV also opened the opportunity to research the role of MCPyV oncogenes in MCC carcinogenesis

Building upon those earlier discoveries, recent research has been aimed at comparing MCPyV-positive and MCPyV-negative MCCs, which despite evidently different etiologies, have similar disease presentation and prognoses (Fischer et al., 2010; Handschel et al., 2010; Schrama et al., 2011). In virus-associated MCC, MCPyV DNA is integrated into the tumor cell genome in a manner that preserves expression of MCPyV genes called tumor (T) antigens (Shuda et al., 2008, 2011; Cheng et al., 2013). Expression of MCPyV T antigens drives oncogenesis in virus-positive MCC tumors and is required for the growth of the tumor cells (Houben et al., 2010, 2012; Shuda et al., 2011, 2014; Spurgeon and Lambert, 2013; Verhaegen et al., 2014; Grundhoff and Fischer, 2015; Wendzicki et al., 2015). MCPyV T antigens can support MCC growth and survival despite otherwise low chromosomal mutation burdens in MCPyV-positive MCCs (Starrett et al., 2017). By contrast, virus-negative MCCs exhibit a high, UV-related, mutation frequency indicating that pro-oncogenic mutations arose as a direct result of chronic exposure to UV-radiation (Harms et al., 2015; Wong et al., 2015; Goh et al., 2016; Starrett et al., 2017). MCPyV-negative MCCs also have higher levels of activation-induced cytidine deaminase (AID) which could contribute to mutagenesis (Matsushita et al., 2017). The gradual selection for transforming mutations may lead to shared traits among MCPyV-negative cancers such as loss-of-function mutations in Rb, NOTCH, PRUNE2, as well as, activating mutations in PI3KCA and HRAS (Sihto et al., 2011; Nardi et al., 2012; Harms et al., 2013, 2015; Cimino et al., 2014; Sahi et al., 2014; Wong et al., 2015; Goh et al., 2016; Harms P. W. et al., 2016).

Disparities between the etiologies of MCPyV-positive and -negative MCCs extend to differences in their morphology. MCPyV-containing malignances are more likely to have regularly-shaped nuclei, low cytoplasm volume, and more homogeneous cell types than those lacking MCPyV (Kuwamoto et al., 2011; Iwasaki et al., 2013). They are also more likely to display classical markers for MCC such as CK20 and neurofilament (Pasternak et al., 2018). Differences in morphological phenotype between the two MCC types could be a reflection of their alternative expression profiles in factors such as cell adhesion molecules or miRNAs (Xie et al., 2014; Iwasaki et al., 2016).

There are also disparities between these two types of cancers that have more immediately discernible implications. Virus-associated MCCs are more likely to occur in non-sun-exposed areas than MCPyV-negative MCC (Dabner et al., 2014; Leroux-Kozal et al., 2015) and on a population scale, virus-negative MCCs occur in greater proportions in Australia, where a significant population of individuals with low-melanin concentrations are exposed to high levels of UV-radiation (Paik et al., 2011). Moreover, MCC tumors in younger patients and females are more likely to be virus-positive (Wang et al., 2017). These trends suggest that while UV-exposure and advanced age increase the incidence of both cancer types, MCPyV oncogenesis is less dependent on these exogenous factors.

Beyond differences in oncogenic mechanism, morphology, and incidence, there are an increasing number of reports that MCPyV-positive MCC patient prognosis is statistically better than those with MCPyV-negative MCC (Sihto et al., 2009;

Laude et al., 2010; Higaki-Mori et al., 2012; Leroux-Kozal et al., 2015; Moshiri et al., 2017). One reason for the improved patient survival associated with MCPyV-LT-expressing MCC tumors may be correlated with the presence of foreign T antigens that enhance immunogenicity (Walsh et al., 2016). In MCC patients undergoing PD-1 treatment, there is a greater degree of B and T cell clonality in MCPyV-positive tumor infiltrates than MCPyV-negative, reflecting the greater diversity of neoantigens in the latter case (Miller et al., 2018). MCPyV-positive MCCs also exhibit elevated expression of prokineticin-2, an inflammatory and angiogenic signaling molecule, resulting in enhanced T cell infiltration (Lauttia et al., 2014). Another reason for better prognoses in MCPyV-positive MCC cases could be that lower frequency of somatic mutations equate to expression of wild type tumor suppressors like p53 that support therapeutic interventions and native immune responses in restricting cancer progression.

The juxtaposition of these two MCC subtypes informs our understanding of both through comparative analysis, and can guide the development of novel treatments. In MCPyV-driven MCC, there exists the promise of truly targeted therapies toward an aggressive solid tumor. What we learn about viral MCCs can be applied to the more complicated and divergent cases of MCPyV-negative MCC. These lessons can, in turn, broaden our understanding of this family of rapidly metastasizing skin cancer.

MCPyV Genome and Encoded Genes

MCPyV Genome

MCPyV has a ~5.4 kb circular dsDNA genome (**Figure 1**). Like other polyomaviruses, existing evidence suggests that the MCPyV genome remains episomal throughout the infectious cycle (Gjoerup and Chang, 2010; Liu et al., 2016a,b). The viral genome is divided into early and late regions by a non-coding control region (NCCR) containing the viral origin of replication and bidirectional promoters that drive early and late gene transcription (Harrison et al., 2011). The early region expresses alternatively spliced tumor antigens, termed large tumor antigen (LT) and small tumor antigen (sT) that support replication, as well as, 57kT and an alternate LT open reading frame (ALTO) with functions that are less defined (Kwun et al., 2009; Carter et al., 2013). Major and minor capsid proteins, VP1 and VP2, respectively, are expressed from the MCPyV late region along with a miRNA that has been proposed to modulate early gene expression (Seo et al., 2009; Schowalter et al., 2011).

In MCPyV-positive MCC, the MCPyV genome is integrated into the host DNA such that the functions of its early promoter and partial expression of its T antigens are preserved (Feng et al., 2008). Point mutations in other regions of the genome and truncations of the MCPyV LT C-terminal domain, however, are common in viral MCCs (Liu et al., 2016a). Expression of the viral oncoproteins is largely driven by the preserved MCPyV promoter rather than endogenous promoters, though there are conflicting reports as to whether MCPyV is more likely to integrate into specific regions of chromatin (Doolittle-Hall et al., 2015; Czech-Sioli et al., 2020). Sequencing of integration sites in multiple MCC tumors reveal that initial recombination of a linearized MCPyV genome with the host genome could lead to transient circularization and amplification of the viral genome and neighboring host DNA (Starrett et al., 2017). The amount of amplification and the site of DNA repair accounts for differences in viral genome copy number and duplications of host sequences.

Large Tumor Antigen

In MCPyV infected cells, LT localizes to the nucleus where it performs functions directly and indirectly supporting MCPyV replication (Nakamura et al., 2010). Like T antigens in other polyomaviruses, LT contains an origin binding domain (OBD) and an ATP-dependent helicase domain by which it unwinds MCPyV DNA for replication (Harrison et al., 2011). LT localizes to replication foci containing high concentrations of nascently synthesized MCPyV genomes (Liu et al., 2016b). In replication foci, LT binds to G(A/G)GGC-like pentanucleotide sequences on the MCPyV genome to initiate efficient replication in a manner that requires the LT DnaJ domain and is supported by the presence of sT (Kwun et al., 2009; Harrison et al., 2011).

Somatic genes also localize to MCPyV replication foci and support LT-mediated replication. Bromodomain protein-4 (BRD4) associates with LT in replication centers where it amplifies MCPyV replication by recruiting replication factor C (RFC) (Wang et al., 2012). Ataxia telangiectasia mutated (ATM) and Rad3-related (ATR) DNA damage response (DDR) factors also co-localize to MCPyV replication centers in a manner dependent on the presence of LT and the MCPyV origin (Tsang et al., 2014). These DDR proteins support efficient viral genomic DNA synthesis, but may also be essential in limiting the transforming potential of MCPyV T antigens. For example, ATM phosphorylates LT in the C-terminal domain at Ser-816, leading to increased apoptosis (Li et al., 2015). Alanine mutagenesis at this site leads to enhanced colony formation in C33A cells. Therefore, this LT-ATM interaction could both promote MCPyV replication and limit rampant cellular growth. The delicate balance of establishing an S-phase-like environment for the production of new virions without causing the terminal fate of cellular transformation can explain the duality of MCPyV traits.

The necessity of MCPyV to avoid terminating its infectious cycle by transforming its host cell is underscored by the fact that unlike other polyomavirus T antigens, LT neither binds nor inhibits p53 (Lilyestrom et al., 2006; Cheng et al., 2013). In fact, the studies by Li and colleagues showed that the helicase activity in full-length LT, in the context of MCPyV DNA synthesis, induces cell cycle arrest in a p53-dependent manner that limits cellular proliferation (Li et al., 2013). This observation provided an evolutionary explanation as to why MCPyV may have lost the ability to inactivate p53, in that allowing p53 to guard cell cycle progression could limit incidental progression to cancer and abortive MCPyV infection. It also suggests why mature MCCs invariably express a truncated variant of LT (LTT) lacking the C-terminal helicase domain. In support of the protective nature of the LT C-terminal domain, expression of LTT, but not full-length LT, sensitizes cells to UV-DNA damage due to impaired cell cycle arrest and DDR (Demetriou et al., 2012). Moreover, expression of LTT promotes cell growth, while expression of the C-terminal domain alone, or full-length LT, negatively regulates cell growth (Cheng et al., 2013).

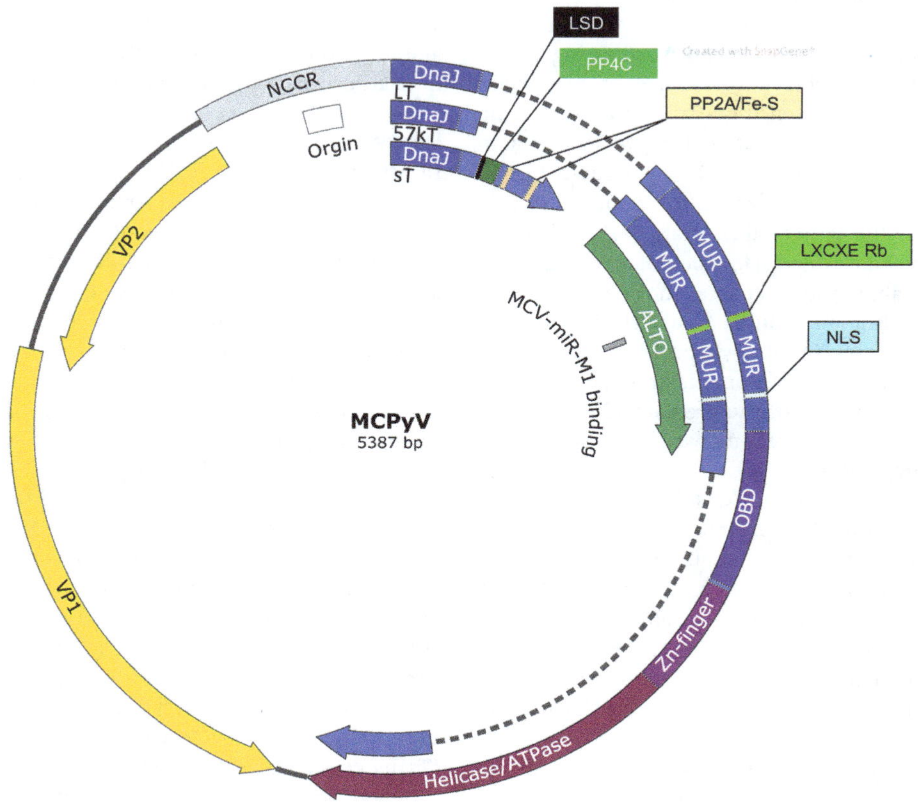

FIGURE 1 | Map of MCPyV genome. NCCR, Non-coding control region; Origin, Origin of replication; LSD, LT stabilization domain; NLS, Nuclear localization signal; MUR, MCPyV unique region; OBD, Origin binding domain.

The ability of MCPyV LTT to promote cellular proliferation has been attributed to its ability to bind and inactivate Rb through an LXCXE domain similar to other polyomaviruses (Houben et al., 2012). This region is present in both wild-type LT and LTT. The LT-Rb interaction results in enhanced E2F-transcriptional activity; promoting growth in MCPyV-positive MCC cells (Sihto et al., 2011; Hesbacher et al., 2016; Schrama et al., 2016). The impact of LT-Rb binding was further illustrated by the fact that silencing LTT expression in a xenograft MCC mouse model resulted in tumor regression in an Rb-binding dependent manner (Houben et al., 2012). The LXCXE-Rb interaction also enhances entry into S-phase, cellular proliferation, and motility in hTERT immortalized BJ human foreskin fibroblasts (BJ-hTERT) (Richards et al., 2015). The functional significance of MCPyV LTT inactivation of Rb in human populations is also supported by the finding that MCPyV-negative MCCs frequently contain mutations in the Rb gene, whereas MCPyV-positive tumors usually express wild type Rb (Sihto et al., 2011).

LT-Rb binding domain could also be responsible for increasing Sox2 and subsequent Atoh expression in MCPyV-positive MCC cells (Harold et al., 2019). This is significant because the activity of these transcription factors can confer cells with markers of the shared phenotype between Merkel cells and MCCs both *in vitro* and *in vivo* (Verhaegen et al., 2017). Though sT has garnered more attention regarding cellular transformation, it may be that LT alters the transcriptional landscape of the original cell of MCC to imbue it with its morphological characteristics.

Recently, it has been shown that the Rb inhibitory domain of LT could indirectly activate p53 by upregulating ARF, an inhibitor of the p53-degrading E3 ubiquitin ligase MDM2 (Park et al., 2019). This assertion suggests that even without the helicase domain, LTT would activate p53 in MCC cells, but the investigators propose that the sT-MYC-EP400 transcriptional complex counteracts p53 activity through upregulation of MDM2 and the related enzyme MDM4 (Park et al., 2019).

Small Tumor Antigen

MCPyV sT consists of 186 amino acids, including a C-terminus that is spliced out of the other MCPyV T antigens that confers it with entirely unique functions. MCPyV sT localizes to the nucleus and is able to support LT-mediated replication though the exact mechanism remains unclear (Kwun et al., 2009). The functions carried out by the C-terminal domain unique to MCPyV sT is of critical importance because its expression is necessary for MCC survival and appears to be the primary driver of cellular transformation (Shuda et al., 2011).

MCPyV sT expression is capable of transforming rat fibroblasts and epithelial cells in an *in vivo* mouse model via a region incorporating amino acids 91–95 termed the LT stabilization domain (LSD) (Shuda et al., 2011; Kwun et al., 2015; Verhaegen et al., 2015). As its name implies, MCPyV sT containing wild-type LSD increases LT protein level, though the underlying mechanism is an area of active investigation (Kwun et al., 2013; Dye et al., 2019). MCPyV sT drives cellular transformation in rat fibroblasts by promoting hyperphosphorylation of eukaryotic translation-initiation factor 4E-binding protein (4E-BP1) (Shuda et al., 2011; Wu et al., 2015; Velasquez et al., 2016). The LSD domain was also linked to activation of the non-canonical NF-κB pathway, induction of a senescence associated secretory phenotype (SASP), and enhanced MCC cell proliferation (Zhao et al., 2020). Besides those functions attributed to the LSD domain, numerous other oncogenic functions have been ascribed to MCPyV sT.

MCPyV sT expression may promote cellular growth by activating c-Jun downstream of MEK/ERK factors (Wu et al., 2016). In addition, MCPyV sT expression in normal fibroblasts elevates aerobic glycolysis via modulation of the host cell transcriptome, including upregulation of monocarboxylate lactate transporter SLC16A1 (MCT1), likely contributing to oncogenic potential (Berrios et al., 2016). Still another way in which sT could enhance metastatic potential is through disruption of inter-cellular junctions via upregulation of A-disintegrase-and-metalloproteinase (ADAM) 10 and 17, which are more highly expressed in MCPyV-positive MCCs (Nwogu et al., 2018). The manner in which MCPyV sT might be affecting transcriptional changes described above is by recruiting a MYCL-MAX heterodimer to the EP400 complex (Cheng et al., 2017). This interaction was elegantly shown to promote cell viability in MCPyV-positive cell lines, MKL-1 and WaGa, as well as, confer a transforming phenotype in keratinocytes (Cheng et al., 2017). Two genes that are upregulated by this transcriptional program are MDM2, which promotes p53 proteasomal degradation, and lysine-specific histone demethylase 1A (LSD1), which is necessary for maintaining plasticity and proliferative capacity of MCC cells (Park et al., 2019, 2020; Leiendecker et al., 2020). Importantly, inhibition of MDM2 and LSD1 induces cell death in MCC cells and reduces the growth of MCC tumor in mice, demonstrating the therapeutic potential of using MDM2 and LSD1 inhibitors in treating this highly aggressive skin cancer (Park et al., 2019, 2020; Leiendecker et al., 2020).

MCPyV sT contains protein phosphatase 2A (PP2A) binding sites similar to other polyomaviruses, but this binding activity is not required for transformation of rat fibroblasts (Kwun et al., 2015). It has been suggested that these PP2A binding sites are involved in the interaction with protein phosphatase 4C (PP4C) (Griffiths et al., 2013; Kwun et al., 2015). In addition to findings mentioned earlier, one group found that sT targets NEMO through interaction with its regulatory subunit (PP4R1) to disrupt NF-κB mediated inflammatory signaling (Griffiths et al., 2013; Abdul-Sada et al., 2017). The sT-PP4C interaction has also been implicated in lowering microtubule stability through altered expression of cellular proteins like stathmin, as well as, Rho GTPase-mediated actin remodeling, leading to an enhanced cell motility phenotype (Knight et al., 2015; Stakaityte et al., 2018). These broad changes resulting from the sT-PP4C interaction have been recently ascribed to upregulated p38 MAPK signaling via MKK4 (Dobson et al., 2020). MCPyV sT related motility might therefore confer transformed cells with invasive and metastatic properties.

Our group found that the proposed PP2A binding sites might also serve as iron-sulfur (Fe/S) cluster domains (Tsang et al., 2015). This discovery had significance because proteins containing Fe/S domains often modulate helicase activity (Pugh et al., 2008; Wu and Brosh, 2012). The function of MCPyV sT Fe/S clusters was linked with its localization to LT-containing replication foci and enhanced MCPyV DNA synthesis without increasing LT protein stability. Moreover, MCPyV sT was able to coordinate Fe/S much more efficiently than sT proteins from SV40, HPyV6, and HPyV7. Another group recently found that expression of MCPyV sT in HEK 293 cells elevated several markers of DNA damage, and at a higher rate than HPyV6 and HPyV7 sT proteins (Wu et al., 2019). Given these findings, the supportive role of sT in LT-mediated MCPyV replication could be direct, through sT activity in replication centers, or indirect, through activation of ATM and subsequent phosphorylation of LT Ser816.

57kT and ALTO

A third alternatively spliced T antigen is that of 57kT (**Figure 1**). 57kT does not appear to support MCPyV replication, and its specific function in infection or in MCC oncogenesis is unclear (Kwun et al., 2009). Because it shares the MCPyV unique region (MUR) with LT, but lacks the helicase and origin-binding domains, it is reasonable to hypothesize that 57kT indirectly supports MCPyV infection, but does not directly support replication as LT does. Similar to LTT, 57kT could bolster pro-oncogenic functions associated with Rb-binding without helicase-related cell cycle arrest or DNA damage.

Carter and colleagues discovered an overprinting gene product expressed from the early region that they termed alternate Large T open reading frame (ALTO) (Carter et al., 2013) (**Figure 1**). This transcript utilizes a start codon that is +1 nucleotide frame-shifted relative to the second exon of LT. The authors hypothesize that overprinting genes such as these evolve in viruses as a strategy to maximize the coding potential of relatively small genomes (Carter et al., 2013). Recently, several ALTO-encoding circular RNAs have been identified in MCPyV-positive MCC cell lines and tumor tissues (Yang et al., 2021). MCPyV ALTO translated from these circular RNAs has the ability to transactivate recombinant promoters, as well as, a number of key cellular genes involved in MCPyV pathogenesis. Therefore MCPyV ALTO protein may be able to modulate MCPyV infectious and tumorigenic potential through transcription regulation (Yang et al., 2021).

VP1, VP2, and miR-M1

The MCPyV late promoter drives expression of the capsid proteins VP1 and VP2, as well as, a miRNA, MCPyV miR-M1 (**Figure 1**). VP1 and VP2 encapsidate MCPyV DNA during packaging and mediate cell surface interactions that activate entry and trafficking (Schowalter et al., 2011; Neu et al., 2012; Schowalter and Buck, 2013). Attachment to cell surfaces is mediated through interactions between VP1 capsomeres and sulphated polysaccharides while subsequent viral entry requires the interaction between VP1 and sialic acid (Neu et al., 2012; Bayer et al., 2020). In A549 cells, MCPyV entry was mediated through caveolar/lipid raft endocytosis (Becker et al., 2019). Subsequent MCPyV trafficking is carried out by the endosomal-to-ER pathway requiring microtubule transport activity (Becker et al., 2019). By comparison, VP2 mediates post-attachment phases of MCPyV entry and is necessary for native MCPyV infection, if not the formation of pseudo-virus particles (Schowalter and Buck, 2013).

Another late region gene product MCPyV miR-M1 likely regulates MCPyV early gene expression. In MCPyV-transfected neuroectodermal tumor (PFSK-1) cells, highly expressed miR-M1 transcripts down-regulated the expression of MCPyV T antigens and MCPyV replication (Theiss et al., 2015). The function of miRNA-M1 to restrain MCPyV replication and gene expression enabled a low level of detectable MCPyV to persist in cells for several months. Thus, the MCPyV miRNA could drive a persistence mechanism by which the virus maintains a limited infection in human hosts for prolonged periods. In addition, it was found that expression of a synthetic MCPyV-miR-M1 in HEK293 or MCC cells targets the cellular host gene SP100 thereby lowering CXCL8 expression and neutrophil chemotaxis (Akhbari et al., 2018). In principle, this anti-inflammatory effect could be protective in the setting of MCPyV infection. Unlike analogous miRNAs in animal polyomavirus tumors, however, the MCPyV miRNA is not highly expressed in MCC tumors, suggesting that the function for which it is selected in MCPyV infection does not, in turn, promote tumor fitness (Chen et al., 2015).

MCPyV Tropism and a Model of Infection

Epidemiological evidence suggests that MCPyV establishes asymptomatic, persistent infections in most people. As many as 88% of healthy adults are positive for MCPyV-specific antibodies (Kean et al., 2009; Pastrana et al., 2009; Tolstov et al., 2009; Touze et al., 2011). Serological activity against the MCPyV major capsid protein increases as populations age, from about 10% in early childhood to about 80% in adults (Chen et al., 2011; Tolstov et al., 2011; Viscidi et al., 2011). MCPyV-specific antibody titers positively correlate with viral load as measured by MCPyV DNA encapsidated in viral particles shed from healthy skin, suggesting that MCPyV positivity rates could also increase as populations age (Schowalter et al., 2010; Pastrana et al., 2012).

Within a given healthy individual, MCPyV antibody titers remain relatively stable over a period of at least 15 months (Pastrana et al., 2012). By comparison, neutralizing antibody titers to MCPyV, but not other human polyomaviruses, are significantly higher in patients with MCPyV-positive MCC despite the fact that MCC tumors do not express capsid protein (Pastrana et al., 2009). Together, these findings suggest that MCPyV has the capacity to persist, and that MCPyV expansion within a host correlates with disease propensity. Inadequate restriction of MCPyV may be a critical factor in enabling MCC development. This hypothesis is supported by the fact that chronic UV-exposure, advanced age, and HIV-related or iatrogenic immunosuppression pose significant risk for MCC (Heath et al., 2008; Bertrand et al., 2013; Ma and Brewer, 2014).

Direct evidence of the natural host reservoir cells that maintain latent MCPyV infection remains elusive. To take steps in establishing the cellular context of MCPyV infection, we discovered that primary human skin dermal fibroblasts support productive MCPyV infection *in vitro* and *ex vivo* (Liu et al., 2016b). While developing the *in vitro* model, we found that the addition of modulatory factors present in the skin could greatly enhance MCPyV proliferation. Specifically, viral entry is stimulated during the first 2 days of infection in the absence of serum and in the presence of collagenase. This is analogous to the inflammatory skin in which matrix metalloproteinases (MMPs) digest collagen fibers and activate chemokines (Werner and Grose, 2003; Gill and Parks, 2008). Subsequently, MCPyV replication is boosted by priming human dermal fibroblasts with epidermal and fibroblast growth factors and a WNT activator, which induce fibroblast proliferation and MMP expression (Liu et al., 2016b). That these same conditions are found in the skin wounding response suggests that the MCPyV infection cycle could be linked to damage to the skin by way of abrasions or UV-damage.

The picture of MCPyV infection is far from complete, yet inferences can be made from distinct sources of evidence. In *ex vivo* skin culture, MCPyV preferentially infects dermal fibroblasts underlying the basal layer of the epidermis and those surrounding hair follicles (Liu et al., 2016b). Furthermore, MCPyV virions are readily detected in eyebrow hair bulbs sampled from healthy human volunteers (Peretti et al., 2014; Bellaud et al., 2015; Hampras et al., 2015). It is possible that MCPyV infects the dermal cells surrounding the hair follicle and subsequently uses the follicular space as a means to disseminate to the skin surface and access new hosts. In addition, migration of MCPyV-infected fibroblasts to wound sites could represent another mode of transmission from reservoir cells into the deeper layers of the skin.

MCPyV may also infect cells at body sites other than the skin to establish a reservoir (Salakova et al., 2016). For instance, MCPyV DNA was detected in buffy coats of healthy blood donors and inflammatory monocytes of MCC patients, indicating that the virus may establish latent infection in peripheral blood leukocytes (Mertz et al., 2010; Pancaldi et al., 2011). In two MCPyV-positive patients with prior history of MCC and active non-melanoma/non-MCC skin cancers respectively, MCPyV DNA was detected in inflammatory, but not resident monocytes (Mertz et al., 2010). Presence of MCPyV in inflammatory monocytes of patients with distinct medical histories suggests that the virus may reside in these cells and use them to spread throughout the body (Mertz et al., 2010).

There is no animal model for MCPyV infection; a goal which has proven to be challenging due to the narrow host range of the virus (Liu et al., 2018). Lack of an animal model for MCPyV infection presents a major obstacle for identifying potential reservoirs and elucidating the MCPyV infectious cycle. Generation of MCPyV chimeras with mammalian polyomaviruses may provide a solution to overcome its narrow host range in the future (Liu et al., 2018).

MCC Cell of Origin

Though named for similarities to Merkel cells, the true original cell of MCC is rigorously debated. The proposition that MCC arises from differentiated Merkel cells is in question because these cells are post-mitotic, and thereby have limited oncogenic potential, and because they arise in the epidermis, while MCCs almost always occur in the dermis or subcutis layers (Toker, 1972). In response, it has been suggested that MCCs could arise from Merkel cell progenitor cells present at the hair follicle (Zur Hausen et al., 2013; Sauer et al., 2017; Narisawa et al., 2019). Similarly, progenitor cells derived from the neural crest have been pointed to since MCPyV-positive MCC cell lines cocultured with keratinocytes undergo neuronal morphological differentiation in a manner dependent on MCPyV LT upregulation of Sox2 and Atoh1 (Harold et al., 2019).

Some also propose that MCC could have an epithelial origin since on rare occasions, epithelial MCCs have been reported (Narisawa et al., 2020; Navarrete-Dechent et al., 2020; Song et al., 2020). One group advocating for an epithelial origin of MCC points to a case of a combined MCC and trichoblastoma tumor that shared somatic mutations (Kervarrec et al., 2019). They propose that this mixed tumor could represent a transition from early to late MCC carcinogenesis in cells with integrated MCPyV genome beginning to predominate. The same group also found that expressing MCPyV sT and GLI1 in keratinocytes results in an MCC-like phenotype, including expression of CK20 (Kervarrec et al., 2020). Another group has developed a mouse model for MCC, by expressing MCPyV sT and Atoh in keratinocytes, that results in the epidermal layer developing several MCC markers and characteristics (Verhaegen et al., 2017).

It has also been argued that pre/pro B cells are the source of MCC because MCC cells consistently express a number of B-lymphoid lineage markers, like Pax5 and TdT (Zur Hausen et al., 2013; Sauer et al., 2017). Cell expression similarities may be coincidental however, since it has also been proposed that epigenetic changes in the cell of origin could lead to a dramatic transcriptional and phenotypic changes culminating in Merkel cell resemblance. It has even been proposed that MCPyV-positive and -negative carcinomas have distinct cells of origin, and that through epigenetic reprogramming they converge on a common phenotype (Sunshine et al., 2018). Under normal developmental conditions, loss of polycomb repressive complex 2 (PRC2) and subsequent reduction H3K27me3 marks enables the differentiation of Merkel cells in mice (Bardot et al., 2013; Perdigoto et al., 2016). Given this information, one group reasoned that the development of MCC may involve a similar change in the epigenome of the unknown cell of origin. They found that pure MCPyV-positive MCCs were more likely to have lower H3K27me3 than MCPyV-negative tumors (Busam et al., 2017). Other researchers, however, found contradicting evidence that virus-negative MCCs, especially those with combined squamous cell carcinomas, had lower H3K27me3 marks than MCPyV-positive MCCs (Matsushita et al., 2019).

Immune Responses to MCC

Immune function is relevant to every aspect of MCC progression. Incidence of MCC is greatly increased in immunocompromised individuals, especially in those who are HIV-positive or recipients of organ transplants (Koljonen et al., 2009; Ma and Brewer, 2014; Cook et al., 2019). Loss of adaptive immune competence increases the risk of both MCPyV-positive and negative tumors, implying that immune surveillance of nascently transformed MCC cells is protective at early stages of the disease. There is also evidence that adequate immune responses can lessen the severity of MCC disease progression. For example, patients with chronic inflammatory disease had higher rates of MCC incidence, and the tumors of those that developed MCC had higher expression of the proliferative marker Ki-67, and a greater tumor size (Sahi et al., 2017). Furthermore, systemic immune suppression has been linked to greater incidence of MCC, as well as, lower rates of survival in MCC patients (Paulson et al., 2013). These epidemiological data suggest that immune restriction of MCC is critical to patient outcomes at each stage of the disease.

Studies of the immunological interface in MCC tumors have revealed further detail regarding the course of disease and the ability of MCC to evade destruction. For example, circulating MCPyV T antigen-specific antibody level positively correlates with MCPyV-positive MCC recurrence and has prognostic value (Samimi et al., 2016; Paulson et al., 2017). In MCC tumors, CD8 T cell and other immune cell infiltration is usually poor, and those cases with better infiltration positively correlate with patient outcomes (Sihto et al., 2012; Lipson et al., 2013; Wheat et al., 2014; Feldmeyer et al., 2016; Miller et al., 2017). Moreover, the MCPyV-specific T cells present in MCC tumors expressed markers of exhaustion like PD-1 and Tim-3 (Afanasiev et al., 2013). The same phenomenon could be found *in vitro* and in a MCC xenograft mouse-model (Dowlatshahi et al., 2013). Histopathology of MCC tumors indicate that immune cells expressing exhaustion markers like PD-1 and CD33 congregate in the areas surrounding the tumors, suggesting that MCC acquires traits that suppress immune cell migration (Mitteldorf et al., 2017).

Observations that tumor-experienced T cells were unable to infiltrate MCC tumors led to recent efforts to introduce immune checkpoint therapies in metastatic cases. A 2015 case study showed a promising response in a patient with metastatic MCC case treated with anti-PD1 antibodies (Mantripragada and Birnbaum, 2015). In the years that followed, clinical trials exploring safety and efficacy of anti-PD1 and anti-PDL-1 infusions yielded significant response rates and relatively low rates of adverse events given the severity of patient prognosis (Iyer et al., 2016; Kaufman et al., 2016; Nghiem et al., 2019). While the durability of responses varied, they could last well over a year (Kaufman et al., 2018; Nghiem et al., 2019).

Given that there are no effective chemotherapeutic treatments available for metastatic MCC, the introduction of immune checkpoint inhibitors greatly benefitted patients (Colunga et al., 2017; Paulson et al., 2018a). Still, a significant portion of patients do not respond or have responses that are short-lived. Moreover, patients with immunosuppression or autoimmune disease may not be eligible for immune-based therapy. It also became clear that loss of durability or relapse is a problem in long term treatment for MCC, even in MCPyV-positive MCC cases where mutagenesis is low. A longitudinal study revealed that HLA-I components were downregulated in resistant tumor cells at the level of transcription as a result of continued interaction with CD8 T cells (Paulson et al., 2018b). These shortcomings necessitate the development of alternative strategies or combination of existing therapies to modulate immunity to MCC.

One such strategy is to augment innate immunity at the primary tumor site in order to enhance adaptive function systemically. One group was able to achieve improved responses at distal MCC metastases by injecting a TLR-4 agonist intratumorally at the primary MCC site followed by standard-of-care surgery and irradiation (Bhatia et al., 2019). They later delivered IL-12 plasmids to MCC tumors via electroporation that led to enhanced immunogenicity at primary and distal tumors in all patients tested; 25% of which had responses in the progression of their disease (Bhatia et al., 2020). Still other means of activating intralesional innate inflammation have proven effective. Administration of an oncolytic herpesvirus that stimulates granulocyte-macrophage colony-stimulating factor has led to durable complete responses in multiple patients (Nguyen et al., 2019; Westbrook et al., 2019). A recent case study involving an advanced-stage MCC patient resulted in complete remission upon receiving a combination of radiation therapy and anti-PD1 therapy (Bloom et al., 2019). This suggests that targeted DNA damage at accessible lesions combined with activation of immunity against a primary tumor could help train immune responses against distant lesions.

While probing the cause of immune suppression characterizing the MCC tumor microenvironment, our group discovered that STING (stimulator of interferon genes) is dramatically repressed in MCC cell lines and tumor cells (Liu et al., 2020). Among these immortalized and primary MCC cells, the marked reduction in STING expression was unique to those that were MCPyV-positive (Liu et al., 2020). Since SV40 LT has been shown to antagonize the STING signaling pathway (Lau et al., 2015), it would be valuable to determine if MCPyV LTT expressed in virus-positive MCC cells downregulates STING expression. We also showed that rescuing STING expression and activation in MCC cells led to greatly induced cytokine expression, T cell migration, and MCC cell death (Liu et al., 2020). Delivery of a mutant STING vector via AAV transduction and subsequent activation with a selective agonist could achieve the same results. Such a strategy has the potential to be highly specific in humans without the danger of systemic inflammatory pathology because the mutant-specific STING agonist does not interact with native human STING (Liu et al., 2020).

Targeting distal MCC metastases is also the aim of researchers activating or genetically engineering immune cells for autologous infusion. For example, one group showed that activation and administration of genetically engineered T cells expressing TCRs specific to naturally processed MCPyV T epitopes led to tumor regression in mouse MCC xenografts (Gavvovidis et al., 2018). In one human case study, a similar infusion procedure using MCPyV T antigen-specific T cells that were expanded *ex vivo* resulted in HLA upregulation, T cell recruitment, and responses in most metastases (Chapuis et al., 2014). A recent study developed a means of improving autologous CD8 T cell therapeutic vaccines for MCC by exposing those T cells to cytokine-conditioned dendritic cells presenting LTT peptides on both MHC-I and II surface receptors (Gerer et al., 2017). MCPyV-positive tumor microenvironments can also be engaged by engineered CD4 T cells that recognize the LXCXE epitope of LTT (Longino et al., 2019).

Immune Responses to MCPyV

Given that the risk factors for developing MCC, including advanced age, UV exposure, and compromised adaptive immunity, can each alter the immune environment in the skin, it is possible that unmitigated proliferation of MCPyV encourages oncogenesis (Stang et al., 2018). The possibility that uncontrolled MCPyV activity leads to MCC cases agrees with the ability of Chang and Moore to predict the viral etiology of MCC due to its greater incidence in immune compromised persons (Feng et al., 2008). The transition from low-level MCPyV persistence to rampant proliferation could promote carcinogenesis by increasing the frequency of integration events or entry into the original host cell of MCC. Because nascently transformed cells are also favored by loss of normal immunity, it would be easy to conflate these two factors. Interestingly though, there is increasing evidence that alterations to systemic and skin immunity can exacerbate MCPyV infections.

A study in Japan found that MCPyV DNA prevalence and viral load on sun-exposed skin increased sharply in individuals over the age of 40 and remained high for the oldest groups (Hashida et al., 2016a). Also, HIV-positive men more frequently have detectable MCPyV DNA on their skin and in their sera, and those with poorly-controlled HIV infection have higher MCPyV antibody titers and DNA loads than those with better-controlled infections (Wieland et al., 2011; Fukumoto et al., 2013; Vahabpour et al., 2017). In kidney transplant recipients, MCPyV DNA was more readily detected in the urine of those with BKPyV-DNAemia and with histologically verified polyomavirus-associated nephropathy (Signorini et al., 2014; Wang et al., 2019). MCPyV DNA detection rates and loads were significantly lower in patients with psoriasis compared to the skin of healthy volunteers suggesting a potential inverse relationship between chronic inflammation in the skin and MCPyV proliferation (Hashida et al., 2019). MCPyV-positive MCC patients, however, have higher MCPyV DNA loads shed from their skin and more frequently produce MCPyV VP1-specific circulating antibodies and at higher titers (Pastrana et al., 2009, 2012; Faust et al., 2011; Touze et al., 2011; Hashida et al., 2016b). More recently, it was found that higher MCPyV DNA load correlates with worse survival outcomes in MCC patients (Von Der Grun et al., 2019).

These findings suggest that sudden loss of normal immune functions could swing the balance between host and virus to favor uncontrolled MCPyV proliferation (**Figure 2**). From the perspective of the virus, however, MCPyV must have evolved mechanisms of its own to evade host immunity since it can persist and remain highly prevalent in the general population asymptomatically (Tolstov et al., 2009; Schowalter et al., 2010; Foulongne et al., 2012). The mechanisms by which MCPyV evades immune detection and/or destruction are not known.

Some examples of MCPyV gene products or transfected MCPyV genomes interacting with cellular immunity have been documented. For instance, LT expression reduces TLR-9 expression via downregulation of C/EBP transcription factors in epithelial and MCC cell lines (Shahzad et al., 2013). This observation agrees with *in vivo* data revealing that TLR-9 expression was significantly lower in MCPyV-positive MCC tumors compared to MCPyV-negative tumors (Jouhi et al., 2015). MCPyV sT expression was shown to inhibit NF-κB inflammatory signaling through its interaction with PP4C and the adapter NEMO (Griffiths et al., 2013; Abdul-Sada et al., 2017). In addition, it has been shown that a MCPyV-miR-M1 mimic specifically targeted SP100 for degradation (Akhbari et al., 2018). This downregulation of SP100 reduced the secretion of CXCL8 in MCC cells treated with TNF-α (Akhbari et al., 2018). Notably, depletion of the nuclear protein SP100 also enhances MCPyV replication in H1299 cells (Neumann et al., 2016).

There are also examples of cells eliciting an immune response to the expression of MCPyV genes and genomes. As mentioned previously, MCPyV LT and sT expression in BJ-hTERT cells led to upregulation of cellular growth and expression of genes that increase motility (Richards et al., 2015). Accompanying this phenotype was the dramatic induction of many inflammatory response genes including interferon-stimulated genes (ISGs) like OAS1 and ISG20; cytokines like IL-1β and IL-6; and chemokines like CXCL1 and CXCL6 (Richards et al., 2015). Whether MCPyV T antigens induce such a response in the context of infection remains undetermined.

Despite the recent progress made in revealing the MCPyV-host interface, the approaches used previously involved transfection or transduction of MCPyV genes into established cancer cell lines. In order to understand how these mechanisms may contribute to MCPyV persistence, our group examined the innate immune response to MCPyV in the context of infection in human dermal fibroblasts, which plausibly model MCPyV infection of human skin (Krump et al., 2021). After establishing the MCPyV gene expression and replication kinetics in infected cells, we found that late events in the infectious cycle activated the cGAS-STING and NF-κB pathways and subsequent expression of anti-viral ISGs as well as innate inflammatory cytokines (Krump et al., 2021). CRISPR knockout of elements of these immune regulatory pathways yielded significantly higher levels of MCPyV replication per cell, suggesting that the innate gene induction has the potential to restrict MCPyV replication, even in the absence of cellular immune factors (Krump et al., 2021).

A Model of MCPyV Dysbiosis Leading to MCC Development

MCPyV infects and sheds from the skin of most people without discernible symptoms (Pastrana et al., 2009; Schowalter et al., 2010). The evolutionary strategies that allow MCPyV to asymptomatically infect a large portion of the population, often for prolonged periods of time, remain a mystery (Chen et al., 2011). The auspicious discovery that human dermal fibroblasts support MCPyV infection enabled our recent characterization of the MCPyV infectious cycle and the consequences it poses for the host cell (Liu et al., 2016b; Krump et al., 2021). By understanding the scenarios in which MCPyV might fail to strike a balance with the host immune system, we may be able to infer the events preceding MCPyV integration and oncogenesis.

While direct observation of the interface between MCPyV and systemic immune responses awaits development of an animal model, it is currently possible to formulate a model of MCPyV infection based on data from several sources: (1) the epidemiology of MCC and MCPyV infections, (2) existing research on fibroblast biology and wounding responses in human skin, and (3) *in vitro* findings that establish the prerequisites for MCPyV replication and gene expression (Liu et al., 2016b; Krump et al., 2021). In a similar manner, by juxtaposing decades of skin pathology research with observed cellular response to MCPyV infection, we may be able to provide new insights regarding dysregulated conditions that might lead to MCPyV-driven MCC (Walder et al., 1971; Hardie et al., 1980; Ahmad et al., 2014; Krump et al., 2021).

If indeed dermal fibroblasts are capable of supporting MCPyV infection *in vivo* as they are *ex vivo* and *in vitro* (Liu et al., 2016b), then a model of the course of MCPyV infection can begin to take shape (**Figure 2**). For instance, healthy human hosts may support a low basal rate of MCPyV activity in fibroblasts that avoids immune recognition, as early events like viral entry and trafficking *in vitro* failed to activate ISGs (Krump et al., 2021). In the event that host skin is abraded or irradiated with UV light, damaged keratinocytes release growth factors and WNT agonists to induce MMP expression and expansion of fibroblasts (Gill and Parks, 2008; Whyte et al., 2012). These tissue changes could stimulate MCPyV early gene expression and DNA synthesis (Liu et al., 2016b). In this scenario, MCPyV PAMPS and/or DAMPs present during later stages of infection upregulate ISGs and inflammatory cytokines in manner that restricts viral replication (Krump et al., 2021). Serological evidence suggests that antibody-related adaptive responses to elevated MCPyV loads could also be a significant restriction factor (Faust et al., 2011). Dermal fibroblasts proliferating and navigating to the wounded tissue or shedding layers of sunburned skin could facilitate MCPyV transmission to new hosts (**Figure 2**). The antiviral state conferred by ISG induction, innate cytokine signaling, and likely recruited immune cells at the wound site would restrict and clear cells with high levels of MCPyV infection. A return to persistent, low-level MCPyV infection could be achieved by those infected resident skin cells that avoid immune detection (**Figure 2**).

Fluctuations in MCPyV load in dynamic equilibrium with insults to the skin and immune responses could be evolutionarily advantageous to MCPyV as it would only risk detection when the opportunity to infect new hosts arises (**Figure 2**). Should MCPyV activity correspond to skin damage and repair, then chronic wounding, inflammation, or altered skin architecture could represent the early events that promote MCPyV DNA amplification and integration into host DNA that lead to MCPyV-associated MCC (**Figures 2, 3**). This

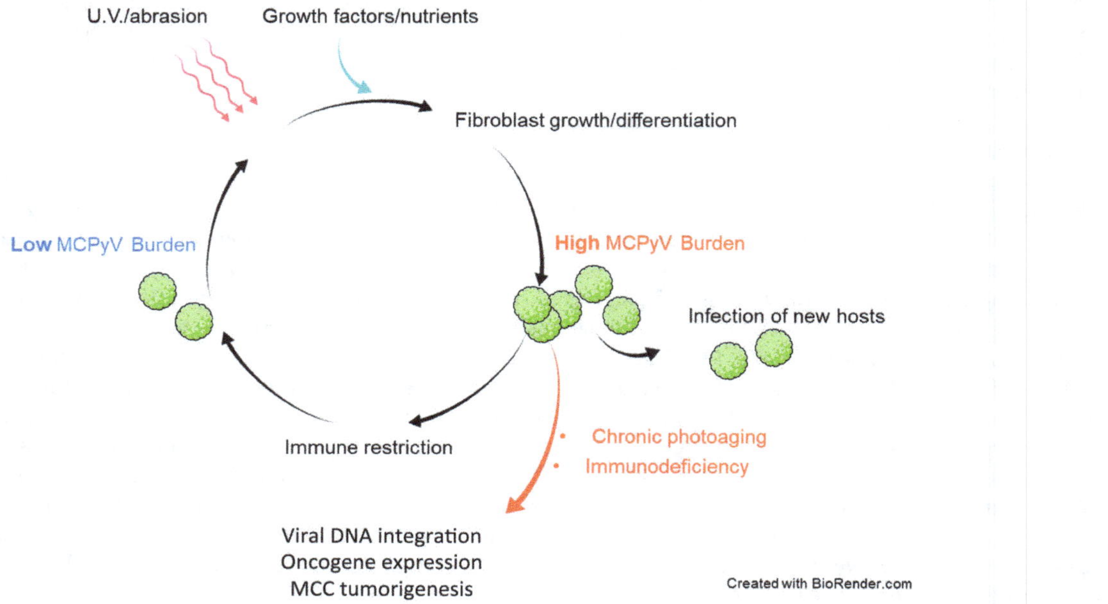

FIGURE 2 | Hypothetical model of *in vivo* MCPyV persistence and dysbiosis leading to MCPyV-positive MCC. Healthy individuals support both low and high MCPyV loads, depending on external factors. U.V. irradiation or abrasion of the skin could cause infected dermal fibroblasts to upregulate MCPyV gene expression and replication. Damaged and repairing skin could be a path by which MCPyV escapes the dermis to infect new hosts. Healthy immune responses may reduce the MCPyV burden asymptomatically. In immunocompromised patients and those with years of chronic U.V. damage, the microenvironment of the skin may be altered in a way that induces MCPyV entry into the original cell of MCC and integration into the host chromatin to drive MCC tumorigenesis.

possibility is supported by epidemiological studies showing a strong correlation between immunosuppression, elevated MCPyV genome loads, and increased risk for MCC (Heath et al., 2008; Wieland et al., 2011). These studies suggest that faulty immune control of MCPyV infection could disturb the balance of MCPyV-host interaction to cause unbridled viral replication, which can increase the chance of incidental integration of viral DNA and MCC oncogenesis (**Figures 2, 3**). These observations would also explain why certain populations have a higher risk of developing MCC.

The molecular events linking MCPyV infection and MCC development are reminiscent of those underlying the malignancies driven by human papillomaviruses (HPVs). In non-malignant human cells, HPVs, like MCPyV, normally replicate and maintain their genomes as episomes (Longworth and Laimins, 2004; You et al., 2004; You, 2010; Wang et al., 2013) (**Figure 3**). During the course of persistent infection, a compromised immune system and/or other pathologic conditions could cause rampant viral replication to promote integration of viral genomes into the host DNA. An additional parallel between MCPyV and HPV oncogenic mechanisms is that the integrated viral genomes typically lose the ability to replicate, but the non-replicating viral genomes retain the capacity to express viral oncogenes, such as LTT/sT (encoded by MCPyV) and E6/E7 (encoded by HPV). These viral oncoproteins stimulate cellular proliferation and malignant transformation by inhibiting host tumor suppressor such as RB and p53 (Gaglia and Munger, 2018) (**Figure 3**). The uncontrolled cellular proliferation could ultimately inflict oncogenesis by allowing virally induced precancerous lesions to persist and expand (**Figure 3**). In addition, viral oncogenes encoded by the integrated MCPyV and HPV genomes also share the ability to induce genomic instability (Li et al., 2013; Gaglia and Munger, 2018), which can introduce more DNA breaks in the host genome to stimulate viral genome integration. Hyperproliferation and DNA damage induced by viral oncogenes and/or U.V. irradiation may allow the emerging tumor cells to accumulate additional genetic mutations needed to develop into invasive tumors (**Figure 3**).

Future Perspective

Over 90% of MCC patients are not immune-compromised by clinical definitions, yet almost all are over the age of 50 and have low melanin content in their skin (Heath et al., 2008). Therefore, unraveling the impact of UV-radiation and aging to the skin could reveal key aspects of early events in MCPyV-associated MCC. Further elucidation of tactics employed by MCPyV to manipulate the host immune system for promoting its own propagation and driving cellular transformation will likely offer new clues for understanding the mechanism driving MCPyV tumorigenesis.

The bourgeoning of cancer therapies aimed at activating and directing immune responses to malignancies give much cause for hope for the treatment of MCC and other viral cancers. Still, gaps in our understanding of the biology driving MCPyV-related

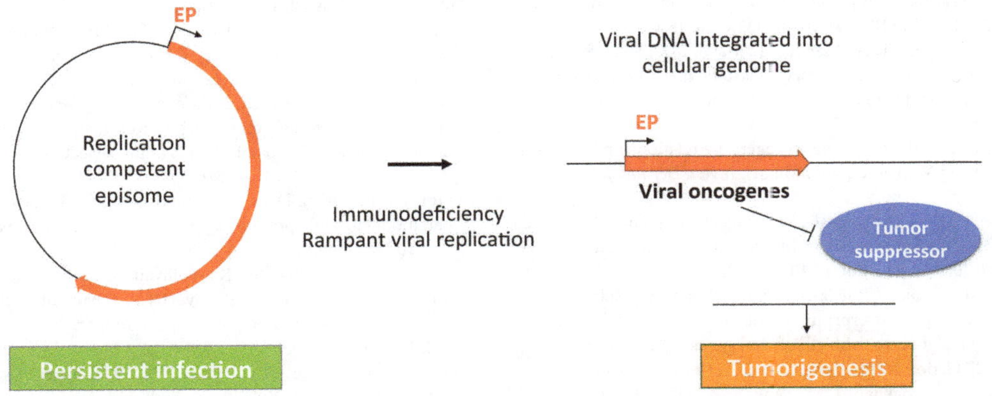

FIGURE 3 | A common theme in MCPyV- and HPV-induced tumorigenesis. MCPyV and HPV both replicate as episomes in persistently infected cell. Failure of host immune system may cause uncontrolled viral replication, which can stimulate viral DNA integration into the host cellular genome. The integrated viral genome expresses viral oncogenes that can inhibit tumor suppressors to induce malignant transformation. Red line indicates the early region of the oncogenic viruses. EP, Early promoter.

oncogenesis and MCC immune escape could widen the breadth of patients that respond to treatments and the durability of those responses. Addressing some of our gaps in knowledge will require technological advances like improved detection of low-copy number viral DNA genomes in tissue isolates or accurate animal models of MCPyV infection. Until that time, we can make strides in our investigation using the wealth of knowledge on human skin and cancer biology, and by expanding the model of *in vitro* MCPyV infection. Applying this knowledge to re-establish asymptomatic equilibrium between host and MCPyV in at-risk individuals has the potential to prevent MCC cases from occurring in the future.

AUTHOR CONTRIBUTIONS

NK and JY: conceptualization and writing—review and editing. NK: writing—original draft preparation and visualization. JY: supervision, project administration, and funding acquisition. Both authors have read and agreed to the published version of the manuscript.

ACKNOWLEDGMENTS

The authors would like to thank all members of the JY's laboratory for their feedback and support throughout the course of this project. We apologize to our colleagues whose primary research results could not be cited due to space constraints.

REFERENCES

Abdul-Sada, H., Muller, M., Mehta, R., Toth, R., Arthur, J. S. C., Whitehouse, A., et al. (2017). The PP4R1 sub-unit of protein phosphatase PP4 is essential for inhibition of NF-kappaB by merkel polyomavirus small tumour antigen. *Oncotarget* 8, 25418–25432. doi: 10.18632/oncotarget.15836

Afanasiev, O. K., Yelistratova, L., Miller, N., Nagase, K., Paulson, K., Iyer, J. G., et al. (2013). Merkel polyomavirus-specific T cells fluctuate with merkel cell carcinoma burden and express therapeutically targetable PD-1 and Tim-3 exhaustion markers. *Clin. Cancer Res.* 19, 5351–5360. doi: 10.1158/1078-0432.CCR-13-0035

Ahmad, I., Simanyi, E., Guroji, P., Tamimi, I. A., Delarosa, H. J., Nagar, A., et al. (2014). Toll-like receptor-4 deficiency enhances repair of UVR-induced cutaneous DNA damage by nucleotide excision repair mechanism. *J. Invest. Dermatol.* 134, 1710–1717. doi: 10.1038/jid.2013.530

Akhbari, P., Tobin, D., Poterlowicz, K., Roberts, W., and Boyne, J. R. (2018). MCV-miR-M1 targets the host-cell immune response resulting in the attenuation of neutrophil chemotaxis. *J. Invest. Dermatol.* 138, 2343–2354. doi: 10.1016/j.jid.2018.03.1527

Bardot, E. S., Valdes, V. J., Zhang, J., Perdigoto, C. N., Nicolis, S., Hearn, S. A., et al. (2013). Polycomb subunits Ezh1 and Ezh2 regulate the Merkel cell differentiation program in skin stem cells. *EMBO J.* 32, 1990–2000. doi: 10.1038/emboj.2013.110

Bayer, N. J., Januliene, D., Zocher, G., Stehle, T., Moeller, A., and Blaum, B. S. (2020). Structure of merkel cell polyomavirus capsid and interaction with its glycosaminoglycan attachment receptor. *J. Virol.* 94, e01664–e01619. doi: 10.1128/JVI.01664-19

Becker, J. C., Stang, A., Hausen, A. Z., Fischer, N., Decaprio, J. A., Tothill, R. W., et al. (2017). Epidemiology, biology and therapy of Merkel cell carcinoma: conclusions from the EU project IMMOMEC. *Cancer Immunol. Immunother.* 67, 341–351. doi: 10.1007/s00262-017-2099-3

Becker, M., Dominguez, M., Greune, L., Soria-Martinez, L., Pfleiderer, M. M., Schowalter, R., et al. (2019). Infectious entry of merkel cell polyomavirus. *J. Virol.* 93, e02004–e02018. doi: 10.1128/JVI.02004-18

Bellaud, G., Gheit, T., Pugin, A., Pretet, J. L., Tommasino, M., Mougin, C., et al. (2015). Prevalence of human polyomavirus DNA in eyebrow hairs plucked from patients with psoriasis treated with TNF inhibitors. *J. Eur. Acad. Dermatol. Venereol.* 29, 1019–1021. doi: 10.1111/jdv.12439

Berrios, C., Padi, M., Keibler, M. A., Park, D. E., Molla, V., Cheng, J., et al. (2016). Merkel cell polyomavirus small t antigen promotes pro-glycolytic metabolic perturbations required for transformation. *PLoS Pathog.* 12:e1006020. doi: 10.1371/journal.ppat.1006020

Bertrand, M., Mirabel, X., Desmedt, E., Vercambre-Darras, S., Martin De Lassalle, E., Bouchindhomme, B., et al. (2013). [Merkel cell carcinoma: a new radiation-induced cancer?]. *Ann. Dermatol. Venereol.* 140, 41–45. doi: 10.1016/j.annder.2012.10.598

Bhatia, S., Longino, N. V., Miller, N. J., Kulikauskas, R., Iyer, J. G., Ibrani, D., et al. (2020). Intratumoral delivery of plasmid IL12 via electroporation leads to regression of injected and noninjected tumors in merkel cell carcinoma. *Clin. Cancer Res.* 26, 598–607. doi: 10.1158/1078-0432.CCR-19-0972

Bhatia, S., Miller, N. J., Lu, H., Longino, N. V., Ibrani, D., Shinohara, M. M., et al. (2019). Intratumoral G100, a TLR4 agonist, induces antitumor immune responses and tumor regression in patients with merkel cell carcinoma. *Clin. Cancer Res.* 25, 1185–1195. doi: 10.1158/1078-0432.CCR-18-0469

Bloom, B. C., Augustyn, A., Pezzi, T. A., Menon, H., Mayo, L. L., Shah, S. J., et al. (2019). Rescue of immunotherapy-refractory metastatic merkel cell carcinoma with conventionally fractionated radiotherapy and concurrent pembrolizumab. *Front. Oncol.* 9:223. doi: 10.3389/fonc.2019.00223

Buck, C. B., and Lowy, D. R. (2009). Getting stronger: the relationship between a newly identified virus and Merkel cell carcinoma. *J. Invest. Dermatol.* 129, 9–11. doi: 10.1038/jid.2008.302

Busam, K. J., Pulitzer, M. P., Coit, D. C., Arcila, M., Leng, D., Jungbluth, A. A., et al. (2017). Reduced H3K27me3 expression in Merkel cell polyoma virus-positive tumors. *Mod. Pathol.* 30, 877–883. doi: 10.1038/modpathol.2017.8

Carter, J. J., Daugherty, M. D., Qi, X., Bheda-Malge, A., Wipf, G. C., Robinson, K., et al. (2013). Identification of an overprinting gene in Merkel cell polyomavirus provides evolutionary insight into the birth of viral genes. *Proc. Natl. Acad. Sci. U.S.A.* 110, 12744–12749. doi: 10.1073/pnas.1303526110

Cassler, N. M., Merrill, D., Bichakjian, C. K., and Brownell, I. (2016). Merkel cell carcinoma therapeutic update. *Curr. Treat. Options Oncol.* 17, 36. doi: 10.1007/s11864-016-0409-1

Chadburn, A., Abdul-Nabi, A. M., Teruya, B. S., and Lo, A. A. (2013). Lymphoid proliferations associated with human immunodeficiency virus infection. *Arch. Pathol. Lab. Med.* 137, 360–370. doi: 10.5858/arpa.2012-0095-RA

Chang, Y., Cesarman, E., Pessin, M. S., Lee, F., Culpepper, J., Knowles, D. M., et al. (1994). Identification of herpesvirus-like DNA sequences in AIDS-associated Kaposi's sarcoma. *Science* 266, 1865–1869. doi: 10.1126/science.7997879

Chapuis, A. G., Afanasiev, O. K., Iyer, J. G., Paulson, K. G., Parvathaneni, U., Hwang, J. H., et al. (2014). Regression of metastatic Merkel cell carcinoma following transfer of polyomavirus-specific T cells and therapi capable of re-inducing HLA class-I. *Cancer Immunol. Res.* 2, 27–36. doi: 10.1158/2326-6066.CIR-13-0087

Chen, C. J., Cox, J. E., Azarm, K. D., Wylie, K. N., Woolard, K. D., Pesavento, P. A., et al. (2015). Identification of a polyomavirus microRNA highly expressed in tumors. *Virology* 476, 43–53. doi: 10.1016/j.virol.2014.11.021

Chen, T., Hedman, L., Mattila, P. S., Jartti, T., Ruuskanen, O., Soderlund-Venermo, M., et al. (2011). Serological evidence of Merkel cell polyomavirus primary infections in childhood. *J. Clin. Virol.* 50, 125–129. doi: 10.1016/j.jcv.2010.10.015

Cheng, J., Park, D. E., Berrios, C., White, E. A., Arora, R., Yoon, R., et al. (2017). Merkel cell polyomavirus recruits MYCL to the EP400 complex to promote oncogenesis. *PLoS Pathog.* 13:e1006668. doi: 10.1371/journal.ppat.1006668

Cheng, J., Rozenblatt-Rosen, O., Paulson, K. G., Nghiem, P., and Decaprio, J. A. (2013). Merkel cell polyomavirus large T antigen has growth-promoting and inhibitory activities. *J. Virol.* 87, 6118–6126. doi: 10.1128/JVI.00385-13

Cimino, P. J., Robirds, D. H., Tripp, S. R., Pfeifer, J. D., Abel, H. J., and Duncavage, E. J. (2014). Retinoblastoma gene mutations detected by whole exome sequencing of Merkel cell carcinoma. *Mod. Pathol.* 27, 1073–1087. doi: 10.1038/modpathol.2013.235

Colunga, A., Pulliam, T., and Nghiem, P. (2017). Merkel cell carcinoma in the age of immunotherapy: facts and hopes. *Clin Cancer Res.* 24, 2035–2043. doi: 10.1158/1078-0432.CCR-17-0439

Cook, M., Baker, K., Redman, M., Lachance, K., Nguyen, M. H., Parvathaneni, U., et al. (2019). Differential outcomes among immunosuppressed patient with merkel cell carcinoma: impact of immunosuppression type on cancer-specific and overall survival. *Am. J. Clin. Oncol.* 42, 82–88. doi: 10.1097/COC.0000000000000482

Cowey, C. L., Mahnke, L., Espirito, J., Helwig, C., Oksen, D., and Bharmal, M. (2017). Real-world treatment outcomes in patients with metastatic Merkel cell carcinoma treated with chemotherapy in the USA. *Future Oncol.* 13, 1699–1710. doi: 10.2217/fon-2017-0187

Czech-Sioli, M., Günther, T., Therre, M., Spohn, M., Indenbirken, D., Theiss, J., et al. (2020). High-resolution analysis of Merkel Cell Polyomavirus in Merkel Cell Carcinoma reveals distinct integration patterns and suggests NHEJ and MMBIR as underlying mechanisms. *PLoS Pathog.* 16:e1008562. doi: 10.1371/journal.ppat.1008562

Dabner, M., Mcclure, R. J., Harvey, N. T., Budgeon, C. A., Beer, T. W., Amanuel, B., et al. (2014). Merkel cell polyomavirus and p63 status in Merkel cell carcinoma by immunohistochemistry: Merkel cell polyomavirus positivity is inversely correlated with sun damage, but neither is correlated with outcome. *Pathology* 46, 205–210. doi: 10.1097/PAT.0000000000000069

D'angelo, S. P., Russell, J., Lebbe, C., Chmielowski, B., Gambichler, T., Grob, J. J., et al. (2018). Efficacy and safety of first-line avelumab treatment in patients with stage iv metastatic merkel cell carcinoma: a preplanned interim analysis of a clinical trial. *JAMA Oncol.* 4:e180077. doi: 10.1001/jamaoncol.2018.0077

De Wolff-Peeters, C., Marien, K., Mebis, J., and Desmet, V. (1980). A cutaneous APUDoma or Merkel cell tumor? a morphologically recognizable tumor with a biological and histological malignant aspect in contrast with its clinical behavior. *Cancer* 46, 1810–1816.

Decaprio, J. A. (2009). Does detection of Merkel cell polyomavirus in Merkel cell carcinoma provide prognostic information? *J. Natl. Cancer Inst.* 101, 905–907. doi: 10.1093/jnci/djp162

Demetriou, S. K., Ona-Vu, K., Sullivan, E. M., Dong, T. K., Hsu, S. W., and Oh, D. H. (2012). Defective DNA repair and cell cycle arrest in cells expressing Merkel cell polyomavirus T antigen. *Int. J. Cancer* 131, 1818–1827. doi: 10.1002/ijc.27440

Dobson, S. J., Anene, A., Boyne, J. R., Mankouri, J., Macdonald, A., and Whitehouse, A. (2020). Merkel cell polyomavirus small tumour antigen activates the p38 MAPK pathway to enhance cellular motility. *Biochem. J.* 477, 2721–2733. doi: 10.1042/BCJ20200399

Doolittle-Hall, J. M., Cunningham Glasspoole, D. L., Seaman, W. T., and Webster-Cyriaque, J. (2015). Meta-analysis of DNA tumor-viral integration site selection indicates a role for repeats, gene expression and epigenetics. *Cancers (Basel)* 7, 2217–2235. doi: 10.3390/cancers7040887

Dowlatshahi, M., Huang, V., Gehad, A. E., Jiang, Y., Calarese, A., Teague, J. E., et al. (2013). Tumor-specific T cells in human Merkel cell carcinomas: a possible role for Tregs and T-cell exhaustion in reducing T-cell responses. *J. Invest. Dermatol.* 133, 1879–1889. doi: 10.1038/jid.2013.75

Duncavage, E. J., Zehnbauer, B. A., and Pfeifer, J. D. (2009). Prevalence of Merkel cell polyomavirus in Merkel cell carcinoma. *Mod. Pathol.* 22, 516–521. doi: 10.1038/modpathol.2009.3

Dye, K. N., Welcker, M., Clurman, B. E., Roman, A., and Galloway, D. A. (2019). Merkel cell polyomavirus Tumor antigens expressed in Merkel cell carcinoma function independently of the ubiquitin ligases Fbw7 and beta-TrCP. *PLoS Pathog.* 15:e1007543. doi: 10.1371/journal.ppat.1007543

Ellerbrock, T. V., Chiasson, M. A., Bush, T. J., Sun, X. W., Sawo, D., Brudney, K., et al. (2000). Incidence of cervical squamous intraepithelial lesions in HIV-infected women. *JAMA* 283, 1031–1037. doi: 10.1001/jama.283.8.1031

Engels, E. A., Frisch, M., Goedert, J. J., Biggar, R. J., and Miller, R. W. (2002). Merkel cell carcinoma and HIV infection. *Lancet* 359, 497–498. doi: 10.1016/S0140-6736(02)07668-7

Faust, H., Pastrana, D. V., Buck, C. B., Dillner, J., and Ekstrom, J. (2011). Antibodies to Merkel cell polyomavirus correlate to presence of viral DNA in the skin. *J. Infect. Dis.* 203, 1096–1100. doi: 10.1093/infdis/jiq173

Feldmeyer, L., Hudgens, C. W., Ray-Lyons, G., Nagarajan, P., Aung, P. P., Curry, J. L., et al. (2016). Density, distribution, and composition of immune infiltrates correlate with survival in merkel cell carcinoma. *Clin. Cancer Res.* 22, 5553–5563. doi: 10.1158/1078-0432.CCR-16-0392

Feng, H., Shuda, M., Chang, Y., and Moore, P. S. (2008). Clonal integration of a polyomavirus in human Merkel cell carcinoma. *Science* 319, 1096–1100. doi: 10.1126/science.1152586

Fischer, N., Brandner, J., Fuchs, F., Moll, I., and Grundhoff, A. (2010). Detection of Merkel cell polyomavirus (MCPyV) in Merkel cell carcinoma cell lines: cell morphology and growth phenotype do not reflect presence of the virus. *Int. J. Cancer* 126, 2133–2142. doi: 10.1002/ijc.24877

Fitzgerald, T. L., Dennis, S., Kachare, S. D., Vohra, N. A., Wong, J. H., and Zervos, E. E. (2015). Dramatic increase in the incidence and mortality from merkel cell carcinoma in the United States. *Am. Surg.* 81, 802–806. doi: 10.1177/000313481508100819

Foulongne, V., Sauvage, V., Hebert, C., Dereure, O., Cheval, J., Gouilh, M. A., et al. (2012). Human skin microbiota: high diversity of dna viruses identified on the human skin by high throughput sequencing. *PLoS ONE* 7:e38499. doi: 10.1371/journal.pone.0038499

Freeman, M. B., Holman, D. M., Qin, J., and Lunsford, N. B. (2019). Merkel cell carcinoma incidence, trends, and survival rates among adults aged ≥50 years from United States Cancer Statistics. *J. Am. Acad. Dermatol.* 80, 1154–1156. doi: 10.1016/j.jaad.2018.10.045

Fukumoto, H., Sato, Y., Hasegawa, H., and Katano, H. (2013). Frequent detection of Merkel cell polyomavirus DNA in sera of HIV-1-positive patients. *Virol. J.* 10:84. doi: 10.1186/1743-422X-10-84

Gaglia, M. M., and Munger, K. (2018). More than just oncogenes: mechanisms of tumorigenesis by human viruses. *Curr. Opin. Virol.* 32, 48–59. doi: 10.1016/j.coviro.2018.09.003

Gavvovidis, I., Leisegang, M., Willimsky, G., Miller, N. J., Nghiem, P., and cells specific to T-antigens of Merkel cell polyomavirus. *Clin. Cancer Res.* 24, 3644–3655. doi: 10.1158/1078-0432.CCR-17-2661

Gerer, K. F., Erdmann, M., Hadrup, S. R., Lyngaa, R., Martin, L. M., Voll, R. E., et al. (2017). Preclinical evaluation of NF-kappaB-triggered dendritic cells expressing the viral oncogenic driver of Merkel cell carcinoma for therapeutic vaccination. *Ther. Adv. Med. Oncol.* 9, 451–464. doi: 10.1177/1758834017712630

Gill, S. E., and Parks, W. C. (2008). Metalloproteinases and their inhibitors: regulators of wound healing. *Int. J. Biochem. Cell Biol.* 40, 1334–1347. doi: 10.1016/j.biocel.2007.10.024

Gjoerup, O., and Chang, Y. (2010). "Chapter 1-update on human polyomaviruses and cancer," in *Advances in Cancer Research*, eds F.V.W. George and K. George (Cambridge, MA: Academic Press), 1–51.

Goh, G., Walradt, T., Markarov, V., Blom, A., Riaz, N., Doumani, R., et al. (2016). Mutational landscape of MCPyV-positive and MCPyV-negative Merkel cell carcinomas with implications for immunotherapy. *Oncotarget* 7, 3403–3415. doi: 10.18632/oncotarget.6494

Griffiths, D. A., Abdul-Sada, H., Knight, L. M., Jackson, B. R., Richards, K., Prescott, E. L., et al. (2013). Merkel cell polyomavirus small T antigen targets the NEMO adaptor protein to disrupt inflammatory signaling. *J. Virol.* 87, 13853–13867. doi: 10.1128/JVI.02159-13

Grundhoff, A., and Fischer, N. (2015). Merkel cell polyomavirus, a highly prevalent virus with tumorigenic potential. *Curr. Opin. Virol.* 14, 129–137. doi: 10.1016/j.coviro.2015.08.010

Gu, J., Polak, J. M., Van Noorden, S., Pearse, A. G., Marangos, P. J., and Azzopardi, J. G. (1983). Immunostaining of neuron-specific enolase as a diagnostic tool for Merkel cell tumors. *Cancer* 52, 1039–1043.

Hampras, S. S., Michel, A., Schmitt, M., Waterboer, T., Kranz, L., Gheit, T., et al. (2015). Merkel cell polyomavirus (MCV) T-antigen seroreactivity, MCV DNA in eyebrow hairs, and squamous cell carcinoma. *Infect. Agents Cancer* 10:35. doi: 10.1186/s13027-015-0030-0

Handschel, J., Muller, D., Depprich, R. A., Ommerborn, M. A., Kubler, N. R., Naujoks, C., et al. (2010). The new polyomavirus (MCPyV) does not affect the clinical course in MCCs. *Int. J. Oral Maxillofac. Surg.* 39, 1086–1090. doi: 10.1016/j.ijom.2010.06.024

Hardie, I. R., Strong, R. W., Hartley, L. C., Woodruff, P. W., and Clunie, G. J. (1980). Skin cancer in Caucasian renal allograft recipients living in a subtropical climate. *Surgery* 87, 177–183.

Harms, K. L., Healy, M. A., Nghiem, P., Sober, A. J., Johnson, T. M., Bichakjian, C. K., et al. (2016). Analysis of Prognostic Factors from 9387 Merkel Cell Carcinoma Cases Forms the Basis for the New 8th Edition AJCC Staging System. *Ann. Surg. Oncol.* 23, 3564–3571. doi: 10.1245/s10434-016-5266-4

Harms, P. W. (2017). Update on Merkel Cell Carcinoma. *Clin. Lab. Med.* 37, 485–501. doi: 10.1016/j.cll.2017.05.004

Harms, P. W., Collie, A. M., Hovelson, D. H., Cani, A. K., Verhaegen, M E., Patel, R. M., et al. (2016). Next generation sequencing of Cytokeratin 20-negative Merkel cell carcinoma reveals ultraviolet-signature mutations and recurrent TP53 and RB1 inactivation. *Mod. Pathol.* 29, 240–248. doi: 10.1038/modpathol.2015.154

Harms, P. W., Patel, R. M., Verhaegen, M. E., Giordano, T. J., Nash, K. T., Johnson, C. N., et al. (2013). Distinct gene expression profiles of viral- and nonviral-associated merkel cell carcinoma revealed by transcriptome analysis. *J. Invest. Dermatol.* 133, 936–945. doi: 10.1038/jid.2012.445

Harms, P. W., Vats, P., Verhaegen, M. E., Robinson, D. R., Wu, Y. M., Dhanasekaran, S. M., et al. (2015). The distinctive mutational spectra of polyomavirus-negative merkel cell carcinoma. *Cancer Res.* 75, 3720–3727. doi: 10.1158/0008-5472.CAN-15-0702

Harold, A., Amako, Y., Hachisuka, J., Bai, Y., Li, M. Y., Kubat, L., et al. (2019). Conversion of Sox2-dependent Merkel cell carcinoma to a differentiated neuron-like phenotype by T antigen inhibition. *Proc. Natl. Acad. Sci. U.S.A.* 116, 20104–20114. doi: 10.1073/pnas.1907154116

Harrison, C. J., Meinke, G., Kwun, H. J., Rogalin, H., Phelan, P. J., Bullock, P. A., et al. (2011). Asymmetric assembly of Merkel cell polyomavirus large T-antigen origin binding domains at the viral origin. *J. Mol. Biol.* 409, 529–542. doi: 10.1016/j.jmb.2011.03.051

Hashida, Y., Higuchi, T., Tanaka, M., Shibata, Y., Nakajima, K., Sano, S., et al. (2019). Prevalence and viral loads of cutaneous human polyomaviruses in the skin of patients with chronic inflammatory skin diseases. *J. Infect. Dis.* 219, 1564–1573. doi: 10.1093/infdis/jiy618

Hashida, Y., Kamioka, M., Tanaka, M., Hosokawa, S., Murakami, M., Nakajima, K., et al. (2016a). Ecology of merkel cell polyomavirus in healthy skin among individuals in an asian cohort. *J. Infect. Dis.* 213, 1708–1716. doi: 10.1093/infdis/jiw040

Hashida, Y., Nakajima, K., Nakajima, H., Shiga, T., Tanaka, M., Murakami, M., et al. (2016b). High load of Merkel cell polyomavirus DNA detected in the normal skin of Japanese patients with Merkel cell carcinoma. *J. Clin. Virol.* 82, 101–107. doi: 10.1016/j.jcv.2016.07.011

Haugg, A. M., Rennspiess, D., Zur Hausen, A., Speel, E. J., Cathomas, G., Becker, J. C., et al. (2014). Fluorescence in situ hybridization and qPCR to detect Merkel cell polyomavirus physical status and load in Merkel cell carcinomas. *Int. J. Cancer* 135, 2804–2815. doi: 10.1002/ijc.28931

Heath, M., Jaimes, N., Lemos B., Mostaghimi, A., Wang, L. C., Penas, P. F., et al. (2008). Clinical characteristics of Merkel cell carcinoma at diagnosis in 195 patients: the AEIOU features. *J. Am. Acad. Dermatol.* 58, 375–381. doi: 10.1016/j.jaad.2007.11.020

Hesbacher, S., Pfitzer, L., Wiedorfer, K., Angermeyer, S., Borst, A., Haferkamp, S., et al. (2016). RB1 is the crucial target of the Merkel cell polyomavirus Large T antigen in Merkel cell carcinoma cells. *Oncotarget* 7, 32956–32968. doi: 10.18632/oncotarget.8793

Higaki-Mori, H., Kuwamoto, S., Iwasaki, T., Kato, M., Murakami, I., Nagata, K., et al. (2012). Association of Merkel cell polyomavirus infection with clinicopathological differences in Merkel cell carcinoma. *Hum. Pathol.* 43, 2282–2291. doi: 10.1016/j.humpath.2012.04.002

Houben, R., Adam, C., Baeurle, A., Hesbacher, S., Grimm, J., Angermeyer, S., et al. (2012). An intact retinoblastoma protein-binding site in Merkel cell polyomavirus large T antigen is required for promoting growth of Merkel cell carcinoma cells. *Int. J. Cancer* 130, 847–856. doi: 10.1002/ijc.26076

Houben, R., Shuda, M., Weinkam, R., Schrama, D., Feng, H., Chang, Y., et al. (2010). Merkel cell polyomavirus-infected Merkel cell carcinoma cells require expression of viral T antigens. *J. Virol.* 84, 7064–7072. doi: 10.1128/JVI.02400-09

Iwasaki, T., Matsushita, M., Kuwamoto, S., Kato, M., Murakami, I., Higaki-Mori, H., et al. (2013). Usefulness of significant morphologic characteristics in distinguishing between Merkel cell polyomavirus-positive and Merkel cell polyomavirus-negative Merkel cell carcinomas. *Hum. Pathol.* 44, 1912–1917. doi: 10.1016/j.humpath.2013.01.026

Iwasaki, T., Matsushita, M., Nonaka, D., Nagata, K., Kato, M., Kuwamoto, S., et al. (2016). Lower expression of CADM1 and higher expression of MAL in Merkel cell carcinomas are associated with Merkel cell polyomavirus infection and better prognosis. *Hum. Pathol.* 48, 1–8. doi: 10.1016/j.humpath.2015.09.030

Iyer, J. G., Blom, A., Doumani, R., Lewis, C., Tarabadkar, E. S., Anderson, A., et al. (2016). Response rates and durability of chemotherapy among 62 patients with metastatic Merkel cell carcinoma. *Cancer Med.* 5, 2294–2301. doi: 10.1002/cam4.815

Jacobs, D., Huang, H., Olino, K., Weiss, S., Kluger, H., Judson, B. L., et al. (2020). Assessment of age, period, and birth cohort effects and trends in merkel cell carcinoma incidence in the United States. *JAMA Dermatol.* 157, 59–65. doi: 10.1001/jamadermatol.2020.4102

Jouhi, L., Koljonen, V., Bohling, T., Haglund, C., and Hagstrom, J. (2015). The expression of Toll-like receptors 2, 4, 5, 7 and 9 in Merkel cell carcinoma. *Anticancer Res.* 35, 1843–1849.

Kaufman, H. L., Russell, J., Hamid, O., Bhatia, S., Terheyden, P., D'angelo, S. P., et al. (2016). Avelumab in patients with chemotherapy-refractory metastatic Merkel cell carcinoma: a multicentre, single-group, open-label, phase 2 trial. *Lancet Oncol.* 17, 1374–1385. doi: 10.1016/S1470-2045(16)30364-3

Kaufman, H. L., Russell, J. S. Hamid, O., Bhatia, S., Terheyden, P., D'angelo, S. P., et al. (2018). Updated efficacy of avelumab in patients with previously treated metastatic Merkel cell carcinoma after >/=1 year of follow-up: JAVELIN Merkel 200, a phase 2 clinical trial. *J. Immunother. Cancer* 6:7. doi: 10.1186/s40425-017-0310-x

Kean, J. M., Rao, S., Wang, M., and Garcea, R. L. (2009). Seroepidemiology of human polyomaviruses. *PLoS Pathog.* 5:e1000363. doi: 10.1371/journal.ppat.1000363

Kervarrec, T., Aljundi, M., Appenzeller, S., Samimi, M., Maubec, E., Cribier, B., et al. (2019). Polyomavirus-positive merkel cell carcinoma derived from a trichoblastoma suggests an epithelial origin of this merkel cell carcinoma. *J. Invest. Dermatol.* 140, 976–985. doi: 10.1016/j.jid.2019.09.026

Kervarrec, T., Samimi, M., Hesbacher, S., Berthon, P., Wobser, M., Sallot, A., et al. (2020). Merkel Cell Polyomavirus T Antigens Induce Merkel Cell-Like Differentiation in GLI1-Expressing Epithelial Cells. *Cancers (Basel)* 12:1989. doi: 10.3390/cancers12071989

Knight, L. M., Stakaityte, G., Wood, J. J., Abdul-Sada, H., Griffiths, D. A., Howell, G. J., et al. (2015). Merkel cell polyomavirus small T antigen mediates microtubule destabilization to promote cell motility and migration. *J. Virol.* 89, 35–47. doi: 10.1128/JVI.02317-14

Koljonen, V., Kukko, H., Pukkala, E., Sankila, R., Bohling, T., Tukiainen, E., et al. (2009). Chronic lymphocytic leukaemia patients have a high risk of Merkel-cell polyomavirus DNA-positive Merkel-cell carcinoma. *Br. J. Cancer* 101, 1444–1447. doi: 10.1038/sj.bjc.6605306

Krump, N. A., Wang, R., Liu, W., Yang, J. F., Ma, T., and You, J. (2021). Merkel cell polyomavirus infection induces an antiviral innate immune response in human dermal fibroblasts. *J. Virol.* 95:e0221120. doi: 10.1128/JVI.02211-20

Kuwamoto, S., Higaki, H., Kanai, K., Iwasaki, T., Sano, H., Nagata, K., et al. (2011). Association of Merkel cell polyomavirus infection with morphologic differences in Merkel cell carcinoma. *Hum. Pathol.* 42, 632–640. doi: 10.1016/j.humpath.2010.09.011

Kwun, H. J., Guastafierro, A., Shuda, M., Meinke, G., Bohm, A., Moore, P. S., et al. (2009). The minimum replication origin of merkel cell polyomavirus has a unique large T-antigen loading architecture and requires small T-antigen expression for optimal replication. *J. Virol.* 83, 12118–12128. doi: 10.1128/JVI.01336-09

Kwun, H. J., Shuda, M., Camacho, C. J., Gamper, A. M., Thant, M., Chang, Y., et al. (2015). Restricted protein phosphatase 2A targeting by Merkel cell polyomavirus small T antigen. *J. Virol.* 89, 4191–4200. doi: 10.1128/JVI.00157-15

Kwun, H. J., Shuda, M., Feng, H., Camacho, C. J., Moore, P. S., and Chang, Y. (2013). Merkel cell polyomavirus small T antigen controls viral replication and oncoprotein expression by targeting the cellular ubiquitin ligase SCFFbw7. *Cell Host Microbe* 14, 125–135. doi: 10.1016/j.chom.2013.06.008

Lau, L., Gray, E. E., Brunette, R. L., and Stetson, D. B. (2015). DNA tumor virus oncogenes antagonize the cGAS-STING DNA-sensing pathway. *Science* 350:568. doi: 10.1126/science.aab3291

Laude, H. C., Jonchere, B., Maubec, E., Carlotti, A., Marinho, E., Couturaud, B., et al. (2010). Distinct merkel cell polyomavirus molecular features in tumour and non tumour specimens from patients with merkel cell carcinoma. *PLoS Pathog.* 6:e1001076. doi: 10.1371/journal.ppat.1001076

Lauttia, S., Sihto, H., Kavola, H., Koljonen, V., Bohling, T., and Joensuu, H. (2014). Prokineticins and Merkel cell polyomavirus infection in Merkel cell carcinoma. *Br. J. Cancer* 110, 1446–1455. doi: 10.1038/bjc.2014.20

Leiendecker, L., Jung, P. S., Krecioch, I., Neumann, T., Schleiffer, A., Mechtler, K., et al. (2020). LSD1 inhibition induces differentiation and cell death in Merkel cell carcinoma. *EMBO Mol. Med.* 12:e12525. doi: 10.15252/emmm.202012525

Leroux-Kozal, V., Leveque, N., Brodard, V., Lesage, C., Dudez, O., Makeieff, M., et al. (2015). Merkel cell carcinoma: histopathologic and prognostic features according to the immunohistochemical expression of Merkel cell polyomavirus large T antigen correlated with viral load. *Hum. Pathol.* 46, 443–453. doi: 10.1016/j.humpath.2014.12.001

Li, J., Diaz, J., Wang, X., Tsang, S. H., and You, J. (2015). Phosphorylation of Merkel cell polyomavirus large tumor antigen at serine 816 by ATM kinase induces apoptosis in host cells. *J. Biol. Chem.* 290, 1874–1884. doi: 10.1074/jbc.M114.594895

Li, J., Wang, X., Diaz, J., Tsang, S. H., Buck, C. B., and You, J. (2013). Merkel cell polyomavirus large T antigen disrupts host genomic integrity and inhibits cellular proliferation. *J. Virol.* 87, 9173–9188. doi: 10.1128/JVI.01216-13

Lilyestrom, W., Klein, M. G., Zhang, R., Joachimiak, A., and Chen, X. S. (2006). Crystal structure of SV40 large T-antigen bound to p53: interplay between a viral oncoprotein and a cellular tumor suppressor. *Genes Dev.* 20, 2373–2382. doi: 10.1101/gad.1456306

Lipson, E. J., Vincent, J. G., Loyo, M., Kagohara, L. T., Luber, B. S., Wang, H., et al. nt: (2013). PD-L1 expression in the Merkel cell carcinoma microenvironmne association with inflammation, Merkel cell polyomavirus and overall survival. *Cancer Immunol Res* 1, 54–63. doi: 10.1158/2326-6066.CIR-13-0034

Liu, W., Kim, G. B., Krump, N. A., Zhou, Y., Riley, J. L., and You, J. (2020). Selective reactivation of STING signaling to target Merkel cell carcinoma. *Proc. Natl. Acad. Sci. U.S.A.* 117, 13730–13739. doi: 10.1073/pnas.1919690117

Liu, W., Krump, N. A., Macdonald, M., and You, J. (2018). Merkel cell polyomavirus infection of animal dermal fibroblasts. *J. Virol.* 92, e01610–e01617. doi: 10.1128/JVI.01610-17

Liu, W., Macdonald, M., and You, J. (2016a). Merkel cell polyomavirus infection and Merkel cell carcinoma. *Curr. Opin. Virol.* 20, 20–27. doi: 10.1016/j.coviro.2016.07.011

Liu, W., Yang, R., Payne, A. S., Schowalter, R. M., Spurgeon, M. E., Lambert, P. F., et al. (2016b). Identifying the target cells and mechanisms of merkel cell polyomavirus infection. *Cell Host Microbe* 19, 775–787. doi: 10.1016/j.chom.2016.04.024

Longino, N. V., Yang, J., Iyer, J. G., Ibrani, D., Chow, I. T., Laing, K. J., et al. (2019). Human CD4(+) T cells specific for merkel cell polyomavirus localize to merkel cell carcinomas and target a required oncogenic domain. *Cancer Immunol. Res.* 7, 1727–1739. doi: 10.1158/2326-6066.CIR-19-0103

Longworth, M. S., and Laimins, L. A. (2004). Pathogenesis of human papillomaviruses in differentiating epithelia. *Microbiol. Mol. Biol. Rev.* 68, 362–372. doi: 10.1128/MMBR.68.2.362-372.2004

Ma, J. E., and Brewer, J. D. (2014). Merkel cell carcinoma in immunosuppressed patients. *Cancers (Basel)* 6, 1328–1350. doi: 10.3390/cancers6031328

Mantripragada, K., and Birnbaum, A. (2015). Response to anti-PD-1 therapy in metastatic merkel cell carcinoma metastatic to the heart and pancreas. *Cureus* 7:e403. doi: 10.7759/cureus.403

Martel-Jantin, C., Pedergnana, V., Nicol, J. T., Leblond, V., Tregouet, D. A., Tortevoye, P., et al. (2013). Merkel cell polyomavirus infection occurs during early childhood and is transmitted between siblings. *J. Clin. Virol.* 58, 288–291. doi: 10.1016/j.jcv.2013.06.004

Matsushita, M., Iwasaki, T., Nonaka, D., Kuwamoto, S., Nagata, K., Kato, M., et al. (2017). Higher expression of activation-induced cytidine deaminase is significantly associated with merkel cell polyomavirus-negative merkel cell carcinomas. *Yonago Acta Med.* 60, 145–153. doi: 10.33160/yam.2017.09.002

Matsushita, M., Iwasaki, T., Wardhani, L. O., Kuwamoto, S., Nonaka, D., Nagata, K., et al. (2019). Decreased H3K27me3 expression is associated with merkel cell polyomavirus-negative merkel cell carcinoma, especially combined with cutaneous squamous cell carcinoma. *Anticancer Res.* 39, 5573–5579. doi: 10.21873/anticanres.13751

Mertz, K. D., Junt, T., Schmid, M., Pfaltz, M., and Kempf, W. (2010). Inflammatory monocytes are a reservoir for Merkel cell polyomavirus. *J. Invest. Dermatol.* 130, 1146–1151. doi: 10.1038/jid.2009.392

Miller, N. J., Church, C. D., Dong, L., Crispin, D., Fitzgibbon, M. P., Lachance, K., et al. (2017). Tumor-infiltrating merkel cell polyomavirus-specific T cells are diverse and associated with improved patient survival. *Cancer Immunol. Res.* 5, 137–147. doi: 10.1158/2326-6066.CIR-16-0210

Miller, N. J., Church, C. D., Fling, S. P., Kulikauskas, R., Ramchurren, N., Shinohara, M. M., et al. (2018). Merkel cell polyomavirus-specific immune responses in patients with Merkel cell carcinoma receiving anti-PD-1 therapy. *J. Immunother. Cancer* 6:131. doi: 10.1186/s40425-018-0450-7

Mitteldorf, C., Berisha, A., Tronnier, M., Pfaltz, M. C., and Kempf, W. (2017). PD-1 and PD-L1 in neoplastic cells and the tumor microenvironment of Merkel cell carcinoma. *J. Cutan. Pathol.* 44, 740–746. doi: 10.1111/cup.12973

Moll, R., Lowe, A., Laufer, J., and Franke, W. W. (1992). Cytokeratin 20 in human carcinomas. a new histodiagnostic marker detected by monoclonal antibodies. *Am. J. Pathol.* 140, 427–447.

Moshiri, A. S., Doumani, R., Yelistratova, L., Blom, A., Lachance, K., Shinohara, M. M., et al. (2017). Polyomavirus-negative merkel cell carcinoma: a more aggressive subtype based on analysis of 282 cases using multimodal tumor virus detection. *J. Invest. Dermatol.* 137, 819–827. doi: 10.1016/j.jid.2016.10.028

Nakamura, T., Sato, Y., Watanabe, D., Ito, H., Shimonohara, N., Tsuji, T., et al. (2010). Nuclear localization of Merkel cell polyomavirus large T antigen in Merkel cell carcinoma. *Virology* 398, 273–279. doi: 10.1016/j.virol.2009.12.024

Nardi, V., Song, Y., Santamaria-Barria, J. A., Cosper, A. K., Lam, Q., Faber, A. C., et al. (2012). Activation of PI3K signaling in Merkel cell carcinoma. *Clin. Cancer Res.* 18, 1227–1236. doi: 10.1158/1078-0432.CCR-11-2308

Narisawa, Y., Inoue, T., and Nagase, K. (2019). Evidence of proliferative activity in human Merkel cells: implications in the histogenesis of Merkel cell carcinoma. *Arch. Dermatol. Res.* 311, 37–43. doi: 10.1007/s00403-018-1877-x

Narisawa, Y., Inoue, T., and Nagase, K. (2020). Dermal and intraepidermal merkel cell carcinoma with squamous cell carcinoma: a report of a rare case with special reference to the touch dome. *Am. J. Dermatopathol.* 43, 15–20. doi: 10.1097/DAD.0000000000001618

Navarrete-Dechent, C., Cordova, M., Aleissa, S., Battle, L. R., Ganly, I., Pulitzer, M., et al. (2020). Dermoscopy and reflectance confocal microscopy of intraepidermal Merkel cell carcinoma. *Australas J. Dermatol.* 62, 238–241. doi: 10.1111/ajd.13513

Neu, U., Hengel, H., Blaum, B. S., Schowalter, R. M., Macejak, D., Gilbert, M., et al. (2012). Structures of Merkel cell polyomavirus VP1 complexes define a sialic acid binding site required for infection. *PLoS Pathog.* 8:e1002738. doi: 10.1371/journal.ppat.1002738

Neumann, F., Czech-Sioli, M., Dobner, T., Grundhoff, A., Schreiner, S., and Fischer, N. (2016). Replication of Merkel cell polyomavirus induces reorganization of promyelocytic leukemia nuclear bodies. *J. Gen. Virol.* 97, 2926–2938. doi: 10.1099/jgv.0.000593

Nghiem, P., Bhatia, S., Lipson, E. J., Sharfman, W. H., Kudchadkar, R. R., Brohl, A. S., et al. (2019). Durable tumor regression and overall survival in patients with advanced merkel cell carcinoma receiving pembrolizumab as first-line therapy. *J. Clin. Oncol.* 37, 693–702. doi: 10.1200/JCO.18.01896

Nguyen, M. H. K., Leong, S. P., Abendroth, R., Kashani-Sabet, M., and Kim, K. B. (2019). Complete clinical response to intralesional talimogene laherparepvec injection in a patient with recurrent, regionally advanced Merkel cell carcinoma. *JAAD Case Rep.* 5, 849–851. doi: 10.1016/j.jdcr.2019.07.006

Nwogu, N., Boyne, J. R., Dobson, S. J., Poterlowicz, K., Blair, G. E., Macdonald, A., et al. (2018). Cellular sheddases are induced by Merkel cell polyomavirus small tumour antigen to mediate cell dissociation and invasiveness. *PLoS Pathog.* 14:e1007276. doi: 10.1371/journal.ppat.1007276

Paik, J. Y., Hall, G., Clarkson, A., Lee, L., Toon, C., Colebatch, A., et al. (2011). Immunohistochemistry for Merkel cell polyomavirus is highly specific but not sensitive for the diagnosis of Merkel cell carcinoma in the Australian population. *Hum. Pathol.* 42, 1385–1390. doi: 10.1016/j.humpath.2010.12.013

Pancaldi, C., Corazzari, V., Maniero, S., Mazzoni, E., Comar, M., Martini, F., et al. (2011). Merkel cell polyomavirus DNA sequences in the buffy coats of healthy blood donors. *Blood* 117, 7099–7101. doi: 10.1182/blood-2010-09-310557

Park, D. E., Cheng, J., Berrios, C., Montero, J., Cortes-Cros, M., Ferretti, S., et al. (2019). Dual inhibition of MDM2 and MDM4 in virus-positive Merkel cell carcinoma enhances the p53 response. *Proc. Natl. Acad. Sci. U.S.A.* 116, 1027–1032. doi: 10.1073/pnas.1818798116

Park, D. E., Cheng, J., Mcgrath, J. P., Lim, M. Y., Cushman, C., Swanson, S. K., et al. (2020). Merkel cell polyomavirus activates LSD1-mediated blockade of non-canonical BAF to regulate transformation and tumorigenesis. *Nat. Cell Biol.* 22, 603–615. doi: 10.1038/s41556-020-0503-2

Pasternak, S., Carter, M. D., Ly, T. Y., Doucette, S., and Walsh, N. M. (2018). Immunohistochemical profiles of different subsets of Merkel cell carcinoma. *Hum. Pathol.* 82, 232–238. doi: 10.1016/j.humpath.2018.07.022

Pastrana, D. V., Tolstov, Y. L., Becker, J. C., Moore, P. S., Chang, Y., and Buck, C. B. (2009). Quantitation of human seroresponsiveness to Merkel cell polyomavirus. *PLoS Pathog.* 5:e1000578. doi: 10.1371/journal.ppat.1000578

Pastrana, D. V., Wieland, U., Silling, S., Buck, C. B., and Pfister, H. (2012). Positive correlation between Merkel cell polyomavirus viral load and capsid-specific antibody titer. *Med. Microbiol. Immunol.* 201, 17–23. doi: 10.1007/s00430-011-0200-7

Paulson, K. G., Iyer, J. G., Blom, A., Warton, E. M., Sokil, M., Yelistratova, L., et al. (2013). Systemic immune suppression predicts diminished Merkel cell carcinoma-specific survival independent of stage. *J. Invest. Dermatol.* 133, 642–646. doi: 10.1038/jid.2012.388

Paulson, K. G., Lewis, C. W., Redman, M. W., Simonson, W. T., Lisberg, A., Ritter, D., et al. (2017). Viral oncoprotein antibodies as a marker for recurrence of Merkel cell carcinoma: a prospective validation study. *Cancer* 123, 1464–1474. doi: 10.1002/cncr.30475

Paulson, K. G., Park, S. Y., Vandeven, N. A., Lachance, K., Thomas, H., Chapuis, A. G., et al. (2018a). Merkel cell carcinoma: current US incidence and projected increases based on changing demographics. *J. Am. Acad. Dermatol.* 78, 457–463.e2. doi: 10.1016/j.jaad.2017.10.028

Paulson, K. G., Voillet, V., Mcafee, M. S., Hunter, D. S., Wagener, F. D., Perdicchio, M., et al. (2018b). Acquired cancer resistance to combination immunotherapy from transcriptional loss of class I HLA. *Nat. Commun.* 9:3868. doi: 10.1038/s41467-018-06300-3

Perdigoto, C. N., Dauber, K. L., Bar, C., Tsai, P. C., Valdes, V. J., Cohen, I., et al. (2016). Polycomb-mediated repression and sonic hedgehog signaling interact to regulate merkel cell specification during skin development. *PLoS Genet.* 12:e1006151. doi: 10.1371/journal.pgen.1006151

Peretti, A., Borgogna, C., Rossi, D., De Paoli, L., Bawadekar, M., Zavattaro, E., et al. (2014). Analysis of human beta-papillomavirus and Merkel cell polyomavirus infection in skin lesions and eyebrow hair bulbs from a cohort of patients with chronic lymphocytic leukaemia. *Br. J. Dermatol.* 171, 1525–1528. doi: 10.1111/bjd.13215

Ponce, R. A., Gelzleichter, T., Haggerty, H. G., Heidel, S., Holdren, M. S., Lebrec, H., et al. (2014). Immunomodulation and lymphoma in humans. *J. Immunotoxicol.* 11, 1–12. doi: 10.3109/1547691X.2013.798388

Pugh, R. A., Honda, M., Leesley, H., Thomas, A., Lin, Y., Nilges, M. J., et al. (2008). The iron-containing domain is essential in Rad3 helicases for coupling of ATP hydrolysis to DNA translocation and for targeting the helicase to the single-stranded DNA-double-stranded DNA junction. *J. Biol. Chem.* 283, 1732–1743. doi: 10.1074/jbc.M707064200

Richards, K. F., Guastafierro, A., Shuda, M., Toptan, T., Moore, P. S., and Chang, Y. (2015). Merkel cell polyomavirus T antigens promote cell proliferation and inflammatory cytokine gene expression. *J. Gen. Virol.* 96, 3532–3544. doi: 10.1099/jgv.0.000287

Sahi, H., Savola, S., Sihto, H., Koljonen, V., Bohling, T., and Knuutila, S. (2014). RB1 gene in Merkel cell carcinoma: hypermethylation in all tumors and concurrent heterozygous deletions in the polyomavirus-negative subgroup. *APMIS* 122, 1157–1166. doi: 10.1111/apm.12274

Sahi, H., Sihto, H., Artama, M., Koljonen, V., Bohling, T., and Pukkala, E. (2017). History of chronic inflammatory disorders increases the risk of Merkel cell carcinoma, but does not correlate with Merkel cell polyomavirus infection. *Br. J. Cancer* 116, 260–264. doi: 10.1038/bjc.2016.391

Salakova, M., Koslabova, E., Vojtechova, Z., Tachezy, R., and Sroller, V. (2016). Detection of human polyomaviruses MCPyV, HPyV6, and HPyV7 in malignant and non-malignant tonsillar tissues. *J. Med. Virol.* 88, 695–702. doi: 10.1002/jmv.24385

Samimi, M., Molet, L., Fleury, M., Laude, H., Carlotti, A., Gardair, C., et al. (2016). Prognostic value of antibodies to Merkel cell polyomavirus T antigens and VP1 protein in patients with Merkel cell carcinoma. *Br. J. Dermatol.* 174, 813–822. doi: 10.1111/bjd.14313

Santos-Juanes, J., Fernandez-Vega, I., Fuentes, N., Galache, C., Coto-Segura, P., Vivanco, B., et al. (2015). Merkel cell carcinoma and Merkel cell polyomavirus: a systematic review and meta-analysis. *Br. J. Dermatol.* 173, 42–49. doi: 10.1111/bjd.13870

Sarma, B., Willmes, C., Angerer, L., Adam, C., Becker, J. C., Kervarrec, T., et al. (2020). Artesunate affects T antigen expression and survival of virus-positive merkel cell carcinoma. *Cancers (Basel)* 12:919. doi: 10.3390/cancers12040919

Sauer, C. M., Haugg, A. M., Chteinberg, E., Rennspiess, D., Winnepenninckx, V., Speel, E. J., et al. (2017). Reviewing the current evidence supporting early B-cells as the cellular origin of Merkel cell carcinoma. *Crit. Rev. Oncol. Hematol.* 116, 99–105. doi: 10.1016/j.critrevonc.2017.05.009

Schadendorf, D., Lebbe, C., Zur Hausen, A., Avril, M. F., Hariharan, S., Bharmal, M., et al. (2017). Merkel cell carcinoma: epidemiology, prognosis, therapy and unmet medical needs. *Eur. J. Cancer* 71, 53–69. doi: 10.1016/j.ejca.2016.10.022

Schowalter, R. M., and Buck, C. B. (2013). The Merkel cell polyomavirus minor capsid protein. *PLoS Pathog.* 9:e1003558. doi: 10.1371/journal.ppat.1003558

Schowalter, R. M., Pastrana, D. V., and Buck, C. B. (2011). Glycosaminoglycans and sialylated glycans sequentially facilitate Merkel cell polyomavirus infectious entry. *PLoS Pathog.* 7:e1002161. doi: 10.1371/journal.ppat.1002161

Schowalter, R. M., Pastrana, D. V., Pumphrey, K. A., Moyer, A. L., and Buck, C. B. (2010). Merkel cell polyomavirus and two previously unknown polyomaviruses are chronically shed from human skin. *Cell Host Microbe* 7, 509–515. doi: 10.1016/j.chom.2010.05.006

Schrama, D., Hesbacher, S., Angermeyer, S., Schlosser, A., Haferkamp, S., Aue, A., et al. (2016). Serine 220 phosphorylation of the Merkel cell polyomavirus large T antigen crucially supports growth of Merkel cell carcinoma cells. *Int. J. Cancer* 138, 1153–1162. doi: 10.1002/ijc.29862

Schrama, D., Peitsch, W. K., Zapatka, M., Kneitz, H., Houben, R., Eib, S., et al. (2011). Merkel cell polyomavirus status is not associated with clinical course of Merkel cell carcinoma. *J. Invest. Dermatol.* 131, 1631–1638. doi: 10.1038/jid.2011.115

Seo, G. J., Chen, C. J., and Sullivan, C. S. (2009). Merkel cell polyomavirus encodes a microRNA with the ability to autoregulate viral gene expression. *Virology* 383, 183–187. doi: 10.1016/j.virol.2008.11.001

Shahzad, N., Shuda, M., Gheit, T., Kwun, H. J., Cornet, I., Saidj, D., et al. (2013). The T antigen locus of Merkel cell polyomavirus downregulates human Toll-like receptor 9 expression. *J. Virol.* 87, 13009–13019. doi: 10.1128/JVI.01786-13

Shuda, M., Chang, Y., and Moore, P. S. (2014). Merkel cell polyomavirus-positive Merkel cell carcinoma requires viral small T-antigen for cell proliferation. *J. Invest. Dermatol.* 134, 1479–1481. doi: 10.1038/jid.2013.483

Shuda, M., Feng, H., Kwun, H. J., Rosen, S. T., Gjoerup, O., Moore, P. S., et al. (2008). T antigen mutations are a human tumor-specific signature for Merkel cell polyomavirus. *Proc. Natl. Acad. Sci. U.S.A.* 105, 16272–16277. doi: 10.1073/pnas.0806526105

Shuda, M., Kwun, H. J., Feng, H., Chang, Y., and Moore, P. S. (2011). Human Merkel cell polyomavirus small T antigen is an oncoprotein targeting the 4E-BP1 translation regulator. *J. Clin. Invest.* 121, 3623–3634. doi: 10.1172/JCI46323

Signorini, L., Belingheri, M., Ambrogi, F., Pagani, E., Binda, S., Ticozzi, R., et al. (2014). High frequency of Merkel cell polyomavirus DNA in the urine of kidney transplant recipients and healthy controls. *J. Clin. Virol.* 61, 565–570. doi: 10.1016/j.jcv.2014.10.012

Sihto, H., Bohling, T., Kavola, H., Koljonen, V., Salmi, M., Jalkanen, S., et al. (2012). Tumor infiltrating immune cells and outcome of Merkel cell carcinoma: a population-based study. *Clin. Cancer Res.* 18, 2872–2881. doi: 10.1158/1078-0432.CCR-11-3020

Sihto, H., Kukko, H., Koljonen, V., Sankila, R., Bohling, T., and Joensuu, H. (2009). Clinical factors associated with Merkel cell polyomavirus infection in Merkel cell carcinoma. *J. Natl. Cancer Inst.* 101, 938–945. doi: 10.1093/jnci/djp139

Sihto, H., Kukko, H., Koljonen, V., Sankila, R., Bohling, T., and Joensuu, H. (2011). Merkel cell polyomavirus infection, large T antigen, retinoblastoma protein and outcome in Merkel cell carcinoma. *Clin. Cancer Res.* 17, 4806–4813. doi: 10.1158/1078-0432.CCR-10-3363

Song, Y., Zheng, S., and Guo, Y. (2020). Intraepidermal merkel cell carcinoma mimicking melanoma *in situ*: a case report. *Am. J. Dermatopathol.* 42, 977–980. doi: 10.1097/DAD.0000000000001793

Spurgeon, M. E., and Lambert, P. F. (2013). Merkel cell polyomavirus: a newly discovered human virus with oncogenic potential. *Virology* 435, 118–130. doi: 10.1016/j.virol.2012.09.029

Stakaityte, G., Nwogu, N., Dobson, S. J., Knight, L. M., Wasson, C. W., Salguero, F. J., et al. (2018). Merkel cell polyomavirus small T antigen drives cell motility via Rho-GTPase-induced filopodium formation. *J. Virol.* 92:e00940-17. doi: 10.1128/JVI.00940-17

Stang, A., Becker, J. C., Nghiem, P., and Ferlay, J. (2018). The association between geographic location and incidence of Merkel cell carcinoma in comparison to melanoma: an international assessment. *Eur. J. Cancer* 94, 47–60. doi: 10.1016/j.ejca.2018.02.003

Starrett, G. J., Marcelus, C., Cantalupo, P. G., Katz, J. P., Cheng, J., Akagi, K., et al. (2017). Merkel cell polyomavirus exhibits dominant control of the tumor genome and transcriptome in virus-associated merkel cell carcinoma. *MBio* 8:e02079-16. doi: 10.1128/mBio.02079-16

Starrett, G. J., Thakuria, M., Chen, T., Marcelus, C., Cheng, J., Nomburg, J., et al. (2020). Clinical and molecular characterization of virus-positive and virus-negative Merkel cell carcinoma. *Genome Med.* 12:30. doi: 10.1186/s13073-020-00727-4

Sunshine, J. C., Jahchan, N. S., Sage, J., and Choi, J. (2018). Are there multiple cells of origin of Merkel cell carcinoma? *Oncogene* 37, 1409–1416. doi: 10.1038/s41388-017-0073-3

Theiss, J. M., Gunther, T., Alawi, M., Neumann, F., Tessmer, U., Fischer, N., et al. (2015). A Comprehensive analysis of replicating merkel cell polyomavirus genomes delineates the viral transcription program and suggests a role for mcv-miR-M1 in episomal persistence. *PLoS Pathog.* 11:e1004974. doi: 10.1371/journal.ppat.1004974

Toker, C. (1972). Trabecular carcinoma of the skin. *Arch. Dermatol.* 105, 107–110. doi: 10.1001/archderm.1972.01620040075020

Tolstov, Y. L., Pastrana, D. V., Feng, H., Becker, J. C., Jenkins, F. J., Moschos, S., et al. (2009). Human Merkel cell polyomavirus infection II. MCV is a common human infection that can be detected by conformational capsid epitope immunoassays. *Int. J. Cancer* 125, 1250–1256. doi: 10.1002/ijc.24509

Tolstov, Y. L., Knauer, A., Chen, J. G., Kensler, T. W., Kingsley, L. A., Moore, P. S., et al. (2011). Asymptomatic primary Merkel cell polyomavirus infection among adults. *Emerging Infect. Dis.* 17, 1371–1380. doi: 10.3201/eid1708.110079

Touze, A., Le Bidre, E., Laude, H., Fleury, M. J., Cazal, R., Arnold, F., et al. (2011). High levels of antibodies against merkel cell polyomavirus identify a subset of patients with merkel cell carcinoma with better clinical outcome. *J. Clin. Oncol.* 29, 1612–1619. doi: 10.1200/JCO.2010.31.1704

Tsang, S. H., Wang, R., Nakamaru-Ogiso, E., Knight, S. A., Buck, C. B., and You, J. (2015). The oncogenic small tumor antigen of merkel cell polyomavirus is an iron-sulfur cluster protein that enhances viral DNA replication. *J. Virol.* 90, 1544–1556. doi: 10.1128/JVI.02121-15

Tsang, S. H., Wang, X., Li, J., Buck, C. B., and You, J. (2014). Host DNA damage response factors localize to merkel cell polyomavirus DNA replication sites to support efficient viral DNA replication. *J. Virol.* 88, 3285–3297. doi: 10.1128/JVI.03656-13

Vahabpour, R., Nasimi, M., Naderi, N., Salehi-Vaziri, M., Mohajel, N., Sadeghi, F., et al. (2017). Merkel cell polyomavirus IgG antibody levels are associated with progression to AIDS among HIV-infected individuals. *Arch. Virol.* 162, 963–969. doi: 10.1007/s00705-016-3186-z

Velasquez, C., Cheng, E., Shuda, M., Lee-Oesterreich, P. J., Pogge Von Strandmann, L., Gritsenko, M. A., et al. (2016). Mitotic protein kinase CDK1 phosphorylation of mRNA translation regulator 4E-BP1 Ser83 may contribute to cell transformation. *Proc. Natl. Acad. Sci. U.S.A.* 113, 8466–8471. doi: 10.1073/pnas.1607768113

Verhaegen, M. E., Mangelberger, D., Harms, P. W., Eberl, M., Wilbert, D. M., Meireles, J., et al. (2017). Merkel cell polyomavirus small T antigen initiates merkel cell carcinoma-like tumor development in mice. *Cancer Res.* 77, 3151–3157. doi: 10.1158/0008-5472.CAN-17-0035

Verhaegen, M. E., Mangelberger, D., Harms, P. W., Vozheiko, T. D., Weick, J. W., Wilbert, D. M., et al. (2014). Merkel cell polyomavirus small T antigen is oncogenic in transgenic mice. *J. Invest. Dermatol.* 135, 1415–1424. doi: 10.1038/jid.2014.446

Verhaegen, M. E., Mangelberger, D., Harms, P. W., Vozheiko, T. D., Weick, J. W., Wilbert, D. M., et al. (2015). Merkel cell polyomavirus small T antigen is oncogenic in transgenic mice. *J. Invest. Dermatol.* 135, 1415–1424.

Viscidi, R. P., Rollison, D. E., Sondak, V. K., Silver, B., Messina, J. L., Giuliano, A. R., et al. (2011). Age-specific seroprevalence of Merkel cell polyomavirus, BK virus, and JC virus. *Clin. Vaccine Immunol.* 18, 1737–1743. doi: 10.1128/CVI.05175-11

Von Der Grun, J., Winkelmann, R., Meissner, M., Wieland, U., Silling, S., Martin, D., et al. (2019). Merkel cell polyoma viral load and intratumoral cd8+ lymphocyte infiltration predict overall survival in patients with merkel cell carcinoma. *Front. Oncol.* 9:20. doi: 10.3389/fonc.2019.00020

Walder, B. K., Robertson, M. R., and Jeremy, D. (1971). Skin cancer and immunosuppression. *Lancet* 2, 1282–1283. doi: 10.1016/S0140-6736(71)90602-7

Walsh, N. M., Fleming, K. E., Hanly, J. G., Dakin Hache, K., Doucette, S., Ferrara, G., et al. (2016). A morphological and immunophenotypic map of the immune response in Merkel cell carcinoma. *Hum. Pathol.* 52, 190–196. doi: 10.1016/j.humpath.2016.02.002

Wang, L., Harms, P. W., Palanisamy, N., Carskadon, S., Cao, X., Siddiqui, J., et al. (2017). Age and Gender associations of virus positivity in merkel cell carcinoma characterized using a novel RNA *in situ* hybridization assay. *Clin. Cancer Res.* 23, 5622–5630. doi: 10.1158/1078-0432.CCR-17-0299

Wang, X., Helfer, C. M., Pancholi, N., Bradner, J. E., and You, J. (2013). Recruitment of Brd4 to the human papillomavirus type 16 DNA replication complex is essential for replication of viral DNA. *J. Virol.* 87, 3871–3884. doi: 10.1128/JVI.03068-12

Wang, X., Li, J., Schowalter, R. M., Jiao, J., Buck, C. B., and You, J. (2012). Bromodomain protein Brd4 plays a key role in Merkel cell polyomavirus DNA replication. *PLoS Pathog.* 8:e1003021. doi: 10.1371/journal.ppat.1003021

Wang, Y., Strassl, R., Helantera, I., Aberle, S. W., Bond, G., Hedman, K., et al. (2019). Multiplex analysis of Human Polyomavirus diversity in kidney transplant recipients with BK virus replication. *J. Clin. Virol.* 120, 6–11. doi: 10.1016/j.jcv.2019.08.012

Weber, R., Sabin, C. A., Friis-Moller, N., Reiss, P., El-Sadr, W. M., Kirk, O., et al. (2006). Liver-related deaths in persons infected with the human immunodeficiency virus: the D:A:D study. *Arch. Intern. Med.* 166, 1632–1641. doi: 10.1001/archinte.166.15.1632

Wendzicki, J. A., Moore, P. S., and Chang, Y. (2015). Large T and small T antigens of Merkel cell polyomavirus. *Curr. Opin. Virol.* 11, 38–43. doi: 10.1016/j.coviro.2015.01.009

Werner, S., and Grose, R. (2003). Regulation of wound healing by growth factors and cytokines. *Physiol. Rev.* 83, 835–870. doi: 10.1152/physrev.2003.83.3.835

Westbrook, B. C., Norwood, T. G., Terry, N. L. J., Mckee, S. B., and Conry, R. M. (2019). Talimogene laherparepvec induces durable response of regionally advanced Merkel cell carcinoma in 4 consecutive patients. *JAAD Case Rep.* 5, 782–786. doi: 10.1016/j.jdcr.2019.06.034

Wheat, R., Roberts, C., Waterboer, T., Steele, J., Marsden, J., Steven, N. M., et al. (2014). Inflammatory cell distribution in primary merkel cell carcinoma. *Cancers (Basel)* 6, 1047–1064. doi: 10.3390/cancers6021047

Whyte, J. L., Smith, A. A., and Helms, J. A. (2012). Wnt signaling and injury repair. *Cold Spring Harb. Perspect. Biol.* 4:a008078. doi: 10.1101/cshperspect.a008078

Wieland, U., Silling, S., Scola, N., Potthoff, A., Gambichler, T., Brockmeyer, N. H., et al. (2011). Merkel cell polyomavirus infection in HIV-positive men. *Arch. Dermatol.* 147, 401–406. doi: 10.1001/archdermatol.2011.42

Wong, S. Q., Waldeck, K., Vergara, I. A., Schroder, J., Madore, J., Wilmott, J. S., et al. (2015). UV-associated mutations underlie the etiology of MCV-negative merkel cell carcinomas. *Cancer Res.* 75, 5228–5234. doi: 10.1158/0008-5472.CAN-15-1877

Wu, J. H., Narayanan, D., Limmer, A. L., Simonette, R. A., Rady, P. L., and Tyring, S. K. (2019). Merkel cell polyomavirus small t antigen induces DNA damage response. *Intervirology* 62, 96–100. doi: 10.1159/000501419

Wu, J. H., Simonette, R. A., Hsiao, T., Doan, H. Q., Rady, P. L., and Tyring, S. K. (2015). Cutaneous human polyomavirus small T antigens and 4E-BP1 targeting. *Intervirology* 58, 382–385. doi: 10.1159/000444921

Wu, J. H., Simonette, R. A., Nguyen, H. P., Rady, P. L., and Tyring, S. K. (2016). Merkel cell polyomavirus in Merkel cell carcinogenesis: small T antigen-mediates c-Jun phosphorylation. *Virus Genes* 52, 397–399. doi: 10.1007/s11262-016-1304-3

Wu, Y., and Brosh, R. M. Jr. (2012). DNA helicase and helicase-nuclease enzymes with a conserved iron-sulfur cluster. *Nucleic Acids Res.* 40, 4247–4260. doi: 10.1093/nar/gks039

Xie, H., Lee, L., Caramuta, S., Hoog, A., Browaldh, N., Bjornhagen, V., et al. (2014). MicroRNA expression patterns related to merkel cell polyomavirus infection in human merkel cell carcinoma. *J. Invest. Dermatol.* 134, 507–517. doi: 10.1038/jid.2013.355

Yang, R., Lee, E. E., Kim, J., Choi, J. H., Kolitz, E., Chen, Y., et al. (2021). Characterization of ALTO-encoding circular RNAs expressed by Merkel cell polyomavirus and trichodysplasia spinulosa polyomavirus. *PLoS Pathog.* 17:e1009582. doi: 10.1371/journal.ppat.1009582

You, J. (2010). Papillomavirus interaction with cellular chromatin. *Biochim. Biophys. Acta* 1799, 192–199. doi: 10.1016/j.bbagrm.2009.09.009

You, J., Croyle, J. L., Nishimura, A., Ozato, K., and Howley, P. M. (2004). Interaction of the bovine papillomavirus E2 protein with Brd4 tethers the viral DNA to host mitotic chromosomes. *Cell* 117, 349–360. doi: 10.1016/S0092-8674(04)00402-7

Zhao, J., Jia, Y., Shen, S., Kim, J., Wang, X., Lee, E., et al. (2020). Merkel cell polyomavirus small T antigen activates noncanonical NF-κB signaling to promote tumorigenesis. *Mol. Cancer Res.* 18, 1623–1637. doi: 10.1158/1541-7786.MCR-20-0587

Zur Hausen, A., Rennspiess, D., Winnepenninckx, V., Speel, E. J., and Kurz, A. K. (2013). Early B-cell differentiation in Merkel cell carcinomas: clues to cellular ancestry. *Cancer Res.* 73, 4982–4987. doi: 10.1158/0008-5472.CAN-13-0616

10

Induction of Tyrosine Phosphorylation of UV-Activated EGFR by the Beta-Human Papillomavirus Type 8 E6 Leads to Papillomatosis

Stefanie Taute, Herbert J. Pfister and Gertrud Steger*

Institute of Virology, University of Cologne, Cologne, Germany

Correspondence:
Gertrud Steger
gertrud.steger@uni-koeln.de

Epidemiological evidence is accumulating that beta-human papillomaviruses (HPV) synergize with UV-light in the development of precancerous actinic keratosis, and cutaneous squamous cell carcinomas (cSCC), one of the most common cancers in the Caucasian population. We previously demonstrated the tumorigenic activity of beta-HPV type 8 (HPV8) in the skin of transgenic mice and its cooperation with UV-light. Analysis of underlying mechanisms now showed that in keratinocytes expressing the HPV8E6 protein a transient increase of tyrosine phosphorylated epidermal growth factor receptor (EGFR) in response to UV-irradiation occurred, while EGFR tyrosine phosphorylation, i.e., receptor tyrosine kinase (RTK)-activity was hardly affected in empty vector control cells. FACS and immunofluorescences revealed that the EGFR was internalized into early endosomes in response to UV-exposure in both, HPV8E6 positive and in control cells, yet with a higher rate in the presence of HPV8E6. Moreover, only in HPV8E6 expressing keratinocytes the EGFR was further sorted into CD63+ intraluminal vesicles, indicative for trafficking to late endosomes. The latter requires the ubiquitination of the EGFR, and in correlation, we could show that only in HPV8E6 positive keratinocytes the EGFR was ubiquitinated upon UV-exposure. HPV8E6 and tyrosine phosphorylated EGFR directly interacted which was enhanced by UV-irradiation. The treatment of K14-HPV8E6 transgenic mice with Canertinib, an inhibitor of the RTK-activity of the EGFR, suppressed skin papilloma growth in response to UV-irradiation. This confirms the crucial role of the RTK-activity of the EGFR in HPV8E6 and UV-mediated papillomatosis in transgenic mice. Taken together, our results demonstrate that HPV8E6 alters the signaling of the UV-activated EGFR and this is a critical step in papilloma formation in response to UV-light in transgenic mice. Our results provide a molecular basis how a beta-HPV type may support early steps of skin tumor formation in cooperation with UV-light.

Keywords: beta-HPV8, E6 oncoprotein, cutaneous squamous cell carcinomas, UV-light, papillomatosis, EGFR signaling and trafficking

INTRODUCTION

The cutaneous squamous cell carcinoma (cSCC) is one of the most prevalent skin tumors in the Caucasian population and particularly frequent after organ transplantation. Since cSCC is a cancer of the elderly population with a mean age of 75 years it is estimated that its incidence will augment in the future due to the increased life expectation (Hillen et al., 2014). The precancerous actinic (solar) keratosis (AK) is an intraepidermal squamous neoplasm of sun-damaged skin. The transition to invasive cSCC is reported in 5–10% and with immunosuppression in 30% of patients. On the other side, 80% of the cSCC have AK with a variable grade of dysplasia in their periphery. Immunosuppressed organ transplant recipients (OTR) have a 100-fold increased risk to develop an invasive cSCC and 250-fold increased risk for AK (Lomas et al., 2012). Most AK and cSCC appear on sun exposed skin areas, which clearly points to the etiologic role of UV-light as initiator and tumor promoter of AK and cSCC. This relies on DNA damage including inactivating mutations of p53, and on effects of UV-light on signal transduction pathways that regulate cell proliferation and survival such as the signaling by the epidermal growth factor receptor (EGFR).

Evidence is accumulating that human papillomaviruses (HPV) belonging to the genus beta (β-HPV) synergize with UV-light in the development of cSCC. This was initially recognized in patients suffering from the rare disease Epidermodysplasia verruciformis (EV). CSCC in EV-patients harbor multiple, extrachromosomal genome copies of specific β-HPV types, especially HPV5 or HPV8 (reviewed in Howley and Pfister, 2015). β-HPVs are wide spread in humans but cause no apparent lesions in the skin of the general population. These viruses replicate in the hair follicles and are regarded as part of the commensal skin flora. Iatrogenic immunosuppression in OTR allows a more active replication of the commensal β-HPV spectrum in the entire skin with the result of higher viral load (Weissenborn et al., 2012). A high β-HPV DNA load in plucked eyebrow hairs was shown to imply a significant risk for the development of cSCC (Neale et al., 2013). The viral load of β-HPV in cSCC of the general population is lower compared to EV with usually less than 1 viral genome per cell (Weissenborn et al., 2005) and no viral transcripts have been detected (Arron et al., 2011). Though, the DNA loads of β-HPVs are higher in the precancerous AK (Weissenborn et al., 2005) and active viral replication and gene expression could be demonstrated (Borgogna et al., 2014). These findings are consistent with a role of β-HPV at early steps in non-melanoma skin cancer development by acting as a co-factor that enhances the carcinogenic potential of UV light.

The tumorigenic activity of β-HPV was demonstrated in transgenic mouse studies. We generated K14-HPV8CER transgenic mice that express the complete early region (CER) of HPV8 in the basal layer of their epidermis. Nearly all K14-HPV8CER transgenic mice spontaneously developed papillomas with varying degrees of epidermal dysplasia within 1 year. CSCC appeared in 6% of the animals (Schaper et al., 2005). After a single UV-irradiation or mechanical wounding, benign skin tumors grew within 3 weeks in all transgenic animals, which was consistently preceded by an enhanced expression of the viral oncogenes (Marcuzzi et al., 2009; Hufbauer et al., 2010). K14-HPV8E6 transgenic animals expressing only the E6 oncoprotein had the same phenotype as the K14-HPV8CER mice, indicating that HPV8E6 is the major oncogene in the murine skin (Marcuzzi et al., 2009). Transgene expression turned out to be crucial for tumor development since siRNA-mediated suppression of HPV8E6 reduced the papilloma incidence in these mice (Hufbauer et al., 2010). Thus, in this mouse model the HPV8 early genes cooperate with UV-light in the induction of skin tumors and the HPV8E6 oncogene is sufficient for this.

UV-irradiation transiently activates the EGFR which leads to increased proliferation, suppression of cell death and hyperplasia (El-Abaseri et al., 2006). Studies on mouse models deciphered the importance of EGFR signaling and downstream targets in the UV-induced skin tumorigenesis (Wan et al., 2001; El-Abaseri et al., 2005) and normal skin homeostasis (reviewed in Schneider et al., 2008). Ligand-, such as EGF, dependent activation initiates EGFR dimerization, which activates the receptor tyrosine kinase (RTK) resulting in the auto-phosphorylation of intracellular localized tyrosine residues of the EGFR. These phospho-tyrosines serve as binding motifs for a number of effectors which initiate the activation of downstream signaling pathways including the phosphatidylinositol 3 kinase (PI3K)/AKT, the Ras/mitogen-activated protein kinase (MAPK) pathways and Rac1 (Zhu et al., 2015) to promote cell survival and proliferation (reviewed in Lemmon and Schlessinger, 2010). Full activation of the EGFR as well as termination of the signaling depends on receptor endocytosis and intracellular trafficking. EGF-activated EGFR is rapidly internalized into early endosomes. Further downstream processing to late endosomes/lysosomes depends on the ubiquitination of the EGFR, which is initiated by binding of the E3 ubiquitin ligase Cbl to phospho-tyrosine residues of the EGFR. Ubiquitination is a prerequisite for the recognition by the endosomal sorting complex required for transport (ESCRT) that drives EGFR sorting from early endosomes via intraluminal vesicles (ILVs) to late endosomes and lysosomes leading to the proteasomal degradation. Dysregulation of this sorting process contributes to oncogenesis (reviewed in Tomas et al., 2014). Many intrinsic and iatrogenic cellular stresses such as UV-light, the cytokine TNFα or the cancer therapeutic cisplatin activate the EGFR in a tyrosine-kinase-independent way. UV-irradiation triggers a rapid clathrin-mediated internalization of the EGFR, which is ligand and RTK-activity independent and results in the accumulation of the UV-activated EGFR within the endosomal compartment without degradation (Zwang and Yarden, 2006).

Here, we addressed the effects of HPV8E6 on the UV-activated EGFR signaling and the implications for HPV8E6 mediated skin tumor formation in transgenic mice.

MATERIALS AND METHODS

Mice

The K14-HPV8E6 mice were in the FVB/N background and express the HPV8E6 oncogene under control of the keratin 14 promoter (Marcuzzi et al., 2009). All mice were irradiated with UV as described previously at a dose of 1 J/cm^{-2} for UVB and 10 J/cm^{-2} for UVA (Marcuzzi et al., 2009). UV-radiation was generated by a UV device (UV 801; Waldmann). Prior to UV-exposure, mice were anesthetized and their back area was shaved with an electric shaver. A 2 cm^2 area was irradiated while the rest of the skin was covered with a UV-impermeable sheet. The Canertinib group was administered once 20 mg/kg Canertinib (CI-1033, Selleckchem, S1019) solved in 150 μl PBS by gavage and the control group obtained 150 μl PBS 4 h prior UV-irradiation. After UV, the Canertinib group was treated with 10 mg/kg Canertinib solved in 150 μl PBS and the control group with 150 μl PBS daily for 24 days, respectively.

Cell Culture

Normal human epithelial keratinocytes (NHEK) were obtained from PromoCell and were cultivated in KGM2 supplemented with growth factors and penicillin and streptomycin (S/P). HaCaT (provided by Professor N. Fusenig, German Cancer Research Center, Heidelberg, Germany) and C33A cells (from ATCC) were grown in DMEM. The immortalized keratinocyte cell line RTS3b [obtained from I. Leigh (Purdie et al., 1993)] and N/TERT (obtained from the ATCC) were cultivated in E-Medium. DMEM and E-medium were supplemented with 10% FCS and S/P. Transduction with pLXSN or pLXSN-HPV8E6 and selection by G418 was performed as previously protocol (Leverrier et al., 2007). RTS3b cells were transiently transfected with the X-treme gene reagent from Roche and C33A cells by the $CaCl_2$ precipitate method. UV irradiation was performed at a dosage of 30 or 40 mJ/cm^2 with UVB light using a UVP CL-1000 ultra-violet cross-linker with F8T5 bulbs giving a spectral peak at 320 nm. Cells were grown in media containing Canertinib, (4 or 7 μM), AG478 (10 μM) (Selleckchem) or vehicle for 2 h before UV-irradiation.

Plasmids

The expression vectors pLXSN, pLXSN-HPV8E6, and pXJ41-FLAG-HPV8E6 have been described previously (Müller-Schiffmann et al., 2006; Leverrier et al., 2007). The expression vector for EGFR-GFP (Addgene Plasmid 32751) was a gift from Alexander Sorkin (Carter and Sorkin, 1998).

Antibodies

The antibodies against the EGFR (D38B1) uncoupled or coupled to sepharose beads or to Alexa Flour (AF) 488, the phospho-EGFR-Y1068 (D7A5) and -Y1045 (#2237), -T669 (#8808) and the K48-polyubiquitin (12805), as well as the rabbit IgG isotype control (DA1E) were from Cell Signaling. The anti-EEA1 (BD Clone 14) and CD63 (BD clone H5C6) were purchased from BD Biosciences and M2-FLAG-affinity Gel and antibodies from Sigma and the GFP-tag antibody from Thermo-Scientific (A-11122). The guinea pig polyclonal antibody against HPV8E6 was kindly provided by Janet L. Brandsma and is described in Hufbauer et al. (2010).

Western Blots and Co-IP

Cells were washed once in ice cold PBS and lyzed in low salt lysis buffer (20% glycerol, 50 mM Tris pH 7.9, 150 mM NaCl, 0.1% Nonidet-P40, 1 mM DTT) supplemented with protease inhibitors PMSF, aprotinin, leupeptin, and pepstatin and the phosphatase inhibitors NaF and Na-orthovanadate on ice for 15 min followed by sonification. IPs, blotting, and WB were done according to standard procedures. Blots were either developed with the use of X-ray films and scanned for digitalization or with the ChemiDoc XRS System (Bio-Rad, Dreieich, Germany), further processed with Adobe Photoshop CS6 (Adobe Systems Inc., Dublin, Ireland). Quantification was done with ImageJ software.

Immunostainings and FACS-Analysis

Skin lesions were excised from transgenic mice, fixed in 4% paraformaldehyde and processed for paraffin embedding. Four micrometers thick sections were mounted and processed. IHC staining was performed with the Vectastain Universal Elite ABC Kit (Vector Laboratories, Peterborough, United Kingdom). Paraffin sections were stained for hematoxylin/eosin (H/E) and Giemsa following standard protocols. Sections were analyzed with the Leica DM4000B light microscope equipped with a KY-F75U digital camera (JVC) and Diskus 4.50 Software. For IFTs, cells were grown on coverslips, fixed in 4% paraformaldehyde for 15 min, washed with PBS three times and blocked for 60 min in PBS/10% horse serum/0.3% Triton-X-100, followed by incubation with the antibodies against EEA1 or CD63 (both diluted 1:200 in PBS, 5% horse serum, 0.15% Triton-X-100) for 2 h at rt. After three PBS washes for 5 min, the anti-mouse-IgG-Rhodamine (Santa Cruz), (1:100) and the anti-EGFR-AF488 (Cell Signaling, 1:150) antibodies were mixed and incubated for 2 h, followed by three PBS wash steps with DAPI being added to the last PBS wash. Coverslips were mounted on object plates and analyzed by a DMI6000B microscope equipped with a fluorescence Leica DFC365FX camera. The overlays were processed by the Leica LASX software. Pictures were further adapted with Adobe Photoshop CS6 (Adobe Systems Inc., Dublin, Ireland). Cells for flow cytometry were trypsinized, washed in PBS and fixed in 4% paraformaldehyde for 10 min at 37°C followed by 1 min on ice. After two washing steps with PBS/0.5% BSA, the cells were incubated with the anti-EGFR antibody (1:100) or the rabbit isotype control, both coupled to AF488 for 1 h at rt. After two times washing, the cells were resuspended in PBS and analyzed by FACS in a MACS Quant analyzer (Miltenyi, Germany) and the FlowJo software.

RNA Processing

Skin samples were stored at −20°C in RNALater until RNA was isolated with the RNeasy kit (Qiagen, Hilden, Germany). One microgram of RNA was reverse transcribed using the GoTaq-RT-PCR System (Promega). Quantitative PCR were performed with the Go-Taq qPCR-Sybr-Green System (Promega) and a LightCycler480 (Roche).

Ethics Statement

The generation of the transgenic mice and the UV irradiation protocols were approved by the governmental animal care office North-Rhine-Westphalia (protocol no. 84-02.04.2014.A087) and were in accordance with the German Animal Welfare Act as well as the German Regulation for the protection of animals used for experimental purposes.

RESULTS

The Expression of HPV8E6 Leads to Increased Tyrosine Phosphorylation of the EGFR in Response to UV-Light in Keratinocytes

To decipher the effects of UV and HPV8E6 on the activation of the EGFR we used keratinocytes expressing the HPV8E6 protein under control of the rather weak long terminal repeat (LTR) promoter of pLXSN-retroviruses to match the low level of the E6 protein as observed during natural HPV infections (Wallace et al., 2014). The expression of HPV8E6 in the stably transduced immortalized keratinocyte lines HaCat, RTS3b, and N/TERT, and in primary NHEK was confirmed by qRT-PCR (data not shown). All types of keratinocytes were kept 24 h under low serum conditions (i.e., 0.2% FBS), followed by UV-irradiation (30 mJ/cm^2) and a recovery period of 30 min prior to be harvested. The stimulation of the RTK-activity in the UV-treated cells was analyzed by detecting the phosphorylation of the EGFR at tyrosine at pos. 1068 (pEGFR-Y1068) by WB. All unirradiated keratinocytes, except HaCat cells, had low, but detectable level pEGFR-Y1068 (**Figure 1A**, lanes 1, 5, and 13). These were hardly affected by UV-irradiation. In HaCat cells, pEGFR-Y1068 was only detectable after UV-irradiation. Importantly, in all four tested keratinocytes the signals corresponding to pEGFR-Y1068 were stronger in the presence of HPV8E6 compared those of empty vector cells 30 min after UV-irradiation (**Figure 1A**, lanes 4, 8, 12, and 16). The quantifications of the ratio of total EGFR versus pEGFR-Y1068 revealed that in the presence of HPV8E6 UV-exposure enhanced the RTK-activity of the EGFR, which ranged from 2.5-fold (in HaCat cells) to more than 4-fold (in RTS3b, N/TERT and primary keratinocytes). This implies that HPV8E6 increases the RTK-activity of the EGFR in response to UV-irradiation. We consistently observed a slight shift in the migration of the EGFR after UV-exposure (**Figure 1A**, compare lanes 1 and 2, 5 and 6, 13 and 14). This may be attributed to the UV-dependent phosphorylations of S or T residues which included the threonine at pos. 669 (T669). These phosphorylations have been found to be required for the internalization of the UV-exposed EGFR (Zwang and Yarden, 2006). The UV-light induced phosphorylation of the EGFR at T669 was confirmed in all four types of keratinocytes we investigated here (**Figure 1A**).

To address the effect of HPV8E6 on the tyrosine phosphorylation of the EGFR in more detail, we performed a kinetic. In empty vector control NHEK the level of pEGFR-Y1068 was hardly affected by UV-light within 60 min following the treatment. We regularly observed an enhanced tyrosine phosphorylation 90 or 120 min after UV-exposure in empty vector cells, which may be triggered by UV-induced p38MAPK activity, as suggested previously (Tomas et al., 2015). In HPV8E6 expressing primary keratinocytes, UV-irradiation led to a marked increase of the level of pEGFR-Y1068 30 min and 45 min after UV-treatment. Then, the amounts declined and finally returned to background level (**Figure 1B**, upper part). A similar

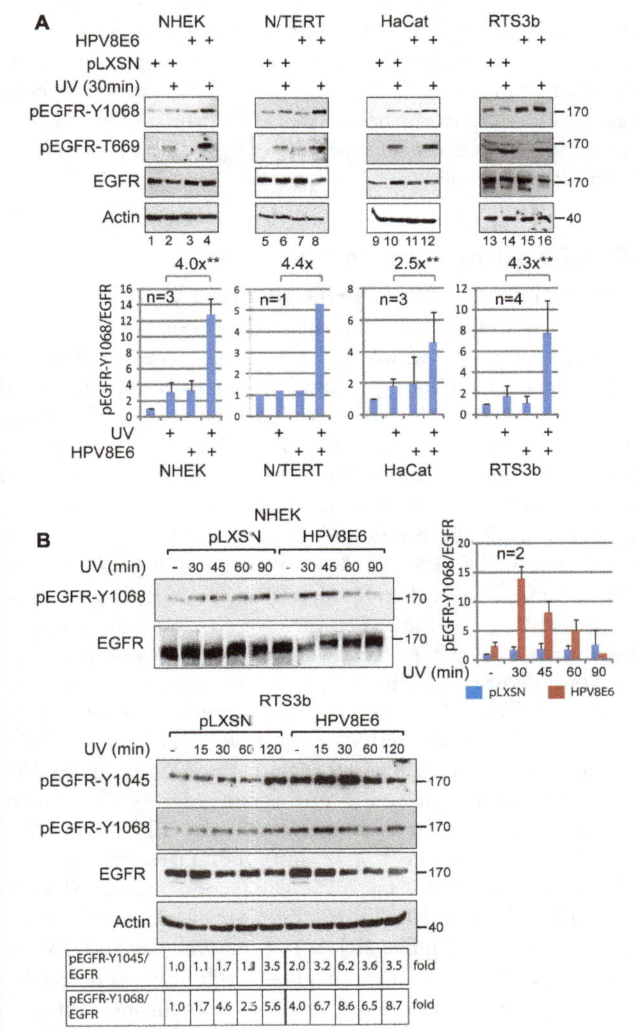

FIGURE 1 | HPV8E6 increases the rate of tyrosine-phosphorylation of the EGFR after UV-irradiation. **(A)** Normal human epithelial keratinocytes (NHEK), N/TERT, HaCat and RTS3b cells, harboring either pLXSN or pLXSN-HPV8E6, respectively, were left untreated or irradiated with UV light and further cultivated for 30 min. Protein extracts were used for a WB developed with antibodies as indicated in the figure. Shown is one representative blot for each cell line. The signals were quantitated and the average ratio of pEGFR-Y1068 versus total EGFR obtained with three to four independent experiments, as indicated, were given in the graph for NHEK, RTS3b, and HaCat cells. The fold changes of the pEGFR-Y1068 versus total EGFR in UV-irradiated cell due to the expression of HPV8E6 are given. The ratios with N/TERTS are from one experiment (**$p < 0.05$). **(B)** pLXSN-HPV8E6 or empty vector harboring NHEK and RTS3b cells were UV-irradiated and harvested at the indicated time points later. The pEGFR-Y1068, (pEGFR-Y1045 in the case of RTS3b) and the total EGFR were detected by WB. Shown is one representative example out of two experiments using NHEK, which both were used for quantifications shown in the figure. The values of the quantification of WB with the RTS3 cells are given as well. The positions of the molecular weight markers are given (in kDa).

kinetic of UV- and HPV8E6-mediated increase of the pEGFR-Y1068 was observed in RTS3b cell (**Figure 1B**, lower part). In addition, UV-irradiation transiently triggered the pEGFR-Y1045 detectable 30 min and 45 min later in HPV8E6 expressing cells. These results support the notion that the expression of HPV8E6 transiently increases the RTK-activity of the EGFR in response to UV-irradiation.

HPV8E6 Alters the Intracellular Trafficking of the UV-Activated EGFR

UV-light induces an RTK independent EGFR transactivation and internalization, which results in an arrest within the early endosome without the ubiquitination and proteasomal degradation of the UV-activated EGFR within the first hour post-UV (reviewed in Tan et al., 2016). In order to investigate whether the internalization and the downstream sorting of the UV-activated EGFR was modulated by the expression of HPV8E6 we initially monitored the cell surface expression of the UV-exposed EGFR by FACS analysis with non-permeabilized N/TERT and HaCat keratinocytes. In both cell types, the amounts of EGFR at the cell surface were reduced 30 min after UV-irradiation, independently whether HPV8E6 was expressed or not (see **Figure 2A**). After a 75 min recovery period, however, in control cells the EGFR surface level returned to those as in untreated cells, while in HPV8E6 positive N/TERT and HaCat the amount of the surface EGFR remained reduced (**Figure 2A**). This implies that the intracellular processing of the UV-activated, internalized EGFR is altered in the presence of HPV8E6.

We further addressed this by immunofluorescence staining of UV-irradiated cells. In unirradiated control and HPV8E6 expressing N/TERT the EGFR was diffusely distributed along the plasma membrane (**Figure 2B**). It is noticeable that in HPV8E6 expressing keratinocytes a specific EGFR staining was detectable particularly at the adhesion sites, which was not further addressed here. Following UV-irradiation a substantial portion of the EGFR was redistributed from the plasma membrane into early endosomes, indicated by a co-localization of the early endosomal associated protein 1 (EEA1) and the EGFR (**Figure 2B**). This was detectable as early as 15 min up to 75 min post-UV exposure in both, control and HPV8E6 expressing cells, respectively (**Figure 2B**). Quantifications by counting the number of yellow spots within the cytoplasm per cell documented, however, that in the presence of HPV8E6 more EGFR was associated with early endosomes which was most obvious early after UV-irradiation (**Figure 2C**), implying that HPV8E6 enhances the internalization of the UV-activated EGFR.

To address the processing of the EGFR downstream of the early endosome we performed co-staining with CD63, also known as Lamp3, a well-established component of intraluminal vesicles (ILVs) and of late endosomal and lysosomal membranes. As early endosomes mature they can accumulate ILVs through inward budding of the membrane. The number of ILVs increases during endosome maturation. These finally fuse with the late endosomes and lysosomes and are then exposed to lysosomal hydrolysis (Oksvold et al., 2001). Interestingly, in the HPV8E6 positive cells a significant co-localization of CD63 positive structures and the EGFR was observed, indicated by the yellow spots which were not detectable in empty vector cells (**Figure 2B**). This was most pronounced 15 min after UV-irradiation, mostly at perinuclear sites. This co-localization progressively decreased 30 min and 75 min post UV, as confirmed by the quantification of the number of yellow spots (**Figures 2B,C**). No significant co-localization was obvious in the empty vector cells. Thus, UV-activated EGFR is further processed to ILVs in UV-irradiated HPV8E6 expressing cells while in control cells the UV-activated EGFR stays within the early endosome, in agreement with the findings described in the literature (Oksvold et al., 2001; Tomas et al., 2015).

The Association of HPV8E6 with the EGFR Is Enhanced by UV-Light and Requires RTK-Activity

Ubiquitination of the EGFR is a prerequisite for ESCRT-mediated sorting into ILVs followed by proteasomal degradation of the tyrosine phosphorylated EGFR (Tomas et al., 2014). Since we observed that in the presence of HPV8E6 the UV-exposed EGFR is processed downstream of the early endosome into CD63 positive structures we analyzed whether the EGFR is ubiquitinated. We used UV-irradiated RTS3b cells, since these immortalized keratinocytes can be transiently transfected to high rate. After the transient transfection of a vector expressing FLAG-HPV8E6 under control of the strong CMV promoter the endogenous EGFR was precipitated. A subsequent WB with an antibody against K48-linked polyubiquitin-chains demonstrates that the EGFR underwent poly-ubiquitination in HPV8E6 positive cells after UV-exposure (**Figure 3A**, lane 4), in contrast to cells transfected with the empty vector. Beyond that, probing the blot with the antibody against HPV8E6 revealed that HPV8E6 specifically co-precipitated with the EGFR after UV-irradiation. This was confirmed by a co-immunoprecipitation of the EGFR with the FLAG-antibody, recognizing the FLAG-tagged HPV8E6 (**Figure 3A**, lanes 5–8). Again, the HPV8E6-associated EGFR was highly ubiquitinated. A specific interaction between the EGFR and HPV8E6 in response to UV-irradiation could also be demonstrated with extracts from the RTS3b-pLXSN-HPV8E6 cell line, which expresses much lower levels of HPV8E6 (**Figure 3B**). These results demonstrate that UV-irradiation enhances the binding of HPV8E6 to the endogenous EGFR and that the HPV8E6-associated EGFR is ubiquitinated. Since the ubiquitination of the EGFR requires its prior tyrosine phosphorylation, we analyzed whether the RTK-activity modulates the interaction with HPV8E6 and cultivated the transiently transfected cells in medium containing the irreversible RTK-pan-ErbB-inhibitor Canertinib, also known as CI-1033 (Smaill et al., 2000). As shown in **Figure 3C**, the binding of HPV8E6 to the EGFR was abolished in a dose dependent manner in the presence of Canertinib even when the cells have been exposed to UV-light. No tyrosine phosphorylated EGFR could be detected in the input confirming the efficiency of the RTK-inhibitor. The amount of total EGFR and HPV8E6 were hardly affected by Canertinib and by UV-irradiation, respectively (**Figure 3C**). We

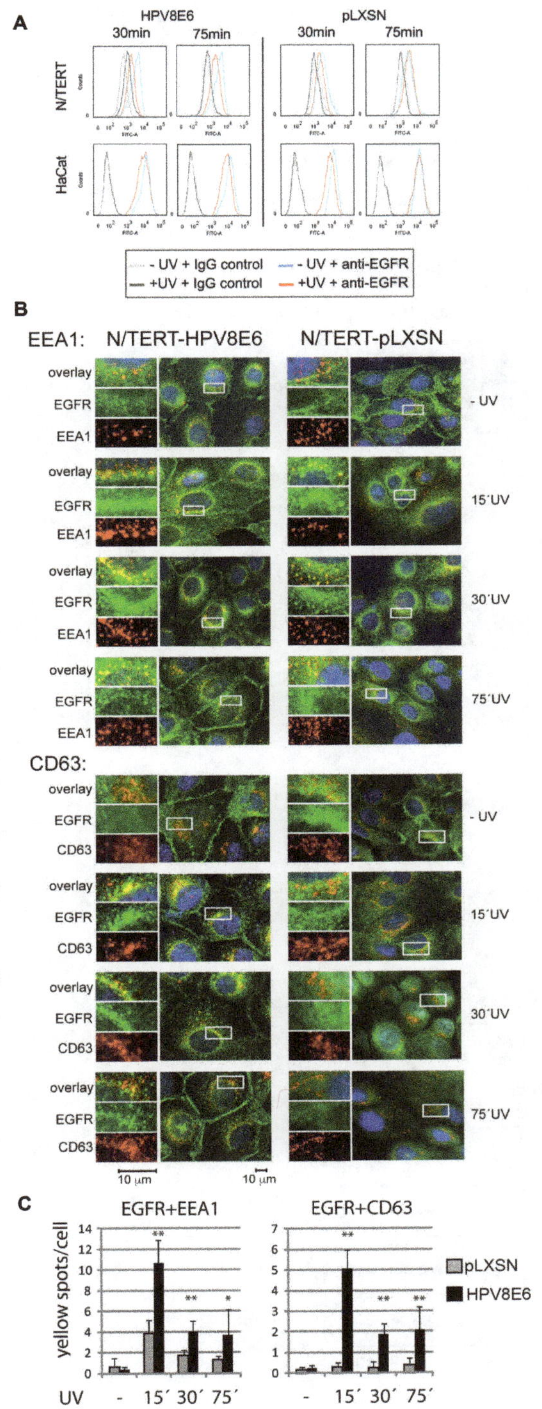

FIGURE 2 | HPV8E6 alters the intracellular trafficking of the EGFR after UV-irradiation. **(A)** FACS analysis of fixed and non-permeabilized pLXSN-empty vector or HPV8E6-NTERT and HaCat cells. Cells were left untreated or irradiated with a dose of UV-light of 40 mJ/cm^2 and harvested 30 or 75 min after UV-exposure. The cells were stained with the anti-EGFR-AF488 or the isotype control IgG-AF488 coupled antibody. The graphs represent the overlays of the EGFR-positive non-irradiated cells (blue line) with those harvested 30 min or 75 min post UV (red line), respectively. *(Continued)*

FIGURE 2 | Continued
The light and dark gray graphs represent the cells stained with the isotype control. **(B)** Immunofluorescence analysis. N/TERT harboring the pLXSN or pLXSN-HPV8E6 were fixed and permeabilized after UV-exposure, as indicated. Immunofluorescence was performed with anti-EGFR-AF488 (green) and with the anti-EEA1 (red, upper part) or the anti-CD63 (red, lower part) antibody. Nuclei were stained with DAPI. The photos represent representative images, respectively. A more detailed section in a higher magnification is provided including the single stains. The scale bars are given at the bottom (magnification 1:1000). **(C)** Quantification of the number of EGFR positive early endosomes (EGFR and EEA1 positive), and of the CD63 and EGFR positive ILVs (in each case indicated by yellow spots). Bar graphs represent the fold changes of the number of yellow spots per cell, indicative for a co-localization of EGFR and EEA1 or CD63 15, 30, and 75 min after UV-irradiation. The values were obtained by counting the yellow spots in a total of 70 to 130 cells, obtained from two independent experiments. Error bars indicate the standard deviations, the asterisks indicate the significance ($^{**}p < 0.001$, $^{*}p = 0.052$).

further confirmed these results with recombinant proteins. C33A cells were transiently transfected with expression vectors for GFP-tagged EGFR and FLAG-HPV8E6 and treated in addition to Canertinib also with the EGFR specific inhibitor tyrphostin AG-1478 followed by UV-irradiation. AG-1478 competitively binds to the ATP pocket of the EGFR to inhibit its RTK-activity (Gan et al., 2007). Here, FLAG-HPV8E6 co-precipitated with the GFP-tagged EGFR. This interaction was clearly reduced in the presence of AG-1478 and abolished by Canertinib. It has to be mentioned that the endogenous EGFR present in C33A cells could not be precipitated and detected under these conditions (data not shown). The residual binding may result from marginal Y-1068 phosphorylation of the overexpressed EGFR in the presence of AG-1478, which was still visible after long exposures (data not shown). Thus, HPV8E6 directly binds to the EGFR, which requires its Y-phosphorylation. From this we conclude that HPV8E6 enhances the RTK-activity of the UV-exposed EGFR, which promotes its interaction with HPV8E6 and leads to ubiquitination and to altered intracellular trafficking of the EGFR.

Inhibition of the RTK-Activity of the EGFR Suppresses UV-Induced Skin Papillomatosis in K14-HPV8E6 Mice

We asked whether the activation of the RTK-activity of EGFR by HPV8E6 is relevant for the induction of papilloma growth in transgenic mice. Initially, we determined the level of pEGFR-Y1068 in hyperplastic skin lesions that appeared 13 days after UV-irradiation in K14-HPV8E6 transgenic mice by immunohistochemistry with the specific antibody. A faint specific staining of the epidermal cells associated with the plasma membranes and intracellular sites was readily visible indicating that the EGFR is in a tyrosine phosphorylated state (**Figure 4A**). To address its functional contribution to HPV8E6 and UV-mediated tumor formation, we treated K14-HPV8E6 transgenic mice with the RTK-inhibitor Canertinib. Seventeen K14-HPV8E6 transgenic mice obtained orally once 20 mg/kg body-weight Canertinib 4 h prior UV-irradiation and then once daily 10 mg/kg Canertinib for a period of 24 days while 12

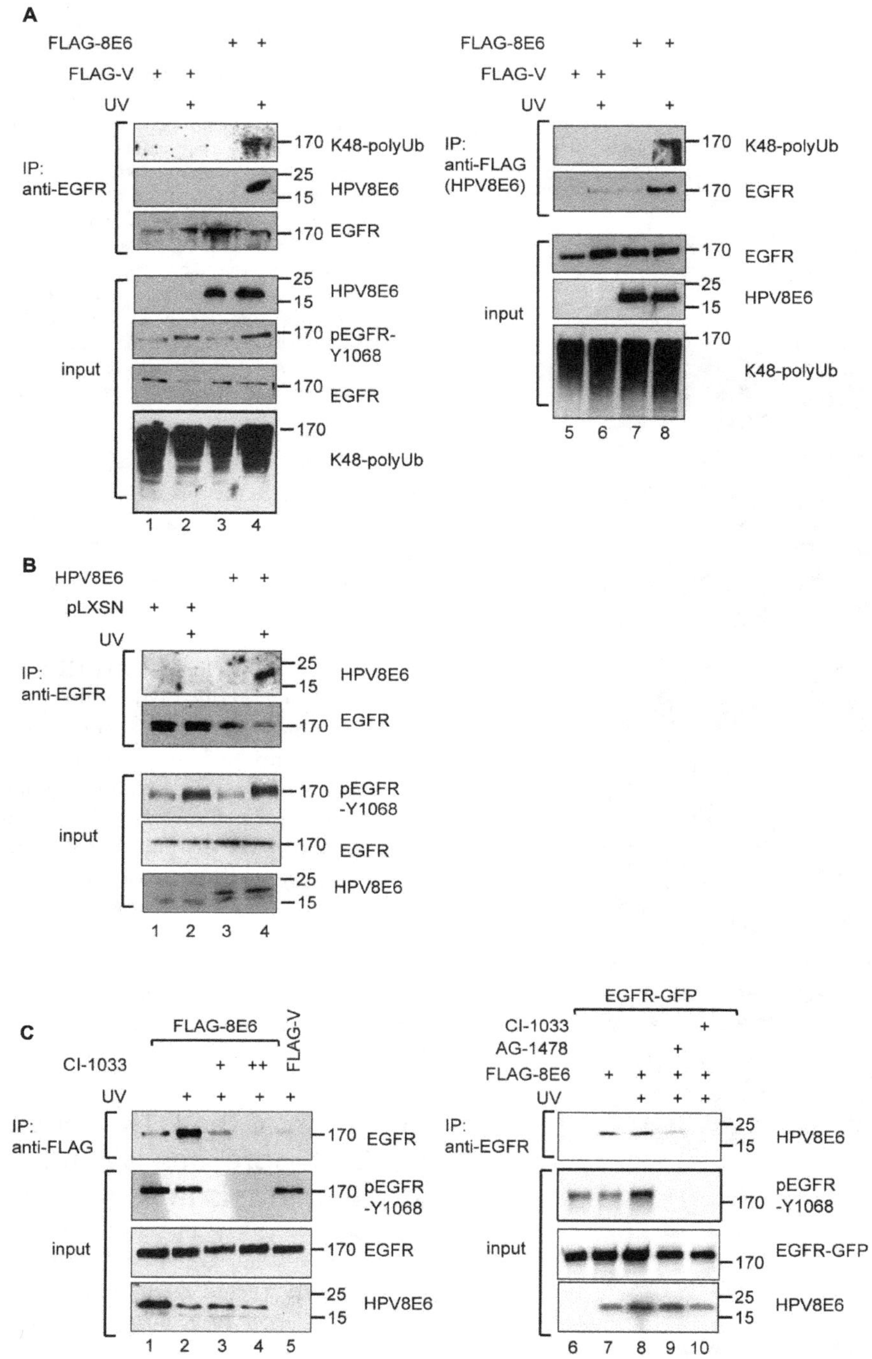

FIGURE 3 | HPV8E6 directly binds to the ubiquitinated EGFR in an UV-dependent manner. **(A)** RTS3b cells were transiently transfected with a vector directing the expression of FLAG-tagged HPV8E6 under control of the CMV-promoter or the empty vector. Where indicated the cells have been irradiated with UV-light 30 min prior harvesting. 400 μg of extracts were incubated with the anti-EGFR-antibody (lanes 1–4) or with the FLAG-antibody (lanes 5–8), both coupled to sepharose, washed four times in 0.3 M KCl-buffer prior analysis by WB and 40 μg of the extracts were used in the input blots. **(B)** IP with anti-EGFR sepharose and 800 μg of extracts derived from the stable RTS3b-pLXSN and RTS3b-HPV8E6 lines, either left untreated or UV-irradiated 30 min prior harvesting. FLAG-HPV8E6 and EGFR present in the precipitate as well as in the input were detected by WB. **(C)** Extracts from UV-irradiated RTS3b cells that have been transiently transfected with the FLAG-HPV8E6 or the FLAG-vector were incubated either with DMSO (lanes 1, 2, 5), 3 μM (lane 3) or 7 μM (lane 4) Canertinib for 30 min. The IP was performed with the FLAG-antibody. All WB were developed with the indicated antibodies. In lanes 6–10, C33A cells were transiently transfected with expression vectors for EGFR-GFP and FLAG-HPV8E6, and UV-irradiated, where indicated, prior harvesting 30 min later. EGFR-GFP was precipitated from 400 μg of extract by the EGFR antibody and bound HPV8E6 was detected by the FLAG-antibody. The input blots were developed with the antibodies against pEGFR-Y1068, GFP, and FLAG. The positions of the molecular weight markers are provided (in kDa).

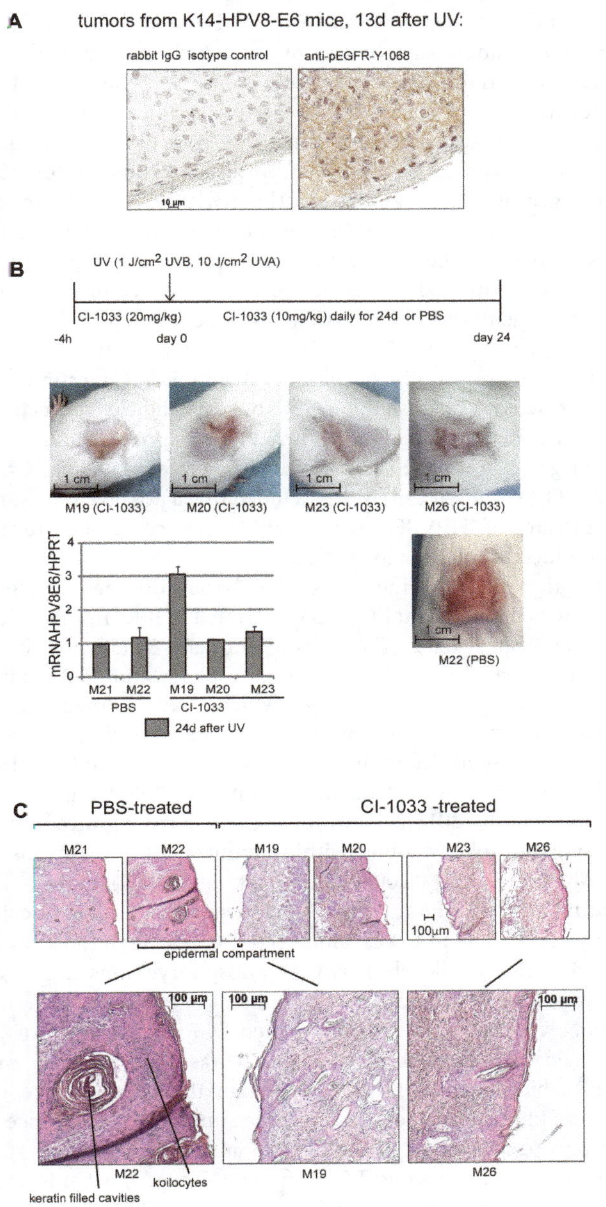

FIGURE 4 | Inhibition of the RTK-activity of the EGFR by the pan-ErbB-inhibitor Canertinib (CI-1033) suppresses UV-induced papillomatosis in K14-HPV8E6 transgenic mice. **(A)** Immunohistochemical staining of paraffin embedded sections obtained from skin of K14-HPV8E6 transgenic mice 13 days after UV-exposure with the anti-pEGFR-Y1068 or rabbit IgG isotype control (magnification 1:400). **(B)** Transgenic mice obtained either Canertinib (CI-1033) (20 mg/kg weight) or the same volume of PBS 4 h prior UV-irradiation followed by applications of Canertinib once daily at a dose of 10 mg/kg weight or 150 µl PBS for 24 days, as given in the time line. The pictures represent examples of the lesions from four mice treated with CI-1033 (M19, 20, 23, and M26) and from one control mouse which obtained PBS (M22). The graph beneath shows the quantification of RT-PCR results with RNA isolated from two PBS and three Canertinib-treated animals to demonstrate the expression of HPV8E6. **(C)** Histology with H/E staining of skin section obtained from two PBS-control (M21 and M22) and four Canertinib (CI-1033)-treated animals (M19, M20, M23, and M26) 24 days after UV-irradiation.

UV-irradiated K14-HPV8E6 transgenic animals, representing the control group, were administered the solvent PBS at the same time points (see the time scale in **Figure 4B**). All K14-HPV8E6 transgenic mice as well as two wt mice (which were included as control) developed a sun burn 2–3 days after UV-irradiation according to our previously established protocol (Marcuzzi et al., 2009). While the sun burn healed after about 7 days in the wt mice, as described previously (Marcuzzi et al., 2009), papillomas started to grow in the transgenic mice demonstrating the effect of HPV8E6 which is expressed in the skin of these animals. After 24 days, all 12 animals in the control group had developed large, exalted papillomas covering the initially irradiated skin sections. In contrast, in all 17 animals treated with Canertinib the initially UV-irradiated skin-areal, which had developed a sun burn, had shrunk and none of the lesions was exalted (**Figure 4B**). The affected skin within the irradiated area appeared to be renewed and tender. RT-PCR with RNA isolated 24 days after UV-treatment from the lesions excluded that the expression of the HPV8E6 was diminished due to the application of Canertinib (**Figure 4B**). H/E-staining of lesions from two PBS treated animals revealed histology of papillomatosis, with multiple cavities filled with lamellated concentric keratin masses in the epidermal compartment In the upper layers, intracytoplasmic keratohyalin granules were present and in some areas koilocytosis occurred, as observed previously (Schaper et al., 2005; Marcuzzi et al., 2009). The histology of the lesions from four animals of the Canertinib group illustrates that the epidermis from three Canertinib treated animals (M19, M23, and M26) was composed of two to three cell layers (**Figure 4C**). In the section of one treated mouse, the epidermal compartment was thickened but was still much thinner compared to the lesions of the control animals (M20, **Figure 4C**). These results demonstrate that the RTK-activity of the EGFR is required for UV-induced papilloma formation in K14-HPV8E6 transgenic mice.

DISCUSSION

We demonstrate here that HPV8E6 transiently increases the RTK-activity of the EGFR shortly after UV-exposure. We observe an increased tyrosine phosphorylation of the EGFR as a consequence of the expression of HPV8E6 in three different immortalized keratinocyte lines as well as in primary keratinocytes. This excludes cell-lineage dependent effects and points to a specific impact of HPV8E6 on the RTK-activity. We provide evidence that the effect of HPV8E6 has consequences on the downstream processing of the EGFR. The UV-activated EGFR is ubiquitinated only in HPV8E6 positive cells indicating that the HPV8E6-dependent increased tyrosine phosphorylation of the UV-exposed EGFR is sufficient to recruit the E3 ubiquitin-ligase Cbl and its associated Grb2. Indeed we observed a co-precipitation of Grb with the UV-stimulated EGFR in the presence of HPV8E6 (data not shown). Moreover, there was an enhanced internalization of the UV-activated EGFR into early endosomes in HPV8E6 cells compared to control cells and the presence of the EGFR in structures downstream of the early endosome even entirely depended on HPV8E6.

Tyrosine phosphorylated, ubiquitinated and endocytosed EGFR was shown to interact with Eps15 and AP-2, two endocytotic adaptor proteins to form clathrin coated endocytic vesicles (Zwang and Yarden, 2009). The complex is then targeted by the ESCRT and further sorted to CD63 positive ILVs beyond the early endosome, which fuse with lysosomes to complete the degradation of the EGFR and attenuate the signaling (Tomas et al., 2014). This supports the notion that UV-activated EGFR is prone to lysosomal degradation in HPV8E6 expressing cells, and indeed we occasionally observed reduced amounts of EGFR in the HPV8E6 cells up to 30 min after UV-irradiation where the highest level of tyrosine phosphorylation was present (see **Figure 1A**, lanes 7, 8, 15, 16 and **Figure 1B**). The distinct mode of endosomal EGFR trafficking induced by HPV8E6 was underlined by the lack of detectable ubiquitination and of co-localization with CD63 of the UV-activated EGFR in HPV8E6 negative cells. Thus, in agreement with previous reports the UV-light resulted in EGFR internalization with an arrest in the early endosome in HPV8E6 negative cells (Tomas et al., 2014; Peng et al., 2016).

The altered intracellular trafficking of the UV-activated EGFR induced by HPV8E6 may prolong the signaling and support cell survival. Activation of EGFR-signaling pathways not only occurs from the plasma-membrane. For instance, EGFR endocytosis to early endosomes was found to be required for the full stimulation of EGF-induced ERK1/2 and PI3K/AKT signaling (Vieira et al., 1996). Particularly, perinuclear endosomes have been shown to provide a spatial compartment for prolonged EGFR signaling (Huang et al., 2016). Our data showing a co-localization of the UV-activated EGFR and CD63 predominantly at perinuclear regions in HPV8E6 N/TERTs may thus reflect a prolonged signaling. A stimulation of the EGFR-mediated MAPK-Ras signaling pathway was suggested to occur from late endosomes and lysosomes as well (Oksvold et al., 2001; Jiang and Sorkin, 2002; Fehrenbacher et al., 2009; German et al., 2011). Moreover, continuous EGFR signaling from late endosomes was shown to contribute to sustained downstream AKT and STAT3 activation and the endosomal accumulation of the activated EGFR increased tumor cell survival (Huang et al., 2016).

In accordance with these observations, we report here that the functional interaction between HPV8E6 and the UV-activated EGFR which we have characterized here has a crucial role in the UV- and HPV8E6-induced skin tumor induction *in vivo* since the pharmacological inhibition of the RTK-activity of the EGFR suppressed papillomatosis in transgenic mice. The contribution of HPV8E6 is reflected by the facts that the UV-induced skin lesions, i.e., sun burn, healed in wt mice, while in HPV8E6 positive mice a massive tumor growth was induced, as observed previously (Marcuzzi et al., 2009). Since these mice have the same phenotype as the K14-HPV8CER mice, expressing all early HPV8 proteins, it is obvious that HPV8 E6 is the major oncogene in the mouse skin and can function on its own to stimulate papilloma growth in cooperation with UV-light. In addition, it is also necessary since its suppression reduced tumor formation in the HPV8CER mice (Hufbauer et al., 2010). Nevertheless, it has to be admitted that with this setting we used here potential interaction between the other early viral proteins E7, E2 and E1 with E6 or with the EGFR or the corresponding signaling pathways, which may occur during natural infections, have not been considered and cannot be excluded.

A previous study suggested that the short lived UV-induced activation of the EGFR is a powerful promoter of skin tumorigenesis of initiated keratinocytes (El-Abaseri et al., 2005). Similarly, the HPV8E6-mediated transient boost of the RTK-activity of the EGFR may support papilloma growth. It has to be mentioned that although our *in vivo* results obtained with transgenic mice imply that the functional stimulation of the EGFR-activity by HPV8E6 is essential for tumor induction, they do not prove it. The pan-ErbB inhibitor Canertinib has highest activity against the EGFR but also blocks the activity of ErbB2/Her2, which was shown to be expressed and to be tumorigenic in mouse skin as well (Kiguchi et al., 2000; Krahn et al., 2001). Thus, it cannot be excluded that a possible functional interaction of HPV8E6 with ErbB2 may contribute to the UV-induced papilloma formation.

What might be the molecular basis for the HPV8E6-mediated enhancement of the UV-activated EGFR? In agreement with published data (Zwang and Yarden, 2006), we found that UV-treatment induced S/T phosphorylations including that of the T in pos. 669, which were shown to be dependent on the UV-activated p38MAPK. These triggered a gradual and weak transient RTK-activation of the internalized EGFR which was detectable within the following 2–4 h (Tomas et al., 2015). However, others have reported weak tyrosine phosphorylations within minutes after UV-exposure (El-Abaseri et al., 2006; Singh et al., 2009). Since the binding of HPV8E6 to the EGFR depended on its tyrosine phosphorylation and was enhanced by UV-light, one might speculate that low level of tyrosine phosphorylations early after UV-exposure will initiate the recruitment of HPV8E6. This may somehow stabilize the phosphorylated EGFR form by a not yet characterized feedback mechanism. It has been reported that EGFR ubiquitination requires a certain threshold of receptor tyrosine phosphorylations, namely the simultaneous presence of two phosphotyrosines, of the pY1045 and either one of pY1068 or pY1086, on the same EGFR moiety. These mechanistically led to the cooperative recruitment of the E3 ligase Cbl in complex with Grb2, to the EGFR (Sigismund et al., 2013). Thus, HPV8E6 might promote to pass the required threshold of tyrosine phosphorylation allowing then EGFR-ubiquitination, with the consequence of altered endosomal trafficking and signaling of the UV-activated EGFR as discussed. Further studies are necessary to elucidate the mechanism how HPV8E6 stimulates the RTK-activity of the EGFR and whether the interaction will affect the activity of E6. Moreover, a functional interaction of HPV8E6 with other ErbB family members may participate, as discussed above, which has to be analyzed as well. The observation that the pharmacological inhibition of the RTK-activity suppressed papillomatosis mediated by HPV8E6 and UV-light was surprising in view of multiple, pleiotropic effects described for β-HPV E6 proteins. In common they have the capacity to inhibit MAML, which acts as co-factor for Notch.

In this way, E6 may suppress keratinocyte differentiation via inhibiting Notch (Tan et al., 2012; Meyers et al., 2013) and thus further amplify the negative effect of EGFR signaling on Notch (Kolev et al., 2008). The E6 proteins of HPV8 and other β-HPV-types are able to inhibit apoptosis (Jackson and Storey, 2000; Jackson et al., 2000; Struijk et al., 2008) and interfere with the repair of UVB-induced DNA damage and repair (Wallace et al., 2012; Hufbauer et al., 2015) and thus favor the accumulation of mutations including UV-induced inactivating mutations of p53, which are thought to be a crucial step in the development of AKs and cSCC also in humans (Brash et al., 1991; Kemp et al., 1993; Jiang et al., 1999). These broader activities of HPV8E6 may support the progression of the benign papillomas, which depend on the RTK-activity of the EGFR as we have demonstrated here, to cSCC (Schaper et al., 2005; Marcuzzi et al., 2009).

Targeting the EGFR signaling seems to be a common theme for HPV. Previously, the E5 and the E6 oncoproteins of the high risk genital HPV16 belonging to the genus alpha were found to interfere with EGF stimulated EGFR signaling pathways and thus protect cells from apoptosis and induce migration, respectively (Zhang et al., 2005; Spangle and Munger, 2013). Here, we demonstrate for the first time, to our best knowledge, a functional interaction of an HPVE6 protein with the UV-activated EGFR. Remarkably, β-HPV types do not encode an E5 protein and E6 may have overtaken the role to modify signaling by UV-activated EGFR. This may reflect the association of β-HPV with the sun exposed cutaneous skin. It will be interesting to analyze whether other β-HPVE6 proteins are able to bind the Y-phosphorylated EGFR and to stimulate the UV-dependent activation of the EGFR as well and whether this is linked to E6 proteins of HPV types that are cancer associated.

Our data obtained with the use of transgenic mice and human keratinocytes provide a molecular basis how HPV8 may cooperate with UV-light in the induction of papillomas and also support a role of β-HPV in the development of proliferative skin lesions in humans, as implied by epidemiological studies. These findings also provide a molecular mechanism explaining the contribution of β-HPVs to the early steps in the cSCC development in human, particularly in immunosuppressed patients. In these patients, higher loads of β-HPV in the skin and the hair follicles due to their immune-suppression will result in elevated levels of E6, which then alter UV-induced EGFR signaling according to our data. Although this effect will be transient, reiterated UV irradiation may lead to sustained activation of the EGFR and downstream signaling pathways and thus trigger hyperproliferation of the epidermis and the development of AK, the precursor lesions of cSCC.

AUTHOR CONTRIBUTIONS

ST, HP, and GS planned and designed the experiments. ST conducted most of the experiments and analyzed the results. GS conducted and analyzed some of the experiments. GS wrote the manuscript. All the authors reviewed the manuscript.

ACKNOWLEDGMENTS

We thank Baki Akgül (Institute of Virology, University of Cologne, Germany) and the members of his group for helpful discussion, and Janet L. Brandsma (Yale University, New Haven, CT, United States) for providing the antibody against HPV8E6.

REFERENCES

Arron, S. T., Ruby, J. G., Dybbro, E., Ganem, D., and Derisi, J. L. (2011). Transcriptome sequencing demonstrates that human papillomavirus is not active in cutaneous squamous cell carcinoma. *J. Invest. Dermatol.* 131, 1745–1753. doi: 10.1038/jid.2011.91

Borgogna, C., Lanfredini, S., Peretti, A., De Andrea, M., Zavattaro, E., Colombo, E., et al. (2014). Improved detection reveals active beta-papillomavirus infection in skin lesions from kidney transplant recipients. *Mod. Pathol.* 27, 1101–1115. doi: 10.1038/modpathol.2013.240

Brash, D. E., Rudolph, J. A., Simon, J. A., Lin, A., McKenna, G. J., Baden, H. P., et al. (1991). A role for sunlight in skin cancer: UV-induced p53 mutations in squamous cell carcinoma. *Proc. Natl. Acad. Sci. U.S.A.* 88, 10124–10128. doi: 10.1073/pnas.88.22.10124

Carter, R. E., and Sorkin, A. (1998). Endocytosis of functional epidermal growth factor receptor-green fluorescent protein chimera. *J. Biol. Chem.* 273, 35000–35007. doi: 10.1074/jbc.273.52.35000

El-Abaseri, T. B., Fuhrman, J., Trempus, C., Shendrik, I., Tennant, R. W., and Hansen, L. A. (2005). Chemoprevention of UV light-induced skin tumorigenesis by inhibition of the epidermal growth factor receptor. *Cancer Res.* 65, 3958–3965. doi: 10.1158/0008-5472.CAN-04-2204

El-Abaseri, T. B., Putta, S., and Hansen, L. A. (2006). Ultraviolet irradiation induces keratinocyte proliferation and epidermal hyperplasia through the activation of the epidermal growth factor receptor. *Carcinogenesis* 27, 225–231. doi: 10.1093/carcin/bgi220

Fehrenbacher, N., Bar-Sagi, D., and Philips, M. (2009). Ras/MAPK signaling from endomembranes. *Mol. Oncol.* 3, 297–307. doi: 10.1016/j.molonc.2009.06.004

Gan, H. K., Walker, F., Burgess, A. W., Rigopoulos, A., Scott, A. M., and Johns, T. G. (2007). The epidermal growth factor receptor (EGFR) tyrosine kinase inhibitor AG1478 increases the formation of inactive untethered EGFR dimers. Implications for combination therapy with monoclonal antibody 806. *J. Biol. Chem.* 282, 2840–2850. doi: 10.1074/jbc.M605136200

German, C. L., Sauer, B. M., and Howe, C. L. (2011). The STAT3 beacon: IL-6 recurrently activates STAT 3 from endosomal structures. *Exp. Cell Res.* 317, 1955–1969. doi: 10.1016/j.yexcr.2011.05.009

Hillen, U., Ulrich, M., Alter, M., Becker, J. C., Gutzmer, R., Leiter, U., et al. (2014). Cutaneous squamous cell carcinoma: a review with consideration of special patient groups. *Hautarzt* 65, 590–599. doi: 10.1007/s00105-013-2734-7

Howley, P. M., and Pfister, H. J. (2015). Beta genus papillomaviruses and skin cancer. *Virology* 479–480, 290–296. doi: 10.1016/j.virol.2015.02.004

Huang, C. C., Lee, C. C., Lin, H. H., and Chang, J. Y. (2016). Cathepsin S attenuates endosomal EGFR signalling: a mechanical rationale for the combination of cathepsin S and EGFR tyrosine kinase inhibitors. *Sci. Rep.* 6:29256. doi: 10.1038/srep29256

Hufbauer, M., Cooke, J., van der Horst, G. T., Pfister, H., Storey, A., and Akgul, B. (2015). Human papillomavirus mediated inhibition of DNA damage sensing and repair drives skin carcinogenesis. *Mol. Cancer* 14:183. doi: 10.1186/s12943-015-0453-7

Hufbauer, M., Lazic, D., Akgul, B., Brandsma, J. L., Pfister, H., and Weissenborn, S. J. (2010). Enhanced human papillomavirus type 8 oncogene expression levels are crucial for skin tumorigenesis in transgenic mice. *Virology* 403, 128–136. doi: 10.1016/j.virol.2010.04.013

Jackson, S., Harwood, C., Thomas, M., Banks, L., and Storey, A. (2000). Role of Bak in UV-induced apoptosis in skin cancer and abrogation by HPV E6 proteins. *Genes Dev.* 14, 3065–3073. doi: 10.1101/gad.182100

Jackson, S., and Storey, A. (2000). E6 proteins from diverse cutaneous HPV types inhibit apoptosis in response to UV damage. *Oncogene* 19, 592–598. doi: 10.1038/sj.onc.1203339

Jiang, W., Ananthaswamy, H. N., Muller, H. K., and Kripke, M. L. (1999). p53 protects against skin cancer induction by UV-B radiation. *Oncogene* 18, 4247–4253. doi: 10.1038/sj.onc.1202789

Jiang, X., and Sorkin, A. (2002). Coordinated traffic of Grb2 and Ras during epidermal growth factor receptor endocytosis visualized in living cells. *Mol. Biol. Cell* 13, 1522–1535. doi: 10.1091/mbc.01-11-0552

Kemp, C. J., Donehower, L. A., Bradley, A., and Balmain, A. (1993). Reduction of p53 gene dosage does not increase initiation or promotion but enhances malignant progression of chemically induced skin tumors. *Cell* 74, 813–822. doi: 10.1016/0092-8674(93)90461-X

Kiguchi, K., Bol, D., Carbajal, S., Beltran, L., Moats, S., Chan, K., et al. (2000). Constitutive expression of erbB2 in epidermis of transgenic mice results in epidermal hyperproliferation and spontaneous skin tumor development. *Oncogene* 19, 4243–4254. doi: 10.1038/sj.onc.1203778

Kolev, V., Mandinova, A., Guinea-Viniegra, J., Hu, B., Lefort, K., Lambertini, C., et al. (2008). EGFR signalling as a negative regulator of Notchl gene transcription and function in proliferating keratinocytes and cancer. *Nat. Cell Biol.* 10, 902–911. doi: 10.1038/ncb1750

Krahn, G., Leiter, U., Kaskel, P., Udart, M., Utikal, J., Bezold, G., et al. (2001). Coexpression patterns of EGFR, HER2, HER3 and HER4 in non-melanoma skin cancer. *Eur. J. Cancer* 37, 251–259. doi: 10.1016/S0959-8049(00)00364-6

Lemmon, M. A., and Schlessinger, J. (2010). Cell signaling by receptor tyrosine kinases. *Cell* 141, 1117–1134. doi: 10.1016/j.cell.2010.06.011

Leverrier, S., Bergamaschi, D., Ghali, L., Ola, A., Warnes, G., Akgul, B., et al. (2007). Role of HPV E6 proteins in preventing UVB-induced release of pro-apoptotic factors from the mitochondria. *Apoptosis* 12, 549–560. doi: 10.1007/s10495-006-0004-1

Lomas, A., Leonardi-Bee, J., and Bath-Hextall, F. (2012). A systematic review of worldwide incidence of nonmelanoma skin cancer. *Br. J. Dermatol.* 166, 1069–1080. doi: 10.1111/j.1365-2133.2012.10830.x

Marcuzzi, G. P., Hufbauer, M., Kasper, H. U., Weissenborn, S. J., Smola, S., and Pfister, H. (2009). Spontaneous tumour development in human papillomavirus type 8 E6 transgenic mice and rapid induction by UV-light exposure and wounding. *J. Gen. Virol.* 90(Pt 12), 2855–2864. doi: 10.1099/vir.0.012872-0

Meyers, J. M., Spangle, J. M., and Munger, K. (2013). The human papillomavirus type 8 E6 protein interferes with NOTCH activation during keratinocyte differentiation. *J. Virol.* 87, 4762–4767. doi: 10.1128/JVI.02527-12

Müller-Schiffmann, A., Beckmann, J., and Steger, G. (2006). The E6 protein of the cutaneous human papillomavirus type 8 can stimulate the viral early and late promoters by distinct mechanisms. *J. Virol.* 80, 8718–8728. doi: 10.1128/JVI.00250-06

Neale, R. E., Weissenborn, S., Abeni, D., Bavinck, J. N., Euvrard, S., Feltkamp, M. C., et al. (2013). Human papillomavirus load in eyebrow hair follicles and risk of cutaneous squamous cell carcinoma. *Cancer Epidemiol. Biomarkers Prev.* 22, 719–727. doi: 10.1158/1055-9965.EPI-12-0917-T

Oksvold, M. P., Skarpen, E., Wierod, L., Paulsen, R. E., and Huitfeldt, H. S. (2001). Re-localization of activated EGF receptor and its signal transducers to multivesicular compartments downstream of early endosomes in response to EGF. *Eur. J. Cell Biol.* 80, 285–294. doi: 10.1078/0171-9335-00160

Peng, K., Dai, Q., Wei, J., Shao, G., Sun, A., Yang, W., et al. (2016). Stress-induced endocytosis and degradation of epidermal growth factor receptor are two independent processes. *Cancer Cell Int.* 16:25. doi: 10.1186/s12935-016-0301-x

Purdie, K. J., Sexton, C. J., Proby, C. M., Glover, M. T., Williams, A. T., Stables, J. N., et al. (1993). Malignant transformation of cutaneous lesions in renal allograft patients: a role for human papillomavirus. *Cancer Res.* 53, 5328–5333.

Schaper, I. D., Marcuzzi, G. P., Weissenborn, S. J., Kasper, H. U., Dries, V., Smyth, N., et al. (2005). Development of skin tumors in mice transgenic for early genes of human papillomavirus type 8. *Cancer Res.* 65, 1394–1400. doi: 10.1158/0008-5472.CAN-04-3263

Schneider, M. R., Werner, S., Paus, R., and Wolf, E. (2008). Beyond wavy hairs: the epidermal growth factor receptor and its ligands in skin biology and pathology. *Am. J. Pathol.* 173, 14–24. doi: 10.2353/ajpath.2008.070942

Sigismund, S., Algisi, V., Nappo, G., Conte, A., Pascolutti, R., Cuomo, A., et al. (2013). Threshold-controlled ubiquitination of the EGFR directs receptor fate. *EMBO J.* 32, 2140–2157. doi: 10.1038/emboj.2013.149

Singh, B., Schneider, M., Knyazev, P., and Ullrich, A. (2009). UV-induced EGFR signal transactivation is dependent on proligand shedding by activated metalloproteases in skin cancer cell lines. *Int. J. Cancer* 124, 531–539. doi: 10.1002/ijc.23974

Smaill, J. B., Rewcastle, G. W., Loo, J. A., Greis, K. D., Chan, O. H., Reyner, E. L., et al. (2000). Tyrosine kinase inhibitors. 17. Irreversible inhibitors of the epidermal growth factor receptor: 4-(phenylamino)quinazoline- and 4-(phenylamino)pyrido[3,2-d]pyrimidine-6-acrylamides bearing additional solubilizing functions. *J. Med. Chem.* 43, 1380–1397. doi: 10.1021/jm990482t

Spangle, J. M., and Munger, K. (2013). The HPV16 E6 oncoprotein causes prolonged receptor protein tyrosine kinase signaling and enhances internalization of phosphorylated receptor species. *PLOS Pathog.* 9:e1003237. doi: 10.1371/journal.ppat.1003237

Struijk, L., van der Meijden, E., Kazem, S., ter Schegget, J., de Gruijl, F. R., Steenbergen, R. D., et al. (2008). Specific betapapillomaviruses associated with squamous cell carcinoma of the skin inhibit UVB-induced apoptosis of primary human keratinocytes. *J. Gen. Virol.* 89(Pt 9), 2303–2314. doi: 10.1099/vir.0.83317-0

Tan, M. J., White, E. A., Sowa, M. E., Harper, J. W., Aster, J. C., and Howley, P. M. (2012). Cutaneous beta-human papillomavirus E6 proteins bind Mastermind-like coactivators and repress Notch signaling. *Proc. Natl. Acad. Sci. U.S.A.* 109, E1473–E1480. doi: 10.1073/pnas.1205991109

Tan, X., Lambert, P. F., Rapraeger, A. C., and Anderson, R. A. (2016). Stress-induced EGFR trafficking: mechanisms, functions, and therapeutic implications. *Trends Cell Biol.* 26, 352–366. doi: 10.1016/j.tcb.2015.12.006

Tomas, A., Futter, C. E., and Eden, E. R. (2014). EGF receptor trafficking: consequences for signaling and cancer. *Trends Cell Biol.* 24, 26–34. doi: 10.1016/j.tcb.2013.11.002

Tomas, A., Vaughan, S. O., Burgoyne, T., Sorkin, A., Hartley, J. A., Hochhauser, D., et al. (2015). WASH and Tsg101/ALIX-dependent diversion of stress-internalized EGFR from the canonical endocytic pathway. *Nat. Commun.* 6:7324. doi: 10.1038/ncomms8324

Vieira, A. V., Lamaze, C., and Schmid, S. L. (1996). Control of EGF receptor signaling by clathrin-mediated endocytosis. *Science* 274, 2086–2089. doi: 10.1126/science.274.5295.2086

Wallace, N. A., Robinson, K., and Galloway, D. A. (2014). Beta human papillomavirus E6 expression inhibits stabilization of p53 and increases tolerance of genomic instability. *J. Virol.* 88, 6112–6127. doi: 10.1128/JVI.03808-13

Wallace, N. A., Robinson, K., Howie, H. L., and Galloway, D. A. (2012). HPV 5 and 8 E6 abrogate ATR activity resulting in increased persistence of UVB induced DNA damage. *PLOS Pathog.* 8:e1002807. doi: 10.1371/journal.ppat.1002807

Wan, Y. S., Wang, Z. Q., Shao, Y., Voorhees, J. J., and Fisher, G. J. (2001). Ultraviolet irradiation activates PI 3-kinase/AKT survival pathway via EGF receptors in human skin in vivo. *Int. J. Oncol.* 18, 461–466. doi: 10.3892/ijo.18.3.461

Weissenborn, S., Neale, R. E., Waterboer, T., Abeni, D., Bavinck, J. N., Green, A. C., et al. (2012). Beta-papillomavirus DNA loads in hair follicles of immunocompetent people and organ transplant recipients. *Med. Microbiol. Immunol.* 201, 117–125. doi: 10.1007/s00430-011-0212-3

Weissenborn, S. J., Nindl, I., Purdie, K., Harwood, C., Proby, C., Breuer, J., et al. (2005). Human papillomavirus-DNA loads in actinic keratoses exceed those in non-melanoma skin cancers. *J. Invest. Dermatol.* 125, 93–97. doi: 10.1111/j.0022-202X.2005.23733.x

Zhang, B., Srirangam, A., Potter, D. A., and Roman, A. (2005). HPV16 E5 protein disrupts the c-Cbl-EGFR interaction and EGFR ubiquitination in human foreskin keratinocytes. *Oncogene* 24, 2585–2588. doi: 10.1038/sj.onc.1208453

Zhu, G., Fan, Z., Ding, M., Zhang, H., Mu, L., Ding, Y., et al. (2015). An EGFR/PI3K/AKT axis promotes accumulation of the Rac1-GEF Tiam1 that is critical in EGFR-driven tumorigenesis. *Oncogene* 34, 5971–5982. doi: 10.1038/onc.2015.45

Zwang, Y., and Yarden, Y. (2006). p38 MAP kinase mediates stress-induced internalization of EGFR: implications for cancer chemotherapy. *EMBO J.* 25, 4195–4206. doi: 10.1038/sj.emboj.7601297

Zwang, Y., and Yarden, Y. (2009). Systems biology of growth factor-induced receptor endocytosis. *Traffic* 10, 349–363. doi: 10.1111/j.1600-0854.2008.00870.x

11

Analysis of the Replication Mechanisms of the Human Papillomavirus Genomes

Lisett Liblekas, Alla Piirsoo, Annika Laanemets, Eva-Maria Tombak, Airiin Laaneväli, Ene Ustav, Mart Ustav and Marko Piirsoo*

Institute of Technology, University of Tartu, Tartu, Estonia

***Correspondence:**
Marko Piirsoo
marko.piirsoo@ut.ee

The life-cycle of human papillomaviruses (HPVs) includes three distinct phases of the viral genome replication. First, the viral genome is amplified in the infected cells, and this amplification is often accompanied by the oligomerization of the viral genomes. Second stage includes the replication of viral genomes in concert with the host cell genome. The viral genome is further amplified during the third stage of the viral-life cycle, which takes place only in the differentiated keratinocytes. We have previously shown that the HPV18 genomes utilize at least two distinct replication mechanisms during the initial amplification. One of these mechanisms is a well-described bidirectional replication *via* theta type of replication intermediates. The nature of another replication mechanism utilized by HPV18 involves most likely recombination-dependent replication. In this paper, we show that the usage of different replication mechanisms is a property shared also by other HPV types, namely HPV11 and HPV5. We further show that the emergence of the recombination dependent replication coincides with the oligomerization of the viral genomes and is dependent on the replicative DNA polymerases. We also show that the oligomeric genomes of HPV18 replicate almost exclusively using recombination dependent mechanism, whereas monomeric HPV31 genomes replicate bi-directionally during the maintenance phase of the viral life-cycle.

Keywords: HPV, virus replication, non-theta replication, 2D, theta replication

INTRODUCTION

Papillomaviruses are small DNA viruses that infect the cutaneous and mucosal epithelium. Persistent infection of a number of different human papillomavirus (HPV) types can lead to various types of malignancies (Graham, 2017). A unique feature of the HPV life-cycle, shared by Epstein-Barr Virus, is that the viral genome is maintained in the infected cells as an extrachromosomal nuclear replicon over a long period of time. The HPV infection-cycle can be divided into three distinct steps based on the behavior of the viral genome in the cell. First, initially following the infection the copy-number of the viral genome increases as it replicates more than once in the cell-cycle. Second, during the latent infection, the copy number of the viral genome is maintained constant over time, and the virus replicates in concert with the host cell genome. Third, the viral copy number increases again, and new virus particles are formed. The latter takes place only in the terminally differentiated keratinocytes (McBride, 2017).

The HPV genomes are replicating using largely the host cell replication machinery. The only viral elements necessary for the HPV replication during the initial amplification stage of the infection cycle, are two viral proteins E1 and E2, and an origin of replication (ori) residing in the non-coding part of the viral genome (McBride, 2017). The viral proteins are necessary for the recognition of the ori and recruitment of the host cell replication machinery to it. In addition, the E1 protein possesses helicase activity and is believed to be present in the replication elongation complex (Bergvall et al., 2013).

It is unclear, however, how the latent phase of the HPV life-cycle is established, why the replication of viral genomes becomes limited to one time per cell cycle, and which viral elements are necessary during this stage of the viral infection. Several indications suggest that the mechanism and determinants of the viral genome replication might differ during the latent infection as compared to that during the initial amplification. First, it has been shown that while the initial amplification of the HPV11 and HPV18 genomes proceeds bi-directionally, *via* theta type of replication intermediates, starting from the viral ori, later another, unknown replication mechanism (referred here as non-theta) gradually replaces it, as assessed by the analysis of the replication intermediates using two-dimensional (2D) gel electrophoresis in the U2OS and HaCat cells (Orav et al., 2015, 2019). The maintenance replication of the HPV18 genomes occurs almost exclusively using this non-theta replication mechanism in the U2OS cells (Piirsoo et al., 2020). Second, in contrast to the initial infection, when a monomeric 8 kb HPV genome infects the cell, the viral genomes tend to form oligomeric concatemeric structures in the beginning or during the stable replication phase of the viral life-cycle (Frattini et al., 1996; Orav et al., 2013; Warburton et al., 2018; Piirsoo et al., 2020; Lototskaja et al., 2021). Third, it has been shown that the viral protein E1 is dispensable for the maintenance replication of various HPV types (Egawa et al., 2012; Murakami et al., 2019; Piirsoo et al., 2020). In addition, we have previously shown that the maintenance replication of the major oligomeric form of the HPV5 genome is independent of the viral E2 protein in U2OS cells (Lototskaja et al., 2021).

The above-described observations have led us to further analyze the nature of the non-theta HPV replication mechanism in an attempt to understand the mechanism of transition from the initial amplification to the stable maintenance phase of the viral life-cycle. In this paper, we show that the non-theta replication mechanism, previously observed only in the case of mucosal alpha HPV types, is present also in the beta HPV5 genome in the U2OS cells. We also show that the non-theta replication of the HPV genomes is not confined to the artificial cellular systems but takes also place in the CIN612 cells, which are natural host cells for HPV and contain stably replicating HPV31 genomes. Finally, we establish that the appearance of non-theta mechanism in the HPV replication is connected with the oligomerization of the viral genomes.

MATERIALS AND METHODS

DNA Constructs

Plasmids containing HPV5, HPV11, HPV18, HPV18E, and HPV18E8-genomes on the basis of the pMC.BESBX minicircle production vector have been described previously (Sankovski et al., 2014; Orav et al., 2015). Minicircle genomes were generated in *Escherichia coli* strain ZYCY10P3S2T using the minicircle DNA technology as previously described (Orav et al., 2015). Plasmids pUCURR18 and pGLURR18 harboring HPV18 URR, and HPV18 E1 (pMH18E1), and E2 (pQM18E2) expression vectors have been described previously (Kadaja et al., 2007; Kurg et al., 2010). pGEXURR18 was constructed by digesting the pGEXGSTFar1 plasmid (kind gift from Dr. Mart Loog) with XbaI to remove the yeast Far1 cDNA, blunting the 5' overhangs with Klenow fragment and cloning the blunted HPV18 URR BamHI fragment (nt 6929-119) into it.

Cell Culture and Transfections

Human osteosarcoma cell line U2OS (ATCC No HTB-96) and SV40 transformed African green monkey kidney cell line Cos1 (ATCC No CRL-1650) were propagated in the normal growth medium containing Iscove's Modified Dulbecco's Medium, 10% fetal calf serum (FCS) and 1% penicillin/streptomycin at 37°C, and 5% CO2. The cells were transfected by electroporation (975 µF and 220 V for U2OS or 180 V for Cos1 and) using a Gene Pulser XCell system (Bio-Rad Laboratories). The following amounts of wt or modified HPV minicircle genomes were used for the transfection of 2 × 106 U2OS cells: HPV5 and HPV18E 2 µg and HPV11 and HPV18E8-0.5 µg. A total of 2 µg of HPV18 URR containing plasmids (pUCURR18, pGLURR18, or pGEXURR18) were transfected together with 50 µg of pMH18E1 and 250 ng of pQM18E2 expression vectors to 2 × 106 U2OS cells. A total of 0.5 µg of pCDNA3 was transfected to 2 × 106 Cos1 cells.

CIN612 cells (kind gift from Dr. Frank Stubenrauch) were grown in the Defined Keratinocyte-SFM Medium (DKSM; Gibco, Thermo Fisher Scientific). Cells were detached using 0.05% Trypsin-EDTA solution, immediately transferred into DKSM containing 2.5% FCS, centrifuged at room temperature (RT) 1200 rpm for 5 min, and plated onto a new culture dish and fresh DKS after every 3–4 days. The cells were allowed to differentiate in the DKSM containing 1.5 mM Ca++ for 72 h.

1D and 2D Analysis of Replication

Episomal or genomic DNA was isolated from cells as described previously (Geimanen et al., 2011). DNA isolated from the transient replication assays was digested with a restriction endonuclease DpnI, to eliminate input, non-replicated DNA. The following enzymes were used to linearize replicons analyzed: BglI (HPV18, HPV18E, and HPV18E8-), SacI (HPV5), BstEII (HPV11), BstXI (HPV31), XbaI (pUCURR18, pGLURR18), NcoI (pGEXURR18), and XmaI (pCDNA3). The following enzymes were used as noncutters for the replicons analyzed: HindIII (HPV18), BamHI (HPV31), BglII (pUCURR18), EcoRI (pGLURR18), and KpnI (pGEXURR18).

One dimensional (1D) and 2D analysis of replication by Southern blotting (SB) was performed as previously described (Orav et al., 2015). A total of 3–5 μg-s of DNA was used for 1D analysis of replication, 120 μg (HPV18E8- and pCDNA3), or 150 μg (all other replicons) of the episomal DNA was used for 2D analysis of replication intermediates.

Signals from Southern blots were manually marked and pixels in the marked areas were counted using ImageQuant software. Background noise was separately substracted from every blot. Data was analyzed using Graphpad software.

Statistical Analysis

The values of *p* for the two-tailed *t*-test were based on assumed equal variances and calculated using Excel software.

Cell Cycle Analysis

Cell cycle profiles of U2OS cells were analyzed using propidium iodide staining and FACS analysis as described previously (Piirsoo et al., 2019).

Immunoblotting

Western blot analysis was performed as previously described (Kauts et al., 2013). The E1 protein was detected using mouse anti-HA antibody (clone HA-7, Sigma-Aldrich) at a dilution 1:3,000. The E2 protein was detected using mouse monoclonal antibody 2E7.1 against HPV18 E2 protein, at a dilution 1: 2,500 (kind gift from Mihkel Allik).

RESULTS

Transient Replication of the HPV Genomes Involves Two Distinct Mechanisms

We and others have previously shown that the initial amplification of the genus alpha HPV11 and -18 genomes proceeds *via* at least two distinct mechanisms, with one involving the theta type of replication intermediates (Orav et al., 2015, 2019). These two mechanisms were observed in both U2OS and HaCat cells, indicating that it is not a cell type specific phenomenon. We were therefore interested, if the replication of the genus beta HPV genomes also involves different mechanisms. We used U2OS cells as a cell culture model permissive for HPV genome replication (Geimanen et al., 2011) and compared the replication mechanisms of HPV5 to those of HPV11 and HPV18. It has been previously shown that all these genomes replicate in the U2OS cells, with HPV5 having the lowest and HPV11 having the highest efficiency of replication (Geimanen et al., 2011).

Mechanisms of replication were elucidated by analyzing the replication intermediates that can be resolved in 2D electrophoresis, followed by SB analysis of the specific signals. Different types of 2D systems can be used to study the replication mechanisms, and depending on the nature of replicon and site of digest relative to the ori, different patterns of the replication intermediates can be observed (Henno et al., 2017). We chose neutral-neutral 2D system and digested HPV genome once in the vicinity of the replication origin, since the migration pattern of replication intermediates arising under these conditions are easy to interpret and explain. Schematic representation of the expected replication intermediates arising from a bi-directionally replicating circular replicon and analyzed under the above-mentioned conditions are depicted in **Figures 1A,B.** Majority of the analyzed replicons are not replicating at a given moment, since only a limited number of cells in a population are in the S phase. Non-replicating molecules run as spots of 1n and 2n. 1n spot is always more prominent, since the G1 phase is the longest and has the highest number of cells. The line between 1n and 2n molecules represents linear arc and probably consists of replicating molecules, where replication fork structure has been broken either in the cells or during the extraction of DNA. Major replication intermediates that can be observed using this type of analysis are called as doubleY and simpleY structures. DoubleY structures represent replication intermediates with two replication forks emanating from the ori and proceeding away from each other (called as converging forks). Circular replicons have often trouble finishing replication, and therefore the most abundant portion of the doubleY structures is almost fully replicated molecules. SimpleY structures indicate either unidirectional replication or result from the bidirectional replication, where one of the replication forks has been stalled early on for some reason. It has also been suggested that simpleY structures might represent the rolling circle type of replication in case of SV40 (Sowd et al., 2013).

The HPV5, HPV11, or HPV18 genomes were transfected into the U2OS cells, and episomal DNA was extracted 72 h post-transfection. Episomal DNA was digested with a restriction endonuclease cutting the respective genome once near the ori, resolved on two dimensions and hybridized with a probe for the specific HPV type.

As seen in **Figure 1C**, all three HPV types analyzed had similar replication intermediates. The signal intensity was proportional to the replication efficiency observed previously (Geimanen et al., 2011), as HPV5 replication was the weakest, and HPV11 replication was the strongest. DoubleY structures were observed in each case (black arrows), with substantial amounts of almost fully replicated molecules present (black arrowheads). Accumulation of almost fully replicated molecules indicates that the finishing of the HPV replication is problematic, which is a common problem among circular replicons.

In addition, all analyzed HPV types contained additional non-theta replication intermediates, as previously observed in the case of HPV11 and HPV18 (white arrows). To the best of our knowledge, the migration pattern of these intermediates does not concur with any type of replication intermediates observed in other systems, where the DNA replication mechanisms have been studied using 2D analysis.

The complete lack of the simpleY structures in the case of HPV theta replication should also be mentioned. This is in sharp contrast with the replication of a related DNA virus SV40 and yeast 2-micron plasmid, where simpleY structures showing unidirectional replication are present along with doubleY structures, if a replicon is cleaved once in the vicinity of the ori (Brewer and Fangman, 1987; Sowd et al., 2013). We also

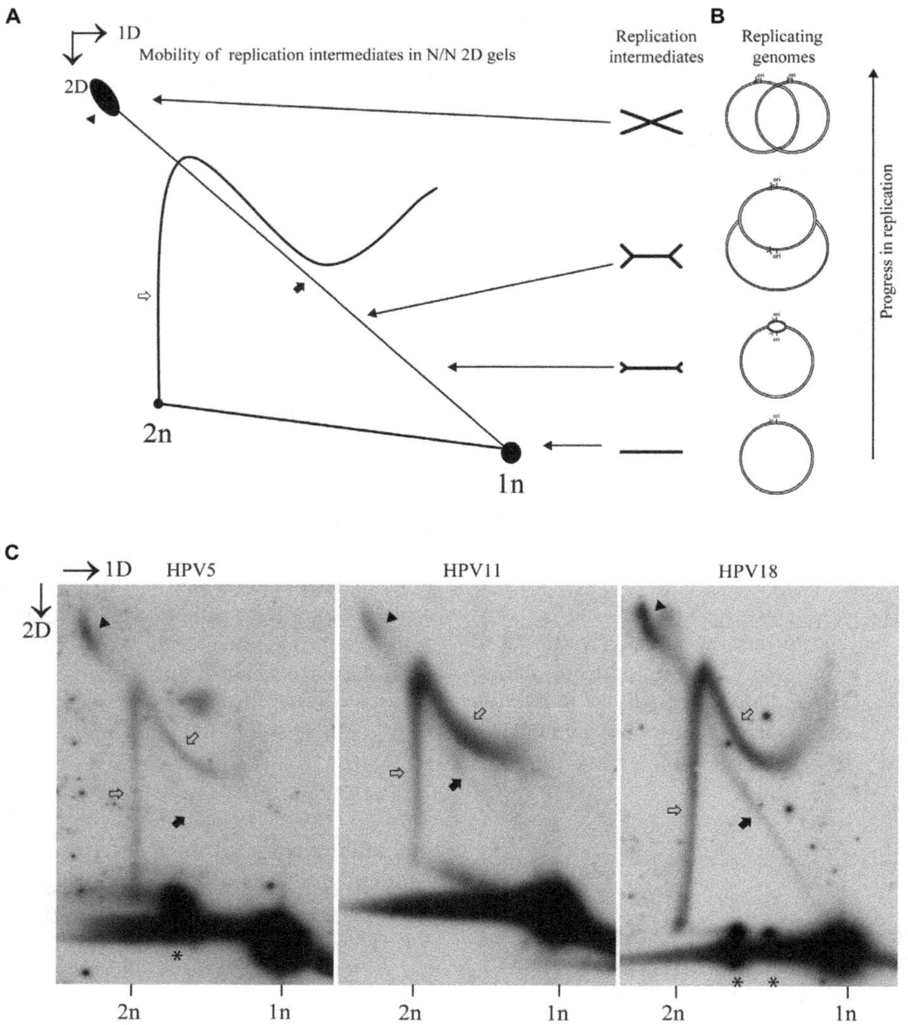

FIGURE 1 | Usage of the non-theta replication mechanism during transient replication is characteristic to different human papillomavirus (HPV) types. **(A)** Schematic representation of the expected mobility of the theta replication intermediates in neutral-neutral two-dimensional (2D) gel in case a circular replicon is linearized near the origin of replication (ori). Almost a straight diagonal line emanating from the spot of 1n linear molecules represents a doubleY structure, with two replication forks that started from the ori to opposite directions advancing as the line retreats from the spot of 1n linear molecules. A non-linear line ending in the 2D spot represents the structure arising from the non-theta type of replication. **(B)** Sketch of the HPV replicon at the different stages of bidirectional replication. Ori represents origin of replication; scissors refer to the position, where the HPV genome is linearized. **(C)** Neutral-neutral 2D analysis of the replication intermediates arising from the HPV5, HPV11, and HPV18 genome replication after transient transfection of the respective genomes into U2OS cells. Episomal DNA was extracted 72 h post-transfection, linearized with a restriction enzyme cutting near ori [HPV5 – SacI (nt 702); HPV11- BstEII (nt 7,899) HPV18 – BglI (nt 7,656)] run on an agarose gel at two dimensions and analyzed by Southern blotting (SB). Black arrows refer to the theta replication intermediates, black arrowheads refer to the almost fully replicated genomes, white arrows refer to the non-theta replication intermediates, asterisks depict the linear HPV genome fragments running between the size of 1n and 2n.

often observed discreet spots running on the linear arc of molecules between the lengths of 1n (8 kb) and 2n (16 kb) molecules (depicted by asterisks in **Figure 1C**). These molecules represent partially replicated HPV genomes, indicating that replication of HPV genomes is inefficient, and collapse of replication forks is frequent.

We have previously shown that the abundance of the non-theta replication intermediates increases over time during the initial amplification of the HPV18 genomes in the U2OS cells (Orav et al., 2015). At the same time, the HPV genomes tend to form oligomers, if transfected into the U2OS cells (Orav et al., 2013). We were therefore interested to analyze if the appearance of the oligomeric HPV genomes coincides with the appearance of the non-theta replication intermediates. To do that, we quantified the amounts of the replicated monomeric and oligomeric HPV18 genomes at 3, 4, and 5 days after transfection and compared that to the abundance of the theta- and non-theta replication intermediates at the same time points (**Figure 2**). The monomeric HPV genomes and the theta intermediates were prevalent at 3 days post-transfection. Four days after the transfection, the amounts of the monomeric and oligomeric genomes were similar, whereas almost 70% of the replication

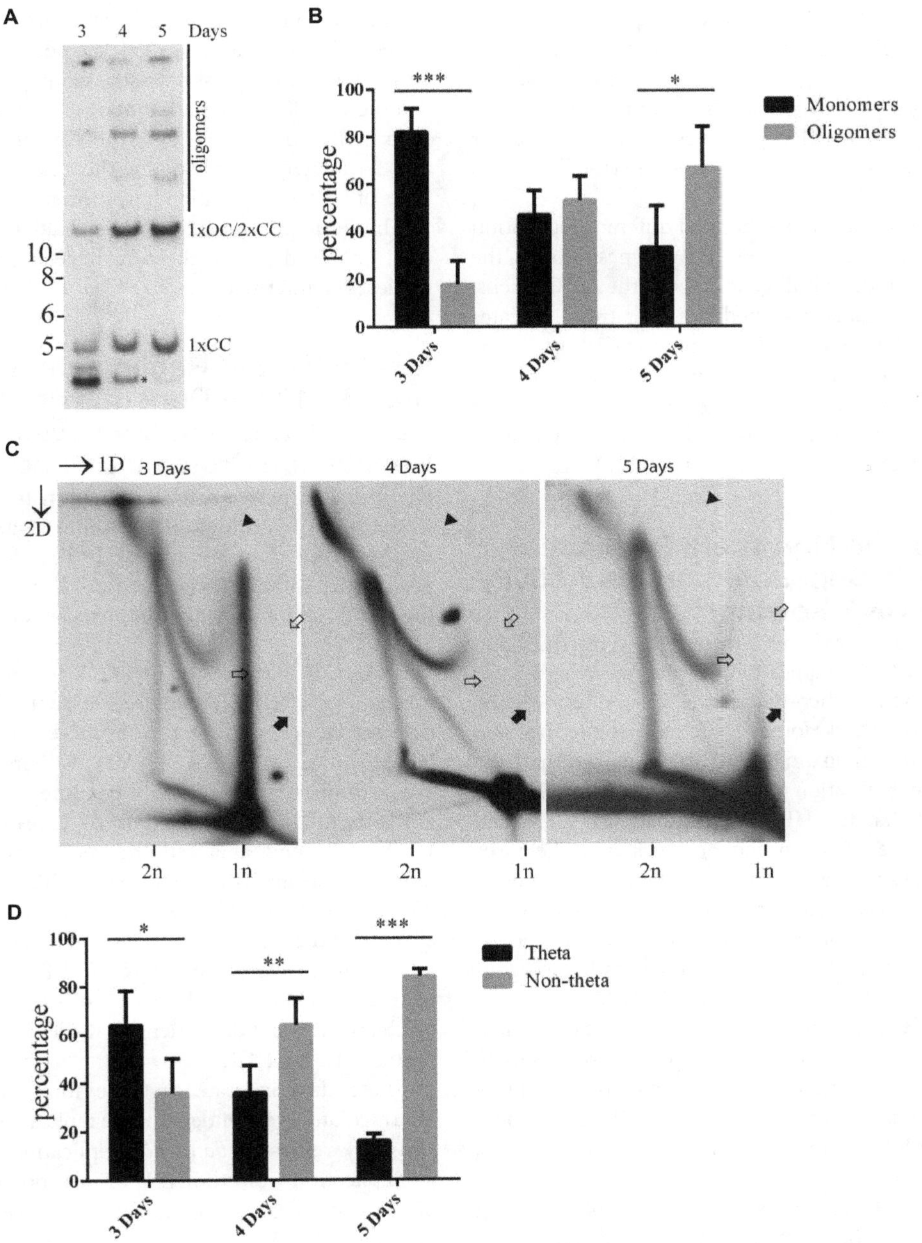

FIGURE 2 | Appearance of the non-theta replication intermediates during the transient replication of the HPV18 genomes in the U2OS cells concurs with the oligomerization of the replicated viral genomes. **(A)** An example of different forms of the HPV18 genome arising as a result of the transient replication in U2OS cells at 3 4, or 5 days after the transfection. Genomic DNA was extracted from the cells at indicated time points, digested with HPV18 non-cutter HindIII and DpnI to separate non-replicated input DNA, resolved on 0.6% gel and analyzed by SB. Migration of the monomeric closed circular (1xCC), monomeric open circular (1XOC), dimeric closed circular (2xCC), and oligomeric forms are shown. Asterisk represents migration of non-replicated, DpnI sensitive fragment of HPV18.
(B) Quantification of the replicated monomeric and oligomeric HPV18 genomes at 3, 4, and 5 days after the transfection in the U2OS cells. The data are expressed as average means ± the SD (*$p<0.05$; **$p<0.01$; and ***$p<0.001$) of four independent experiments. Monomeric open circular and dimeric closed circular genomes migrate together under the conditions used to resolve DNA and were therefore omitted from calculation. **(C)** An example of different types of the replication intermediates arising during the transient replication of the HPV18 genome in U2OS cells at 3, 4, and 5 days post-transfection. Black arrows refer to the theta replication intermediates, black arrowheads refer to the almost fully replicated genomes, white arrows refer to the non-theta replication intermediates.
(D) Quantification of the theta- and non-theta replication intermediates arising during the transient replication of the HPV18 genomes at 3, 4, and 5 days after the transfection in the U2OS cells. The data are expressed as average means ± the SD (*$p<0.05$; **$p<0.01$; and ***$p<0.001$) of four independent experiments.

intermediates were of non-theta type. It should be noted, however, that the amounts of the oligomeric genomes may be underestimated in our quantitation, since it is virtually impossible to separate monomeric open circular and dimeric closed circular genomes under these gel conditions. At 5 days post-transfection more than 60% of the replicated HPV18 genomes were oligomeric and more than 80% of the replication intermediates were of non-theta type (**Figures 2B,D**). Representative images of 1D (used for quantification of the monomeric and oligomeric HPV genomes) and 2D (used for quantification of the theta and non-theta intermediates) SB are shown in **Figures 2A,C**.

Taken together, these data show that two different replication mechanisms are utilized by different HPV types during the initial amplification of the viral genomes in the U2OS cells. Appearance of the non-theta intermediates over time indicates their relation with the formation of the oligomeric HPV genomes. In addition, the accumulation of almost fully replicated genomes in the doubleY arc and partially replicated genomes in the linear arc indicates that the HPV replication is inefficient in both elongation and termination (or partitioning) phases.

Appearance of the Non-theta Replication Intermediates Is Dependent on the Activity of Replicative DNA Polymerases

One possible explanation for the non-theta type of intermediates observed during the HPV replication is that these structures represent recombination, rather than replication intermediates. It has been shown in yeast that Holliday junctions, as intermediates of the homologous recombination, can occur at least partially independently of the replication (Zou and Rothstein, 1997). It is widely established that the HPV infection induce ATM and ATR mediated DDR response in the host cell and the virus utilizes homologous recombination mediated replication, although the exact molecular details of this process are poorly understood (Sakakibara et al., 2013). Moreover, it has been shown that the HPV genomes tend to form oligomeric structures *via* homologous recombination in the U2OS cells (Orav et al., 2013).

If the formation of the recombining structures is not dependent on the DNA polymerases, inhibiting DNA polymerase activity should not prevent their formation. We tested this possibility by challenging U2OS cells transfected with the HPV18 genome with a reversible inhibitor of replicative DNA polymerases, aphidicolin.

Exposure of the U2OS cells to aphidicolin for 24 h, starting the treatment 48 h after the transfection, induced substantial cell cycle arrest, with 62% of the cells residing in G1, 14% in S and 24% in the G2/M phase (**Figure 3A**). As expected, this arrest was reversed, when aphidicolin was removed. Within 3 h in the normal growth medium, the cell cycle profile was changed dramatically, and cells entered successfully into the S phase (36% in G1, 39% in S, and 25% in G2/M). At 7.5 h after the release into the cell cycle, majority of the cells had reached G2/M phase of the cell cycle (21% in G1, 24% in S, and 55% in G2/M). After 24 h the normal distribution of the cell cycle was recovered (44% in G1, 25% in S, and 32% in G2/M; **Figure 3A**).

Two-dimensional analysis of the HPV18 genome replication showed that almost all recognizable replication intermediates were missing in the cells challenged with aphidicolin, with only small amounts of almost fully replicated molecules present (black arrowhead; **Figure 3B**, left panel). Majority of the HPV molecules were retained in the 1n spot or migrated as branched structures above 1n spot (asterisk in **Figure 3A**). We believe that these molecules represent the open structures with replication forks stalled due to the DNA polymerase inhibition. At 3, 7.5, and 24 h after the release of the cells into the cell cycle, all types of HPV18 replication intermediates reappeared (**Figure 3B**).

These data indicate that replicative DNA polymerase(s) are involved in the formation of the non-theta replication intermediates.

Mechanism of Replication Initiated From the HPV18 Ori Depends on the Size of the Replicon and Not the Levels of the Viral Replication Proteins E1 and E2

One possible prerequisite for the non-theta type of replication is the virus specific transcriptional regulation, which results in the production of correct levels of the viral replication proteins E1 and E2. These levels can be altered by co-transfecting the viral genome with the expression vectors coding for E1 and E2.

To test, if the levels of E1 and E2 could alter the replication mechanism of HPV18, we used mutant HPV18 genome, which does not express E8/E2 repressor protein, and therefore replicates better than the wt HPV18 (Reinson et al., 2013). We co-transfected the mutant genome together with increasing amounts of the HPV18 E1 or E2 expression vectors into the U2OS cells and analyzed the mechanisms of replication by 2D gel electrophoresis followed by SB. Results of this analysis are shown in the **Figure 4**. We could not detect any major changes in the relative distribution of different types of replication intermediates even at high levels of E1 or E2 present. Therefore, we can conclude that the usage of distinct type of replication mechanisms is not dependent on the levels of the viral replication proteins E1 and E2.

These data indicate that the formation of the non-theta intermediates is dependent on the replicative DNA polymerase(s), and they represent *bona fide* replication intermediates.

Replication from the HPV ori can proceed also, if the origin of replication is cloned into a heterologous plasmid and the viral proteins E1 and E2 are provided in trans from the expression vectors. We used this set-up to analyze, if any other viral protein or cis-elements lying outside the viral ori, might influence the mechanism of HPV replication. We used replicons of different sizes containing HPV18 URR (nt 6929-119). This 1.1 kb fragment contains all the necessary cis elements for replication (Remm et al., 1992). This fragment was cloned into pUC (pUCURR18), resulting in a 4-kb replicon, pGL4 (pGL4URR18), resulting in a 6.5-kb replicon, and into pGEXFar1 (pGEXFarURR18), resulting in a 8.2-kb replicon. The plasmids were transfected into the U2OS cells together with the HPV18 E1 and E2 expression vectors, and their replication was analyzed 72 h after the transfection. For the analysis of the replication, we extracted episomal DNA and digested it with the restriction endonucelases that either linearize the replicon or do not cut

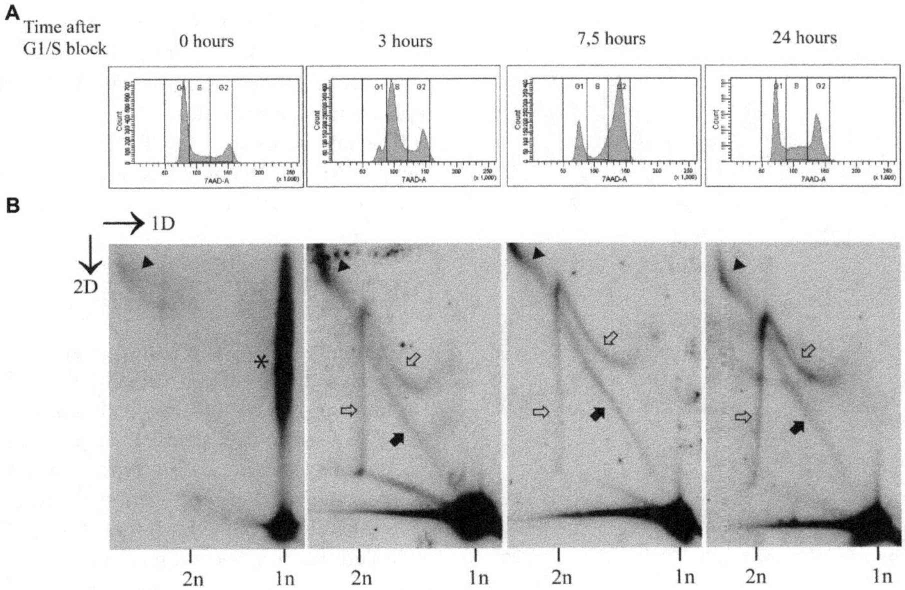

FIGURE 3 | The non-theta replication of the HPV18 genomes is dependent on the replicative DNA polymerase(s). **(A)** The cell cycle profile of the aphidicolin arrested cells (0 h), followed by the release into the cell cycle at various time points (3, 7.5, and 24 h) post-arrest. The U2OS cells were transfected with the HPV18 genome, 48 h after the transfection the cells were arrested at G1/S phase using aphidicolin treatment (2 µg/ml) for 24 h, followed by the removal of the drug and release of the cells to cycling conditions for the indicated periods of time. **(B)** Neutral-neutral 2D analysis of the replication intermediates arising from the HPV18 genome replication after the transfection into the U2OS cells at various time points after the G1/S block using aphidicolin. Nearly all replication intermediates are absent at the end of 24-h block by aphidicolin (0 h). Instead, the collapsed intermediates migrate above the 1n linear molecule spot (indicated by asterisk). At 3 h post-release, when majority of the cells have entered the S-phase, both theta and non-theta type of replication intermediates are present. About 7.5 h after the release majority of the cells have entered G2/M phase, and still both type of replication intermediates are detectable. At 24 h post-release, the cells have restored the normal distribution of the cell cycle and both theta- and non-theta replication intermediates can be seen. Black arrows refer to the theta replication intermediates, black arrowheads refer to the almost fully replicated genomes, and white arrows refer to the non-theta replication intermediates.

the replicon. All digestions were performed in the presence of DpnI enzyme to cut transfected, non-replicated DNA and expression vectors.

Southern blotting analysis showed that all three constructs were able to replicate in the U2OS cells given that the HPV18 E1 and E2 expression vectors were co-transfected (**Figure 5A**). Analysis of the linearized replicons showed that all replicated plasmids were of the expected sizes (**Figure 5A**, right panel). Analysis on the noncut replicons showed that all plasmids formed oligomeric structures in the cell (**Figure 5A**, left panel).

Two-dimensional analysis of the respective replicons was performed by linearizing the replicons once near the HPV18 ori. The analysis showed that the 4 kb pUCURR18 plasmid replicated strictly *via* theta type of intermediates, with substantial amounts of singleY structures present, indicating unidirectional replication (**Figure 5B**, left panel). This distribution of the replication intermediates was almost indistinguishable from the replication of SV40 origin containing 5.4 kb pcDNA3 plasmid in Cos1 cells (**Figure 5B**, upper panel).

The pattern of the replication intermediates was different in the case of 6.5 kb pGLURR18 and 8.2 kb pGEXURR18 replicons (**Figure 5B**, lower panel). Both replicons had the non-theta replication as a prevailing mechanism, while the start of the non-theta intermediate differed between them. By start, we mean the tail of the intermediate that migrates at the size of 1n molecules. The start of the 6.5 kb pGLURR18 replicon was directed toward linear 1n molecules, while the start of 8.2 kb pGEXURR18 molecules was directed away from it.

These data show that the non-theta replication of the HPV genomes is not dependent on the E1 and E2 levels, or any cis element lying in the coding region of the genome, but rather is a function of the replicon size.

Maintenance Replication of the HPV31 Genomes in CIN612 Keratinocytes Proceeds *via* Two Distinct Mechanisms

In order to corroborate our results about distinct replication mechanisms utilized by the HPV genomes obtained from U2OS based cell systems, we used a different cell type, CIN612 keratinocytes, which is permissive for HPV replication. These cells harbor stably replicating HPV31 genomes as extrachromosomal plasmids. In sharp contrast to the U2OS based stable HPV positive cell lines, majority of HPV genomes are monomeric in CIN612 cells (**Figure 6A**).

Analysis of the replication mechanisms utilized by HPV31 genomes in CIN612 cells showed that a dominating mechanism of replication is that of theta type (**Figure 6B**, black arrows). However, we could also detect the non-theta replication intermediates that are similar to those observed in U2OS cells for other HPV types (**Figure 6B**, white arrows).

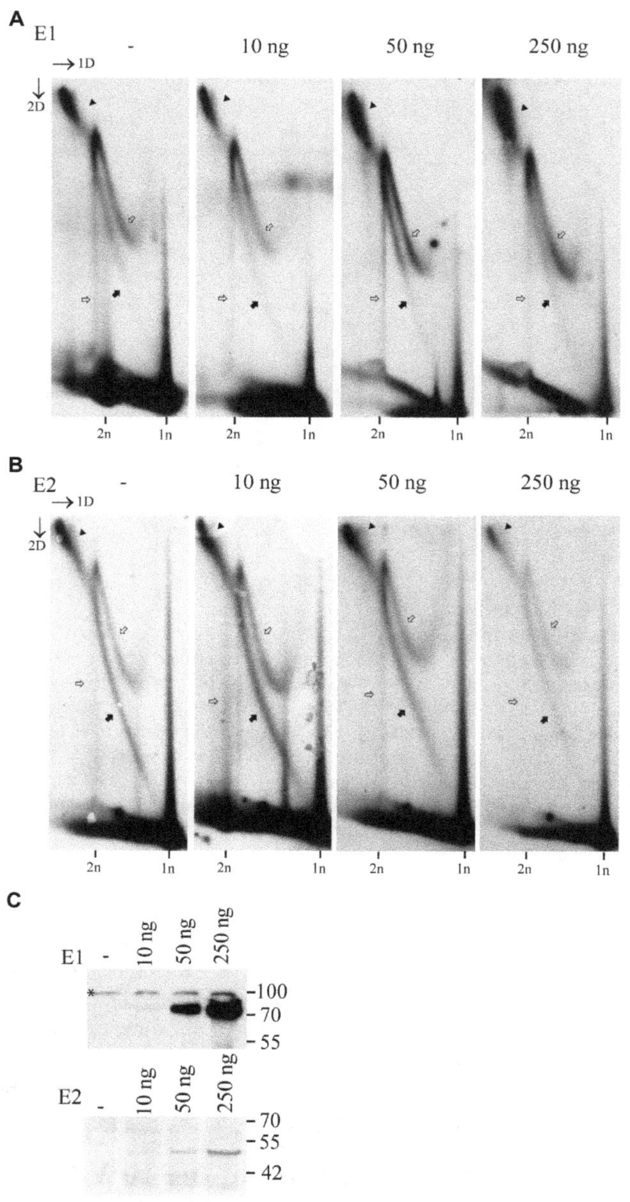

FIGURE 4 | Mechanism of replication initiated from the HPV18 ori does not depend on the E1 and E2 protein levels. **(A)** Neutral-neutral 2D analysis of the replication intermediates arising from the HPV18 E8-genome replication in the presence of growing amounts of the E1 expression vector. **(B)** Neutral-neutral 2D analysis of the replication intermediates arising from the HPV18 E8-genome replication in the presence of growing amounts of the E2 expression vector. Episomal DNA was extracted 72 h after the transfection, linearized with a restriction enzyme BglII cutting near the ori, run on an agarose gel at two dimensions and analyzed by SB. Black arrows refer to the theta replication intermediates, black arrowheads refer to the almost fully replicated genomes, white arrows refer to the non-theta replication intermediates. **(C)** Western blot analysis showing the expression levels of the HPV18 E1 and E2 proteins, when co-transfected together with the HPV18 E8-genome.

As a comparison, we used HPV5+ and HPV18+ U2OS cells (previously referred as clone 15 and clone 1.13 in Geimanen et al., 2011). These cells have oligomeric HPV genomes stably replicating in the cells (Geimanen et al., 2011; Piirsoo et al., 2020). As shown in the **Figure 6B**, these oligomeric genomes replicate exclusively using the non-theta type of the replication intermediates.

The low abundance of the non-theta type of replication in the CIN612 cells coincides with the amounts of oligomeric forms of the HPV31 genomes in these cells.

DISCUSSION

DNA replication in the mammalian cell nuclei can take place *via* at least three different mechanisms. The most widely used mechanism utilizes the classical semiconservative synthesis of new DNA strands starting from specific sequences, called as origins of replication. This type of replication is essential for the maintenance of the genome integrity, and it has been believed for a long time that the HPV genomes are also replicated this way. Second mechanism of nuclear DNA replication involves break induced replication (BIR), that is activated upon stress conditions to repair the double strand breaks and collapsed classical replication forks (Malkova, 2018). This type of DNA replication does not need specific start sites and leads to the genomic rearrangements. Yet another type of replication, that also does not start from the specific origins, called as rolling circle replication, can take place in the mammalian cell nuclei (Wawrzyniak et al., 2017). This replication mode is utilized by some DNA viruses, including adeno-associated virus and human herpesvirus 6, and results in the concatemeric multimers of the initial replicon (Tattersall and Ward, 1976; Astell et al., 1985; Borenstein and Frenkel, 2009).

All these above-mentioned replication mechanisms have been implicated to be operating during the HPV replication. Semiconservative bidirectional replication has been shown to be the HPV replication mechanism using the analysis of the replication intermediates in 2D gels in the case of HPV11, HPV16, and HPV31 in laryngeal papillomas, W12 and CIN612 cell lines, respectively (Auborn et al., 1994; Flores and Lambert, 1997). Rolling circle type of HPV16 and HPV31 replication has been proposed to take place upon keratinocyte differentiation and could therefore represent the replication mode in the last, vegetative phase of the viral life cycle (Flores and Lambert, 1997). However, these studies actually analyzed subgenomic fragments the whole HPV replicon, which could affect the interpretation of the results. We have shown previously that when the whole HPV18 replicons, extracted from transiently transfected U2OS cells, are investigated using the analysis of the replication intermediates in 2D gels, mixed type of replication could be observed (Orav et al., 2015). Initially most of the HPV18 replication proceeds *via* bidirectional mechanism, but later it is gradually replaced by another mode, which we believe to be BIR. It has been shown that expression of HPV oncoproteins induce replication stress, which in turn activate BIR (Malkova, 2018; Moody, 2019). In the present article, we extend these findings and show that other HPV types, HPV5 and HPV11, also utilize similar mixed replication mechanism upon the

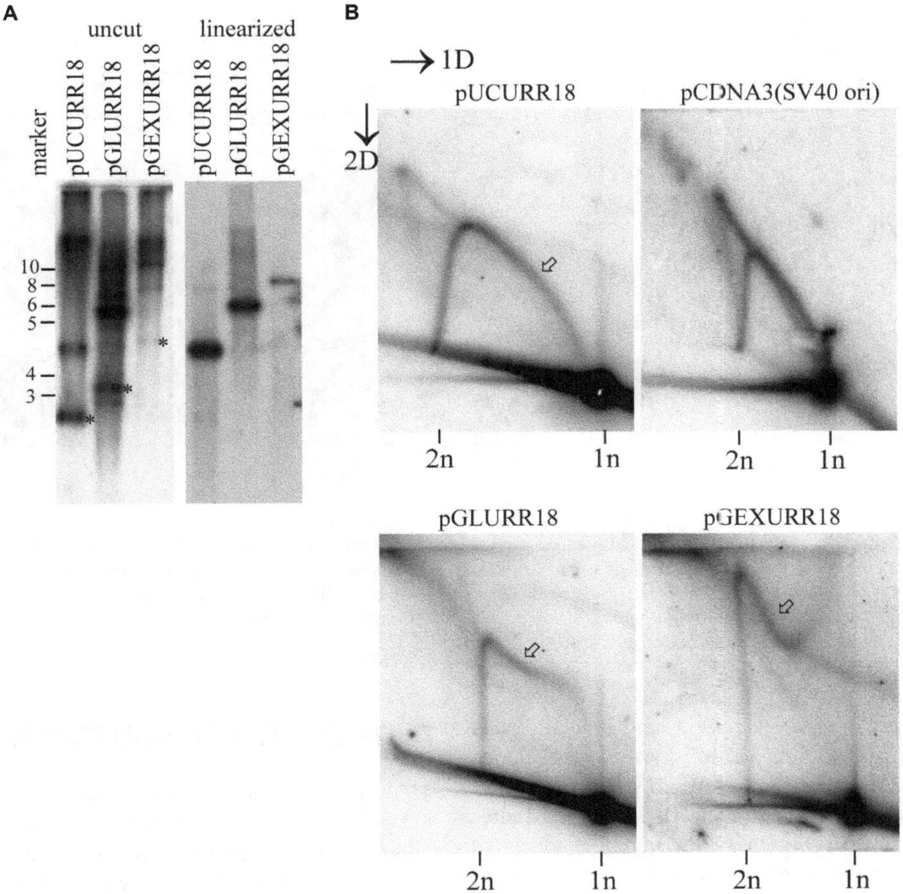

FIGURE 5 | Mechanism of replication initiated from the HPV18 ori depends on the size of the replicon. **(A)** Transient replication of the HPV18 ori harboring replicons with different sizes in the U2OS cells. pUCURR18 (4 kb), pGLURR18 (6 kb), or pGEXURR18 (8,2 kb) were transfected together with the HPV18 E1 and E2 expression vectors into the U2OS cells. Episomal DNA was extracted 72 h after the transfection, digested with replicon non-cutter (left panel) or single cutter enzyme (right panel), combined with DpnI to digest the non-replicated plasmids, resolved in 0.8% agarose gel and analyzed by SB. Asterisks represent migration of the monomeric closed circular forms of the respective replicons. **(B)** Neutral-neutral 2D analysis of the replication intermediates arising from the HPV18 harboring replicons of different sizes during the transient replication in the U2OS cells and the SV40 origin containing pCDNA3 replicon in Cos1 cells. The replication intermediate structure that varies between different HPV replicons is indicated with an arrow.

initial amplification in the U2OS cells. We also show that HPV31 utilizes RDR during maintenance replication in keratinocytes, similarly to the maintenance replication of HPV18 in the U2OS derived cell-lines (Piirsoo et al., 2020).

One of the questions we have tried to answer in this article is what distinguishes the HPV18 genomes replicating in a bidirectional manner vs. those replicating *via* BIR. It has been previously shown, that the HPV genomes form oligomeric structures through homologous recombination (Orav et al., 2013). We observed that BIR type of replication starts to occur only after the oligomeric HPV18 genomes appear in the cells. Furthermore, the abundance of BIR is proportional to the abundance of the oligomeric HPV genomes in the transiently transfected U2OS cells, and in the stable cell lines carrying episomal HPV31 genomes. Therefore, we hypothesize that while monomeric HPV genomes replicate bi-directionally in an E1 and E2 dependent manner, oligomeric HPV genomes replicate using BIR that does not require viral trans factors. Further support to this hypothesis comes from the studies showing that viral the E1 protein is dispensable for the maintenance replication of the HPV genomes (Hubert and Laimins, 2002; Fradet-Turcotte et al., 2010; Egawa et al. 2012; Murakami et al., 2019). We have also recently shown that the maintenance replication of the major topological forms of HPV18 genomes in the U2OS cells is independent of the E1 function (Piirsoo et al., 2020). Furthermore, the major topological forms of the HPV5 genomes do not require the function of E2 protein during the maintenance replication in the U2OS cells (Lototskaja et al., 2021).

One of the possibilities, why the bidirectional HPV replication is replaced by BIR, is poor expression of E1 and E2 from the viral genomes, so that the viral origins of replication are insufficiently fired. To test this possibility, we investigated if the balance between bidirectional replication mode and BIR can be altered by forced expression of the E1 or E2 proteins

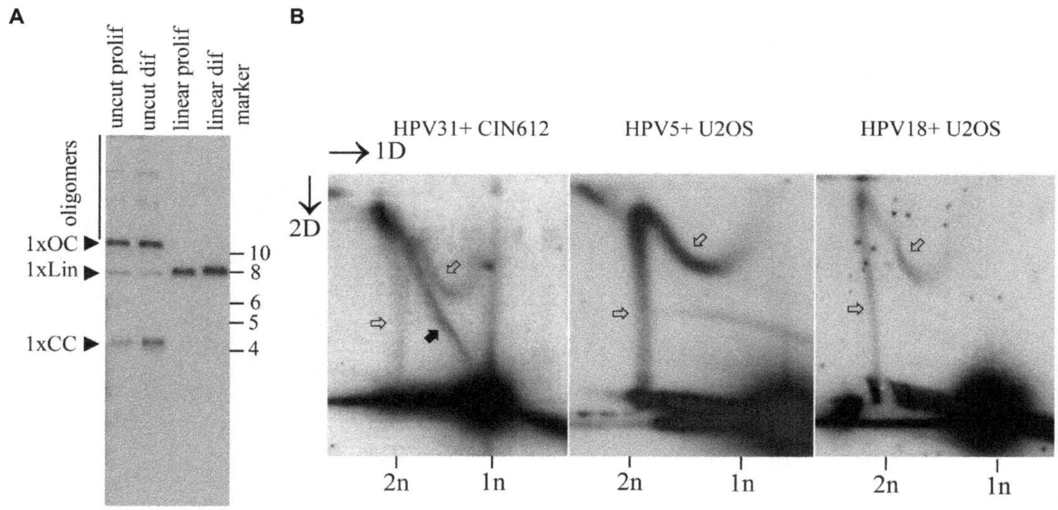

FIGURE 6 | Maintenance replication of the HPV31 genomes proceeds *via* distinct mechanisms in the CIN612 keratinocytes. **(A)** SB showing the status of the HPV31 genomes in CIN612 cells. HPV31 noncutter (BamHI) or single cutter (BstXI) enzymes were used to digest episomal DNA. Migration of the monomeric closed circular (1xCC), monomeric open circular (1XOC), linear (1xLin) and oligomeric forms are shown. **(B)** Neutral-neutral 2D analysis of the replication intermediates arising from the HPV31 maintenance replication in the CIN216 cells, HPV5 and HPV18 maintenance replication in the U2OS cells. Black arrows refer to the theta replication intermediates; white arrows refer to the non-theta replication intermediates.

from the expression vectors. However, we found that the overexpression of neither E1 nor E2 could change this balance toward the bidirectional replication mode. Instead, we found that the distance between two HPV replication oris could alter the replication mechanism. Oligomeric concatemer forms of the HPV genomes have the spacing between the two oris of around 8 kb. These molecules replicate using BIR. When an 8-kb plasmid containing HPV18 URR was transfected into the U2OS cells together with E1 and E2 expression vector, it also formed oligomeric structures and replicated using BIR. However, when a 4-kb plasmid with HPV18 URR was used in a similar experiment, it formed oligomers but continued to replicate in a bidirectional manner. These data suggest that smaller spacing between HPV oris could allow the oligomeric molecules to replicate in a bidirectional manner. The reasons why spacing between the HPV origins of replication is important in determining the replication mode remains to be investigated. One possibility is that the HPV E1 protein, the only viral factor present in the replication elongation complex, is not a very efficient helicase and causes stalling and collapse of the replication forks, which in turn creates substrates for BIR replication. With shorter distances between two oris, however, there is higher chance of completing the bidirectional replication.

Taken together, we propose that a general course of the HPV infection involves the initial E1 and E2 dependent amplification of the viral genomes after the infection, which is accompanied by the replication stress. The replication stress is induced by the expression of HPV oncogenes E6 and E7 (Moody and Laimins, 2009; Moody, 2019) and the inability to fully duplicate the viral genomes using bi-directional replication mechanism. The replication stress leads to the oligomerization of the viral genomes, which start to replicate using the BIR dependent mechanism.

AUTHOR CONTRIBUTIONS

MP and MU designed the experiments. MP, AP, MU, and EU guided the work. LL, AP, AnL, E-MT, and AiL performed the experiments. MP and AP wrote the manuscript. LL, AP, AnL, E-MT, AiL, EU, MU, and MP edited the manuscript. All authors contributed to the article and approved the submitted version.

FUNDING

This research was funded by the European Regional Development Fund through the Centre of Excellence in Molecular Cell Engineering, Estonia (2014-2020.4.01.15-013), an institutional research funding grant (IUT20-27) from the Estonian Research Council, and a personal research funding team grant (PRG198; awarded to MU) from the Estonian Research Council. The funders had no role in study design, data collection and analysis, decision to publish, or preparation of the manuscript.

ACKNOWLEDGMENTS

The authors would like to thank Mart Loog, Frank Stubenrauch, and Mihkel Allik for sharing the reagents.

REFERENCES

Astell, C. R., Chow, M. B., and Ward, D. C. (1985). Sequence analysis of the termini of virion and replicative forms of minute virus of mice DNA suggests a modified rolling hairpin model for autonomous parvovirus DNA replication. *J. Virol.* 54, 171–177. doi: 10.1128/jvi.54.1.171-177.1985

Auborn, K. J., Little, R. D., Platt, T. H. K., Vaccariello, M. A., and Schildkraut, C. L. (1994). Replicative intermediates of human papillomavirus type 11 in laryngeal papillomas: site of replication initiation and direction of replication. *Proc. Natl. Acad. Sci. U. S. A.* 91, 7340–7344. doi: 10.1073/pnas.91.15.7340

Bergvall, M., Melendy, T., and Archambault, J. (2013). The E1 proteins. *Virology* 445, 35–56. doi: 10.1016/j.virol.2013.07.020

Borenstein, R., and Frenkel, N. (2009). Cloning human herpes virus 6A genome into bacterial artificial chromosomes and study of DNA replication intermediates. *Proc. Natl. Acad. Sci. U. S. A.* 106, 19138–19143. doi: 10.1073/pnas.0908504106

Brewer, B. J., and Fangman, W. L. (1987). The localization of replication origins on ARS plasmids in *S. cerevisiae*. *Cell* 51, 463–471. doi: 10.1016/0092-8674(87)90642-8

Egawa, N., Nakahara, T., Ohno, S. I., Narisawa-Saito, M., Yugawa, T., Fujita, M., et al. (2012). The E1 protein of human papillomavirus type 16 is dispensable for maintenance replication of the viral genome. *J. Virol.* 86, 3276–3283. doi: 10.1128/JVI.06450-11

Flores, E. R., and Lambert, P. F. (1997). Evidence for a switch in the mode of human papillomavirus type 16 DNA replication during the viral life cycle. *J. Virol.* 71, 7167–7179. doi: 10.1128/jvi.71.10.7167-7179.1997

Fradet-Turcotte, A., Moody, C., Laimins, L. A., and Archambault, J. (2010). Nuclear export of human papillomavirus type 31 E1 is regulated by Cdk2 phosphorylation and required for viral genome maintenance. *J. Virol.* 84, 11747–11760. doi: 10.1128/JVI.01445-10

Frattini, M. G., Lim, H. B., and Laimins, L. A. (1996). In vitro synthesis of oncogenic human papillomaviruses requires episomal genomes for differentiation-dependent late expression. *Proc. Natl. Acad. Sci. U. S. A.* 93, 3062–3067. doi: 10.1073/pnas.93.7.3062

Geimanen, J., Isok-Paas, H., Pipitch, R., Salk, K., Laos, T., Orav, M., et al. (2011). Development of a cellular assay system to study the genome replication of high- and low-risk mucosal and cutaneous human papillomaviruses. *J. Virol.* 85, 3315–3329. doi: 10.1128/JVI.01985-10

Graham, S. V. (2017). The human papillomavirus replication cycle, and its links to cancer progression: a comprehensive review. *Clin. Sci.* 131, 2201–2221. doi 10.1042/CS20160786

Henno, L., Tombak, E. M., Geimanen, J., Orav, M., Ustav, E., and Ustav, M. (2017). Analysis of human papillomavirus genome replication using two and three-dimensional agarose gel electrophoresis. *Curr. Protoc. Microbiol.* 45, 14B.10.1–14B.10.37. doi: 10.1002/cpmc.28

Hubert, W. G., and Laimins, L. A. (2002). Human papillomavirus type 31 replication modes during the early phases of the viral life cycle depend on transcriptional and posttranscriptional regulation of E1 and E2 expression. *J. Virol.* 76, 2263–2273. doi: 10.1128/JVI.76.9.4678.2002

Kadaja, M., Sumerina, A., Verst, T., Ojarand, M., Ustav, E., and Ustav, M. (2007). Genomic instability of the host cell induced by the human papillomavirus replication machinery. *EMBO J.* 26, 2180–2191. doi: 10.1038/sj.emboj.7601665

Kauts, M. L., Pihelgas, S., Orro, K., Neuman, T., and Piirsoo, A. (2013). CCL5/CCR1 axis regulates multipotency of human adipose tissue derived stromal cells. *Stem Cell Res.* 10, 166–178. doi: 10.1016/j.scr.2012.11.004

Kurg, R., Uusen, P., Võsa, L., and Ustav, M. (2010). Human papillomavirus E2 protein with single activation domain initiates HPV18 genome replication, but is not sufficient for long-term maintenance of virus genome. *Virology* 408, 159–166. doi: 10.1016/j.virol.2010.09.010

Lototskaja, E., Sahharov, O., Piirsoo, M., Kala, M., Ustav, M., and Piirsoo, A. (2021). Cyclic AMP-dependent protein kinase exhibits antagonistic effects on the replication efficiency of different human papillomavirus types. *J. Virol.* 95:e0025121. doi: 10.1128/JVI.00251-21

Malkova, A. (2018). Break-induced replication: the where, the why, and the how. *Trends Genet.* 34, 518–531. doi: 10.1016/j.tig.2018.04.002

McBride, A. A. (2017). Mechanisms and strategies of papillomavirus replication. *Biol. Chem.* 398, 919–927. doi: 10.1515/hsz-2017-0113

Moody, C. A. (2019). Impact of replication stress in human papillomavirus pathogenesis. *J. Virol.* 93, e01012–e01017. doi: 10.1128/JVI.01012-17

Moody, C. A., and Laimins, L. A. (2009). Human papillomaviruses activate the ATM DNA damage pathway for viral genome amplification upon differentiation. *PLoS Pathog.* 5:e1000605. doi: 10.1371/journal.ppat.1000605

Murakami, I., Egawa, N., Griffin, H., Yin, W., Kranjec, C., Nakahara, T., et al. (2019). Roles for E1-independent replication and E6-mediated p53 degradation during low-risk and high-risk human papillomavirus genome maintenance. *PLoS Pathog.* 15:e1007755. doi: 10.1371/journal.ppat.1007755

Orav, M., Gagnon, D., and Archambault, J. (2019). Interaction of the human papillomavirus E1 helicase with UAF1-USP1 promotes unidirectional theta replication of viral genomes. *mBio* 10, e00152–e00119. doi: 10.1128/mBio.00152-19

Orav, M., Geimanen, J., Sepp, E. M., Henno, L., Ustav, E., and Ustav, M. (2015). Initial amplification of the HPV18 genome proceeds via two distinct replication mechanisms. *Sci. Rep.* 5:15952. doi: 10.1038/srep15952

Orav, M., Henno, L., Isok-Paas, H., Geimanen, J., Ustav, M., and Ustav, E. (2013). Recombination-dependent oligomerization of human papillomavirus genomes upon transient DNA replication. *J. Virol.* 87, 12051–12068. doi: 10.1128/JVI.01798-13

Piirsoo, A., Kala, M., Sankovski, E., Ustav, M., and Piirsoo, M. (2020). Uncovering the role of the E1 protein in different stages of human papillomavirus 18 genome replication. *J. Virol.* 94, e00674–e00620. doi: 10.1128/JVI.00674-20

Piirsoo, A., Piirsoo, M., Kala, M., Sankovski, E., Lototskaja, E., Levin, V., et al. (2019). Activity of CK2α protein kinase is required for efficient replication of some HPV types. *PLoS Pathog.* 15:e1007788. doi: 10.1371/journal.ppat.1007788

Reinson, T., Toots, M., Kadaja, M., Pipitch, R., Allik, M., Ustav, E., et al. (2013). Engagement of the ATR-dependent DNA damage response at the human papillomavirus 18 replication centers during the initial amplification. *J. Virol.* 87, 951–964. doi: 10.1128/JVI.01943-12

Remm, M., Brain, R., and Jenkins, J. R. (1992). The E2 binding sites determine the efficiency of replication for the origin of human papillomavirus type 18. *Nucleic Acids Res.* 20, 6015–6021. doi: 10.1093/nar/20.22.6015

Sakakibara, N., Chen, D., and McBride, A. A. (2013). Papillomaviruses use recombination-dependent replication to vegetatively amplify their genomes in differentiated cells. *PLoS Pathog.* 9:e1003321. doi: 10.1371/journal.ppat.1003321

Sankovski, E., Mannik, A., Geimanen, J., Ustav, E., and Ustav, M. (2014). Mapping of betapapillomavirus human papillomavirus 5 transcription and characterization of viral-genome replication function. *J. Virol.* 88, 961–973. doi: 10.1128/JVI.01841-13

Sowd, G. A., Li, N. Y., and Fanning, E. (2013). ATM and ATR activities maintain replication fork integrity during SV40 chromatin replication. *PLoS Pathog.* 9:e1003283. doi: 10.1371/journal.ppat.1003283

Tattersall, P., and Ward, D. C. (1976). Rolling hairpin model for replication of parvovirus and linear chromosomal DNA. *Nature* 263, 106–109. doi: 10.1038/263106a0

Warburton, A., Redmond, C. J., Dooley, K. E., Fu, H., Gillison, M. L., Akagi, K., et al. (2018). HPV integration hijacks and multimerizes a cellular enhancer to generate a viral-cellular super-enhancer that drives high viral oncogene expression. *PLoS Genet.* 14:e1007179. doi: 10.1371/journal.pgen.1007179

Wawrzyniak, P., Plucienniczak, G., and Bartosik, D. (2017). The different faces of rolling-circle replication and its multifunctional initiator proteins. *Front. Microbiol.* 8:2353. doi: 10.3389/fmicb.2017.02353

Zou, H., and Rothstein, R. (1997). Holliday junctions accumulate in replication mutants via a RecA homolog-independent mechanism. *Cell* 90, 87–96. doi: 10.1016/S0092-8674(00)80316-5

12

Characterization of a Merkel Cell Polyomavirus-Positive Merkel Cell Carcinoma Cell Line CVG-1

Celestino Velásquez[1†], Yutaka Amako[1,2], Alexis Harold[1], Tuna Toptan[1,3], Yuan Chang[1,3] and Masahiro Shuda[1,2]*

[1] Cancer Virology Program, University of Pittsburgh Medical Center Hillman Cancer Center, Pittsburgh, PA, United States, [2] Department of Microbiology and Molecular Genetics, University of Pittsburgh, Pittsburgh, PA, United States, [3] Department of Pathology, University of Pittsburgh, Pittsburgh, PA, United States

***Correspondence:**
Masahiro Shuda
mas253@pitt.edu

†Present address:
Celestino Velásquez,
Department of Biology and Chemistry,
Oral Roberts University, Tulsa, OK,
United States*

Merkel cell polyomavirus (MCV) plays a causal role in ~80% of Merkel cell carcinomas (MCC). MCV is clonally integrated into the MCC tumor genome, which results in persistent expression of large T (LT) and small T (sT) antigen oncoproteins encoded by the early locus. In MCV-positive MCC tumors, LT is truncated by premature stop codons or deletions that lead to loss of the C-terminal origin binding (OBD) and helicase domains important for replication. The N-terminal Rb binding domain remains intact. MCV-positive cell lines derived from MCC explants have been valuable tools to study the molecular mechanism of MCV-induced Merkel cell carcinogenesis. Although all cell lines have integrated MCV and express truncated LT antigens, the molecular sizes of the LT proteins differ between cell lines. The copy number of integrated viral genome also varies across cell lines, leading to significantly different levels of viral protein expression. Nevertheless, these cell lines share phenotypic similarities in cell morphology, growth characteristics, and neuroendocrine marker expression. Several low-passage MCV-positive MCC cell lines have been established since the identification of MCV. We describe a new MCV-positive MCV cell line, CVG-1, with features distinct from previously reported cell lines. CVG-1 tumor cells grow in more discohesive clusters in loose round cell suspension, and individual cells show dramatic size heterogeneity. It is the first cell line to encode an MCV sT polymorphism resulting in a unique leucine (L) to proline (P) substitution mutation at amino acid 144. CVG-1 possesses a LT truncation pattern near identical to that of MKL-1 cells differing by the last two C-terminal amino acids and also shows an LT protein expression level similar to MKL-1. Viral T antigen knockdown reveals that, like other MCV-positive MCC cell lines, CVG-1 requires T antigen expression for cell proliferation.

Keywords: Merkel cell polyomavirus, MCV, Merkel cell carcinoma, MCC, cell line

INTRODUCTION

Merkel cell carcinoma (MCC) is an aggressive skin cancer associated with immunosuppression and ultraviolet exposure (Lemos and Nghiem, 2007; Heath et al., 2008). The incidence of MCC is approximately 1,500 cases per year in the United States, which has increased threefold over the past two decades. The discovery of Merkel cell polyomavirus (MCV) in 2008 from MCC lead to a more precise understanding of the pathogenesis of these tumors (Feng et al., 2008).

Merkel cell polyomavirus was discovered by digital transcriptome sequencing of MCC and was found to be clonally integrated in 70–80% of these tumors. While the viral integration sites in the tumor genome are random (Feng et al., 2008; Sastre-Garau et al., 2009; Martel-Jantin et al., 2012), MCC tumor cells express the viral T antigen early gene. The MCV early locus is essential for virus replication and encodes four viral proteins: (1) large T (LT), (2) small T (sT), and (3) 57kT, which are expressed by alternative splicing mechanisms (Shuda et al., 2008), and (4) alternate frame of the large T open reading frame (ALTO) produced through alternative translation initiation (Carter et al., 2013). The MCV LT protein directly replicates the viral genome through its carboxyl (C)-terminal DNA origin binding domain (OBD) and DNA helicase activities, while sT enhances viral DNA replication by stabilizing LT (Kwun et al., 2009, 2013). The functions of 57kT and ALTO in the viral lifecycle have not been determined. Viral sequence analyses in MCC consistently show that tumor-derived LT antigens contain mutations that prematurely truncate the C-terminal helicase domain, while preserving the N-terminal tumor suppressor targeting domains for Rb-binding and DnaJ chaperone-binding functions (Grundhoff and Fischer, 2015; Wendzicki et al., 2015; DeCaprio, 2017). Most MCC tissues, if not all, express the truncated LT and intact sT proteins, whereas 57kT and ALTO have never been detected in tumor tissues (Shuda et al., 2009; Rodig et al., 2012).

These viral features in MCC tissues – clonal integration, LT helicase ablation, and T antigen expression - are also observed in the MCV-positive MCC cell lines. Since the first description of the MCV-positive MKL-1 cell line (Rosen et al., 1987; Shuda et al., 2008), 16 additional cell lines, including MKL-2, WaGa, BroLi, LoKe (Houben et al., 2010, 2012), MCCL-3, MCCL-11, MCCL-12 (Fischer et al., 2010), PeTa, AIDo, WoWe, HeRo, KaRi (Houben et al., 2013), MS-1 (Guastafierro et al., 2013), UM-MCC13, UM-MCC29, and UM-MCC565 (Verhaegen et al., 2014) have been established. The complete viral sequence has been only determined in nine MCC cell lines. The use of MCV-positive cell lines in T antigen knockdown studies revealed that T antigen expression is essential for cell proliferation in most MCV-positive MCC cell lines, consistent with the oncogenic role of T antigens in Merkel cell carcinogenesis (Houben et al., 2010).

Both MCC and small-cell lung carcinoma (SCLC) are neuroendocrine tumors, and MCC cell lines share cytological and histochemical similarities (Carney et al., 1985; Leonard et al., 1993). According to SCLC cell line classification, MCC cell lines can be divided into two groups: (1) classic and (2) variant, as defined by their immunohistochemical expression of markers including neuron-specific enolase and chromogranin A. In addition, cell lines can be classified further into four subtypes (type I-IV) based on growth morphology, colony shape, and aggregation (Leonard et al., 1995). Interestingly, with rare exceptions (Fischer et al., 2010), most MCV-positive MCC cell lines identified to date conform to the classic type with high neuroendocrine marker expression and exhibit type III morphology in which cells grow in loosely aggregated clusters. Gene expression analyses in MCV-positive MCC cell lines demonstrated that classic virus-positive cell lines such as MKL-1 and WaGa mirror the transcriptome profile of MCC tumors (Daily et al., 2015).

Despite their similarities, MCV-positive MCC cell lines show variability in morphology, growth characteristics, and tumorigenicity. Mouse xenograft studies using four MCV-positive MCC cell lines have demonstrated significant differences in the latency required for grafted tumor cell lines to grow (Dresang et al., 2013). In the same study, Dresang et al. also showed that response to the survivin inhibitor YM155 varies between cell lines (Dresang et al., 2013). While individual cancer cell lines possess unique host genetic mutations, phenotypic differences seen in the cell lines may be dependent, in part, on viral factors including the copy number of integrated viral genome and viral T antigen expression levels (Houben et al., 2010; Guastafierro et al., 2013). Further, each MCC tumor and MCV-positive cell line contains unique LT truncation mutations that produce LT proteins of different sizes.

Here, we describe the characteristics of a novel early passage MCV-positive MCC cell line, CVG-1, derived from a metastatic MCC explant and that exhibits LT truncation pattern and integrated viral copy number similar to that of the previously established MKL-1. While we found a unique leucine (L) to proline (P) missense mutation in the CVG-1-derived sT, this substitution mutation did not affect the transformation activity of CVG-1 sT in rodent fibroblasts. In fact, CVG-1 cell proliferation shows oncogenic addiction to viral T antigen expression similar to other MCV-positive MCC cell lines. Despite these similarities in virological features, a striking difference in tumor cell morphology was seen in CVG-1. Thus, establishment of CVG-1 not only extends the repertoire of MCV-positive cell lines but also serves as a tool to investigate host cell factors that contribute to the variations in growth morphology and tumorigenicity observed in other MCC cell lines.

MATERIALS AND METHODS

Tissues and Cell Lines

Metastatic MCC to the left cervical lymph nodes was surgically resected from a 70-year-old female with a previous history of MCC. After surgical resection, the tissue [Collaborative Human Tissue Network (CHTN)] was placed in the RPMI1640 medium. All specimens were tested under University of Pittsburgh Institutional Review Board-approved guidelines. Patient informed consent was obtained by the participating CHTN hospitals in accordance with the Declaration of Helsinki. Tumor tissue was minced to disaggregate tumor cells. To adapt cells to cell culture, cells were initially cultured in the RPMI medium containing 20% heat-inactivated fetal bovine serum (FBS), 0.01% penicillin/streptomycin, 0.01% fungizone, 0.01% insulin–transferrin–selenium, 50 μM bathocuproine disulfate, and 1 mM L-cysteine. After 9 days, cells were transferred into RPMI medium containing 10% FBS and non-essential amino acids (NEAA, Mediatech). CVG-1 cells of passage <10 were cryopreserved in 10% DMSO in FBS. The experimental analyses in this study were carried out using cells at low passage (<40).

Other MCC cell lines (MKL-1, MKL-2, and MS-1) were cultured in the RPMI medium supplemented with 10% FBS and NEAA.

Immunohistochemistry

Formalin-fixed paraffin-embedded tumor tissue was stained according to a previously published protocol (Shuda et al., 2009). Briefly, slides were deparaffinized in xylene and rehydrated through a series of ethanol solutions. Endogenous peroxidase activity was blocked with 3% hydrogen peroxide for 15 min. Epitope retrieval was performed using 1 mM EDTA buffer, pH 8.0, at 125°C for 3 min and 90°C for 15 s in an antigen retrieval chamber (Decloaking Chamber, Biocare Medical). Following blocking with serum-free Protein Block (Dako), MCV large T antigen was immunostained with mouse monoclonal antibody CM2B4 (1 μg/ml) diluted in antibody buffer (1% BSA, 0.1% gelatin, 0.5% Triton-X, 0.05% sodium azide in PBS, pH 7.4) for 1 h at room temperature. After extensive rinsing in 1X tris-buffered saline solution (TBS), sections were incubated with mouse Envision Polymer (Dako) for 30 min at room temperature, reacted with diaminobenzidine (Dako), and counterstained with hematoxylin (Dako).

Immunoblotting

Cells were lysed in RIPA buffer (50 mM Tris–HCl, 150 mM NaCl, 0.1% SDS, 0.5% Triton X, 0.5% sodium deoxycholate, pH 7.0) containing proteinase inhibitor cocktail (Roche). Lysates were sonicated to shear genomic DNA, and protein concentration was determined by the colorimetric DC-Protein Assay kit (Bio-Rad). After protein lysates were mixed with Laemmli buffer and heat-denatured, 30 and 50 μg of total protein were resolved in 12% SDS-polyacrylamide gel for LT and sT detection, respectively. MCV LT protein was detected by CM2B4 (Shuda et al., 2009). MCV sT was detected by CM5E1 (Shuda et al., 2011; **Figure 2C**) or by CM8E6 (Kwun et al., 2009; **Figures 3B,C**).

MCV Genomic Sequencing

Genomic DNA was extracted from CVG-1 cells using standard phenol-chloroform extraction methods. The MCV DNA in CVG-1 cells was then amplified using polymerase chain reaction (PCR) primer sets (Contigl to Contigl3 primers) as described previously (Feng et al., 2008). PCR reactions in this study were performed by Q5 Hot Start High-FIdelity DNA polymerase (NEB). Sanger sequencing was performed by MCLAB (San Francisco, CA, United States).

Viral Copy Number Analysis and Quantitative Reverse Transcription (RT)-Polymerase Chain Reaction (PCR)

Subcellular fractionation was performed to isolate nuclei from MCC cells prior to genomic DNA extraction by Proteinase K/SDS buffer (10 mM Tris/HCl pH 8.0, 100 mM NaCl, 25 mM EDTA, 0.5% SDS, 0.1 mg/mL Proteinase K). After overnight incubation at 50°C, 100 ng/mL of RNaseA was added to the lysates and incubated for 1 h at 37°C. Extracted DNA was further purified by phenol-chloroform extraction and ethanol precipitation prior to quantitative PCR (qPCR). The obtained genomic DNA was dissolved in water and quantified by UV-Vis spectrophotometry. qPCR was performed to obtain absolute quantification using the aforementioned total T antigen primer set. In order to determine the absolute copy number, a dilution series of plasmid MCV-HF was used as a reference template DNA (1 ng MCV-HF plasmid is equivalent to 1.13×10^8 molecules).

Total cellular RNA was extracted and purified from MCV-positive MCC cells using Purezol (Bio-Rad) per manufacturer's instructions, treated with RNase-free DNaseI (NEB), and extracted again with Purezol reagent prior to cDNA synthesis. For cDNA synthesis, 500 ng of total RNA was subjected to first strand synthesis using the iScript cDNA synthesis kit (Bio-Rad). Subsequently, real-time PCR was performed using PowerUP SYBR Green Master mix to quantify total T antigen mRNA (sense: 5′-GCT CCT AAT TGT TAT GGC AAC AT-3′ and antisense: 5′-CAA CAT CCC TCT GAT GAA AGC-3′), sT mRNA (sense: 5′-TCC TTG GGA AGA ATA TGG AAC T-3′ and antisense: 5′-GCG AGA CAA CTT ACA GCT AAT AC-3′), and 18S rRNA (sense: 5′-GGA CAC GGA CAG GAT TGA CA-3′ and antisense: 5′-ACC CAC GGA ATC GAG AAA GA-3′). Real-time PCR reactions were triplicated for each sample and performed on the QuantiStudio 3 system (Applied Biosystems). The determined threshold cycle (Ct) values were used to calculate the mRNA abundance relative to CVG-1 using the delta-delta Ct method. The Ct values of 18S rRNA were used as reference.

Transformation Assays

Rat-1 cell transformation assays were performed as described previously (Shuda et al., 2011). For doxycycline-inducible transgene expression, pLenti TRE.MCS EF.Puro-2A-rTet was modified from TLCV2 by removing the U6 promoter-stuffer fragment by *Kpn*I and *EcoR*I digestion, followed by displacing Cas9-2A-eGFP fragment with double strand DNA linker containing unique restriction sites using *Age*I and *Nhe*I restriction sites. TLCV2 was a gift from Adam Karpf (Addgene #87360). Then, codon-optimized wild-type MCV sT and the amino acid substitution mutants including L114P, LSD, as well as L142A were inserted into pLenti TRE.MCS EF.Puro-2A-rTet by unique *Age*I and *Sbf*I restriction sites. For lentivirus production, 293FT cells (Invitrogen) were transfected with pLenti TRE MCV sT, psPax2, and pMD2.G using Lipofectamine 2000 (Invitrogen). The medium was changed at 12 h after transfection, and the lentivirus produced in the culture supernatant was harvested at 72 h after transfection.

For the foci formation assay, Rat-1 cells were seeded in 6-well plate and infected with 150 μL of lentiviruses encoding multiple MCV sT variants. At day 3 post-infection, fresh growth medium with or without 0.5 μg/mL of doxycycline was added. Rat-1 cells were cultured for 11 days, and cell culture medium was refreshed every 3 days to maintain transgene expression. Cells were stained by 0.5% crystal violet to visualize transformation-associated foci. For soft agar colony formation assays, Rat-1 cells transduced with the aforementioned lentivirus constructs were treated with puromycin (3 μg/mL). After puromycin-resistant cells were selected, 1.0 mL (1.25×10^4) of the cells containing 0.3% noble agar (Sigma) was overlaid on the 2 mL of growth medium containing 0.6% agar. Cells were cultured for 2 weeks to observe colony formation in the soft agar. Colony numbers were counted under a microscope. The data is presented as mean ± standard deviation (SD) ($N = 3$).

shRNA Knockdown of the Viral T Antigen and Cell Proliferation Assays

A modified version of the enhanced 7SK Pol III promoter (e7SK) was used as described previously (Haraguchi et al., 2016). In order to express short-hairpin (sh) RNA under the strong e7SK promoter, we synthesized a DNA fragment of the e7SK promoter (gBlock, IDT) and inserted it into the pENTR1A vector (Addgene plasmid #17398) to generate the pENTR e7SK-Pro construct using *Dra*I and *Eco*RV restriction sites. Oligonucleotides used to generate previously described shpanT (5′-CCG GAA GAG AGG CTC TCT GCA AGC TCT CGA GAG CTT GCA GAG AGC CTC TCT TTT TTG-3′ and 5′-AAT TCA AAA AAG AGA GGC TCT CTG CAA GCT CTC GAG AGC TTG CAG AGA GCC TCT CTT-3′) or control shRNA (5′-CCG GCC TAA GGT TAA GTC GCC CTC GCT CGA GCG AGG GCG ACT TAA CCT TAG GTT TTT G-3′ and 5′-AAT TCA AAA ACC TAA GGT TAA GTC GCC CTC GCT CGA GCG AGG GCG ACT TAA CCT TAG G-3′) (Houben et al., 2010) were annealed and inserted into pENTR e7SK-Pro using *Age*I and *Eco*RI restriction sites to generate pENTR1A-e7SK-shpanT and pENTR1A-e7SK-shCtrl, respectively. These entry vectors were inserted into the pLenti Dest-puro lentiviral vector using LR-clonase II (Invitrogen) to produce pLenti e7SK-shpanT-puro and pLenti e7SK-shCtrl-puro. pLenti Dest-puro was constructed from pMuLE Lenti Dest-Neo (Addgene plasmid #62178) by replacing the neomycin phosphotransferase gene with the puromycin N-acetyltransferase gene containing *Sbf*I and *Xho*I restriction sites. Lentivirus production was performed as described in transformation assays section. pENTR1A no ccdB (w48-1) and pLenti Dest Neo were a gift from Eric Campeau and Paul Kaufman and from Ian Frew, respectively.

For cell proliferation assays, CVG-1 cells were transduced with e7SK-shpanT-puro and pLenti e7SK-shCtrl-puro lentiviruses in the presence of 1 μg/mL polybrene for 2 days and selected for 4 days by puromycin treatment (1 μg/mL) as previously described (Houben et al., 2010). At day 6 post-transduction, 2.5×0^4 cells were seeded in a 96-well plate (day 0). Cell proliferation was measured using WST-8 (Wako) at days 1, 3, 5, 7, 9, and 11. OD values were normalized by values from day 1. The WST-8 formazan product was measured at 440 nm with a reference filter at 600 nm using a Synergy 2™ Multi-Mode Microplate Reader (BioTek).

RESULTS

Establishment of the MCV-Positive MCC CVG-1 Cell Line

A small piece of the metastatic MCC tissue used to establish MCC cell line CVG-1, was formalin-fixed and embedded in paraffin for hematoxylin/eosin (H&E) staining and immunohistochemistry. MCC tumor cell generally exhibit cytological features of monomorphic small round cells with high nuclear to cytoplasmic ratio. However, H&E staining of CVG-1 showed a heterogeneous cell population accentuated by large tumor cells (**Figure 1A**, Top panel). Immunohistochemistry using the MCV LT antibody (CM2B4) showed strong nuclear staining in both large and small tumor cells (**Figure 1A**, Bottom panel) confirming the presence of virus in each tumor cell.

Similar to the morphologic features of the parental MCC tumor, the CVG-1 cell line also displayed tumor cell size variation, having a mixture of large and small round cells (**Figure 1B**). We attempted to single-cell subclone large and small CVG-1 cells to demonstrate that both cells are LT-positive MCC but were unsuccessful. Nevertheless, since MCC tumor tissues are uniformly positive for LT protein, both large and small cells are likely to be MCV infected. CVG-1 cells grow in loose clusters in culture, whereas most MCC cells including MKL-1, MKL-2,

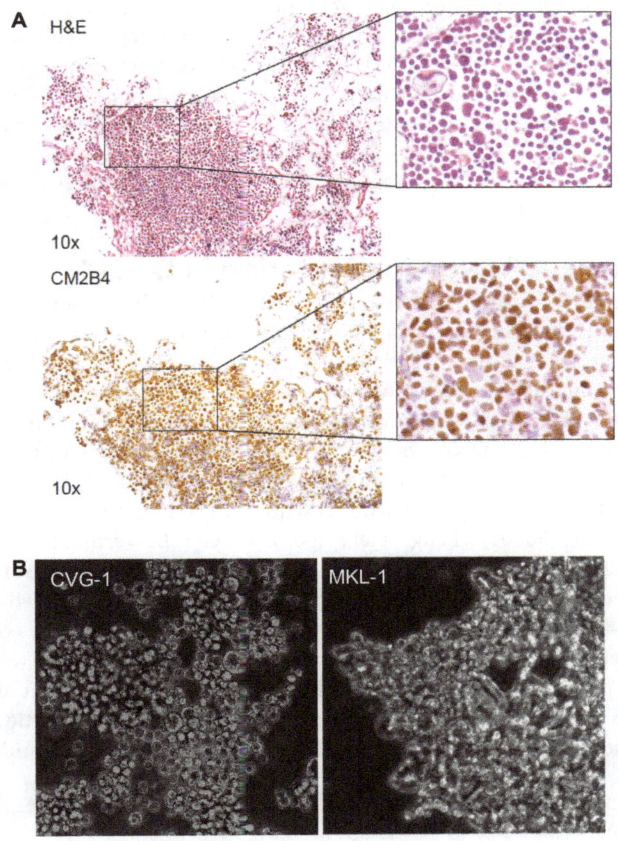

FIGURE 1 | Establishment of the Merkel cell polyomavirus (MCV)-positive CVG-1 cell line from metastatic Merkel cell carcinomas (MCC). **(A)** Hematoxylin/eosin (H&E) staining (top) and MCV large T (LT) immunohistochemistry (bottom) of the metastatic MCC tissue that the CVG-1 cell line was established from MCV LT-positive MCC tumor cells (brown nuclei) demonstrate significant variation in cell size (inset). **(B)** Morphology of the CVG-1 cell line under phase contrast microscopy. CVG-1 exhibits cell size variation and a small round appearance resembling lymphoid cell lines, as opposed to other MCV-positive MCC cell lines, such as MKL-1, which usually grow in loosely aggregated clusters.

and MS-1 grow in large, tightly cohesive aggregates (Guastafierro et al., 2013; **Figure 1B**). CVG-1 cells make contact with each other, but their contact involves only a small segment of the periphery of each cell.

MCV Copy Number and Viral T Antigen Gene Expression in CVG-1

To determine the sequence of the MCV genome in CVG-1 cells, we amplified the viral DNA from CVG-1 using 13 pairs of contiguous primer sets that span the entire region of the MCV genome (Feng et al., 2008). The expected DNA fragments were successfully amplified with all primer sets used, indicating that the whole viral genome is present in CVG-1 cells. Next, the viral genome copy number was determined by qPCR using the previously characterized MKL-1, MKL-2, and MS-1 cell lines for comparison. CVG-1 contains the highest copy number of integrated MCV genome similar to MKL-1 (approximately 7 copies per cell), whereas MS-1 and MKL-2 contained relatively low copy numbers of MCV genome (4 copies and 2 copies per cell, respectively) (**Table 1**). Although genome copy numbers are similar between CVG-1 and MKL-1, analyses using qRT-PCR demonstrated that total T antigen mRNA and sT mRNA expression levels approximately 2.5-fold higher in CVG-1 than in MKL-1 (**Figure 2A**). MKL-2 expressed the lowest levels of T antigen mRNAs, consistent with previous results (Guastafierro et al., 2013; **Figure 2A**).

Viral LT Truncation Mutation in CVG-1

Merkel cell carcinoma tissue-derived MCV harbors mutations that prematurely truncate the DNA helicase domain of LT (Shuda et al., 2008). These truncation mutations have also been identified in MCV-positive MCC cell lines (Guastafierro et al., 2013). Thus, we sought to map the LT truncation mutations in CVG-1. MCV DNA was amplified by the contiguous primers from genomic DNA extracted from CVG-1 cells, and the PCR products were subjected to direct sequencing (GenBank accession no. MH136801) (Feng et al., 2008). CVG-1 LT terminated at nucleotide position 1617 as a result of an A–T transversion mutation, generating a premature termination codon. In the DNA sequencing, while the CVG-1 cell contains ~3.6 copies of integrated viral genomes per haploid cell (**Table 1**), there was no presence of multiple peaks/mixed signals, suggesting that all the copies of integrated MCV possess the identical truncation mutation. On the other hand, MKL-1 LT terminates at nucleotide position 1618 due to a 46-bp deletion that causes a frameshift. This frameshift mutation results in the addition of two unrelated amino acids prior to the termination codon. As their coding regions suggest, both CVG-1 and MKL-1 LTs are composed of 330 amino acids (**Figure 2B**), and the only difference between these was found to be two amino acids at their C-terminal ends—Ser-Asn for CVG-1 and Lys-Leu for MKL-1. As observed in the MKL-1 LT, the premature truncation mutation found in the CVG-1 LT resulted in the complete deletion of the OBD and helicase domains without the affecting Rb-binding domain (**Figure 2B**). The CVG-1 and MKL-1 cell lines are the first pair of cell lines that express the same length LT protein out of the nine MCV-positive MCC cell lines characterized to date. Next, we determined that the LT genetic truncation in CVG-1 has the same migration pattern as MKL-1 in SDS–PAGE (**Figure 2C**). Consistent with the LT truncation pattern observed in the MKL-1 cell line, the CVG-1 LT migrated at 50 kDa. The mobility of CVG-1 LT, however, was marginally slower than that of MKL-1. Furthermore, LT levels in CVG-1 were slightly lower than those in MKL-1, whereas the T antigen mRNA levels in MKL-1 were higher than those in MKL-1 cells (**Figure 2A**).

CVG-1 contains a unique missense mutation in the sT coding sequence (nucleotide position 536) that generates a Leu(L)-to-Pro(P) substitution at the amino acid position 114 of the sT protein. In the nine MCV-positive MCC cell lines in which the viral sequence has been defined, only one amino acid substitution has been found in three cell lines (MKL-2, PeTa, and WoWe), all at position 20 of the sT protein (Ala (A) to Ser(S)). This position corresponds to a common exon1 of the T antigen gene, and thus, both LT and sT proteins are affected by the A20S substitution. Thus, L114P is a unique MCV sT amino acid substitution found in CVG-1. In contrast to LT, sT protein expression is relatively comparable across all the cell lines tested, irrespective of differences in mRNA expression (**Figure 2C**). These results suggest that LT and sT protein expression may be regulated at the post-transcriptional level.

While no precise correlation was observed between T antigen mRNA and protein expression, MKL-1 and CVG-1 cells harboring higher copy numbers of the integrated MCV genome (**Table 1**) tend to express higher LT protein than MKL-2 and MS-1 cell lines, which contain lower copy numbers of viral genome (**Figure 2C**). We also confirmed protein expression of MCC marker CK20 by immunoblot. Consistent with previous results (Houben et al., 2010), all cell lines including CVG-1 express similar levels of CK20 except for MKL-1 which expresses significantly lower levels of CK20.

TABLE 1 | MCV copy numbers in MCV-positive MCC cell lines.

Cell line	Absolute copy number/ng nuclear DNA	Copy number per cell (*N*)*
CVG-1	1007.6 ± 30.1	3.63 ± 0.11
MKL-1	1014.6 ± 72.6	3.65 ± 0.26
MKL-2	280.2 ± 17.0	1.01 ± 0.06
MS-1	553.6 ± 18.3	1.99 ± 0.07

**Merkel cell polyomavirus (MCV) copy number per genome was calculated based on the assumption that 100 ng of nuclear DNA from merkel cell carcinomas (MCC) cells contains 27,777 copies of single human genome (3.6 pg per haploid cell).*

Transforming Activity of CVG-1 sT With L114P Missense Mutation

Merkel cell polyomavirus sT is the major MCV oncoprotein that causes loss of contact inhibition and confers anchorage-independent growth capabilities in immortalized rodent fibroblasts (Shuda et al., 2011). This viral oncoprotein is a well-conserved protein across different isolates. In CVG-1 cells, we found a unique mutation that gives rise to a L114P amino acid substitution in the sT specific region. To date, this is the

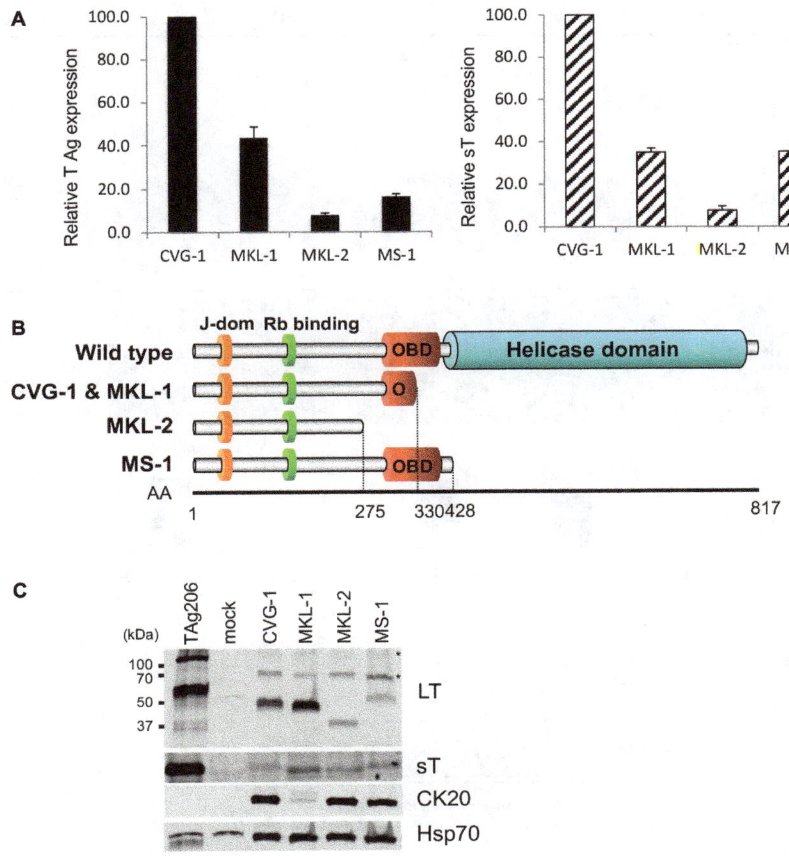

FIGURE 2 | Expression of truncated MCV LT and small T (sT) antigens in CVG-1. **(A)** qRT-PCR analysis of T antigen transcripts in CVG-1 and three previously described MCV-positive MCC cell lines. The levels of total T antigen transcripts and sT transcript expressed in MCC cell lines were analyzed by the delta-delta Ct method to compare abundance of total T antigen (Left) and small T antigen transcripts (Right) relative to CVG-1 cells. Ct values from 18S rRNA amplification were utilized as an internal control. **(B)** Schematic representation of the LT truncation mutation in CVG-1, showing the ablation of the entire helicase domain. **(C)** Immunoblotting analysis of MCV LT and sT protein expression. MCV LT and sT protein expression was detected by CM2B4 and CM5E1 antibodies, respectively. CM2B4 detects full length LT (~110 kDa) and multiply spliced 57kT (~60 kDa) proteins in a positive control prepared from 293FT cells transfected with genomic MCV T antigen expression vector (TAg206), but not in a mock-transfected negative control. Cytokeratin 20 (CK20) expression was also detected as a marker of MCC. Hsp70 was used as a loading control. Asterisks indicate non-specific reactivities of CM2B4 antibody.

second substitution mutation identified in the sT protein in MCV-positive MCC cell lines. In a previous study, we found that the large T stabilization domain (LSD), a domain critical for the transformation activity of sT, is localized to amino acids 91–95 of the sT protein and is part of a disordered loop structure based on the predicted MCV sT structure (Kwun et al., 2013, 2015). Because the L114P mutation is in close proximity to LSD and proline is an amino acid that introduces sharp kinks in the polypeptide backbone, we wondered whether this newly identified sT mutation affects CVG-1 sT transformation activity. We used a previously described rodent cell transformation assay (Shuda et al., 2011). Rat-1 cells were transduced with lentiviruses expressing wild type sT and various sT mutants in the presence of doxycycline (500 ng/mL). Induction of L114P sT mutant expression in cells resulted in dense foci formation similar to that observed in cells expressing wild-type MCV sT and L142A PP2A-binding mutant, whereas cells expressing the non-transforming LSD mutant LSD_{A91-95} did not form dense foci (**Figure 3A**, Top). In parallel with the foci formation assay, we performed a soft agar colony formation assay and observed anchorage-independent growth in cells expressing the L114P sT mutant (**Figure 3A**, Bottom). Colony size and numbers were comparable between L114P and the other transforming MCV sT variants tested, suggesting that the L114P mutation does not affect the transforming activity of MCV sT. Comparable sT protein expression in lentivirus-transduced cells was confirmed by immunoblotting (**Figure 3B**).

CVG-1 Requires Viral T Antigen for Cell Proliferation

While most MCV-positive MCC cell lines established to date require viral T antigen oncogene expression for proliferation, T antigen expression is dispensable only in one MCV-positive MCC cell line, LoKe (Houben et al., 2012). We examined whether CVG-1 also requires T antigen expression by using shRNA panT1

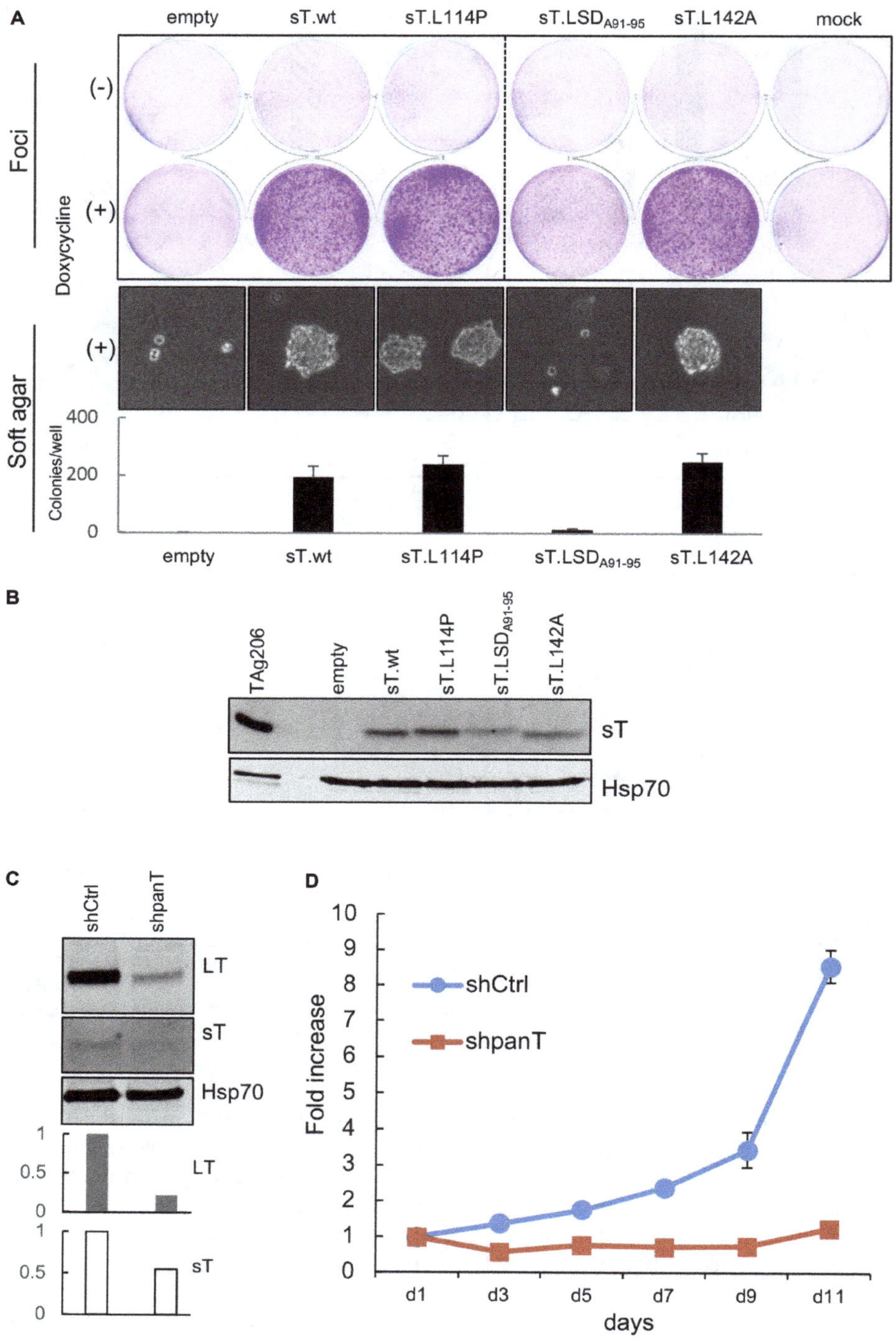

FIGURE 3 | CVG-1 encodes transforming MCV sT and requires viral T antigen expression for cell proliferation. **(A)** Transformation activities of MCV sT L114P substitution mutant expressed in CVG-1. Foci-formation assay was performed in Rat-1 cells transduced with doxycycline-inducible lentiviral vectors that encode MCV sT and various substitution mutants in the presence or absence of 0.5 μg/mL doxycycline (Top). Soft agar colony formation assay was also performed in the presence of 0.5 μg/mL doxycycline (Bottom). The graph shows the average ± standard deviation (SD) of the number of soft agar colonies counted in triplicate wells. **(B)** Immunoblotting analysis confirming MCV sT protein expression in Rat-1 cells. A positive control lysates used in **Figure 2B** was loaded in the first lane. sT was detected by the CM8E6 antibody. Hsp70 was used as a loading control. **(C)** CVG-1 requires MCV T antigen expression for cell proliferation. CVG-1 cells were transduced with shRNA lentiviral vector targeting both LT and sT (shpanT) and control shRNA (shCtrl). After transduced cells were selected by puromycin, knockdown activity was confirmed by immunoblotting for LT, sT, and Hsp70 proteins. Graphs demonstrate knockdown activities of sT relative to shCtrl quantified for LT and sT proteins by LI-COR immunoblotting. T antigen protein expression was normalized by the Hsp70 protein expression. **(D)** CVG-1 cell proliferation requires viral T antigen expression. After knockdown was confirmed, cells were seeded in a 96-well plate, and the proliferation was assessed using the WST-8 assay.

(shpanT) targeting common T antigen exon1 and control shRNA (shCtrl) (Shuda et al., 2011). After shRNA-transduced CVG-1 cells were selected by puromycin, knockdown was examined by quantitative LI-COR immunoblotting. Expression of LT and sT proteins in CVG-1 cells was reduced by 79% and by 46%, respectively, by knockdown with shpanT, as compared to cells transduced with shCtrl (**Figure 3C**). In addition, cell proliferation assays performed with WST-8 showed that T antigen knockdown by shpanT completely ablated the cell proliferation activity of CVG-1 cells (**Figure 3D**). Thus, similar to most MCV-positive cell lines, tumorigenicity of CVG-1 also depends on the viral T antigen expression.

DISCUSSION

Here we report the establishment of a new, early passage MCV-positive MCC cell line CVG-1. As seen in other MCV-positive MCC cell lines MKL-1(Shuda et al., 2008) and MCCL12 (Fischer et al., 2010), CVG-1 harbors multiple copies of the integrated MCV genome with a uniform LT truncation mutation, which may have resulted from the multiplication of a mutated single genome by rolling circle DNA replication (Starrett et al., 2017). Unlike most other MCV-positive MCC cell lines that grow in clusters, CVG-1 cells remain more disaggregated, and trypsin digestion was not required to isolate single cells. The CVG-1 cell line uniquely shows remarkable cell-size variation including large cells, even though MCC is defined as a small cell neoplasia. While we still do not know the specific cause of the size variation in CVG-1 cells, many type of cancers display morphological, proliferative, and functional heterogeneity, which arise from genetic mutations or cancer cell differentiation seen in cancer initiating cells or cancer stem cells. The former could be caused by the MCV sT antigen, which induces aneuploidy by compromising cell cycle checkpoint functions (Kwun et al., 2017). SCLC, another neuroendocrine cancer composed of cells capable of differentiating into neuronal and endocrine lineages, displays comparable morphologic heterogeneity and a gene expression signature similar to MCC (Salcido et al., 2010; Codony-Servat et al., 2016). Thus, self-renewal and cancer cell differentiation may also contribute to MCC tumorigenicity and give rise to morphological heterogeneity.

While the morphology of CVG-1 was unique among previously reported MCV-positive MCC cell lines, CVG-1 tumorigenicity is still dependent on MCV T antigen expression as in other MCV-positive cell lines. Out of seven cell lines tested for T antigen knockdown, only the LoKe cell line does not require T antigen expression for growth (Houben et al., 2012). Characterization of LoKe demonstrated that tumor cells harbor an Rb gene deletion that compensates for the oncogenic function of MCV LT expression in MCC (Houben et al., 2012; Hesbacher et al., 2016). However, it has been shown that Rb gene deletions/mutations are rare in MCV-positive MCC (Gonzalez-Vela et al., 2017; Harms et al., 2017). Thus, it remains likely that most MCV-positive MCC cell lines including CVG-1 require MCV T antigen expression to maintain their tumorigenicity.

The cell of origin in MCC remains unknown. It has been thought to be the epidermal Merkel cells based on the similarities in ultrastructure and gene expression between normal Merkel cells and MCC (Tang and Toker, 1978; Green et al., 1984; Battifora and Silva, 1986) However, it has recently been proposed that the cellular origin of MCV-positive cells may not be the Merkel cells (Zur Hausen et al., 2013; Sauer et al., 2017; Sunshine et al., 2018). Liu et al. (2016) have shown that MCV can infect dermal fibroblasts *in vitro*, but infection of Merkel cells has never been confirmed. Merkel cells are epidermal cells localized in the basal layer of the epidermis. While Merkel cells originate in the epidermis (Van Keymeulen et al., 2009), cutaneous MCCs typically involve only the dermis, and MCCs that develop in the epidermis are rare (<10%) (Smith et al., 1993). Recently, Verhaegen et al. (2017) reported transgenic mice that develop MCC-like tumors by expressing MCV sT and a Merkel cell lineage factor Atoh1 under the keratin 5 (KRT5) promoter, the activity of which is restricted to the basal layer of the epidermis (Ramirez et al., 1994). Interestingly, the pathogenesis of MCC-like tumors in this mouse model was restricted to epidermal layers, consistent with MCC-*in situ* or Merkel cell hyperplasia (McFalls et al., 2017). These data suggest the posibility that most MCV-positive dermal MCCs may originate from non-Merkel cells while MCC-*in situ*, which is confined to the epidermis, may arise from Merkel cells (Ferringer et al., 2005).

Since an animal model that mimics dermal MCC carcinogenesis has not been developed, MCC cell lines are useful tools to study the cellular origin of MCC. It has been shown that SV40 T antigen and human papilloma virus E6/E7 oncoproteins can reversibly transform primary human hepatocytes and human pancreatic duct epithelial cells without affecting normal diploid status (Kobayashi et al., 2000; Inagawa et al., 2014). The MCV-positive MCCs usually contain fewer genetic mutations and sustain normal karyotypes when compared to virus negative MCCs (Harms et al., 2017). Thus, some MCC cell lines may preserve normal genetic components that allow tumor cells to redifferentiate into untransformed, post-mitotic state cells with inhibition of T antigen expression. While most MCV-positive MCC cell lines become arrested after T antigen knockdown, a portion of cells commit non-apoptotic cell death as seen in MKL-1 (Houben et al., 2010). In early-passage cell lines like CVG-1 and MS-1 cells, however, many cells remain viable after T antigen knockdown and are arrested in G0/G1 (unpublished observation). Further molecular and cellular analyses in these early passage cell lines may lead to the identification of host genetic or functional features that represent the cellular origin of MCC.

Studies using MCC cell lines have revealed critical oncogenic pathways regulated by sT and LT. A recent study demonstrated that MCV sT binds to L-Myc and the EP400 histone acetyltransferase complex to activate L-Myc-mediated gene expression in MCC cells critical for MCC cell proliferation (Cheng et al., 2017). MCV LT expression in MCC activates the genes downstream of the E2F transcription factor by inhibiting the function of Rb through its LxCxE Rb-binding domain (Hesbacher et al., 2016). MCV-positive MCC is a unique cancer that has a gene expression signature similar to neuroendocrine Merkel cells. Because MCV T antigens alone are not sufficient to transform normal human fibroblasts (Cheng et al., 2017), MCC-specific oncogenic factors that are amplified in MCC such as L-Myc, may also play important roles in MCV-induced MCC carcinogenesis (Paulson et al., 2009; Cheng et al., 2017). Thus, MCC cell lines are essential tools to study the interplay between viral T antigens and MCC-specific host cell factors.

CONCLUSION

We established a new, early passage MCV-positive MCC cell line CVG-1 from a patient with metastatic MCC. CVG-1 displays different morphologic features from other MCV-positive MCC cell lines, but nevertheless requires MCV T antigen for cell proliferation. While CVG-1 sT antigen contains a unique missense mutation, the mutant sT demonstrated similar transformation activity to prototypic sT in rodent cells. CVG-1 shows similarities to MKL-1 in viral copy numbers and LT truncation patterns. Further analyses of CVG-1 and MKL-1 may lead to the identification of critical host factors beyond the viral T antigen that contribute to the variations observed in MCC cell lines.

AUTHOR CONTRIBUTIONS

CV, YC, and MS established the CVG-1 cell line. MS conceived and designed the experiments. YA performed the qPCR experiments. MS performed the sequencing experiments. YA, AH, and MS performed the immunoblot and cell transformation experiments. TT performed the immunohistochemistry. MS, YA, and YC analyzed the data. MS, YC, CV, and YA wrote the paper.

ACKNOWLEDGMENTS

We thank Cailyn Hall for her technical assistance.

REFERENCES

Battifora, H., and Silva, E. G. (1986). The use of antikeratin antibodies in the immunohistochemical distinction between neuroendocrine (Merkel cell) carcinoma of the skin, lymphoma, and oat cell carcinoma. *Cancer* 58, 1040–1046. doi: 10.1002/1097-0142(19860901)58:5<1040::AID-CNCR282058 0511>3.0.CO;2-L

Carney, D. N., Gazdar, A. F., Bepler, G., Guccion, J. G., Marangos, P. J., Moody, T. W., et al. (1985). Establishment and identification of small cell lung cancer cell lines having classic and variant features. *Cancer Res.* 45, 2913–2923.

Carter, J. J., Daugherty, M. D., Qi, X., Bheda-Malge, A., Wipf, G. C., Robinson, K., et al. (2013). Identification of an overprinting gene in Merkel cell polyomavirus provides evolutionary insight into the birth of viral genes. *Proc. Natl. Acad. Sci. U.S.A.* 110, 12744–12749. doi: 10.1073/pnas.1303526110

Cheng, J., Park, D. E., Berrios, C., White, E. A., Arora, R., Yoon, R., et al. (2017). Merkel cell polyomavirus recruits MYCL to the EP400 complex to promote oncogenesis. *PLoS Pathog.* 13:e1006668. doi: 10.1371/journal.ppat.1006668

Codony-Servat, J., Verlicchi, A., and Rosell, R. (2016). Cancer stem cells in small cell lung cancer. *Transl. Lung Cancer Res.* 5, 16–25. doi: 10.3978/j.issn.2218-6751.2016.01.01

Daily, K., Coxon, A., Williams, J. S., Lee, C. R., Coit, D. G., Busam, K. J., et al. (2015). Assessment of cancer cell line representativeness using microarrays for Merkel cell carcinoma. *J. Invest. Dermatol.* 135, 1138–1146. doi: 10.1038/jid.2014.518

DeCaprio, J. A. (2017). Merkel cell polyomavirus and Merkel cell carcinoma. *Philos. Trans. R. Soc. Lond. B Biol. Sci.* 372:20160276.

Dresang, L. R., Guastafierro, A., Arora, R., Normolle, D., Chang, Y., and Moore, P. S. (2013). Response of Merkel cell polyomavirus-positive merkel cell carcinoma xenografts to a survivin inhibitor. *PLoS One* 8:e80543. doi: 10.1371/journal.pone.0080543

Feng, H., Shuda, M., Chang, Y., and Moore, P. S. (2008). Clonal integration of a polyomavirus in human Merkel cell carcinoma. *Science* 319, 1096–1100. doi: 10.1126/science.1152586

Ferringer, T., Rogers, H. C., and Metcalf, J. S. (2005). Merkel cell carcinoma in situ. *J. Cutan. Pathol.* 32, 162–165. doi: 10.1111/j.0303-6987.2005.00270.x

Fischer, N., Brandner, J., Fuchs, F., Moll, I., and Grundhoff, A. (2010). Detection of Merkel cell polyomavirus (MCPyV) in Merkel cell carcinoma cell lines: cell morphology and growth phenotype do not reflect presence of the virus. *Int. J. Cancer* 126, 2133–2142. doi: 10.1002/ijc.24877

Gonzalez-Vela, M. D., Curiel-Olmo, S., Derdak, S., Beltran, S., Santibanez, M., Martinez, N., et al. (2017). Shared oncogenic pathways implicated in both virus-positive and UV-induced Merkel cell carcinomas. *J. Invest. Dermatol.* 137, 197–206. doi: 10.1016/j.jid.2016.08.015

Green, W. R., Linnoila, R. I., and Triche, T. J. (1984). Neuroendocrine carcinoma of skin with simultaneous cytokeratin expression. *Ultrastruct. Pathol.* 6, 141–152. doi: 10.3109/01913128409018568

Grundhoff, A., and Fischer, N. (2015). Merkel cell polyomavirus, a highly prevalent virus with tumorigenic potential. *Curr. Opin. Virol.* 14, 129–137. doi: 10.1016/j.coviro.2015.08.010

Guastafierro, A., Feng, H., Thant, M., Kirkwood, J. M., Chang, Y., Moore, P. S., et al. (2013). Characterization of an early passage Merkel cell polyomavirus-positive Merkel cell carcinoma cell line, MS-1, and its growth in NOD scid gamma mice. *J. Virol. Methods* 187, 6–14. doi: 10.1016/j.jviromet.2012.10.001

Haraguchi, T., Kondo, M., Uchikawa, R., Kobayashi, K., Hiramatsu, H., Kobayashi, K., et al. (2016). Dynamics and plasticity of the epithelial to mesenchymal transition induced by miR-200 family inhibition. *Sci. Rep.* 6:21117. doi: 10.1038/srep21117

Harms, K. L., Lazo, De La Vega, L., Hovelson, D. H., Rahrig, S., Cani, A. K., et al. (2017). Molecular profiling of multiple primary Merkel cell carcinoma to distinguish genetically distinct tumors from clonally related metastases. *JAMA Dermatol.* 153, 505–512. doi: 10.1001/jamadermatol.2017.0507

Heath, M., Jaimes, N., Lemos, B., Mostaghimi, A., Wang, L. C., Penas, P. F., et al. (2008). Clinical characteristics of Merkel cell carcinoma at diagnosis in 195 patients: the AEIOU features. *J. Am. Acad. Dermatol.* 58, 375–381. doi: 10.1016/j.jaad.2007.11.020

Hesbacher, S., Pfitzer, L., Wiedorfer, K., Angermeyer, S., Borst, A., Haferkamp, S., et al. (2016). RB1 is the crucial target of the Merkel cell polyomavirus Large T antigen in Merkel cell carcinoma cells. *Oncotarget* 7, 32956–32968. doi: 10.18632/oncotarget.8793

Houben, R., Dreher, C., Angermeyer, S., Borst, A., Utikal, J., Haferkamp, S., et al. (2013). Mechanisms of p53 restriction in Merkel cell carcinoma cells are independent of the Merkel cell polyoma virus T antigens. *J. Invest. Dermatol.* 133, 2453–2460. doi: 10.1038/jid.2013.169

Houben, R., Grimm, J., Willmes, C., Weinkam, R., Becker, J. C., and Schrama, D. (2012). Merkel cell carcinoma and Merkel cell polyomavirus: evidence for hit-and-run oncogenesis. *J. Invest. Dermatol.* 132, 254–256. doi: 10.1038/jid.2011.260

Houben, R., Shuda, M., Weinkam, R., Schrama, D., Feng, H., Chang, Y., et al. (2010). Merkel cell polyomavirus-infected Merkel cell carcinoma cells require expression of viral T antigens. *J. Virol.* 84, 7064–7072. doi: 10.1128/JVI.02400-09

Inagawa, Y., Yamada, K., Yugawa, T., Ohno, S., Hiraoka, N., Esaki, M., et al. (2014). A human cancer xenograft model utilizing normal pancreatic duct epithelial cells conditionally transformed with defined oncogenes. *Carcinogenesis* 35, 1840–1846. doi: 10.1093/carcin/bgu112

Kobayashi, N., Fujiwara, T., Westerman, K. A., Inoue, Y., Sakaguchi, M., Noguchi, H., et al. (2000). Prevention of acute liver failure in rats with reversibly immortalized human hepatocytes. *Science* 287, 1258–1262. doi: 10.1126/science.287.5456.1258

Kwun, H. J., Guastafierro, A., Shuda, M., Meinke, G., Bohm, A., Moore, P. S., et al. (2009). The minimum replication origin of merkel cell polyomavirus has a unique large T-antigen loading architecture and requires small T-antigen expression for optimal replication. *J. Virol.* 83, 12118–12128. doi: 10.1128/JVI.01336-09

Kwun, H. J., Shuda, M., Camacho, C. J., Gamper, A. M., Thant, M., Chang, Y., et al. (2015). Restricted protein phosphatase 2A targeting by Merkel cell polyomavirus small T antigen. *J. Virol.* 89, 4191–4200. doi: 10.1128/JVI.00157-15

Kwun, H. J., Shuda, M., Feng, H., Camacho, C. J., Moore, P. S., and Chang, Y. (2013). Merkel cell polyomavirus small T antigen controls viral replication and oncoprotein expression by targeting the cellular ubiquitin ligase SCFFbw7. *Cell Host Microbe* 14, 125–135. doi: 10.1016/j.chom.2013.06.008

Kwun, H. J., Wendzicki, J. A., Shuda, Y., Moore, P. S., and Chang, Y. (2017). Merkel cell polyomavirus small T antigen induces genome instability by E3 ubiquitin ligase targeting. *Oncogene* 36, 6784–6792. doi: 10.1038/onc.2017.277

Lemos, B., and Nghiem, P. (2007). Merkel cell carcinoma: more deaths but still no pathway to blame. *J. Invest. Dermatol.* 127, 2100–2103. doi: 10.1038/sj.jid.5700925

Leonard, J. H., Bell, J. R., and Kearsley, J. H. (1993). Characterization of cell lines established from Merkel-cell ("small-cell") carcinoma of the skin. *Int. J. Cancer* 55, 803–810. doi: 10.1002/ijc.2910550519

Leonard, J. H., Dash, P., Holland, P., Kearsley, J. H., and Bell, J. R. (1995). Characterisation of four Merkel cell carcinoma adherent cell lines. *Int. J. Cancer* 60, 100–107. doi: 10.1002/ijc.2910600115

Liu, W., Yang, R., Payne, A. S., Schowalter, R. M., Spurgeon, M. E., Lambert, P. F., et al. (2016). Identifying the target cells and mechanisms of Merkel cell polyomavirus infection. *Cell Host Microbe* 19, 775–787. doi: 10.1016/j.chom.2016.04.024

Martel-Jantin, C., Filippone, C., Cassar, O., Peter, M., Tomasic, G., Vielh, P., et al. (2012). Genetic variability and integration of Merkel cell polyomavirus in Merkel cell carcinoma. *Virology* 426, 134–142. doi: 10.1016/j.virol.2012.01.018

McFalls, J., Okon, L., Cannon, S., and Lee, J. B. (2017). Intraepidermal proliferation of Merkel cells within a seborrheic keratosis: Merkel cell carcinoma in situ or Merkel cell hyperplasia? *J. Cutan. Pathol.* 44, 480–485. doi: 10.1111/cup.12908

Paulson, K. G., Lemos, B. D., Feng, B., Jaimes, N., Penas, P. F., Bi, X., et al. (2009). Array-CGH reveals recurrent genomic changes in Merkel cell carcinoma including amplification of L-Myc. *J. Invest. Dermatol.* 129, 1547–1555. doi: 10.1038/jid.2008.365

Ramirez, A., Bravo, A., Jorcano, J. L., and Vidal, M. (1994). Sequences 5′ of the bovine keratin 5 gene direct tissue- and cell-type-specific expression of a lacZ gene in the adult and during development. *Differentiation* 58, 53–64. doi: 10.1046/j.1432-0436.1994.5810053.x

Rodig, S. J., Cheng, J., Wardzala, J., Dorosario, A., Scanlon, J. J., Laga, A. C., et al. (2012). Improved detection suggests all Merkel cell carcinomas harbor Merkel polyomavirus. *J. Clin. Invest.* 122, 4645–4653. doi: 10.1172/JCI64116

Rosen, S. T., Gould, V. E., Salwen, H. R., Herst, C. V., Le Beau, M. M., Lee, I., et al. (1987). Establishment and characterization of a neuroendocrine skin carcinoma cell line. *Lab. Invest.* 56, 302–312.

Salcido, C. D., Larochelle, A., Taylor, B. J., Dunbar, C. E., and Varticovski, L. (2010). Molecular characterisation of side population cells with cancer stem cell-like characteristics in small-cell lung cancer. *Br. J. Cancer* 102, 1636–1644. doi: 10.1038/sj.bjc.6605668

Sastre-Garau, X., Peter, M., Avril, M. F., Laude, H., Couturier, J., Rozenberg, F., et al. (2009). Merkel cell carcinoma of the skin: pathological and molecular evidence for a causative role of MCV in oncogenesis. *J. Pathol.* 218, 48–56. doi: 10.1002/path.2532

Sauer, C. M., Haugg, A. M., Chteinberg, E., Rennspiess, D., Winnepenninckx, V., Speel, E. J., et al. (2017). Reviewing the current evidence supporting early B-cells as the cellular origin of Merkel cell carcinoma. *Crit. Rev. Oncol. Hematol.* 116, 99–105. doi: 10.1016/j.critrevonc.2017.05.009

Shuda, M., Arora, R., Kwun, H. J., Feng, H., Sarid, R., Fernandez-Figueras, M. T., et al. (2009). Human Merkel cell polyomavirus infection I. MCV T antigen expression in Merkel cell carcinoma, lymphoid tissues and lymphoid tumors. *Int. J. Cancer* 125, 1243–1249. doi: 10.1002/ijc.24510

Shuda, M., Feng, H., Kwun, H. J., Rosen, S. T., Gjoerup, O., Moore, P. S., et al. (2008). T antigen mutations are a human tumor-specific signature for Merkel cell polyomavirus. *Proc. Natl. Acad. Sci. U.S.A.* 105, 16272–16277. doi: 10.1073/pnas.0806526105

Shuda, M., Kwun, H. J., Feng, H., Chang, Y., and Moore, P. S. (2011). Human Merkel cell polyomavirus small T antigen is an oncoprotein targeting the 4E-BP1 translation regulator. *J. Clin. Invest.* 121, 3623–3634. doi: 10.1172/JCI46323

Smith, K. J., Skelton, HG 3rd., Holland, T. T., Morgan, A. M., and Lupton, G. P. (1993). Neuroendocrine (Merkel cell) carcinoma with an intraepidermal component. *Am. J. Dermatopathol.* 15, 528–533. doi: 10.1097/00000372-199312000-00002

Starrett, G. J., Marcelus, C., Cantalupo, P. G., Katz, J. P., Cheng, J., Akagi, K., et al. (2017). Merkel cell polyomavirus exhibits dominant control of the tumor genome and transcriptome in virus-associated Merkel cell carcinoma. *mBio* 8, e2079–e2016.

Sunshine, J. C., Jahchan, N. S., Sage, J., and Choi, J. (2018). Are there multiple cells of origin of Merkel cell carcinoma? *Oncogene* 37, 1409–1416.

Tang, C. K., and Toker, C. (1978). Trabecular carcinoma of the skin: an ultrastructural study. *Cancer* 42, 2311–2321. doi: 10.1002/1097-0142(197811)42:5<2311::AID-CNCR2820420531>3.0.CO;2-L

Van Keymeulen, A., Mascre, G., Youseff, K. K., Harel, I., Michaux, C., De Geest, N., et al. (2009). Epidermal progenitors give rise to Merkel cells during embryonic development and adult homeostasis. *J. Cell Biol.* 187, 91–100. doi: 10.1083/jcb.200907080

Verhaegen, M. E., Mangelberger, D., Harms, P. W., Eberl, M., Wilbert, D. M., Meireles, J., et al. (2017). Merkel cell polyomavirus small T antigen initiates Merkel cell carcinoma-like tumor development in mice. *Cancer Res.* 77, 3151–3157. doi: 10.1158/0008-5472.CAN-17-0035

Verhaegen, M. E., Mangelberger, D., Weick, J. W., Vozheiko, T. D., Harms, P. W., Nash, K. T., et al. (2014). Merkel cell carcinoma dependence on bcl-2 family members for survival. *J. Invest. Dermatol.* 134, 2241–2250. doi: 10.1038/jid.2014.138

Wendzicki, J. A., Moore, P. S., and Chang, Y. (2015). Large T and small T antigens of Merkel cell polyomavirus. *Curr Opin Virol* 11, 38–43. doi: 10.1016/j.coviro.2015.01.009

Zur Hausen, A., Rennspiess, D., Winnepenninckx, V., Speel, E. J., and Kurz, A. K. (2013). Early B-cell differentiation in Merkel cell carcinomas: clues to cellular ancestry. *Cancer Res.* 73, 4982–4987. doi: 10.1158/0008-5472.CAN-13-0616

13

The Human Polyomavirus Middle and Alternative T-Antigens; Thoughts on Roles and Relevance to Cancer

Els van der Meijden* and Mariet Feltkamp

Department of Medical Microbiology, Leiden University Medical Center, Leiden, Netherlands

***Correspondence:**
Els van der Meijden
p.z.van_der_meijden@lumc.nl

Approximately 15–20% of human cancer is related to infection, which renders them potentially preventable by antimicrobial or antiviral therapy. Human polyomaviruses (PyVs) are relevant in this regard, as illustrated by the involvement of Merkel cell polyomavirus (MCPyV) in the development of Merkel cell carcinoma. The polyomavirus Small and Large tumor antigen (ST and LT) have been extensively studied with respect to their role in oncogenesis. Recently it was shown that a number of human PyVs, including MCPyV and the trichodysplasia spinulosa polyomavirus (TSPyV), express additional T-antigens called Middle T (MT) and alternative T (ALT). ALT is encoded by ORF5, also known as the alternative T open reading frame (ALTO), which also encodes the second exon of MT, and overlaps out-of-frame with the second exon of LT. Previously, MT was considered unique for oncogenic rodent polyomaviruses, and ALT was still unknown. In this mini-review, we want to point out there are important reasons to explore the involvement of MT and ALT in human cellular transformation. First, just like their rodent equivalents, MT and ALT probably disrupt cellular pathways that control signaling and proliferation. Second, expression of the MT and ALT-encoding ORF5/ALTO characterizes a monophyletic polyomavirus clade that includes human and animal PyVs with known oncogenic potential. And third, ORF5/ALTO is subject to strong positive selection aimed specifically at a short linear motif within MT and ALT that overlaps completely with the RB-binding motif in LT. The latter suggests tight interplay between these T-antigens with possible consequences for cell transformation.

Keywords: polyomavirus, T-antigens, oncogenesis, cell-signaling, evolution

BACKGROUND

An established causal relationship between a certain cancer and a particular infection provides ample opportunities to study oncogenesis in detail, and identify unique targets for cancer prevention and treatment. The best example in this regard is probably cervical cancer and human papillomavirus (HPV) infection. The E6 and E7 oncoproteins encoded by high risk HPV types are directly involved in tumorigenesis and maintenance of the transformed state (McLaughlin-Drubin and Munger, 2009). Such knowledge has contributed directly to development of preventive HPV vaccines that reduce the incidence of HPV-related (pre)malignancies (Harper and DeMars, 2017).

The rapidly expanding group of human polyomaviruses (PyVs) is also relevant in this regard. For one human PyV, the Merkel cell polyomavirus (MCPyV), causal involvement in the development of Merkel cell carcinoma (MCC) has been established (Feng et al., 2008;

Shuda et al., 2008; Houben et al., 2010). Consequently, MCPyV has been defined as a group 2A carcinogenic biological agent (Bouvard et al., 2012). The polyomavirus Small and Large T-antigens (ST and LT) that resemble HPV E6 and E7 in several ways, are the usual suspects when it comes to cellular transformation, as they are known to deregulate cellular pathways controlling the cell cycle, DNA repair, and apoptosis. The focus of this mini-review, however, will be on two other T-antigens, Middle T (MT) and Alternative T (ALT), both encoded by the Alternate T-antigen open reading frame (ALTO), also known as ORF5, depending on the polyomavirus in which the open reading frame was recognized (Carter et al., 2013; van der Meijden et al., 2013b; Lauber et al., 2015). ORF5/ALTO is expressed by MCPyV (Carter et al., 2013) and by the trichodysplasia spinulosa polyomavirus (TSPyV) that causes dysplasia of human hair inner root sheath cells and follicular spine formation of the skin (van der Meijden et al., 2010, 2015). While for MCPyV ALTO only ALT expression has been demonstrated, TSPyV ORF5 was shown to express both MT and ALT. This mini-review will address what is currently known about the human PyV MT and ALT products and speculate about their role in human cellular transformation.

THE POLYOMAVIRUS T-ANTIGENS, ESPECIALLY THE ORF5/ALTO-ENCODED MT AND ALT PRODUCTS

Because the human PyVs cause rare diseases observed only in specific immunocompromised patient groups, they are less known. Nevertheless they have striking similarities with HPV, including inactivation of the tumorsuppressor proteins p53 and RB through the T-antigens (DeCaprio and Garcea, 2013). Until recently human PyVs were believed to express only two major T-antigens, ST and LT, next to some smaller splice products thereof (Gjoerup and Chang, 2010). Rodent PyVs, including some oncogenic ones (Gross, 1953; Eddy et al., 1962; Girardi et al., 1962), are known to express an additional T-antigen called MT (Ito et al., 1977; Courtneidge et al., 1991; Fluck and Schaffhausen, 2009; Schaffhausen and Roberts, 2009).

Until the discovery of MCPyV in 2008, the T-antigens were merely seen as viral oncoproteins useful to study oncogenesis *in vitro* and in animal models, for instance the murine polyomavirus (MPyV) in the mouse mammary tumor virus (MMTV) breast cancer model (Fluck and Schaffhausen, 2009). This situation changed considerably with the identification of MCPyV in human MCCs (Feng et al., 2008). MCC is a rare but aggressive skin tumor of neuroendocrine origin, although early B-cells have also been proposed as cells of origin (Sauer et al., 2017). The majority of MCCs harbor clonally integrated MCPyV genome copies that express ST and preliminary truncated versions of LT (Feng et al., 2008; Shuda et al., 2008, 2009; Houben et al., 2010). Studies have shown that MCPyV-positive MCC tumor cell growth depends on the interaction of LT with RB (Houben et al., 2012), while ST promotes cell proliferation by deregulation of the mTOR signaling pathway via inactivation of 4E-BP1 (Shuda et al., 2011; Velasquez et al., 2016). The contribution of ALT and MT to development of MCC or any other human tumor type, respectively, is not known at the moment. Below, we summarize some recent findings that should prompt the interest in MT and ALT as potential viral oncoproteins that merit further study.

ONCOGENIC POLYOMAVIRUSES EXPRESSING ORF5/ALTO PHYLOGENETICALLY CLUSTER TOGETHER

Recently, the Polyomaviridae Study Group of the International Committee on Taxonomy of Viruses (ICTV) (Polyomaviridae Study Group of the International Committee on Taxonomy of Viruses et al., 2016; Moens et al., 2017a) established a new phylogeny-based taxonomy based on conserved regions in LT. This resulted in the demarcation of four genera (*alpha–delta*) within the polyomavirus family (**Figure 1**, right part), and the recognition of 13 human PyV *species* found among three genera (*alpha, beta,* and *delta).* The *alpha* genus contains many (if not all) known naturally oncogenic PyVs, underlined in **Figure 1**, including MCPyV (*Human polyomavirus 5*), the raccoon polyomavirus (RacPyV, *Procyon lotor polyomavirus 1*) (Dela Cruz et al., 2013), MPyV (*Mus musculus polyomavirus 1*) and hamster PyV (*Mesocricetus auratus polyomavirus 1*) (Gross, 1953; Graffi et al., 1969). The dysplasia-inducing TSPyV (*Human polyomavirus 8*) also belongs to the *alpha* genus (van der Meijden et al., 2010; Kazem et al., 2012). The BK and JC polyomaviruses (*Human polyomavirus 1 and 2*), which are sometimes implied in bladder and colon cancer, respectively (Dalianis and Hirsch, 2013), do not belong to the alpha genus (**Figure 1**, in blue).

As far as reported, *alpha* PyVs, including three additional human PyVs so far without attributable disease (HPyV9, HPyV12, and New Jersey PyV), are prevalent in the general population, with a seroprevalence up to 80% (Kean et al., 2009; Nicol et al., 2013; van der Meijden et al., 2013a; Gossai et al., 2016). In our laboratory and elsewhere it was shown that only *alphapolyomaviruses* contain a full length ORF5/ALTO open reading frame (Carter et al., 2013; Lauber et al., 2015; van der Meijden et al., 2015; Moens et al., 2017b) (**Figures 1, 2A**, arrow). The ORF5/ALTO-like shorter open reading frame in PyVs from other genera contains a premature stop codon and does not encode the hydrophobic C-terminus. Full length ORF5/ALTO was previously recognized only in the (oncogenic) hamster and murine PyVs. It is also found in RacPyV causing brain tumors in raccoons (Brostoff et al., 2014).

ALTERNATIVE EXPRESSION OF ORF5/ALTO INVOLVES LT TRANSCRIPTION

The location and context of ORF5/ALTO in the PyV genome is shown in **Figures 2A,B**. ORF5/ALTO overlaps entirely (out

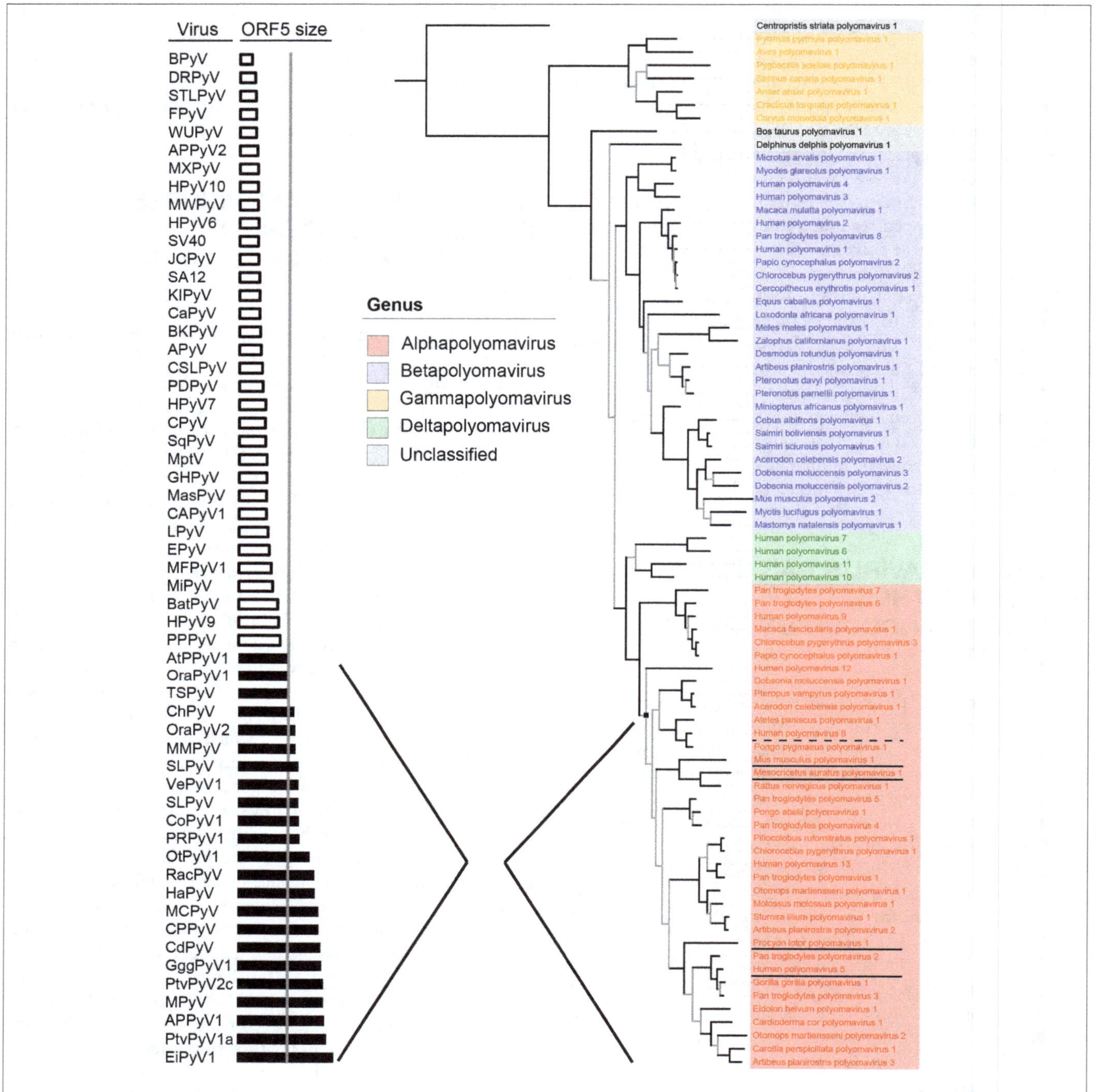

FIGURE 1 | Evolutionary conservation of Middle T and ALT (ORF5) Bayesian phylogeny based on conserved regions in LT, as used by the Study Group of the ICTV for the demarcation of genera (adapted from Moens et al., 2017b) is shown on the right. On the left, polyomaviruses are ordered by ORF5 size. Shown in black bars are intact versions of ORF5, containing the characteristic disordered domains, SLIMs, proline-rich areas and a C-terminal transmembrane domain, that define the major clade (node) of the *alphapolyomaviruses* shown in red on the right. *Alphapolyomaviruses* with known oncogenic or dysplastic properties are respectively underlined or with dashed line.

of frame) with the second exon of LT, which is encoded by ORF2. As shown by us for TSPyV (van der Meijden et al., 2015), ORF5/ALTO is expressed in two different ways to encode MT or ALT. MT is expressed through alternative splicing resulting in a transcript that combines exon 1, which largely overlaps with ST and the first exon of LT, with exon 2 encoded by ORF5/ALTO. Next to this regular expression pattern seen in many more PyVs and HPVs, ORF5/ALTO can be expressed also on its own to encode ALT. For this purpose, the major T-transcript encoding LT is used (van der Meijden et al., 2015). *In vitro*

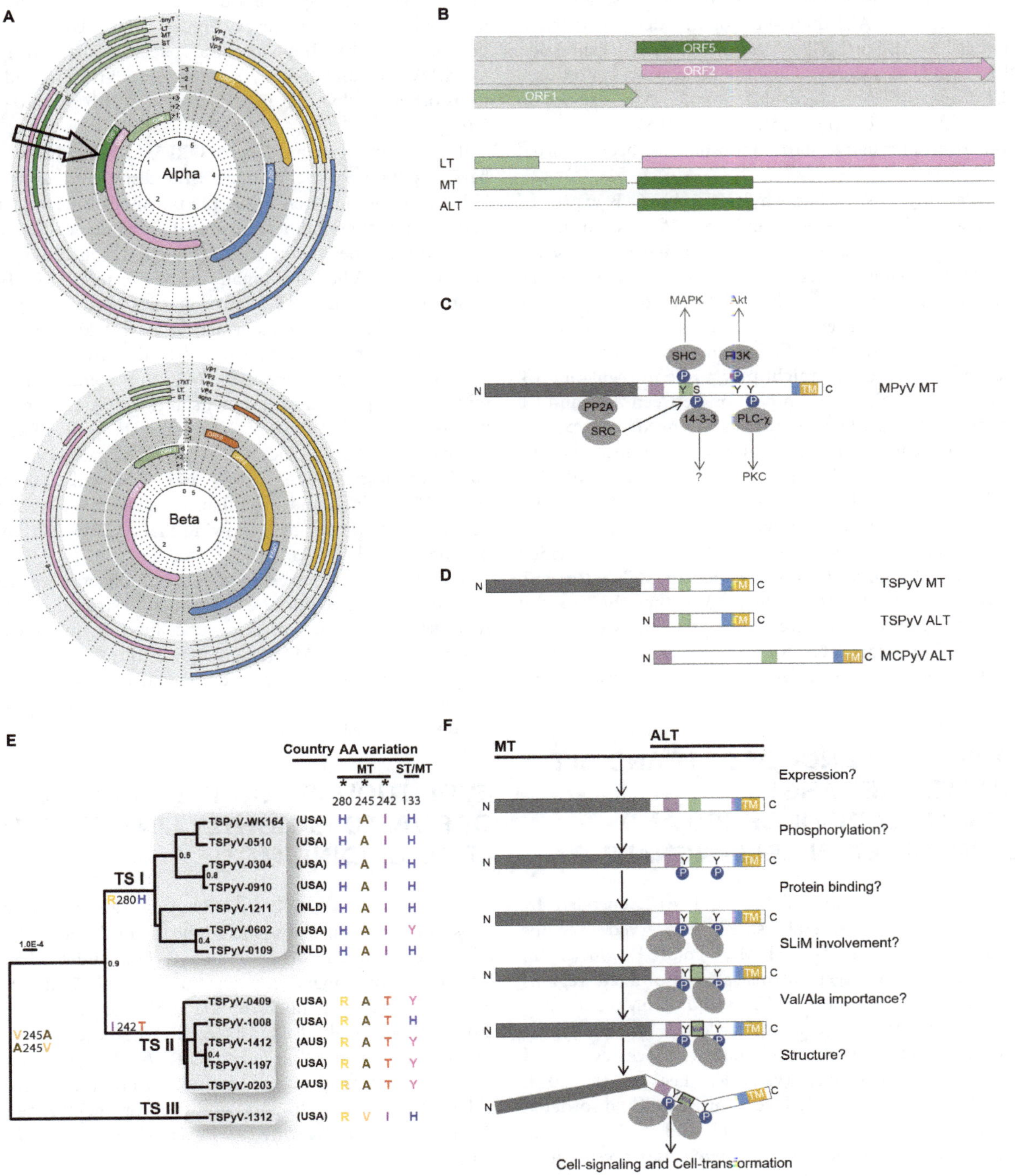

FIGURE 2 | Expression, evolution, and putative role of ORF5 and MT/ALT in cell-signaling and transformation. **(A)** Genomes of an *alpha* and *betapolyomavirus* are shown (adapted from Moens et al., 2017b). Notice the presence of ORF5 in the *alphapolyomavirus* genome (arrow). **(B)** ORF5 encodes the second exon of MT and ALT, and overlaps with the second exon of LT. The colors of the (spliced) T-antigens correspond to the encoding ORF. **(C)** Phosphorylation of mouse polyomavirus (MPyV) MT by Src tyrosine kinase interacting with PP2A-bound by the N-terminal part of MT shown in gray. Phosphorylated MT induces docking and activation of members of the signal transduction pathway, SHK, PI3K, 14-3-3, and PLC (Dilworth, 2002). The colored blocks represent SLiMs present in the intrinsically disordered region (IRD) shown in white (Lauber et al., 2015). The C-terminal transmembrane domain (TM) is shown in yellow. Phosphorylation (P-spheres) of tyrosines (Y) and protein interactions (gray ovals) are depicted. **(D)** Schematic representation of human MT and ALT expressed by TSPyV and MCPyV (colors and shapes as explained in **C**). **(E)** TSPyV phylogeny adapted with permission from Kazem et al. (2016) showing three lineages of TSPyV defined by predominant non-synonymous substitutions in MT/ALT during evolution. **(F)** Schematic overview of HPyV MT/ALT related issues regarding its state, structure and role (colors and shapes as explained in **C**).

at least, the latter route seems to generate the most abundant product, as much more ALT than MT protein is detected (van der Meijden et al., 2015). For MCPyV thus far only ALT expression from ORF5/ALTO was shown. How the major start codon used by the LT transcript is avoided and whether ALT expression involves an internal ribosome entry site (IRES) and the use of a downstream alternative start codon has not been resolved yet.

It is challenging to speculate why ORF5/ALTO is expressed in different ways, from different transcripts. We are not aware of any other viral product that is encoded like this. Possibly ORF5/ALTO expression, either as MT or as ALT, is of crucial importance to the virus life cycle and therefore needs to be ensured at all times, for example during different stages of the host cell cycle or in differentiating host cells. Alternatively, alternating ALTO expression might play a role in regulating LT expression, as there might be competition between ALT and LT for the same transcript. Further studies are needed to explore this possible regulatory process, which might impact on the transforming potential of LT as well. In the case of MCPyV, there might be a correlation with the truncation of MCPyV LT observed in MCC cells, which might call for ALT expression, for instance to supplement a necessary factor normally provided by LT. It should be noticed, however, that in MCC also ALT is often truncated (Carter et al., 2013). Whether the capacity to express both MT and ALT (e.g., TSPyV) opposed to only ALT (e.g., MCPyV) correlates with the capacity to integrate in the host genome as shown for MCPyV is unknown at the moment.

THE ORF5/ALTO ENCODED MT AND ALT PRODUCTS ARE LARGELY INTRINSICALLY DISORDERED AND LIKELY INVOLVED IN CELL-SIGNALING

The shared C-terminal part of MT and ALT encoded by ORF5/ALTO contains several small conserved regions called short linear motifs (SLiMs, colored blocks in **Figures 2C,D**) within larger intrinsically disordered regions (IDRs) (Lauber et al., 2015). IDR and SLiM-containing unstructured proteins are frequently encoded by overlapping ORFs and involved in numerous biologic processes related to disease, including cancer (van der Lee et al., 2014; Xue et al., 2014). As expected for intrinsically disordered proteins, comparison of the shared MT and ALT encoding sequences between different *alphapolyomaviruses* reveals little homology.

From murine studies we know that the second part of MT is proline-rich, contains phosphotyrosine and phosphoserine residues and harbors a transmembrane domain at the very C-terminal end (**Figure 2C**) (Dilworth, 2002; Cheng et al., 2009; Fluck and Schaffhausen, 2009). Functionally, MT acts as an engaged transmembrane growth factor receptor (Dilworth, 2002; Fluck and Schaffhausen, 2009). Upon membrane and PP2A binding, MT interacts with Src tyrosine kinase, which results in phosphorylation of MT and subsequent activation of important phosphokinases, such as PI3K and MAPK involved in cell-signaling (**Figure 2C**) (Dilworth, 2002). Furthermore, the Hippo pathway effectors Taz and Yap, bind to MPyV MT and thereby support Src activation and cellular transformation by MT (Rouleau et al., 2016; Shanzer et al., 2017).

Expression of a full-length ORF5/ALTO (**Figure 1**, black bars), containing the characteristic disordered domains, the SLIMs, the proline-rich areas, the phosphoamino acid residues and the transmembrane domain, defines the vast majority of PyVs within the *alpha* genus (**Figure 1**), including MCPyV and TSPyV. Whether human PyV MT and ALT also show established rodent MT-like properties and are potentially involved in cellular transformation is not known yet. From sequence comparisons showing that the involved motifs are present, for example PP2A in MT, this seems likely. In co-immunoprecipitation experiments and with mutational analysis it was shown that TSPyV MT interacts with PP2A, which involves activation of the MAPK signaling pathway (Wu et al., 2017), as described for MPyV MT (Dilworth, 2002; Cheng et al., 2009; Fluck and Schaffhausen, 2009). We have recently obtained preliminary data showing that MCPyV ALT indeed is phosphorylated.

For MCPyV it was shown that an intact transmembrane domain is required for the subcellular distribution pattern of ALT, comparable to discrete subcellular membrane binding observed for MPyV MT (Zhou et al., 2011; Carter et al., 2013). MPyV MT mutant studies showed that membrane association is required for MT-induced transformation (Novak and Griffin, 1981; Carmichael et al., 1982).

EVOLUTIONARY CONSERVATION OF ORF5/ALTO IS TIGHTLY LINKED TO THE LT RB-BINDING MOTIF

As illustrated above, ORF5/ALTO expression seems important for specific human PyVs, including MCPyV and TSPyV. This relevance is underscored by two recent studies that looked into the evolutionary conservation of ORF5/ALTO among PyVs, especially members of the *alpha* genus (Carter et al., 2013; Lauber et al., 2015). Especially the latter study showed that expression of a full-length ORF5/ALTO (**Figure 1**, black bars), containing the characteristic disordered domains, the SLIMs, the proline-rich areas and the transmembrane domain, defines the vast majority of PyVs within the *alpha* genus (**Figure 1**).

Single nucleotide polymorphism and evolutionary analyses of TSPyV revealed that ORF5/ALTO is the predominant site of non-synonymous substitutions during PyV evolution (**Figure 2E**) (Kazem et al., 2016), subject to strong positive selection (Lauber et al., 2015). Analysis of the entire PyV family showed this pressure is focused on a single amino acid position (MT245/ALT44 for TSPyV, **Figure 2E**) located within a conserved SLiM (green block in **Figures 2C,D**) allowing only two SLiM variants. The latter is highly unusual among conserved residues and results in binary toggling between

Valine and Alanine. Particular interesting in this regard is the information that this restriction is imposed by the highly conserved RB-binding motif (LXCXE) within LT, which completely overlaps with the relevant SLiM (Lauber et al., 2015).

The impact of this finding might seem trivial, since no preference for either a Valine or an Alanine residue is observed among oncogenic PyVs or on the (human) *alphapolyomaviruses* as a whole. However, a dynamic analysis among PyV species taking into account the binary exchange rate of the second codon position corresponding to either Valine–Alanine clearly showed that codon-constrained Valine–Alanine (COCO-VA) toggling is significantly accelerated in ORF5-containing *(alpha)polyomaviruses* compared to ORF5-less viruses (Lauber et al., 2015).

Comparison of 13 TSPyV genomes showed one divergent isolate with a Valine instead of an Alanine residue at position 245 (TSPyV-1312, **Figure 2E**) (Kazem et al., 2016). Adaptation within one species is not observed for any other PyV. For instance in MCPyV, an Alanine residue at position 245 is present in all GenBank-deposited genome isolates regardless of expression of full-length or truncated ALT.

The finding of two overlapping, extremely conserved motifs (the MT/ALT SLiM and the LT RB-binding motif), again suggests that the functional roles of MT/ALT and LT are mutually connected. Since the highly conserved RB-binding motif is also present in the E7 gene of HPV (McLaughlin-Drubin and Munger, 2009), and in the E1A gene of adenoviruses (Munger et al., 2004), we looked for a comparable situation in these related virus families. However, in both of these virus families the RB-binding motif is located in a non-overlapping coding region of the genome, highlighting the unique constellation of the ORF5/ALTO-expressing PyVs.

In general, the presence of two overlapping conserved motifs is rare. More often the organization of functional motifs is such that critical functional residues in one protein overlap with highly mutable regions of the other protein, like observed in the overlapping E2 and E4 genes, and the tat and rev genes of HPV and HIV1, respectively (Hughes and Hughes, 2005; Narechania et al., 2005; Fernandes et al., 2016).

CONCLUSION, DISCUSSION, AND PERSPECTIVE

So far, searches into the role of polyomaviruses in human cancer have focused on the traditional T-antigens LT and ST. Since expression of full length ORF5/ALTO characterizes members of the 'oncogenic' *alphapolyomavirus* genus, we consider it important to study the transforming properties of MT and ALT as well. Next to straightforward approaches investigating involvement of MT and ALT in human cell-signaling and cell cycle regulation through phosphorylation (**Figure 2F**), the relevance of the identified MT/ALT SLiM and Valine–Alanine variants on cell-signaling and cell cycle regulation merits further study. Since SLiMs are involved in (transient) protein interactions and folding of disordered proteins (Davey et al., 2012) (COCO-VA) SLiM variants might impact on the structure, protein-binding and role of MT and ALT (**Figure 2F**). These investigations should take into account the role of the overlapping, possibly competing or supplementing, LT product with known transforming properties that contains the MT/ALT SLiM-overlapping RB-binding motif. Altogether, we believe studying MT and ALT in conjunction with LT will provide valuable insight in the biology of PyV, which will further reveal the involvement of PyV infection in human cancer and possibly provide new targets for cancer prevention and treatment.

AUTHOR CONTRIBUTIONS

All authors listed have made a substantial, direct and intellectual contribution to the work and approved it for publication.

ACKNOWLEDGMENTS

We would like to thank Prof. Dr. A. E. Gorbalenya for useful discussions regarding polyomavirus phylogeny, speciation, and evolution.

REFERENCES

Bouvard, V., Baan, R. A., Grosse, Y., Lauby-Secretan, B., El Ghissassi, F., Benbrahim-Tallaa, L., et al. (2012). Carcinogenicity of malaria and of some polyomaviruses. *Lancet Oncol.* 13, 339–340. doi: 10.1016/S1470-2045(12)70125-0

Brostoff, T., Dela Cruz, F. N. J., Church, M. E., Woolard, K. D., and Pesavento, P. A. (2014). The raccoon polyomavirus genome and tumor antigen transcription are stable and abundant in neuroglial tumors. *J. Virol.* 88, 12816–12824. doi: 10.1128/JVI.01912-14

Carmichael, G. G., Schaffhausen, B. S., Dorsky, D. I., Oliver, D. B., and Benjamin, T. L. (1982). Carboxy terminus of polyoma middle-sized tumor antigen is required for attachment to membranes, associated protein kinase activities, and cell transformation. *Proc. Natl. Acad. Sci. U.S.A.* 79, 3579–3583. doi: 10.1073/pnas.79.11.3579

Carter, J. J., Daugherty, M. D., Qi, X., Bheda-Malge, A., Wipf, G. C., Robinson, K., et al. (2013). Identification of an overprinting gene in Merkel cell polyomavirus provides evolutionary insight into the birth of viral genes. *Proc. Natl. Acad. Sci. U.S.A.* 110, 12744–12749. doi: 10.1073/pnas.1303526110

Cheng, J., Decaprio, J. A., Fluck, M. M., and Schaffhausen, B. S. (2009). Cellular transformation by Simian Virus 40 and Murine Polyoma Virus T antigens. *Semin. Cancer Biol.* 19, 218–228. doi: 10.1016/j.semcancer.2009.03.002

Courtneidge, S. A., Goutebroze, L., Cartwright, A., Heber, A., Scherneck, S., and Feunteun, J. (1991). Identification and characterization of the hamster polyomavirus middle T antigen. *J. Virol.* 65, 3301–3308.

Dalianis, T., and Hirsch, H. H. (2013). Human polyomaviruses in disease and cancer. *Virology* 437, 63–72. doi: 10.1016/j.virol.2012.12.015

Davey, N. E., Van Roey, K., Weatheritt, R. J., Toedt, G., Uyar, B., Altenberg, B., et al. (2012). Attributes of short linear motifs. *Mol. Biosyst.* 8, 268–281. doi: 10.1039/c1mb05231d

DeCaprio, J. A., and Garcea, R. L. (2013). A cornucopia of human polyomaviruses. *Nat. Rev. Microbiol.* 11, 264–276. doi: 10.1038/nrmicro2992

Dela Cruz, F. N. J., Giannitti, F., Li, L., Woods, L. W., Del, V. L., Delwart, E., et al. (2013). Novel polyomavirus associated with brain tumors in free-ranging raccoons, western United States. *Emerg. Infect. Dis.* 19, 77–84. doi: 10.3201/eid1901.121078

Dilworth, S. M. (2002). Polyoma virus middle T antigen and its role in identifying cancer-related molecules. *Nat. Rev. Cancer* 2, 951–956. doi: 10.1038/nrc946

Eddy, B. E., Borman, G. S., Grubbs, G. E., and Young, R. D. (1962). Identification of the oncogenic substance in rhesus monkey kidney cell culture as simian virus 40. *Virology* 17, 65–75. doi: 10.1016/0042-6822(62)90082-X

Feng, H., Shuda, M., Chang, Y., and Moore, P. S. (2008). Clonal integration of a polyomavirus in human Merkel cell carcinoma. *Science* 319, 1096–1100. doi: 10.1126/science.1152586

Fernandes, J. D., Faust, T. B., Strauli, N. B., Smith, C., Crosby, D. C., Nakamura, R. L., et al. (2016). Functional segregation of overlapping genes in HIV. *Cell* 167, 1762.e12–1773.e12. doi: 10.1016/j.cell.2016.11.031

Fluck, M. M., and Schaffhausen, B. S. (2009). Lessons in signaling and tumorigenesis from polyomavirus middle T antigen. *Microbiol. Mol. Biol. Rev.* 73, 542–563. doi: 10.1128/MMBR.00009-09

Girardi, A. J., Sweet, B. H., Slotnick, V. B., and Hilleman, M. R. (1962). Development of tumors in hamsters inoculated in the neonatal period with vacuolating virus, SV-40. *Proc. Soc. Exp. Biol. Med.* 109, 649–660. doi: 10.3181/00379727-109-27298

Gjoerup, O., and Chang, Y. (2010). Update on human polyomaviruses and cancer. *Adv. Cancer Res.* 106, 1–51. doi: 10.1016/S0065-230X(10)06001-X

Gossai, A., Waterboer, T., Nelson, H. H., Michel, A., Willhauck-Fleckenstein, M., Farzan, S. F., et al. (2016). Seroepidemiology of human polyomaviruses in a US population. *Am. J. Epidemiol.* 183, 61–69. doi: 10.1093/aje/kwv155

Graffi, A., Bender, E., Schramm, T., Kuhn, W., and Schneiders, F. (1969). Induction of transmissible lymphomas in Syrian hamsters by application of DNA from viral hamster papovavirus-induced tumors and by cell-free filtrates from human tumors. *Proc. Natl. Acad. Sci. U.S.A.* 64, 1172–1175. doi: 10.1073/pnas.64.4.1172

Gross, L. (1953). A filterable agent, recovered from Ak leukemic extracts, causing salivary gland carcinomas in C3H mice. *Proc. Soc. Exp. Biol. Med.* 83, 414–421. doi: 10.3181/00379727-83-20376

Harper, D. M., and DeMars, L. R. (2017). HPV vaccines - A review of the first decade. *Gynecol. Oncol.* 146, 196–204. doi: 10.1016/j.ygyno.2017.04.004

Houben, R., Adam, C., Baeurle, A., Hesbacher, S., Grimm, J., Angermeyer, S., et al. (2012). An intact retinoblastoma protein-binding site in Merkel cell polyomavirus large T antigen is required for promoting growth of Merkel cell carcinoma cells. *Int. J. Cancer* 130, 847–856. doi: 10.1002/ijc.26076

Houben, R., Shuda, M., Weinkam, R., Schrama, D., Feng, H., Chang, Y., et al. (2010). Merkel cell polyomavirus-infected Merkel cell carcinoma cells require expression of viral T antigens. *J. Virol.* 84, 7064–7072. doi: 10.1128/JVI.02400-09

Hughes, A. L., and Hughes, M. A. (2005). Patterns of nucleotide difference in overlapping and non-overlapping reading frames of papillomavirus genomes. *Virus Res.* 113, 81–88. doi: 10.1016/j.virusres.2005.03.030

Ito, Y., Brocklehurst, J. R., and Dulbecco, R. (1977). Virus-specific proteins in the plasma membrane of cells lytically infected or transformed by pol-oma virus. *Proc. Natl. Acad. Sci. U.S.A.* 74, 4666–4670. doi: 10.1073/pnas.74.10.4666

Kazem, S., Lauber, C., Van Der Meijden, E., Kooijman, S., Kravchenko, A. A., Trichspin, N., et al. (2016). Limited variation during circulation of a polyomavirus in the human population involves the COCO-VA toggling site of middle and alternative T-antigen(s). *Virology* 487, 129–140. doi: 10.1016/j.virol.2015.09.013

Kazem, S., Van Der Meijden, E., Kooijman, S., Rosenberg, A. S., Hughey, L. C., Browning, J. C., et al. (2012). Trichodysplasia spinulosa is characterized by active polyomavirus infection. *J. Clin. Virol.* 53, 225–230. doi: 10.1016/j.jcv.2011.11.007

Kean, J. M., Rao, S., Wang, M., and Garcea, R. L. (2009). Seroepidemiology of human polyomaviruses. *PLoS Pathog.* 5:e1000363. doi: 10.1371/journal.ppat.1000363

Lauber, C., Kazem, S., Kravchenko, A. A., Feltkamp, M. C., and Gorbalenya, A. E. (2015). Interspecific adaptation by binary choice at de novo polyomavirus T antigen site through accelerated codon-constrained Val-Ala toggling within an intrinsically disordered region. *Nucleic Acids Res.* 43, 4800–4813. doi: 10.1093/nar/gkv378

McLaughlin-Drubin, M. E., and Munger, K. (2009). Oncogenic activities of human papillomaviruses. *Virus Res.* 143, 195–208. doi: 10.1016/j.virusres.2009.06.008

Moens, U., Calvignac-Spencer, S., Lauber, C., Ramqvist, T., Feltkamp, M. C. W., Daugherty, M. D., et al. (2017a). ICTV virus taxonomy profile: Polyomaviridae. *J. Gen. Virol.* 98, 1159–1160. doi: 10.1099/jgv.0.000839

Moens, U., Krumbholz, A., Ehlers, B., Zell, R., Johne, R., Calvignac-Spencer, S., et al. (2017b). Biology, evolution, and medical importance of polyomaviruses: an update. *Infect. Genet. Evol.* 54, 18–38. doi: 10.1016/j.meegid.2017.06.011

Munger, K., Baldwin, A., Edwards, K. M., Hayakawa, H., Nguyen, C. L., Owens, M., et al. (2004). Mechanisms of human papillomavirus-induced oncogenesis. *J. Virol.* 78, 11451–11460. doi: 10.1128/JVI.78.21.11451-11460.2004

Narechania, A., Terai, M., and Burk, R. D. (2005). Overlapping reading frames in closely related human papillomaviruses result in modular rates of selection within E2. *J. Gen. Virol.* 86, 1307–1313. doi: 10.1099/vir.0.80747-0

Nicol, J. T., Robinot, R., Carpentier, A., Carandina, G., Mazzoni, E., Tognon, M., et al. (2013). Age-specific seroprevalences of Merkel cell polyomavirus, human polyomaviruses 6, 7 and 9 and trichodysplasia spinulosa-associated polyomavirus. *Clin. Vaccine Immunol.* 20, 363–368. doi: 10.1128/CVI.00438-12

Novak, U., and Griffin, B. E. (1981). Requirement for the C-terminal region of middle T-antigen in cellular transformation by polyoma virus. *Nucleic Acids Res.* 9, 2055–2073. doi: 10.1093/nar/9.9.2055

Polyomaviridae Study Group of the International Committee on Taxonomy of Viruses Calvignac-Spencer, S., Feltkamp, M. C., Daugherty, M. D., Moens, U., Ramqvist, T., et al. (2016). A taxonomy update for the family Polyomaviridae. *Arch. Virol.* 161, 1739–1750. doi: 10.1007/s00705-016-2794-y

Rouleau, C., Pores Fernando, A. T., Hwang, J. H., Faure, N., Jiang, T., White, E. A., et al. (2016). Transformation by polyomavirus middle T antigen involves a unique bimodal interaction with the hippo effector YAP. *J. Virol.* 90, 7032–7045. doi: 10.1128/JVI.00417-16

Sauer, C. M., Haugg, A. M., Chteinberg, E., Rennspiess, D., Winnepenninckx, V., Speel, E. J., et al. (2017). Reviewing the current evidence supporting early B-cells as the cellular origin of Merkel cell carcinoma. *Crit. Rev. Oncol. Hematol.* 116, 99–105. doi: 10.1016/j.critrevonc.2017.05.009

Schaffhausen, B. S., and Roberts, T. M. (2009). Lessons from polyoma middle T antigen on signaling and transformation: a DNA tumor virus contribution to the war on cancer. *Virology* 384, 304–316. doi: 10.1016/j.virol.2008.09.042

Shanzer, M., Adler, J., Ricardo-Lax, I., Reuven, N., and Shaul, Y. (2017). The nonreceptor tyrosine kinase c-Src attenuates SCF(beta-TrCP) E3-ligase activity abrogating Taz proteasomal degradation. *Proc. Natl. Acad. Sci. U.S.A.* 114, 1678–1683. doi: 10.1073/pnas.1610223114

Shuda, M., Arora, R., Kwun, H. J., Feng, H., Sarid, R., Fernandez-Figueras, M. T., et al. (2009). Human Merkel cell polyomavirus infection I. MCV T antigen expression in Merkel cell carcinoma, lymphoid tissues and lymphoid tumors. *Int. J. Cancer* 125, 1243–1249. doi: 10.1002/ijc.24510

Shuda, M., Feng, H., Kwun, H. J., Rosen, S. T., Gjoerup, O., Moore, P. S., et al. (2008). T antigen mutations are a human tumor-specific signature for Merkel cell polyomavirus. *Proc. Natl. Acad. Sci. U.S.A.* 105, 16272–16277. doi: 10.1073/pnas.0806526105

Shuda, M., Kwun, H. J., Feng, H., Chang, Y., and Moore, P. S. (2011). Human Merkel cell polyomavirus small T antigen is an oncoprotein targeting the 4E-BP1 translation regulator. *J. Clin. Invest.* 121, 3623–3634. doi: 10.1172/JCI46323

van der Lee, R., Buljan, M., Lang, B., Weatheritt, R. J., Daughdrill, G. W., Dunker, A. K., et al. (2014). Classification of intrinsically disordered regions and proteins. *Chem. Rev.* 114, 6589–6631. doi: 10.1021/cr400525m

van der Meijden, E., Bialasiewicz, S., Rockett, R. J., Tozer, S. J., Sloots, T. P., and Feltkamp, M. C. (2013a). Different serologic behavior of MCPyV, TSPyV, HPyV6, HPyV7 and HPyV9 polyomaviruses found on the skin. *PLoS One* 8:e81078. doi: 10.1371/journal.pone.0081078

van der Meijden, E., Dargel, C. A., Kazem, S., and Feltkamp, M. C. W. (2013b). Characterization of T antigens encoded by TSPyV; evidence for middle T expression. *J. Neurovirol.* 19, 306–307.

van der Meijden, E., Janssens, R. W., Lauber, C., Bouwes Bavinck, J. N., Gorbalenya, A. E., and Feltkamp, M. C. (2010). Discovery of a new human polyomavirus associated with trichodysplasia spinulosa in an immunocompromized patient. *PLoS Pathog.* 6:e1001024. doi: 10.1371/journal.ppat.1001024

van der Meijden, E., Kazem, S., Dargel, C. A., Van Vuren, N., Hensbergen, P. J., and Feltkamp, M. C. (2015). Characterization of T antigens, including middle T and alternative T, expressed by the human polyomavirus associated with trichodysplasia spinulosa. *J. Virol.* 89, 9427–9439. doi: 10.1128/JVI.00911-15

Velasquez, C., Cheng, E., Shuda, M., Lee-Oesterreich, P. J., Pogge Von Strandmann, L., Gritsenko, M. A., et al. (2016). Mitotic protein kinase CDK1 phosphorylation of mRNA translation regulator 4E-BP1 Ser83 may contribute to cell transformation. *Proc. Natl. Acad. Sci. U.S.A.* 113, 8466–8471. doi: 10.1073/pnas.1607768113

Wu, J. H., Narayanan, D., Simonette, R. A., Rady, P. L., and Tyring, S. K. (2017). Dysregulation of the MEK/ERK/MNK1 signalling cascade by middle T antigen of the trichoydsplasia spinulosa polyomavirus. *J. Eur. Acad. Dermatol. Venereol.* 31, 1338–1341. doi: 10.1111/jdv.14326

Xue, B., Ganti, K., Rabionet, A., Banks, L., and Uversky, V. N. (2014). Disordered interactome of human papillomavirus. *Curr. Pharm. Des.* 20, 1274–1292. doi: 10.2174/13816128113199990072

Zhou, A. Y., Ichaso, N., Adamarek, A., Zila, V., Forstova, J., Dibb, N. J., et al. (2011). Polyomavirus middle T-antigen is a transmembrane protein that binds signaling proteins in discrete subcellular membrane sites. *J. Virol.* 85, 3046–3054. doi: 10.1128/JVI.02209-10

14

Inhibition of TGF-β and NOTCH Signaling by Cutaneous Papillomaviruses

Jordan M. Meyers[1,2†], Miranda Grace[2], Aayushi Uberoi[3], Paul F. Lambert[3] and Karl Munger[2]*

[1] Program in Virology, Harvard Medical School, Boston, MA, United States, [2] Department of Developmental, Molecular and Chemical Biology, Tufts University School of Medicine, Boston, MA, United States, [3] McArdle Laboratory for Cancer Research, Department of Oncology, School of Medicine and Public Health, University of Wisconsin–Madison, Madison, WI, United States

***Correspondence:**
Karl Munger
karl.munger@tufts.edu

†Present address:
Jordan M. Meyers,
Program in Epithelial Biology, Stanford University School of Medicine, Stanford, CA, United States

Infections with cutaneous papillomaviruses have been linked to cutaneous squamous cell carcinomas that arise in patients who suffer from a rare genetic disorder, epidermodysplasia verruciformis, or those who have experienced long-term, systemic immunosuppression following organ transplantation. The E6 proteins of the prototypical cutaneous human papillomavirus (HPV) 5 and HPV8 inhibit TGF-β and NOTCH signaling. The *Mus musculus* papillomavirus 1, MmuPV1, infects laboratory mouse strains and causes cutaneous skin warts that can progress to squamous cell carcinomas. MmuPV1 E6 shares biological and biochemical activities with HPV8 E6 including the ability to inhibit TGF-β and NOTCH signaling by binding the SMAD2/SMAD3 and MAML1 transcription factors, respectively. Inhibition of TGF-β and NOTCH signaling is linked to delayed differentiation and sustained proliferation of differentiating keratinocytes. Furthermore, the ability of MmuPV1 E6 to bind MAML1 is necessary for wart and cancer formation in experimentally infected mice. Hence, experimental MmuPV1 infection in mice will be a robust and valuable experimental system to dissect key aspects of cutaneous HPV infection, pathogenesis, and carcinogenesis.

Keywords: viral oncogenesis, squamous cell carcinoma, epidermodysplasia verruciformis, keratinocyte differentiation, hit-and-run carcinogenesis

INTRODUCTION

As of January 2018, more than 300 human papillomavirus (HPV) genotypes are listed in the PAVE database[1] (Van Doorslaer et al., 2017). HPVs have ~8 kb circular double stranded DNA genomes, do not generally infect heterologous hosts and exhibit a preference for infecting either mucosal or cutaneous epithelia. Mucosal HPVs are generally transmitted by sexual contact and mucosal infections with α-genus HPVs are the most common sexually transmitted disease with a prevalence of 70 million cases and an annual incidence of 14 million new transmissions in the United States (CDC, 2015). Mucosal HPVs mostly include members of the α-genus. Clinically, α-HPVs can be designated either as "low-risk" or "high-risk." Low-risk α-HPV infections trigger

[1] pave.niaid.nih.gov

benign genital warts, whereas high-risk α-HPVs cause intraepithelial lesions that can undergo malignant progression. Almost 100% of cervical carcinoma are caused by high-risk HPVs and infections with these viruses also contribute to a large percentage of anogenital tract as well as oral cancers (Schiffman et al., 2007). Globally, high-risk α-HPVs infections cause approximately 5% of all human cancers. Despite the availability of efficacious prophylactic vaccines for the most abundant high-risk α-HPVs, there will be approximately 4,170 cervical cancer deaths in 2018 in the United States alone, which means that approximately every 2 h one woman will succumb to cervical cancer (Siegel et al., 2018). Because cancers arise years to decades after the initial infection, a significant impact of these prophylactic vaccines on cervical cancer rates is not expected for another 20 years (Frazer, 2004; Schiller and Lowy, 2012). Unfortunately, there are no antiviral compounds to combat HPV infections (Hellner and Munger, 2011).

Cutaneous HPVs include the β-, γ-, μ-, and ν-genera and some α-HPVs also have a preference for infecting cutaneous epithelia. Cutaneous HPV infections are very frequent and have been linked to development of warts, actinic keratosis, keratoacanthoma, psoriasis, and non-melanoma skin cancers. In Australia, up to 24% of 16- to 18-year-olds have skin warts (Kilkenny et al., 1998). The prevalence of actinic keratosis in the United States is ~20% and resulted in 47 million dermatology visits in 2006 (Del Rosso et al., 2014). Keratoacanthoma are low grade, rapidly growing skin tumors that, unlike squamous cell carcinomas, are derived from cells located in the hair follicle. Cutaneous HPV genomes are readily detected in hair follicle cells harvested by plucking hair, and a high viral load is a predictor of cancer development (Neale et al., 2013). Keratoacanthoma mostly occur in sun-exposed skin in middle aged patients. The incidence has been estimated at approximately 1:1,000 (Chuang et al., 1993). Cutaneous HPVs have also been frequently detected in psoriasis patients (Mahe et al., 2003). In patients suffering from a rare inherited disease, *epidermodysplasia verruciformis* (EV), and in the rapidly increasing population of chronically immune-suppressed individuals, such as organ transplant patients, lesions caused by cutaneous HPV infections can progress to cutaneous squamous cell carcinomas (cSCCs) (Pass et al., 1977; Orth et al., 1978; Neale et al., 2013). Indeed, cSCCs arising in EV patients were the first human tumors that were conclusively linked to HPV infections. More recently, β- and γ-HPV genomes have also been detected at mucosal sites, suggesting the possibility that these viruses may also infect mucosal epithelia (Bottalico et al., 2011; Hampras et al., 2017; Smelov et al., 2017).

The incidence of cSCCs in the general population has been linked to UV exposure and is rising rapidly with more than 700,000 cases and 8,000 deaths yearly in the United States (Alam and Ratner, 2001; Deady et al., 2014). The estimated annual costs for cSCC treatments in the United States are at $3.8 billion (Guy et al., 2015). Whether and how HPVs may be involved in cSCCs development in immunocompetent individuals, however, remains a matter of debate (Feltkamp et al., 2008), even though a recent meta-analysis provided evidence for a modestly increased overall risk of 1.42 (1.18–1.72) for β-HPV infection and cSCC development (Chahoud et al., 2016).

Hence, β-HPV infections are highly associated with cSCC development in EV patients, correlated in the case of cSCCs arising in immune suppressed patients, and only slightly or sporadically associated with cSCCs in immune competent patients. HPV sequences are not retained and expressed in every cSCC cell. This indicates that, unlike what has been shown for high-risk α-HPV-associated cancers, cutaneous HPVs may not be necessary for tumor maintenance. Cutaneous HPV genomes are almost universally detected in asymptomatic patients (Antonsson et al., 2003a; Kohler et al., 2007), but it is not clear whether this is reflective of active and/or persistent infection. Detection of HPV RNA or protein expression may provide a better estimation of the frequency of active HPV infection in non-neoplastic skin (Borgogna et al., 2012, 2014) and it has been debated whether cutaneous HPVs function as carcinogenic drivers, or if they appear as innocuous passengers in cSCCs that arise in immunocompetent individuals (Quint et al., 2015). A recent study with a transgenic mouse model, has provided evidence for the alternative model that some cutaneous HPVs are drivers of cancer initiation but are not necessary for tumor maintenance (Viarisio et al., 2017).

CARCINOGENIC ACTIVITIES OF β-HPVs

Because of their isolation from cSCCs in EV patients, much of the early research efforts with the β-HPVs focused on HPV5 and HPV8. Somewhat surprisingly, HPV5 and HPV8 scored as only weakly transforming or non-transforming in standard cell-based assays (Yamashita et al., 1993; Tommasino, 2017). However, experiments with genetically engineered mice where HPV8 sequences were expressed in basal epithelial cells, impressively demonstrated the oncogenic activity of this HPV. While these mice spontaneously develop skin cancer without the requirement of any additional treatment, they also recapitulated the co-carcinogenic effect of UV exposure (reviewed in Howley and Pfister, 2015). These experiments showed that HPV8 E6, E7 and, uniquely, also E2 could each independently contribute to skin cancer formation when ectopically expressed in basal epithelial cells of a transgenic mouse (Schaper et al., 2005; Pfefferle et al., 2008; Marcuzzi et al., 2009).

The β-HPVs are phylogenetically diverse and as of January 2018, 64 β-HPVs are listed in the PAVE database (see text footnote 1; Van Doorslaer et al., 2017). These are further classified into phylogenetic species. HPV5 and HPV8 together with 19 additional HPVs are classified as species 1, there are 22 members classified as species 2, four are species 3, one is species 4, three are species 5, and 13 have not yet been classified by the HPV reference center.

The E6 and E7 proteins of other β-HPVs, including HPV types 20, 38, and 48 also exhibit carcinogenic activities in transgenic mouse models. Mice expressing β1-HPV20 E6 or E7 from keratin K10 promoter and mice with β2-HPV38 E6/E7 expression from a keratin K14 promoter developed skin cancers when exposed to UV. In contrast, mice expressing the β3-HPV49 E6/E7 genes from a keratin 14 promoter were not susceptible to skin carcinogenesis after UV exposure but developed upper digestive tract carcinomas when treated with the chemical carcinogen 4-nitroquinoline 1-oxide (Michel et al., 2006; Viarisio et al., 2011, 2016). Some of these more recently detected β-HPVs also exhibit transforming activities in cell-based assays. Ectopic expression of the β1 HPV24 or HPV36 E6/E7 proteins causes life span extension of primary human foreskin keratinocytes (HFKs), whereas expression of the β2 HPV38 and β3 HPV49 E6/E7 proteins can trigger HFK immortalization (Cornet et al., 2012).

Despite similar genomic organization, there are some differences between the β- and high-risk α-HPVs (McLaughlin-Drubin et al., 2012). Most strikingly, β-HPVs do not encode E5 proteins, which are oncogenic in high-risk α-HPVs (Genther et al., 2003; Maufort et al., 2007, 2010). Moreover, while high-risk α-HPV-associated cervical carcinomas are generally non-productive, cSCCs arising in EV patients are productive infections. Despite these differences, early mechanistic analyses of the oncogenic activities of β-HPVs were modeled after studies with high-risk α-HPV E6 and E7 proteins. Like high-risk α-HPV E6 and E7 proteins, β-HPV E6 and E7s are low molecular weight, cysteine-rich, metal binding proteins of approximately 150 and 100 amino acids, respectively. They lack intrinsic enzymatic activities, are not known to directly bind specific DNA sequences and presumably exert their biological activities by interacting with and functionally modifying cellular regulatory proteins (Munger et al., 2004; Roman and Munger, 2013; Vande Pol and Klingelhutz, 2013). The best studied cellular targets of the high-risk α-HPV E6 and E7 proteins are the TP53 and RB1 tumor suppressors, respectively. The transforming activities of papillomaviruses are a reflection of their life cycles, specifically their need to secure the availability of cellular replication factors in terminally differentiated epithelial cells that would have normally withdrawn from the cell division cycle (Harden and Munger, 2017). Papillomaviruses need to uncouple cell-cycle withdrawal from epithelial differentiation, effectively allowing for unlicensed proliferation in suprabasal keratinocytes. Aberrant DNA synthesis can be sensed by cells and triggers cell abortive responses, which will need to be inhibited by the virus. The strategies that specific papillomaviruses have evolved to enable their productive replication cycles largely determine their oncogenic potential (McLaughlin-Drubin and Munger, 2009; Moody and Laimins, 2010).

The high-risk HPV E7 proteins cause S-phase competence in differentiating cells by targeting the retinoblastoma tumor suppressor, RB1, for degradation. Uncontrolled S-phase entry as a consequence of RB1 inactivation causes activation of the TP53 tumor suppressor, which triggers a transcriptional program to eliminate such rogue cells by apoptosis. This simple, albeit likely not entirely correct, model (Munger et al., 2004; Munger and Jones, 2015) also served as a blueprint for many studies with the EV-associated β-HPVs, even though it became clear very quickly that it was unlikely to apply to these viruses (McLaughlin-Drubin et al., 2012; Meyers and Munger, 2014; Tommasino, 2017). HPV8 E6 does not detectably interact with TP53 or the UBE3A (E6AP) E3 ubiquitin ligase that is necessary for high-risk α-HPV E6 mediated TP53 degradation (Elbel et al., 1997; White et al., 2012a; Brimer et al., 2017). HPV5 and HPV8 E7s weakly bind and do not degrade RB1, similar to the low-risk α-HPV E7s (Yamashita et al., 1993).

All known β-HPV E7 proteins contain canonical LXCXE (L, leucine; C, cysteine; E, glutamate; X, any amino acid)-based binding sites for the retinoblastoma tumor suppressor family of proteins and many have been documented to bind RB1, RBL1 (p107), and RBL2 (p130). Some β-HPV E6 and E7 in fact interfere with RB1 and TP53 stability, reminiscent of cervical cancer associated, high-risk α-HPVs (Caldeira et al., 2003; Accardi et al., 2006; Cornet et al., 2012; White et al., 2014). The interactions described for β-HPV E6 proteins with TP53 are particularly complex as some have been reported to stabilize TP53 (HPV17, HPV38, and HPV92), while others destabilize it (HPV49) and some have been reported to interfere with TP53 activation and/or TP53 mediated activation of certain target genes (HPV5, HPV8, and HPV38) (Cornet et al., 2012; Wallace et al., 2014; White et al., 2014). Whether humans infected with cutaneous HPVs that target RB1 and TP53 similar to the high-risk α-HPVs are at a particularly high risk for developing cSCC, remains to be determined.

Given the fact that most β-HPV-associated tumors arise in sun exposed areas, it was investigated whether these viruses might interfere with UV-induced apoptosis and/or DNA damage repair. Consistent with expectations, several groups reported that β-HPV E6 proteins cause degradation of BAK, a pro-apoptotic BCL2 family member that is released from the mitochondria following UV exposure (Jackson et al., 2000). BAK degradation by β-HPV E6 proteins is predicted to inhibit apoptosis and allow for survival of UV-damaged cells that may have possibly acquired oncogenic mutations (Leverrier et al., 2007; Hufbauer et al., 2015).

Other studies showed that the repair of UV-damaged DNA damage is inhibited in HPV8 E6 expressing cells. HPV5 and HPV8 E6 proteins were reported to bind the EP300/CREBBP acetyltransferases and target them for degradation thereby inhibiting the Ataxia Telangiectasia Mutated (ATM) and Ataxia Telangiectasia and Rad3-Related (ATR) kinases, key sensors, and mediators of double strand DNA break repair. By abrogating ATM/ATR mediated sensing and/or repair of double strand DNA breaks, cellular mutations may accumulate in β-HPV infected cells, thereby driving carcinogenesis (Howie et al., 2011; Wallace et al., 2012; Wendel and Wallace, 2017). These findings support a "hit-and-run" mechanism for β-HPV carcinogenesis where viral gene expression contributes to cancer initiation by increasing the mutational burden caused by UV exposure but is not necessary for tumor maintenance. This would explain why viral gene expression is not maintained in all tumor cells (Arron et al., 2011). Such a model was recently recapitulated with HPV38 transgenic mice (Viarisio et al., 2018). Interestingly, unbiased proteomic analyses of the HPV38 E6 associated proteins provided no evidence for EP300/CREBBP binding to HPV38 E6 (White et al., 2012a), suggesting that inhibition of DNA break repair by β-HPV E6 proteins may not be necessarily linked to EP300/CREBBP degradation.

As mentioned previously, β-HPV genomes have been detected in hair follicles, which contain epithelial stem cells and HPV8 has been reported to increase the number of keratinocytes with stem cell characteristics both in cell- and animal-based model systems (Hufbauer et al., 2013; Lanfredini et al., 2017; Marthaler et al., 2017). Several studies have shown that the TP53 family member and epithelial stem cell marker TP63 is dysregulated in HPV8 E6 expressing keratinocytes. Specifically, higher levels of the amino terminally truncated ΔNp63α and lower levels of full-length TAp63 isoforms were detected in HPV8 E6 expressing human and murine keratinocytes (Lanfredini et al., 2017; Marthaler et al., 2017). NOTCH inhibition decreased TP63 levels in HPV8 E6 expressing undifferentiated keratinocytes, but TP63 expression remained high in differentiating HPV8 E6 expressing keratinocytes, suggesting that there are NOTCH independent pathways that cause deregulated TP63 expression (Meyers et al., 2013). One of these pathways involves down-regulation of microRNA-203 (miR-203) by HPV8 E6 by inhibiting EP300 which in turn affects CCAAT/enhancer-binding protein a (CEBPA) transcription factor activity that controls miR-203 expression. Significantly, up-regulation of miR-203 during calcium-induced differentiation is abrogated in HPV8 E6 expressing keratinocytes (Marthaler et al., 2017). High-level TP63 and low levels of miR-203 were also detected throughout the lesional tissue of an HPV8 positive EV patient (Marthaler et al., 2017). Since EP300 binding is not shared by all β-HPV E6 (White et al., 2012a) it remains to be determined whether this pathway is universally targeted by β-HPV E6 proteins.

THE γ-HPVs; BENIGN FLORA OR DANGEROUS VILLAINS?

As of January 2018, a total of 171 γ-HPVs have been detected, which are classified into 27 different species. The number of species may increase, since 93 γ-HPVs have not yet been classified into species by the HPV reference center (see text footnote 1; Van Doorslaer et al., 2017). The enormous phylogenetic diversity of γ-HPVs is also reflected in their genome organization; members of the γ6 species, for example, do not encode recognizable E6 proteins and some γ-HPVs encode E7 proteins that lack the canonical LXCXE binding site for the RB1 tumor suppressor and the related p107 (RBL1) and p130 (RBL2) proteins. The γ-HPVs were initially isolated from cutaneous epithelia and are often regarded as components of the normal skin viral flora (Antonsson et al., 2003a,b; Forslund, 2007; Chen et al., 2008; Foulongne et al., 2012). More recent studies also detected γ-HPV DNA at mucosal sites (Bottalico et al., 2011; Smelov et al., 2017).

A "deep sequencing" study of human skin cancers and matched normal tissues showed that HPV197, a γ24-HPV, was the most frequently detected HPV genome in cSCCs and was not present in normal skin (Arroyo Muhr et al., 2015). HPV197 could not have been previously detected because the genome is not recognized by the "consensus" PCR primers that are frequently used for HPV analysis of clinical specimens (Arroyo Muhr et al., 2015). To this date, however, there is no evidence that HPV197 sequences are actively expressed in skin cancers and/or that HPV197 or potentially other γ-HPVs contribute to cSCC development in immunosuppressed or immunocompetent individuals.

Analysis of potential cellular targets by affinity purification followed by mass spectrometry (AP/MS) revealed that HPV197 E6 shares many cellular targets with β-HPV E6 proteins, particularly the β1 HPVs that include HPV5 and HPV8 (Grace and Munger, 2017). The HPV197 E7 protein lacks an LXCXE-based RB1 binding site, yet, consistent with earlier work with the γ1 HPV4 E7 protein (Wang et al., 2010), HPV197 E7 interacts with RB1 (Grace and Munger, 2017). Interestingly, however, HPV197 E7 does not bind to RBL1 or RBL2 (Grace and Munger, 2017). The detection of HPV197 DNA in human skin cancers but not normal skin, and the interactions of the E6 and E7 proteins with human tumor suppressor proteins are consistent with the possibility that HPV197 and potentially other γ-HPVs may be associated with skin cancer development. Currently, however, only very few studies have explored the biological activities of γ-HPVs in cell-based or animal models.

MmuPV1, AN ANIMAL MODEL FOR CUTANEOUS HPV INFECTIONS

Papillomaviruses are species specific and generally do not infect heterologous hosts (Knipe and Howley, 2013). This has severely hindered the study of PV pathogenesis *in vivo*. Research has also been stymied by the lack of a papillomavirus that naturally infects and replicates in a genetically tractable laboratory animal. The isolation of *Mus musculus* papillomavirus 1, MmuPV1, from skin warts on immunodeficient nude mice promises to revolutionize PV pathogenesis studies (Ingle et al., 2011; Joh et al., 2011). The ability to cause wart formation upon experimental infection with quasivirus or by naked DNA inoculation was originally observed in mouse strains that have T-cell deficiencies or are temporarily immune suppressed (Handisurya et al., 2014; Joh et al., 2016; Uberoi et al., 2016). Lesions arising due to MmuPV1 infection have malignant potential and can progress to cSCCs. Upon UVB-exposure, experimental MmuPV1 infection also causes skin warts that can progress to cSCCs in immunocompetent, standard laboratory mouse strains (Uberoi and Lambert, 2017). Importantly, there is a correlation between immunosuppression due to UV irradiation and onset of MmuPV1 dependent cutaneous papillomas (Uberoi et al., 2016).

MmuPV1 is a member of the Pi genus, which encompasses rodent PVs (Van Doorslaer et al., 2017) and is related to γ- and β-HPVs (Joh et al., 2011). Consistent with these phylogenetic relationships, the MmuPV1 E6 protein has similar cellular targets as the β-HPV8 E6 protein (Meyers et al., 2017). The MmuPV1 E7 protein is related to the γ-HPV197 E7 protein in that it lacks the canonical LXCXE-based RB1 binding site (Joh et al., 2011; Grace and Munger, 2017). Moreover, transcriptomic analyses revealed that similar to cutaneous HPVs, MmuPV1 expresses E6 and E7 from two separate early promoters (Xue et al., 2017).

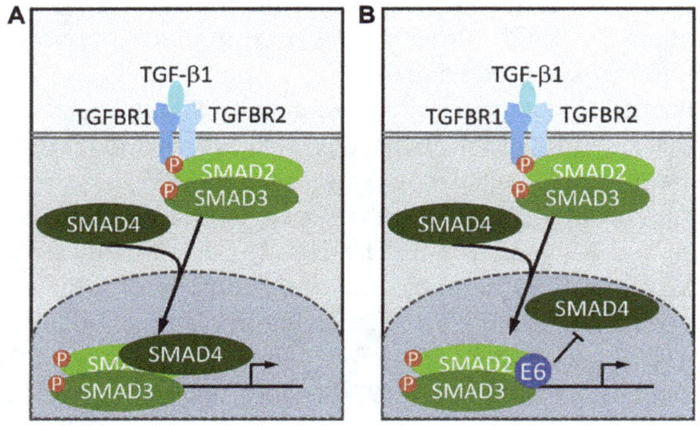

FIGURE 1 | Subversion of TGF-β signaling by HPV8 and MmuPV1 E6. In normal cells, TGF-β binding to the heterotetrameric serine/threonine kinase receptor complex triggers a phosphorylation cascade resulting in phosphorylation of receptor the SMADs, SMAD2, and SMAD3. Phosphorylated receptor SMADs disassociate from the receptor, form a complex with the co-SMAD, SMAD4, and enter the nucleus. The SMAD2/SMAD3/SMAD4 complex then binds to SMAD binding sites to stimulate target gene transcription **(A)**. HPV8 and MmuPV1 E6 proteins bind SMAD2 and SMAD3 and inhibit TGF-β signaling by preventing the formation of the active DNA bound SMAD2/SMAD3/SMAD4 complex **(B)**.

Because of its ability to infect cutaneous epithelia and cause lesions capable of malignant progression upon UV exposure, MmuPV1 may be an important model for determining the potential roles of β- and some γ-HPVs in skin cancer development.

Interestingly, MmuPV1 can productively infect both cutaneous and mucosal tissues (Cladel et al., 2013, 2016; Hu et al., 2015) and thus may also model aspects of mucosal pathogenesis. In any case, results from infection experiments with mutant MmuPV1 genomes can be combined with infection studies of relevant, genetically engineered mouse models. This will enable studies to define mechanisms of action of viral proteins and to determine how viral targeting of specific cellular signaling pathways contribute to the life cycle, pathogenesis and carcinogenicity of a papillomavirus in a natural host.

SUBVERSION OF TGF-β AND NOTCH SIGNALING BY CUTANEOUS PAPILLOMAVIRUSES

While inhibition of UV-mediated apoptosis and/or DNA damage sensing/repair provides a satisfying model to mechanistically support a hit-and-run mechanism of cutaneous HPV mediated carcinogenesis, it does not explain how these viruses may cause warts, a necessary precursor to cSCCs. Moreover, studies with MmuPV1 showed that UV-mediated immune suppression rather than mutagenesis was important for pathogenesis and tumor development (Uberoi et al., 2016).

Inhibition of TGF-β Signaling

Multiple developmental and cellular processes are regulated by TGF-β signaling. The core components of this signal transduction pathway consist of the ligand, TGF-β, heterotetrameric receptors with serine/threonine kinase activity, receptor associated SMAD (R-SMADs) proteins, and co-activator SMADs (co-SMADs). The tetrameric receptor consists of one dimer of the ligand interacting TGF-β type II receptor (TGFBR2), and one dimer of TGF-β type I receptor (TGFBR1). TGF-β binding triggers a phosphorylation cascade from TGFBR2 to TGFBR1 to R-SMADs (Chaikuad and Bullock, 2016). Activin/Nodal and TGFBR1 receptors phosphorylate the R-SMAD pair SMAD2 and SMAD3, whereas the Bone Morphogenetic Protein (BMP) type I receptors activate the R-SMADs SMAD1, SMAD5, and SMAD8 (Miyazawa et al., 2002). After phosphorylation, R-SMADs complex with the co-SMAD, SMAD4, enter the nucleus, bind specific DNA sequences, and activate target gene transcription (**Figure 1A**). Transcriptional activation of the CDK2 inhibitors $p21^{CIP1}$ (CDKN1A) and $p27^{KIP1}$ (CDKN1B), and the CDK4/CDK6 inhibitor $p15^{INK4B}$ (CDKN2B) have been linked to TGF-β mediated G1 cell cycle arrest (Datto et al., 1995; Reynisdottir et al., 1995). Hence, TGF-β functions as a tumor suppressor in epithelial cells, and TGF-β pathway loss of function mutations are frequent in epithelial tumors (Wang et al., 2000; Qiu et al., 2007; Fleming et al., 2013). Importantly, however, TGF-β signaling also induces expression of factors involved in epithelial to mesenchymal transition (EMT) and causes increased production of matrix metalloproteases, which results in enhanced migration and invasion (Valcourt et al., 2016). This is consistent with an oncogenic activity of TGF-β as was originally discovered in fibroblasts (Roberts et al., 1985). Hence, the NOTCH and TGF-β signaling pathways each have tumor suppressor activities at early stages of carcinogenesis and can function as oncogenes during later stages of carcinogenesis.

The first evidence that cutaneous HPVs inhibit TGF-β signaling was provided by Michel Favre's group who reported that HPV5 E6 could target SMAD3 for proteasomal degradation (Mendoza et al., 2006). Consistent with this report, AP/MS experiments provided evidence for SMAD2 and SMAD3 association with HPV8 E6 (Meyers et al., 2017). Similarly, the MmuPV1 E6 protein was also shown to bind SMAD2 and SMAD3 (Meyers et al., 2017). Unlike many other papillomavirus E6 binding cellular proteins, SMAD2 and SMAD3 do not contain helical LXXLL (L, leucine; X, any amino acid) motifs (Chen et al., 1998). There is no evidence for SMAD2, SMAD3, or SMAD4 destabilization by HPV8 E6 or MmuPV1 E6 either under basal or TGF-β stimulated conditions (Meyers et al., 2017). Moreover, there is no defect in SMAD2/SMAD3 phosphorylation and nuclear translocation following TGF-β stimulation in HPV8 or MmuPV1 E6 expressing human keratinocytes. The HPV8 and MmuPV1 E6 proteins, however, were shown to reduce SMAD4 association with SMAD2 and SMAD3 after TGF-β stimulation and to inhibit SMAD2/3 and SMAD4 binding to target DNA. Hence cutaneous papillomavirus E6 proteins inhibit TGF-β signaling by blocking productive binding of the SMAD2/3/4 complex to TGF-β responsive promoters (Meyers et al., 2017; **Figure 1B**). It will be interesting to determine whether these E6 proteins can also inhibit signaling by TGF-β related cytokines. Interestingly, TGF-β signaling is also inhibited by α-HPVs and

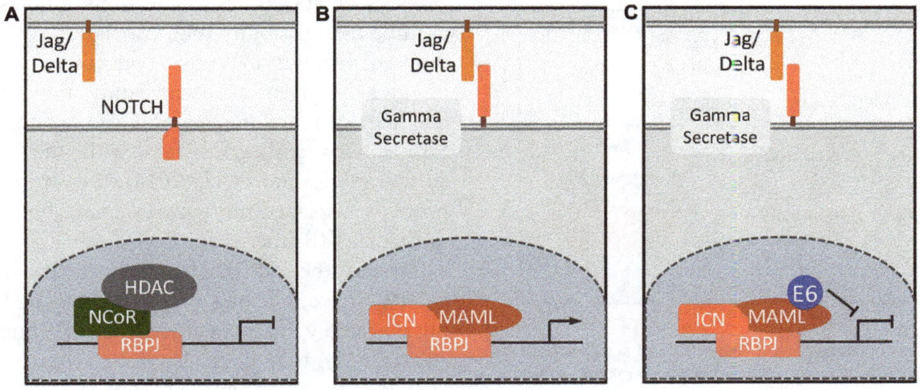

FIGURE 2 | Schematic of NOTCH target gene expression. In the absence of ligand binding, NOTCH responsive genes remain repressed and RBPJ is in a DNA bound, nuclear complex with repressors such as the N-CoR complex **(A)**. Ligand binding leads to NOTCH cleavage and ICN enters the nucleus, displaces repressors and recruits MAML and other co-activators such EP300/CREBBP **(B)**. HPV8 and MmuPV1 E6 proteins inhibit NOTCH signaling by forming a complex with the DNA bound ICN/MAML1 complex thereby preventing formation of a functional transcriptional activator complex **(C)**.

high-risk HPV16 has been reported to inhibit TGF-β through E7 (Pietenpol et al., 1990; Lee et al., 2002) as well as E5 (French et al., 2013), but not through E6. Hence the cutaneous and mucosal HPVs share the ability to inhibit TGF-β signaling although they have evolved different mechanisms.

Inhibition of NOTCH Signaling

Similar to TGF-β, NOTCH regulates multiple processes during embryogenesis and in the adult organism. Of particular interest to papillomavirus biology, NOTCH signaling drives epithelial differentiation and is required for proper formation of the skin barrier (Rangarajan et al., 2001). NOTCH signaling is triggered through cell-to-cell contact where membrane anchored ligands of the Delta or Jagged family bind to NOTCH family receptors. In humans there are four NOTCH receptors (NOTCH1–4), which exhibit some overlapping functions, though this may be context specific (Kojika and Griffin, 2001). Receptor–ligand binding induces conformational changes in NOTCH that result in a series of proteolytic cleavages ultimately releasing an intracellular fragment of the NOTCH receptor, termed Intracellular NOTCH (ICN; De Strooper et al., 1999). ICN translocates to the nucleus where it associates with Recombination Signal Binding Protein for Immunoglobulin Kappa J Region (RBPJ), which binds to specific DNA sequences. In the absence of ICN, RBPJ is bound to the DNA in association with co-repressors, thus repressing target gene expression (Oswald et al., 2002; **Figure 2A**). ICN displaces these co-repressors and the ICN–RBPJ complex recruits a member of the transcriptional co-activators mastermind-like (MAML) family (Nam et al., 2006). The ICN/RBPJ/MAML complex represents the core NOTCH transcriptional activator complex and MAML then recruits additional co-activators (**Figure 2B**; Saint Just Ribeiro and Wallberg, 2009). Classical NOTCH targets include the Hairy and Enhancer of Split (HES) gene, which belongs to a family of basic helix-loop-helix transcriptional repressors, which are particularly important for lateral inhibition and patterning during development (Iso et al., 2003). NOTCH also regulates other targets such as c-myc (MYC; Weng et al., 2006), cyclin D1 (CCND1; Cohen et al., 2010), and the p21^{CIP1} (CDKN1A) cyclin dependent kinase inhibitor (Rangarajan et al., 2001). Due to the variety of cell types where NOTCH signaling is important, NOTCH target genes are lineage specific and critical NOTCH targets that drive keratinocyte differentiation have not been well-characterized.

Human cSCCs frequently harbor loss of function mutations in the NOTCH pathway, implicating NOTCH activity as tumor suppressive in epithelial cells (Nicolas et al., 2003; Agrawal et al., 2011; Stransky et al., 2011; Wang et al., 2011; South et al., 2014). The tumor suppressive effects of NOTCH in keratinocytes are largely thought to be due to a differentiation-induced block of cell proliferation and the activation of keratinocyte cell death (Zhang et al., 2016; Aster et al., 2017). NOTCH, however, also functions as an oncogenic driver in a number of human tumors, particularly hematopoietic cancers such as T-cell acute lymphoblastic leukemia (T-ALL) where gain of function mutations are commonly observed (Demarest et al., 2008).

MAML1 was originally identified in a yeast-two hybrid screen with HPV16 E6 as a bait (Wu et al., 2000). Like many cellular E6 binding proteins, MAML1 contains LXXLL sequence motifs and several groups detected MAML1 as a cellular interactor of β-HPV E6 proteins in AP/MS experiments (Brimer et al., 2012; Rozenblatt-Rosen et al., 2012; Tan et al., 2012; White et al., 2012a). Similarly, the bovine papillomavirus type 1 (BPV1) E6 protein was also shown to bind MAML1 (Brimer et al., 2012; Tan et al., 2012). Despite the original identification as an HPV16 E6 associated cellular protein (Wu et al., 2000), there is no evidence that mucosal α-HPV E6 proteins detectably associate with MAML1 in mammalian cells (Brimer et al., 2017).

Biological Consequences of TGF-β and NOTCH Inhibition by Cutaneous Papillomaviruses

Given that the TGF-β and NOTCH pathways are critical in regulating epithelial differentiation and function as tumor

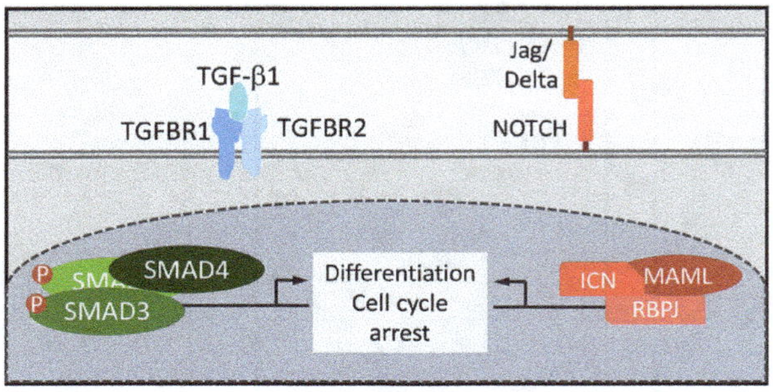

FIGURE 3 | Functional consequences of NOTCH and TGF-β signaling by HPV8 E6 and MmuPV1 E6. TGF-β and NOTCH signaling are critical for cell cycle arrest and keratinocyte differentiation that are tightly coupled in normal squamous epithelial cells. Functional uncoupling of these two processes is a necessary prerequisite for papillomavirus progeny formation in terminally differentiated epithelial cells.

suppressors in a variety of epithelial cancers, inhibition of these two pathways by cutaneous papillomavirus E6 proteins may be key to the transforming activities of these viruses.

Consistent with this model, it was shown that keratinocyte differentiation is inhibited in HPV8 E6 expressing epithelial cells. Chromatin immunoprecipitation experiments showed that E6 binds to and inhibits the DNA bound RBPJ/ICN/MAML1 activator complex (Meyers et al., 2013). HPV8 E6 binds to an LXXLL motif within the C-terminal transactivation domain (TAD) 2 of MAML1 (Tan et al., 2012; Meyers et al., 2017). The mechanism of action of TAD2 is unknown; EP300 and related co-activators associate with MAML through its TAD1 domain (Saint Just Ribeiro and Wallberg, 2009; Gerhardt et al., 2014). The MmuPV1 E6 protein also interacts with MAML1 and inhibits NOTCH signaling thereby inhibiting keratinocyte differentiation (Meyers et al., 2017; **Figure 2C**). MAML1 binding defective HPV8 and MmuPV1 E6 mutants were identified using a structure guided approach (Meyers et al., 2017). Of note, many of the HPV8 E6 mutants that were previously used to characterize the biological relevance of the interaction between cutaneous HPV E6 protein and EP300/CREBBP, were found to be MAML1 binding defective, thus further complicating the interpretation of published studies investigating the biological consequences of the EP300/CREBBP interactions with HPV5 and HPV8 E6 (Meyers et al., 2017). Association of E6 with MAML and inhibition of NOTCH signaling is independent of EP300/CREBBP binding, however, since MAML1 binding defective HPV8 E6 mutants retained EP300/CREBBP association and MmuPV1 E6 does not detectably bind EP300/CREBBP (Meyers et al., 2017). Indeed, the notable absence of EP300/CREBBP peptides in AP/MS experiments with MmuPV1 E6 is consistent with a model whereby E6 binding to TAD2 of MAML1 may inhibit expression of NOTCH transcriptional targets by interfering with recruitment or by displacing EP300/CREBBP from MAML1 TAD1. This model, however, awaits experimental validation.

The presence of an intact binding site for MAML1 in MmuPV1 E6 was shown to be necessary for formation of papillomas and carcinomas in experimentally infected mice (Meyers et al., 2017). While these studies cannot definitively exclude the possibility that association of E6 with other LXXLL domain proteins may also contribute to this phenotype, this is unlikely given a recent study that showed that UBE3A and MAML1 are the major LXXLL targets of papillomavirus E6 proteins and, consistent with the published E6/LXXLL structures (Zanier et al., 2013), the various papillomavirus E6 proteins displayed mutually exclusive binding to either UBE3A or MAML1 (Brimer et al., 2017).

Despite the fact that the E6 proteins of mucosal, high-risk α-HPVs have a strong preference for UBE3A binding and do not detectably interact with MAML1 (White et al., 2012a; Brimer et al., 2017), they have also been reported to inhibit NOTCH. HPV16 E6 can inhibit NOTCH signaling indirectly through degradation of the TP53 tumor suppressor (Dotto, 2009) and/or the TAp63β protein (Ben Khalifa et al., 2011). More recent studies showed that NOTCH inhibition is relevant to the biology of these viruses as HPV16 E6 mediated NOTCH inhibition was shown to decrease the commitment of keratinocytes to differentiation (Kranjec et al., 2017).

Hence, similar to TGF-β, inhibition of keratinocyte differentiation by targeting NOTCH signaling by cutaneous HPVs is shared with mucosal HPVs but is mediated through different mechanisms. Conceptually this is rather satisfying as papillomaviruses all had to evolve to render normally postmitotic, terminally differentiated epithelial cells conducive for supporting the viral life cycle (**Figure 3**). Interestingly however, different papillomaviruses have evolved mechanistically distinct strategies to solve this problem.

"Hit and Run" Carcinogenesis: A Consequence of E6 Mediated NOTCH and TGF-β Inhibition?

Hit and run carcinogenesis is a concept that historically has generated some skepticism, also with the authors of this article. The failure to detect viral gene expression in the majority of cancer cells may also imply that β- and γ-HPVs are biologically innocuous passengers that do not drive the carcinogenic process. Given, however, that at least some of these papillomaviruses are carcinogenic in transgenic mouse models and inhibit TGF-β and NOTCH signaling as well as other tumor suppressor pathways, it is more likely that these viruses provide oncogenic hits that drive at least some early aspects of epithelial carcinogenesis. In addition to many other biological activities of cutaneous HPVs, which include stem cell expansion, abrogating apoptosis, sensing and repair of UV-induced double strand DNA breaks, inhibition of the TGF-β and NOTCH tumor suppressors provide plausible oncogenic "hits" during early phases of carcinogenesis. Since the NOTCH and TGF-β pathways are oncogenic at later stages and drive malignant progression (Massague, 2008; Aster et al., 2017) loss of papillomavirus gene expression will re-activate NOTCH and TGF-β. This may drive malignant progression, thereby providing the mechanistic underpinnings for the "run" component of hit and run carcinogenesis.

It is important to note that the β- and γ-HPVs are phylogenetically and biologically diverse (Cornet et al., 2012;

Van Doorslaer et al., 2017) and that this diversity is also reflected in the cellular interactomes of their E6 and E7 proteins (White et al., 2012a,b). Hence, findings with one specific β- or γ-HPV type may not be applicable to other HPVs, even within the same genus. The accumulation of UV-induced mutations in a recently published HPV38 transgenic skin cancer model that recapitulates hit-and-run carcinogenesis, for example, is unlikely to be caused through an EP300/CREBBP dependent mechanism as no EP300/CREBBP binding has been detected in unbiased AP/MS studies with HPV38 E6 (White et al., 2012a; Viarisio et al., 2018).

The wide application of AP/MS to define cellular interactomes of papillomavirus proteins has already generated interesting hypotheses, many of which await rigorous validation (White and Howley, 2013; McBride, 2017). Next generation sequencing experiments may detect HPV DNA and/or RNA sequences in unexpected anatomic locations and tentatively link them to unanticipated pathologies (Chen et al., 2017). Such studies may also lead to the identification of HPVs that evaded detection by standard PCR-based techniques. The frequent detection of the novel γ-HPV197 genome in a deep sequencing study of human skin cancers, but not in normal skin, while not implying an etiologic link, should provide at least an impetus to study the biology of γ-HPVs in greater detail (Arroyo Muhr et al., 2015). Given that the HPV197 E7 protein, similar to MmuPV1, lacks an LXCXE-based canonical RB1 binding domain, and binds RB1 through a different sequence, suggest that some aspects of HPV197 E7 can be studied with the MmuPV1 animal model. These and other studies might also reveal whether HPV197, and potentially other γ-HPVs, have oncogenic activities.

AUTHOR CONTRIBUTIONS

JM and KM drafted the manuscript. AU, PL, and MG provided editorial and substantive input. KM wrote the final version of the manuscript.

REFERENCES

Accardi, R., Dong, W., Smet, A., Cui, R., Hautefeuille, A., Gabet, A. S., et al. (2006). Skin human papillomavirus type 38 alters p53 functions by accumulation of deltaNp73. *EMBO Rep.* 7, 334–340. doi: 10.1038/sj.embor.7400615

Agrawal, N., Frederick, M. J., Pickering, C. R., Bettegowda, C., Chang, K., Li, R. J., et al. (2011). Exome sequencing of head and neck squamous cell carcinoma reveals inactivating mutations in NOTCH1. *Science* 333, 1154–1157. doi: 10.1126/science.1206923

Alam, M., and Ratner, D. (2001). Cutaneous squamous-cell carcinoma. *N. Engl. J. Med.* 344, 975–983. doi: 10.1056/NEJM200103293441306

Antonsson, A., Erfurt, C., Hazard, K., Holmgren, V., Simon, M., Kataoka, A., et al. (2003a). Prevalence and type spectrum of human papillomaviruses in healthy skin samples collected in three continents. *J. Gen. Virol.* 84, 1881–1886.

Antonsson, A., Karanfilovska, S., Lindqvist, P. G., and Hansson, B. G. (2003b). General acquisition of human papillomavirus infections of skin occurs in early infancy. *J. Clin. Microbiol.* 41, 2509–2514.

Arron, S. T., Ruby, J. G., Dybbro, E., Ganem, D., and Derisi, J. L. (2011). Transcriptome sequencing demonstrates that human papillomavirus is not active in cutaneous squamous cell carcinoma. *J. Invest. Dermatol.* 131, 1745–1753. doi: 10.1038/jid.2011.91

Arroyo Muhr, L. S., Hultin, E., Bzhalava, D., Eklund, C., Lagheden, C., Ekstrom, J., et al. (2015). Human papillomavirus type 197 is commonly present in skin tumors. *Int. J. Cancer* 136, 2546–2555. doi: 10.1002/ijc.29325

Aster, J. C., Pear, W. S., and Blacklow, S. C. (2017). The varied roles of notch in cancer. *Annu. Rev. Pathol.* 12, 245–275. doi: 10.1146/annurev-pathol-052016-100127

Ben Khalifa, Y., Teissier, S., Tan, M. K., Phan, Q. T., Daynac, M., Wong, W. Q., et al. (2011). The human papillomavirus E6 oncogene represses a cell adhesion pathway and disrupts focal adhesion through degradation of TAp63beta upon transformation. *PLoS Pathog.* 7:e1002256. doi: 10.1371/journal.ppat.1002256

Borgogna, C., Lanfredini, S., Peretti, A., De Andrea, M., Zavattaro, E., Colombo, E., et al. (2014). Improved detection reveals active beta-papillomavirus infection in skin lesions from kidney transplant recipients. *Mod. Pathol.* 27, 1101–1115. doi: 10.1038/modpathol.2013.240

Borgogna, C., Zavattaro, E., De Andrea, M., Griffin, H. M., Dell'oste, V., Azzimonti, B., et al. (2012). Characterization of beta papillomavirus E4 expression in tumours from Epidermodysplasia Verruciformis patients and in experimental models. *Virology* 423, 195–204. doi: 10.1016/j.virol.2011.11.029

Bottalico, D., Chen, Z., Dunne, A., Ostoloza, J., Mckinney, S., Sun, C., et al. (2011). The oral cavity contains abundant known and novel human papillomaviruses from the Betapapillomavirus and Gammapapillomavirus genera. *J. Infect. Dis.* 204, 787–792. doi: 10.1093/infdis/jir383

Brimer, N., Drews, C. M., and Vande Pol, S. B. (2017). Association of papillomavirus E6 proteins with either MAML1 or E6AP clusters E6 proteins by structure, function, and evolutionary relatedness. *PLoS Pathog.* 13:e1006781. doi: 10.1371/journal.ppat.1006781

Brimer, N., Lyons, C., Wallberg, A. E., and Vande Pol, S. B. (2012). Cutaneous papillomavirus E6 oncoproteins associate with MAML1 to repress transactivation and NOTCH signaling. *Oncogene* 31, 4639–4646. doi: 10.1038/onc.2011.589

Caldeira, S., Zehbe, I., Accardi, R., Malanchi, I., Dong, W., Giarre, M., et al. (2003). The E6 and E7 proteins of the cutaneous human papillomavirus type 38 display transforming properties. *J. Virol.* 77, 2195–2206. doi: 10.1128/JVI.77.3.2195-2206.2003

CDC (2015). *Epidemiology and Prevention of Vaccine-Preventable Diseases.* Washington, DC: Public Health Foundation.

Chahoud, J., Semaan, A., Chen, Y., Cao, M., Rieber, A. G., Rady, P., et al. (2016). Association between beta-genus human papillomavirus and cutaneous squamous cell carcinoma in immunocompetent individuals-A meta-analysis. *JAMA Dermatol.* 152, 1354–1364. doi: 10.1001/jamadermatol.2015.4530

Chaikuad, A., and Bullock, A. N. (2016). Structural basis of intracellular TGF-β signaling: receptors and smads. *Cold Spring Harb. Perspect. Biol.* 8:a022111. doi: 10.1101/cshperspect.a022111

Chen, A. A., Gheit, T., Stellin, M., Lupato, V., Spinato, G., Fuson, R., et al. (2017). Oncogenic DNA viruses found in salivary gland tumors. *Oral Oncol.* 75, 106–110. doi: 10.1016/j.oraloncology.2017.11.005

Chen, A. C., Mcmillan, N. A., and Antonsson, A. (2008). Human papillomavirus type spectrum in normal skin of individuals with or without a history of frequent sun exposure. *J. Gen. Virol.* 89, 2891–2897. doi: 10.1099/vir.0.2008/003665-0

Chen, J. J., Hong, Y., Rustamzadeh, E., Baleja, J. D., and Androphy, E. J. (1998). Identification of an alpha helical motif sufficient for association with papillomavirus E6. *J. Biol. Chem.* 273, 13537–13544. doi: 10.1074/jbc.273.22.13537

Chuang, T. Y., Reizner, G. T., Elpern, D. J., Stone, J. L., and Farmer, E. R. (1993). Keratoacanthoma in Kauai, Hawaii. The first documented incidence in a defined population. *Arch. Dermatol.* 129, 317–319. doi: 10.1001/archderm.1993.01680240057005

Cladel, N. M., Budgeon, L. R., Balogh, K. K., Cooper, T. K., Hu, J., and Christensen, N. D. (2016). Mouse papillomavirus MmuPV1 infects oral mucosa and preferentially targets the base of the tongue. *Virology* 488, 73–80. doi: 10.1016/j.virol.2015.10.030

Cladel, N. M., Budgeon, L. R., Cooper, T. K., Balogh, K. K., Hu, J., and Christensen, N. D. (2013). Secondary infections, expanded tissue tropism, and evidence for malignant potential in immunocompromised mice infected with *Mus musculus* papillomavirus 1 DNA and virus. *J. Virol.* 87, 9391–9395. doi: 10.1128/JVI.00777-13

Cohen, B., Shimizu, M., Izrailit, J., Ng, N. F., Buchman, Y., Pan, J. G., et al. (2010). Cyclin D1 is a direct target of JAG1-mediated Notch signaling in breast cancer. *Breast Cancer Res. Treat.* 123, 113–124. doi: 10.1007/s10549-009-0621-9

Cornet, I., Bouvard, V., Campo, M. S., Thomas, M., Banks, L., Gissmann, L., et al. (2012). Comparative analysis of transforming properties of E6 and E7 from different beta human papillomavirus types. *J. Virol.* 86, 2366–2370. doi: 10.1128/JVI.06579-11

Datto, M. B., Li, Y., Panus, J. F., Howe, D. J., Xiong, Y., and Wang, X. F. (1995). Transforming growth factor beta induces the cyclin-dependent kinase inhibitor p21 through a p53-independent mechanism. *Proc. Natl. Acad. Sci. U.S.A.* 92, 5545–5549. doi: 10.1073/pnas.92.12.5545

De Strooper, B., Annaert, W., Cupers, P., Saftig, P., Craessaerts, K., Mumm, J. S., et al. (1999). A presenilin-1-dependent gamma-secretase-like protease mediates release of Notch intracellular domain. *Nature* 398, 518–522. doi: 10.1038/19083

Deady, S., Sharp, L., and Comber, H. (2014). Increasing skin cancer incidence in young, affluent, urban populations: a challenge for prevention. *Br. J. Dermatol.* 171, 324–331. doi: 10.1111/bjd.12988

Del Rosso, J. Q., Kircik, L., Goldenberg, G., and Brian, B. (2014). Comprehensive management of actinic keratoses: practical integration of available therapies with a review of a newer treatment approach. *J. Clin. Aesthet. Dermatol.* 7, S2–S12.

Demarest, R. M., Ratti, F., and Capobianco, A. J. (2008). It's T-ALL about Notch. *Oncogene* 27, 5082–5091. doi: 10.1038/onc.2008.222

Dotto, G. P. (2009). Crosstalk of Notch with p53 and p63 in cancer growth control. *Nat. Rev. Cancer* 9, 587–595. doi: 10.1038/nrc2675

Elbel, M., Carl, S., Spaderna, S., and Iftner, T. (1997). A comparative analysis of the interactions of the E6 proteins from cutaneous and genital papillomaviruses with p53 and E6AP in correlation to their transforming potential. *Virology* 239, 132–149. doi: 10.1006/viro.1997.8860

Feltkamp, M. C., De Koning, M. N., Bavinck, J. N., and Ter Schegget, J. (2008). Betapapillomaviruses: innocent bystanders or causes of skin cancer. *J. Clin. Virol.* 43, 353–360. doi: 10.1016/j.jcv.2008.09.009

Fleming, N. I., Jorissen, R. N., Mouradov, D., Christie, M., Sakthianandeswaren, A., Palmieri, M., et al. (2013). SMAD2, SMAD3 and SMAD4 mutations in colorectal cancer. *Cancer Res.* 73, 725–735. doi: 10.1158/0008-5472.CAN-12-2706

Forslund, O. (2007). Genetic diversity of cutaneous human papillomaviruses. *J. Gen. Virol.* 88, 2662–2669. doi: 10.1099/vir.0.82911-0

Foulongne, V., Sauvage, V., Hebert, C., Dereure, O., Cheval, J., Gouilh, M. A., et al. (2012). Human skin microbiota: high diversity of DNA viruses identified on the human skin by high throughput sequencing. *PLoS One* 7:e38499. doi: 10.1371/journal.pone.0038499

Frazer, I. H. (2004). Prevention of cervical cancer through papillomavirus vaccination. *Nat. Rev. Immunol.* 4, 46–54. doi: 10.1038/nri1260

French, D., Belleudi, F., Mauro, M. V., Mazzetta, F., Raffa, S., Fabiano, V., et al. (2013). Expression of HPV16 E5 down-modulates the TGFbeta signaling pathway. *Mol. Cancer* 12:38. doi: 10.1186/1476-4598-12-38

Genther, S. M., Sterling, S., Duensing, S., Munger, K., Sattler, C., and Lambert, P. F. (2003). Quantitative role of the human papillomavirus type 16 E5 gene during the productive stage of the viral life cycle. *J. Virol.* 77, 2832–2842. doi: 10.1128/JVI.77.5.2832-2842.2003

Gerhardt, D. M., Pajcini, K. V., D'altri, T., Tu, L., Jain, R., Xu, L., et al. (2014). The Notch1 transcriptional activation domain is required for development and reveals a novel role for Notch1 signaling in fetal hematopoietic stem cells. *Genes Dev.* 28, 576–593. doi: 10.1101/gad.227496.113

Grace, M., and Munger, K. (2017). Proteomic analysis of the gamma human papillomavirus type 197 E6 and E7 associated cellular proteins. *Virology* 500, 71–81. doi: 10.1016/j.virol.2016.10.010

Guy, G. P. Jr., Machlin, S. R., Ekwueme, D. U., and Yabroff, K. R. (2015). Prevalence and costs of skin cancer treatment in the U.S., 2002-2006 and 2007-2011. *Am. J. Prev. Med.* 48, 183–187. doi: 10.1016/j.amepre.2014.08.036

Hampras, S. S., Rollison, D. E., Giuliano, A. R., Mckay-Chopin, S., Minoni, L., Sereday, K., et al. (2017). Prevalence and concordance of cutaneous beta human papillomavirus infection at mucosal and cutaneous sites. *J. Infect. Dis.* 216, 92–96. doi: 10.1093/infdis/jix245

Handisurya, A., Day, P. M., Thompson, C. D., Bonelli, M., Lowy, D. R., and Schiller, J. T. (2014). Strain-specific properties and T cells regulate the susceptibility to papilloma induction by *Mus musculus* papillomavirus 1. *PLoS Pathog.* 10:e1004314. doi: 10.1371/journal.ppat.1004314

Harden, M. E., and Munger, K. (2017). Human papillomavirus molecular biology. *Mutat. Res. Rev. Mutat. Res.* 772, 3–12. doi: 10.1016/j.mrrev.2016.07.002

Hellner, K., and Munger, K. (2011). Human papillomaviruses as therapeutic targets in human cancer. *J. Clin. Oncol.* 29, 1785–1794. doi: 10.1200/JCO.2010.28.2186

Howie, H. L., Koop, J. I., Weese, J., Robinson, K., Wipf, G., Kim, L., et al. (2011). Beta-HPV 5 and 8 E6 promote p300 degradation by blocking AKT/p300 association. *PLoS Pathog.* 7:e1002211. doi: 10.1371/journal.ppat.1002211

Howley, P. M., and Pfister, H. J. (2015). Beta genus papillomaviruses and skin cancer. *Virology* 479–480, 290–296. doi: 10.1016/j.virol.2015.02.004

Hu, J., Budgeon, L. R., Cladel, N. M., Balogh, K., Myers, R., Cooper, T. K., et al. (2015). Tracking vaginal, anal and oral infection in a mouse papillomavirus infection model. *J. Gen. Virol.* 96, 3554–3565. doi: 10.1099/jgv.0.000295

Hufbauer, M., Biddle, A., Borgogna, C., Gariglio, M., Doorbar, J., Storey, A., et al. (2013). Expression of Betapapillomavirus oncogenes increases the number of keratinocytes with stem cell-like properties. *J. Virol.* 87, 12158–12165. doi: 10.1128/JVI.01510-13

Hufbauer, M., Cooke, J., Van Der Horst, G. T., Pfister, H., Storey, A., and Akgul, B. (2015). Human papillomavirus mediated inhibition of DNA damage sensing and repair drives skin carcinogenesis. *Mol. Cancer* 14:183. doi: 10.1186/s12943-015-0453-7

Ingle, A., Ghim, S., Joh, J., Chepkoech, I., Bennett Jenson, A., and Sundberg, J. P. (2011). Novel laboratory mouse papillomavirus (MusPV) infection. *Vet. Pathol.* 48, 500–505. doi: 10.1177/0300985810377186

Iso, T., Kedes, L., and Hamamori, Y. (2003). HES and HERP families: multiple effectors of the Notch signaling pathway. *J. Cell. Physiol.* 194, 237–255. doi: 10.1002/jcp.10208

Jackson, S., Harwood, C., Thomas, M., Banks, L., and Storey, A. (2000). Role of Bak in UV-induced apoptosis in skin cancer and abrogation by HPV E6 proteins. *Genes Dev.* 14, 3065–3073. doi: 10.1101/gad.182100

Joh, J., Ghim, S. J., Chilton, P. M., Sundberg, J. P., Park, J., Wilcher, S. A., et al. (2016). MmuPV1 infection and tumor development of T cell-deficient mice is prevented by passively transferred hyperimmune sera from normal congenic mice immunized with MmuPV1 virus-like particles (VLPs). *Exp. Mol. Pathol.* 100, 212–219. doi: 10.1016/j.yexmp.2016.01.003

Joh, J., Jenson, A. B., King, W., Proctor, M., Ingle, A., Sundberg, J. P., et al. (2011). Genomic analysis of the first laboratory-mouse papillomavirus. *J. Gen. Virol.* 92, 692–698. doi: 10.1099/vir.0.026138-0

Kilkenny, M., Merlin, K., Young, R., and Marks, R. (1998). The prevalence of common skin conditions in Australian school students: 1. Common, plane and plantar viral warts. *Br. J. Dermatol.* 138, 840–845. doi: 10.1046/j.1365-2133.1998.02222.x

Knipe, D. M., and Howley, P. M. (2013). *Fields Virology*. Philadelphia, PA: Wolters Kluwer.

Kohler, A., Forschner, T., Meyer, T., Ulrich, C., Gottschling, M., Stockfleth, E., et al. (2007). Multifocal distribution of cutaneous human papillomavirus types in hairs from different skin areas. *Br. J. Dermatol.* 156, 1078–1080. doi: 10.1111/j.1365-2133.2007.07809.x

Kojika, S., and Griffin, J. D. (2001). Notch receptors and hematopoiesis. *Exp. Hematol.* 29, 1041–1052. doi: 10.1016/S0301-472X(01)00676-2

Kranjec, C., Holleywood, C., Libert, D., Griffin, H., Mahmood, R., Isaacson, E., et al. (2017). Modulation of basal cell fate during productive and transforming HPV-16 infection is mediated by progressive E6-driven depletion of Notch. *J. Pathol.* 242, 448–462. doi: 10.1002/path.4917

Lanfredini, S., Olivero, C., Borgogna, C., Calati, F., Powell, K., Davies, K. J., et al. (2017). HPV8 field cancerization in a transgenic mouse model is due to Lrig1+ keratinocyte stem cell expansion. *J. Invest. Dermatol.* 137, 2208–2216. doi: 10.1016/j.jid.2017.04.039

Lee, D. K., Kim, B. C., Kim, I. Y., Cho, E. A., Satterwhite, D. J., and Kim, S. J. (2002). The human papilloma virus E7 oncoprotein inhibits transforming growth factor-beta signaling by blocking binding of the Smad complex to its target sequence. *J. Biol. Chem.* 277, 38557–38564. doi: 10.1074/jbc.M206786200

Leverrier, S., Bergamaschi, D., Ghali, L., Ola, A., Warnes, G., Akgul, B., et al. (2007). Role of HPV E6 proteins in preventing UVB-induced release of pro-apoptotic factors from the mitochondria. *Apoptosis* 12, 549–560. doi: 10.1007/s10495-006-0004-1

Mahe, E., Bodemer, C., Descamps, V., Mahe, I., Crickx, B., De Prost, Y., et al. (2003). High frequency of detection of human papillomaviruses associated with epidermodysplasia verruciformis in children with psoriasis. *Br. J. Dermatol.* 149, 819–825. doi: 10.1046/j.1365-2133.2003.05587.x

Marcuzzi, G. P., Hufbauer, M., Kasper, H. U., Weissenborn, S. J., Smola, S., and Pfister, H. (2009). Spontaneous tumour development in human papillomavirus type 8 E6 transgenic mice and rapid induction by UV-light exposure and wounding. *J. Gen. Virol.* 90, 2855–2864. doi: 10.1099/vir.0.012872-0

Marthaler, A. M., Podgorska, M., Feld, P., Fingerle, A., Knerr-Rupp, K., Grasser, F., et al. (2017). Identification of C/EBPalpha as a novel target of the HPV8 E6 protein regulating miR-203 in human keratinocytes. *PLoS Pathog.* 13:e1006406. doi: 10.1371/journal.ppat.1006406

Massague, J. (2008). TGFbeta in Cancer. *Cell* 134, 215–230. doi: 10.1016/j.cell.2008.07.001

Maufort, J. P., Shai, A., Pitot, H. C., and Lambert, P. F. (2010). A role for HPV16 E5 in cervical carcinogenesis. *Cancer Res.* 70, 2924–2931. doi: 10.1158/0008-5472.CAN-09-3436

Maufort, J. P., Williams, S. M., Pitot, H. C., and Lambert, P. F. (2007). Human papillomavirus 16 E5 oncogene contributes to two stages of skin carcinogenesis. *Cancer Res.* 67, 6106–6112. doi: 10.1158/0008-5472.CAN-07-0921

McBride, A. A. (2017). Perspective: the promise of proteomics in the study of oncogenic viruses. *Mol. Cell Proteomics* 16, S65–S74. doi: 10.1074/mcp.O116.065201

McLaughlin-Drubin, M. E., Meyers, J., and Munger, K. (2012). Cancer associated human papillomaviruses. *Curr. Opin. Virol.* 2, 459–466. doi: 10.1016/j.coviro.2012.05.004

McLaughlin-Drubin, M. E., and Munger, K. (2009). Oncogenic activities of human papillomaviruses. *Virus Res.* 143, 195–208. doi: 10.1016/j.virusres.2009.06.008

Mendoza, J. A., Jacob, Y., Cassonnet, P., and Favre, M. (2006). Human papillomavirus type 5 E6 oncoprotein represses the transforming growth factor beta signaling pathway by binding to SMAD3. *J. Virol.* 80, 12420–12424. doi: 10.1128/JVI.02576-05

Meyers, J. M., and Munger, K. (2014). The viral etiology of skin cancer. *J. Invest. Dermatol.* 134, E29–E32. doi: 10.1038/skinbio.2014.6

Meyers, J. M., Spangle, J. M., and Munger, K. (2013). The human papillomavirus type 8 E6 protein interferes with NOTCH activation during keratinocyte differentiation. *J. Virol.* 87, 4762–4767. doi: 10.1128/JVI.02527-12

Meyers, J. M., Uberoi, A., Grace, M., Lambert, P. F., and Munger, K. (2017). Cutaneous HPV8 and MmuPV1 E6 proteins target the NOTCH and TGF-β tumor suppressors to inhibit differentiation and sustain keratinocyte proliferation. *PLoS Pathog.* 13:e1006171. doi: 10.1371/journal.ppat.1006171

Michel, A., Kopp-Schneider, A., Zentgraf, H., Gruber, A. D., and De Villiers, E. M. (2006). E6/E7 expression of human papillomavirus type 20 (HPV-20) and HPV-27 influences proliferation and differentiation of the skin in UV-irradiated SKH-hr1 transgenic mice. *J. Virol.* 80, 11153–11164. doi: 10.1128/JVI.00954-06

Miyazawa, K., Shinozaki, M., Hara, T., Furuya, T., and Miyazono, K. (2002). Two major Smad pathways in TGF-β superfamily signalling. *Genes Cells* 7, 1191–1204. doi: 10.1046/j.1365-2443.2002.00599.x

Moody, C. A., and Laimins, L. A. (2010). Human papillomavirus oncoproteins: pathways to transformation. *Nat. Rev. Cancer* 10, 550–560. doi: 10.1038/nrc2886

Munger, K., Baldwin, A., Edwards, K. M., Hayakawa, H., Nguyen, C. L., Owens, M., et al. (2004). Mechanisms of human papillomavirus-induced oncogenesis. *J. Virol.* 78, 11451–11460. doi: 10.1128/JVI.78.21.11451-11460.2004

Munger, K., and Jones, D. L. (2015). Human papillomavirus carcinogenesis: an identity crisis in the retinoblastoma tumor suppressor pathway. *J. Virol.* 89, 4708–4711. doi: 10.1128/JVI.03486-14

Nam, Y., Sliz, P., Song, L., Aster, J. C., and Blacklow, S. C. (2006). Structural basis for cooperativity in recruitment of MAML coactivators to Notch transcription complexes. *Cell* 124, 973–983. doi: 10.1016/j.cell.2005.12.037

Neale, R. E., Weissenborn, S., Abeni, D., Bavinck, J. N., Euvrard, S., Feltkamp, M. C., et al. (2013). Human papillomavirus load in eyebrow hair follicles and risk of cutaneous squamous cell carcinoma. *Cancer Epidemiol. Biomarkers Prev.* 22, 719–727. doi: 10.1158/1055-9965.EPI-12-0917-T

Nicolas, M., Wolfer, A., Raj, K., Kummer, J. A., Mill, P., Van Noort, M., et al. (2003). Notch1 functions as a tumor suppressor in mouse skin. *Nat. Genet.* 33, 416–421. doi: 10.1038/ng1099

Orth, G., Jablonska, S., Favre, M., Croissant, O., Jarzabek-Chorzelska, M., and Rzesa, G. (1978). Characterization of two types of human papillomaviruses in lesions of epidermodysplasia verruciformis. *Proc. Natl. Acad. Sci. U.S.A.* 75, 1537–1541. doi: 10.1073/pnas.75.3.1537

Oswald, F., Kostezka, U., Astrahantseff, K., Bourteele, S., Dillinger, K., Zechner, U., et al. (2002). SHARP is a novel component of the Notch/RBP-Jkappa signalling pathway. *EMBO J.* 21, 5417–5426. doi: 10.1093/emboj/cdf549

Pass, F., Reissig, M., Shah, K. V., Eisinger, M., and Orth, G. (1977). Identification of an immunologically distinct papillomavirus from lesions of epidermodysplasia verruciformis. *J. Natl. Cancer Inst.* 59, 1107–1112. doi: 10.1093/jnci/59.4.1107

Pfefferle, R., Marcuzzi, G. P., Akgul, B., Kasper, H. U., Schulze, F., Haase, I., et al. (2008). The human papillomavirus type 8 E2 protein induces skin tumors in transgenic mice. *J. Invest. Dermatol.* 128, 2310–2315. doi: 10.1038/jid.2008.73

Pietenpol, J. A., Stein, R. W., Moran, E., Yaciuk, P., Schlegel, R., Lyons, R. M., et al. (1990). TGF-β 1 inhibition of c-myc transcription and growth in keratinocytes is abrogated by viral transforming proteins with pRB binding domains. *Cell* 61, 777–785. doi: 10.1016/0092-8674(90)90188-K

Qiu, W., Schonleben, F., Li, X., and Su, G. H. (2007). Disruption of transforming growth factor beta-Smad signaling pathway in head and neck squamous cell carcinoma as evidenced by mutations of SMAD2 and SMAD4. *Cancer Lett.* 245, 163–170. doi: 10.1016/j.canlet.2006.01.003

Quint, K. D., Genders, R. E., De Koning, M. N., Borgogna, C., Gariglio, M., Bouwes Bavinck, J. N., et al. (2015). Human Beta-papillomavirus infection and keratinocyte carcinomas. *J. Pathol.* 235, 342–354. doi: 10.1002/path.4425

Rangarajan, A., Talora, C., Okuyama, R., Nicolas, M., Mammucari, C., Oh, H., et al. (2001). Notch signaling is a direct determinant of keratinocyte growth arrest and entry into differentiation. *EMBO J.* 20, 3427–3436. doi: 10.1093/emboj/20.13.3427

Reynisdottir, I., Polyak, K., Iavarone, A., and Massague, J. (1995). Kip/Cip and Ink4 Cdk inhibitors cooperate to induce cell cycle arrest in response to TGF-β. *Genes Dev.* 9, 1831–1845. doi: 10.1101/gad.9.15.1831

Roberts, A. B., Anzano, M. A., Wakefield, L. M., Roche, N. S., Stern, D. F., and Sporn, M. B. (1985). Type beta transforming growth factor: a bifunctional regulator of cellular growth. *Proc. Natl. Acad. Sci. U.S.A.* 82, 119–123. doi: 10.1073/pnas.82.1.119

Roman, A., and Munger, K. (2013). The papillomavirus E7 proteins. *Virology* 445, 138–168. doi: 10.1016/j.virol.2013.04.013

Rozenblatt-Rosen, O., Deo, R. C., Padi, M., Adelmant, G., Calderwood, M. A., Rolland, T., et al. (2012). Interpreting cancer genomes using systematic host network perturbations by tumour virus proteins. *Nature* 487, 491–495. doi: 10.1038/nature11288

Saint Just Ribeiro, M., and Wallberg, A. E. (2009). Transcriptional mechanisms by the coregulator MAML1. *Curr. Protein Pept. Sci.* 10, 570–576. doi: 10.2174/138920309789630543

Schaper, I. D., Marcuzzi, G. P., Weissenborn, S. J., Kasper, H. U., Dries, V., Smyth, N., et al. (2005). Development of skin tumors in mice transgenic for early genes of human papillomavirus type 8. *Cancer Res.* 65, 1394–1400. doi: 10.1158/0008-5472.CAN-04-3263

Schiffman, M., Castle, P. E., Jeronimo, J., Rodriguez, A. C., and Wacholder, S. (2007). Human papillomavirus and cervical cancer. *Lancet* 370, 890–907. doi: 10.1016/S0140-6736(07)61416-0

Schiller, J. T., and Lowy, D. R. (2012). Understanding and learning from the success of prophylactic human papillomavirus vaccines. *Nat. Rev. Microbiol.* 10, 681–692. doi: 10.1038/nrmicro2872

Siegel, R. L., Miller, K. D., and Jemal, A. (2018). Cancer statistics, 2018. *CA Cancer J. Clin.* 68, 7–30. doi: 10.3322/caac.21442

Smelov, V., Hanisch, R., Mckay-Chopin, S., Sokolova, O., Eklund, C., Komyakov, B., et al. (2017). Prevalence of cutaneous beta and gamma human papillomaviruses in the anal canal of men who have sex with women. *Papillomavirus Res.* 3, 66–72. doi: 10.1016/j.pvr.2017.02.002

South, A. P., Purdie, K. J., Watt, S. A., Haldenby, S., Den Breems, N. Y., Dimon, M., et al. (2014). NOTCH1 mutations occur early during cutaneous squamous cell carcinogenesis. *J. Invest. Dermatol.* 134, 2630–2638. doi: 10.1038/jid.2014.154

Stransky, N., Egloff, A. M., Tward, A. D., Kostic, A. D., Cibulskis, K., Sivachenko, A., et al. (2011). The mutational landscape of head and neck squamous cell carcinoma. *Science* 333, 1157–1160. doi: 10.1126/science.1208130

Tan, M. J., White, E. A., Sowa, M. E., Harper, J. W., Aster, J. C., and Howley, P. M. (2012). Cutaneous beta-human papillomavirus E6 proteins bind Mastermind-like coactivators and repress Notch signaling. *Proc. Natl. Acad. Sci. U.S.A.* 109, E1473–E1480. doi: 10.1073/pnas.1205991109

Tommasino, M. (2017). The biology of beta human papillomaviruses. *Virus Res.* 231, 128–138. doi: 10.1016/j.virusres.2016.11.013

Uberoi, A., and Lambert, P. F. (2017). Rodent Papillomaviruses. *Viruses* 9:E362. doi: 10.3390/v9120362

Uberoi, A., Yoshida, S., Frazer, I. H., Pitot, H. C., and Lambert, P. F. (2016). Role of ultraviolet radiation in papillomavirus-induced disease. *PLoS Pathog.* 12:e1005664. doi: 10.1371/journal.ppat.1005664

Valcourt, U., Carthy, J., Okita, Y., Alcaraz, L., Kato, M., Thuault, S., et al. (2016). Analysis of epithelial-mesenchymal transition induced by transforming growth factor beta. *Methods Mol. Biol.* 1344, 147–181. doi: 10.1007/978-1-4939-2966-5_9

Van Doorslaer, K., Li, Z., Xirasagar, S., Maes, P., Kaminsky, D., Liou, D., et al. (2017). The papillomavirus episteme: a major update to the papillomavirus sequence database. *Nucleic Acids Res.* 45, D499–D506. doi: 10.1093/nar/gkw879

Vande Pol, S. B., and Klingelhutz, A. J. (2013). Papillomavirus E6 oncoproteins. *Virology* 445, 115–137. doi: 10.1016/j.virol.2013.04.026

Viarisio, D., Gissmann, L., and Tommasino, M. (2017). Human papillomaviruses and carcinogenesis: well-established and novel models. *Curr. Opin. Virol.* 26, 56–62. doi: 10.1016/j.coviro.2017.07.014

Viarisio, D., Muller-Decker, K., Accardi, R., Robitaille, A., Durst, M., Beer, K., et al. (2018). Beta HPV38 oncoproteins act with a hit-and-run mechanism in ultraviolet radiation-induced skin carcinogenesis in mice. *PLoS Pathog.* 14:e1006783. doi: 10.1371/journal.ppat.1006783

Viarisio, D., Mueller-Decker, K., Kloz, U., Aengeneyndt, B., Kopp-Schneider, A., Grone, H. J., et al. (2011). E6 and E7 from beta HPV38 cooperate with ultraviolet light in the development of actinic keratosis-like lesions and squamous cell carcinoma in mice. *PLoS Pathog.* 7:e1002125. doi: 10.1371/journal.ppat.1002125

Viarisio, D., Muller-Decker, K., Zanna, P., Kloz, U., Aengeneyndt, B., Accardi, R., et al. (2016). Novel ß-HPV49 transgenic mouse model of upper digestive tract cancer. *Cancer Res.* 76, 4216–4225. doi: 10.1158/0008-5472.CAN-16-0370

Wallace, N. A., Robinson, K., and Galloway, D. A. (2014). Beta human papillomavirus E6 expression inhibits stabilization of p53 and increases tolerance of genomic instability. *J. Virol.* 88, 6112–6127. doi: 10.1128/JVI.03808-13

Wallace, N. A., Robinson, K., Howie, H. L., and Galloway, D. A. (2012). HPV 5 and 8 E6 abrogate ATR activity resulting in increased persistence of UVB induced DNA damage. *PLoS Pathog.* 8:e1002807. doi: 10.1371/journal.ppat.1002807

Wang, D., Kanuma, T., Mizunuma, H., Takama, F., Ibuki, Y., Wake, N., et al. (2000). Analysis of specific gene mutations in the transforming growth factor-beta signal transduction pathway in human ovarian cancer. *Cancer Res.* 60, 4507–4512.

Wang, J., Zhou, D., Prabhu, A., Schlegel, R., and Yuan, H. (2010). The canine papillomavirus and gamma HPV E7 proteins use an alternative domain to bind and destabilize the retinoblastoma protein. *PLoS Pathog.* 6:e1001089. doi: 10.1371/journal.ppat.1001089

Wang, N. J., Sanborn, Z., Arnett, K. L., Bayston, L. J., Liao, W., Proby, C. M., et al. (2011). Loss-of-function mutations in Notch receptors in cutaneous and lung squamous cell carcinoma. *Proc. Natl. Acad. Sci. U.S.A.* 108, 17761–17766. doi: 10.1073/pnas.1114669108

Wendel, S. O., and Wallace, N. A. (2017). Loss of genome fidelity: Beta HPVs and the DNA damage response. *Front. Microbiol.* 8:2250. doi: 10.3389/fmicb.2017.02250

Weng, A. P., Millholland, J. M., Yashiro-Ohtani, Y., Arcangeli, M. L., Lau, A., Wai, C., et al. (2006). c-Myc is an important direct target of Notch1 in T-cell acute lymphoblastic leukemia/lymphoma. *Genes Dev.* 20, 2096–2109. doi: 10.1101/gad.1450406

White, E. A., and Howley, P. M. (2013). Proteomic approaches to the study of papillomavirus-host interactions. *Virology* 435, 57–69. doi: 10.1016/j.virol.2012.09.046

White, E. A., Kramer, R. E., Tan, M. J., Hayes, S. D., Harper, J. W., and Howley, P. M. (2012a). Comprehensive analysis of host cellular interactions with human papillomavirus E6 proteins identifies new E6 binding partners and reflects viral diversity. *J. Virol.* 86, 13174–13186. doi: 10.1128/JVI.02172-12

White, E. A., Sowa, M. E., Tan, M. J., Jeudy, S., Hayes, S. D., Santha, S., et al. (2012b). Systematic identification of interactions between host cell proteins and E7 oncoproteins from diverse human papillomaviruses. *Proc. Natl. Acad. Sci. U.S.A.* 109, E260–E267. doi: 10.1073/pnas.1116776109

White, E. A., Walther, J., Javanbakht, H., and Howley, P. M. (2014). Genus beta human papillomavirus E6 proteins vary in their effects on the transactivation of p53 target genes. *J. Virol.* 88, 8201–8212. doi: 10.1128/JVI.01197-14

Wu, L., Aster, J. C., Blacklow, S. C., Lake, R., Artavanis-Tsakonas, S., and Griffin, J. D. (2000). MAML1, a human homologue of Drosophila mastermind, is a transcriptional co-activator for NOTCH receptors. *Nat. Genet.* 26, 484–489. doi: 10.1038/82644

Xue, X. Y., Majerciak, V., Uberoi, A., Kim, B. H., Gotte, D., Chen, X., et al. (2017). The full transcription map of mouse papillomavirus type 1 (MmuPV1) in mouse wart tissues. *PLoS Pathog.* 13:e1006715. doi: 10.1371/journal.ppat.1006715

Yamashita, T., Segawa, K., Fujinaga, Y., Nishikawa, T., and Fujinaga, K. (1993). Biological and biochemical activity of E7 genes of the cutaneous human papillomavirus type 5 and 8. *Oncogene* 8, 2433–2441.

Zanier, K., Charbonnier, S., Sidi, A. O., Mcewen, A. G., Ferrario, M. G., Poussin-Courmontagne, P., et al. (2013). Structural basis for hijacking of cellular LxxLL motifs by papillomavirus E6 oncoproteins. *Science* 339, 694–698. doi: 10.1126/science.1229934

Zhang, M., Biswas, S., Qin, X., Gong, W., Deng, W., and Yu, H. (2016). Does Notch play a tumor suppressor role across diverse squamous cell carcinomas? *Cancer Med.* 5, 2048–2060. doi: 10.1002/cam4.731

15

HPV8-E6 Interferes with Syntenin-2 Expression through Deregulation of Differentiation, Methylation and Phosphatidylinositide-Kinase Dependent Mechanisms

Benjamin Marx[1], Daliborka Miller-Lazic[1], John Doorbar[2], Slawomir Majewski[3], Kay Hofmann[4], Martin Hufbauer[1] and Baki Akgül[1]*

[1] Institute of Virology, University of Cologne, Cologne, Germany, [2] Department of Pathology, University of Cambridge, Cambridge, United Kingdom, [3] Department of Dermatology and Venereology, Medical University of Warsaw, Warsaw, Poland, [4] Institute for Genetics, University of Cologne, Cologne, Germany

***Correspondence:**
Baki Akgül
baki.akguel@uk-koeln.de

The E6 oncoproteins of high-risk human papillomaviruses (HPV) of genus alpha contain a short peptide sequence at the carboxy-terminus, the PDZ binding domain, with which they interact with the corresponding PDZ domain of cellular proteins. Interestingly, E6 proteins from papillomaviruses of genus beta (betaPV) do not encode a comparable PDZ binding domain. Irrespective of this fact, we previously showed that the E6 protein of HPV8 (betaPV type) could circumvent this deficit by targeting the PDZ protein Syntenin-2 through transcriptional repression (Lazic et al., 2012). Despite its high binding affinity to phosphatidylinositol-4,5-bisphosphate (PI(4,5)P_2), very little is known about Syntenin-2. This study aimed to extend the knowledge on Syntenin-2 and how its expression is controlled. We now identified that Syntenin-2 is expressed at high levels in differentiating and in lower amounts in keratinocytes cultured in serum-free media containing low calcium concentration. HPV8-E6 led to a further reduction of Syntenin-2 expression only in cells cultured in low calcium. In the skin of patients suffering from Epidermodysplasia verruciformis, who are predisposed to betaPV infection, Syntenin-2 was expressed in differentiating keratinocytes of non-lesional skin, but was absent in virus positive squamous tumors. Using 5-Aza-2′-deoxycytidine, which causes DNA demethylation, Syntenin-2 transcription was profoundly activated and fully restored in the absence and presence of HPV8-E6, implicating that E6 mediated repression of Syntenin-2 transcription is due to promoter hypermethylation. Since Syntenin-2 binds to PI(4,5)P_2, we further tested whether the PI(4,5)P_2 metabolic pathway might govern Syntenin-2 expression. PI(4,5)P_2 is generated by the activity of phosphatidylinositol-4-phosphate-5-kinase type I (PIP5KI) or phosphatidylinositol-5-phosphate-4-kinase type II (PIP4KII) isoforms α, β and γ. Phosphatidylinositide kinases have recently been identified as regulators of gene transcription. Surprisingly, transfection of siRNAs directed against PIP5KI and PIP4KII resulted in higher Syntenin-2 expression with the highest effect mediated by siPIP5KIα. HPV8-E6 was able to counteract siPIP4KIIα, siPIP4KIIβ and siPIP5KIγ mediated Syntenin-2 re-expression but not siPIP5KIα. Finally, we identified Syntenin-2 as a key factor regulating PIP5KIα expression. Collectively, our data demonstrates that Syntenin-2 is regulated through multiple mechanisms and that downregulation of Syntenin-2 expression may contribute to E6 mediated dedifferentiation of infected skin cells.

Keywords: human papillomavirus (HPV), E6 oncoprotein, Syntenin-2, methylation, differentiation, phosphatidylinositol-4,5-bisphosphate

INTRODUCTION

Papillomaviruses are a family of non-enveloped DNA tumor viruses that infect the skin or mucosa of their vertebrate hosts (Bravo et al., 2010). Human papillomaviruses (HPV) are associated with the development of epithelial cancers and high-risk HPV of genus alpha (alphaPV) have been proven to be a necessary causative factor for cervical and oropharyngeal cancer (Hübbers and Akgül, 2015). HPV types of genus beta (betaPV) have been implicated in the development of cutaneous squamous cell carcinomas (SCC) and actinic keratosis. The association between betaPV and skin cancer was first reported in patients with Epidermodysplasia verruciformis (EV) (Majewski and Jablonska, 2006). Patients suffering from this condition have a specific susceptibility to infections with betaPV, which is characterized by virus-positive cutaneous lesions. These lesions mainly occur in sun-exposed areas and harbor a considerable risk of malignant transformation into SCC in affected individuals (Akgül et al., 2006; Borgogna et al., 2012; Howley and Pfister, 2015). Viral gene expression and replication proceed in a tightly controlled fashion regulated by keratinocyte differentiation, and lead to the expression of several non-structural viral early (E) proteins. Expression of the viral E4 protein during a productive infection contributes to virus release by perturbing the cytokeratin network. However, it may also represent a marker for viral infection during betaPV-associated skin cancer progression in EV patients (Borgogna et al., 2012; Quint et al., 2015). The HPV E6 and E7 oncoproteins are necessary for malignant conversion (Wallace and Galloway, 2015). A main feature of E6 oncoproteins from high-risk alphaHPV, e.g., HPV16, is their PDZ binding motif [identified as a domain interacting with PSD-95, Dlg, and ZO-1 proteins (hence the name PDZ (Ganti et al., 2015))], through which they promote the proteasomal degradation of a variety of cellular substrates harboring PDZ domains. Such PDZ proteins play a major role in maintenance of cell polarity, growth and differentiation as well as scaffolding proteins in multi-protein signaling complexes (Pim et al., 2012). Their degradation by the HPV E6 protein may cause loss of cell polarity and morphological conversion accompanied by an epithelial-mesenchymal transition, leading to transformation and carcinogenesis (Yugawa and Kiyono, 2009). The ability of E6 to bind to PDZ proteins correlates with its oncogenic potential (James and Roberts, 2016). In addition, the interactions between E6 and PDZ proteins also results in a significant stabilization of the E6 protein, which may ensure that sufficient E6 levels are maintained (Nicolaides et al., 2011). As previously mentioned, E6 of betaPV, e.g., HPV8, do not encode for a PDZ binding motif. We recently found, that the PDZ protein Syntenin-2, but not Syntenin-1, is transcriptionally downregulated in primary human keratinocytes by HPV8-E6. These results identified Syntenin-2 as the first PDZ protein being controlled by a betaHPV at mRNA level (Lazic et al., 2012). The PDZ protein family of Syntenins comprises Syntenin-1 and Syntenin-2. Syntenin-1 was originally identified as a protein that binds directly to the cytoplasmic domain of the syndecan family of heparan sulfate proteoglycans (Grootjans et al., 1997). These are implicated in cell adhesion and several growth factor signaling pathways (Zimmermann and David, 1999; Couchman, 2003; Egea-Jimenez et al., 2016; Fares et al., 2016). Although Syntenin-1 and -2 show different preferences, as far as protein binding is concerned, both proteins share the ability to interact with phosphatidylinositol-4,5-bisphosphate ($PI(4,5)P_2$) (Mortier et al., 2005). However, the precise mechanism by which Syntenin-2 is physiologically regulated and how transcription is modulated by HPV8-E6 remained elusive.

This study aimed to extend the understanding of transcriptional regulation controlling Syntenin-2 expression and how E6 interferes with these mechanisms. Our results suggest an interaction of E6 with Syntenin-2 expression through interference of cell differentiation, promoter-methylation and $PI(4,5)P_2$ generating kinases.

MATERIALS AND METHODS

Syntenin Sequence Analysis

For generation of the Syntenin evolutionary trees, representative Syntenin sequences were obtained from The UniProt Consortium (2017), aligned by the L-Ins-I algorithm of the MAFFT package (Katoh et al., 2002), and subjected to tree calculation by the T-Rex server (Boc et al., 2012) using the RAxML method (Stamatakis, 2006). Uniprot accession numbers for sequences analysis: human Syntenin-1 (SDCB1_HUMAN), human Syntenin-2 (SDCB2_HUMAN), murine Syntenin-1 (SDCB1_MOUSE), murine Syntenin-2 (SDCB2_MOUSE), zebrafish Syntenin-1 (Q6PUR1_DANRE), zebrafish Syntenin-2 (Q803J6_DANRE), xenopus Syntenin-1 (Q66JA3_XENLA), xenopus Syntenin-2 (Q801P2_XENLA), anolis Syntenin-1 (G1KE37_ANOCA), anolis Syntenin-2 (H9GDS9_ANOCA), chicken Syntenin-1 (Q5ZHM8_CHICK), chicken Syntenin-2 (R4GGF6_CHICK), mosquito Syntenin (Q7PK99_ANOGA), tick Syntenin (B7PNL5_IXOSC), nematostella Syntenin (A7S2D9_NEMVE), sponge Syntenin (I1FJB9_AMPQE), capsaspora Syntenin (A0A0D2VN74_CAPO3), monosiga Syntenin (A9UPR7_MONBE).

Retroviral Expression Vectors and Infection of Keratinocytes

We have previously described the generation of the pLXSN-based retroviral vectors coding for HPV8-E6 (Akgül et al., 2010). PLXSN-HPV8-E6 based mutants were generated by site-directed mutagenesis using specific primers. For retroviral infection, 3×10^5 cells were seeded into 6 cm dishes and treated as described in Hufbauer et al. (2013). Selection of infected cells was started 2 days later using 250 μg/ml G418. Positive clones were pooled and expanded.

Cell Lines and Treatments

RTS3b (Purdie et al., 1993) and PM1 keratinocytes (Proby et al., 2000) were maintained in RM+ media [consisting of a 3:1 ratio of DMEM:F12 with 10% fetal bovine serum (FBS), 1% glutamine, 0.4 μg hydrocortisone, 10^{-10}M cholera toxin, 5 μg/ml transferrin, 2×10^{-11}M liothyronine, 5 μg/ml insulin, 10 ng/ml epidermal growth factor, 1× Penicillin/Streptomycin mixture] (Akgül et al., 2003). HaCaT cells (Boukamp et al., 1988) were grown in DMEM with 10% FBS. N/TERT cells (Dickson et al., 2000) were either cultivated in KGM-Gold (which contains low concentrations of calcium to prevent differentiation) or in RM+ media. All cell lines were cultivated at 37°C and 6% CO_2. For global demethylation of DNA, N/TERT cells were treated with 5-aza-2′-deoxycytidine (5-Aza) (Sigma-Aldrich, Steinheim, Germany) diluted in dimethyl sulfoxide (DMSO) with different final concentrations of 0 or 10 μM for 72 h with media renewal every 24 h. Differentiation of N/TERT cells grown in KGM-Gold media was accomplished by treatment with 2 mM $CaCl_2$ for up to 8 days with 24 h media renewal.

siRNA Transfection

Silencing of $PI(4,5)P_2$ generating kinase gene expression was achieved through transfection of siRNA-SMARTpools (Dharmacon, GE Healthcare, Freiburg, Germany) with the RNAiMAX kit (Thermo Scientific, Waltham, MA, United States) according to the manufacturer's protocol (siPIP4KIIα: M-006778-01; siPIP4KIIβ: M-006779-03; siPIP5KIα: M-004780-02; siPIP5KIγ: M-004782-00). These siRNAs have previously been successfully used to decrease kinase expression (Bultsma et al., 2010; Chao et al., 2010). The siRNA against Syntenin-2 had the following sequence: siSyn-2: GCAACGGGCTCCTCACCAATT. Cells transfected with a scramble siRNA (Cat. Nr.: 98129_A, Biospring, Frankfurt, Germany) were used as controls.

Western Blotting

For Western blot analysis, cells were trypsinized, pelleted by centrifugation and lysed on ice in LSDB buffer [50 mM Tris/HCl (pH 8.0), 20% Glycerol, 100 mM KCl, 0,1% NP40, 1 mM DTT, 50 mM NaF, 1 mM orthovanadate, 1 mM PMSF] supplemented with 1× Cocktail Protease Inhibitors (Roche Diagnostics, Mannheim, Germany). The resulting extracts were sonicated, and protein concentration was determined using the Biorad Protein Assay (Biorad, Munich, Germany). Cell extracts were resolved by SDS–PAGE and transferred to a nitrocellulose membrane. After the membrane had been blocked with 5% skimmed milk in TBST [10 mM Tris/HCl (pH 8.0), 150 mM NaCl, 0.05% Tween 20] for 1 h, the blots were probed with antibodies against Syntenin-2 (rabbit polyclonal, Cat. no. 10407-1-AP, diluted 1:1500; Proteintech, Chicago, IL, United States), Loricrin (rabbit polyclonal, Cat. no. ab85679, diluted: 1:1000, Abcam, Cambridge, United Kingdom), PIP5K1α (rabbit polyclonal, Cat. no. PA5-29405, diluted 1:500, Thermo Scientific) and Tubulin (rat monoclonal, Cat. no. YL1/2, diluted 1:10,000; Abcam), which was used as loading control. Immunoreactive proteins were visualized using horseradish peroxidase-coupled IgG secondary antibodies (Dako, Hamburg, Germany) and the BM Chemiluminescence Blotting Substrate Detection System (Roche Diagnostics). The blots were exposed to autoradiographic films and signals were quantified using the ImageJ software.

Immunofluorescence Staining of Skin Samples

Anonymized EV skin lesions were obtained from routine surgical excisions. The use of the EV tissue for "studies on the mechanisms of HPV oncoprotein action in cutaneous oncogenesis" was approved by the local ethics-committee at the Medical University of Warsaw. HPV typing of these lesions was performed as described in Heuser et al. (2016). Four-micrometer formalin-fixed, paraffin-embedded sections were deparaffinized with xylene. Samples were hydrated through a descending alcohol series (100, 90, and 70%; 5 min each) and endogenous peroxidases were inactivated by incubation in 3% H_2O_2 in Methanol for 20 min. Antigen unmasking was performed by boiling the tissue sections in 10 mM citric acid buffer for 3 min in a beaker in a microwave followed by 15 min resting at RT. Further incubation steps were performed in a humid chamber to prevent drying-out. Blocking of unspecific antigen sites was achieved with 50% goat serum (Thermo Scientific) in PBS for 1 h at RT. Incubation with primary antibody against rabbit-anti-Syntenin-2 (ProteinTech) was done in a dilution of 1:250 in 2% goat serum over night at 4°C, followed by three washes with PBS. Sections of EV lesions were stained with rabbit anti-HPV8 E4 antibodies raised against a glutathione S-transferase (GST)-E1^E4 fusion protein (Borgogna et al., 2012). Detection of primary Syntenin-2 antibody was achieved by incubating the sections with a HRP-conjugated goat-anti-rabbit-IgG antibody (Dako, Santa Clara, CA, United States) diluted 1:2000 in 2% goat serum for 1 h at RT, followed by three washes with PBS. The fluorescence staining was performed with the "TSA™-Plus Fluorescein System" (PerkinElmer, Waltham, MA, United States). For E4 detection, sections were incubated with anti-rabbit secondary antibody conjugated with Alexa Fluor 488 (1:500 dilution in 2% FCS; Invitrogen) for 1 h at room temperature. The sections were counterstained with DAPI and embedded with Immumount (Thermo Fisher Scientific, St. Leon-Rot, Germany). Specific signals were visualized on the Leica DMI 6000B fluorescence microscope.

Quantitative Reverse Transcription-PCR (qRT-PCR)

RNA was isolated from cells using the RNeasy kit, and DNase digestion was performed on-column using RNase-free DNase according to the manufacturer's instructions (Qiagen, Hilden, Germany) (Lazic et al., 2011; Hufbauer et al., 2015). One microgram of total RNA was reverse transcribed using the Omniscript RT kit (Qiagen, Hilden, Germany) with 10 μM random nonamers (TIB MOLBIOL, Berlin, Germany) and 1 μM oligo(dT_{23}) primer (Sigma), as well as 10 units of RNase inhibitor (Thermo Fisher Scientific). Quantitative PCR (qPCR) was performed using the Light-Cycler system (Roche Diagnostics). The total copy number of target genes was normalized to the total copy number of the housekeeping gene encoding hypoxanthine phosphoribosyltransferase 1 (HPRT1). One PCR mixture contained 2 μl of 1:10 diluted cDNA in a total volume of 20 μl, 1.25 units Platinum *Taq* polymerase and the buffer provided in the kit (Invitrogen, Karlsruhe, Germany), 4 mM $MgCl_2$, 1.6 μl of a 1:1000 dilution of SYBR® Green (Sigma), 5% DMSO, 0.5 μM each forward and backward primer, 500 ng/μl non-acetylated bovine serum albumin (Thermo Fisher Scientific), and 0.2 mM deoxynucleotide triphosphate. To generate absolute standards, PCR fragments, amplified with primers also used for subsequent qPCR analysis, were cloned into pJET1.2 (Thermo Fisher Scientific). Samples were analyzed in duplicates together with a 10-fold dilution series of standard plasmid. The cycling protocol conditions were 60 s at 95°C, followed by 40 cycles of 1 s at 95°C (20°C/s), 5 s at annealing temperature (melting temperature of primer minus 5°C) (20°C/s), and 15 s at 72°C (20°C/s). The primers used in this study had the following 5′-to-3′ sequences:

Syntenin-2-fw: GTGGACGGGCAGAATGTTAT,
Syntenin-2-bw: ATGGAGATTCTGGCCACG;
HPRT1-fw: CCTAAGATGAGCGCAAGTTGAA,
HPRT1-bw: CCACAGGACTAGAACACCTGCTAA;
PIP4KIIα-fw: ATGGAATTAAGTGCCATGAAAAC,
PIP4KIIα-bw: GCATCATAATGAGTAAGGATGTCAAT;
PIP4KIIβ-fw: TGCATGTGGGAGAGGAGAGT,
PIP4KIIβ-bw: TCAGCTGTGCCAAGAACTCA;
PIP5KIα-fw: CCAACATAAAGAGGCGGAAT,
PIP5KIα-bw: AGGGTTCTGGTTGAGGTTCAT;
PIP5KIγ-fw: AAGGAGGCCGAGTTCCTG,
PIP5KIγ-bw: CGGGTTCTGGTTGAGGTTC;
HPV8-E6-fw: CCGCAACGTTTGAATTTAATG,
HPV8-E6-bw: ATTGAACGTCCTGTAGCTAATTCA.

Immunocytochemistry

Cells were seeded on coverslips and fixed in 4% paraformaldehyde for 10 min at RT and further permeabilized with 0.1% Triton X-100 for 5 min at RT. After blocking in 10% goat serum (diluted in PBS) for 30 min at RT, cells were incubated with primary antibodies against Syntenin-2 (ProteinTech) diluted 1:250 in 2% goat serum over night at 4°C. On the following day cells were incubated with corresponding fluorescently labeled secondary antibodies, counterstained with DAPI and embedded using Immumount (Thermo Fisher Scientific). Fluorescent signals were visualized on a Leica DMI 6000B fluorescence microscope.

Statistical Analysis

All qRT-PCR experiments were repeated a minimum of three times in duplicates. The results are expressed as mean ± SEM. Western blots were repeated in $n = 3$ independent experiments. The data presented as immunoblots or images of immunofluorescence analysis are from a representative experiment, which was qualitatively similar in the replicate experiments. Statistical significance was determined with unpaired 2-tailed Student's *t*-test. The asterisks shown in the figures indicate significant differences of experimental groups ($^{*}p < 0.05$; $^{**}p < 0.01$; $^{***}p < 0.001$). Non-significant changes are labeled as "ns."

RESULTS

Papillomavirus Evolution Corresponds with Syntenin Gene Duplication

The PDZ protein family of Syntenins is comprised of two family members, Syntenin-1 and Syntenin-2. Retrieving Syntenin sequences from UniProt and constructing phylogenetic trees, we identified that both genes are the result of a gene duplication event that occurred during vertebrate evolution from a single ancestral Syntenin gene. Since the host range of papillomaviruses seems to be restricted to vertebrates (Rector and Van Ranst, 2013; Lopez-Bueno et al., 2016), the proposed timing of Syntenin gene duplication correlates with the evolution of the first papillomaviruses (**Figure 1A**). In addition, Syntenin-1 and Syntenin-2 show extensive structural similarity within the different vertebrate lineages (**Figure 1B**). Thus, Syntenin gene duplication may have contributed to both divergent and convergent evolution of Syntenin-1 and Syntenin-2 during vertebrate evolution.

Differentiation Dependent Syntenin-2 Expression Is Repressed by betaPV

To address the mechanisms through which HPV8-E6 regulates gene expression in a cell line model, Syntenin-2 protein levels were determined in different keratinocyte cell lines. Total cell extracts of the HPV-negative PM1, HaCaT and RTS3b cells were analyzed by Western blotting in addition to N/TERT cells grown either in RM+ ($N/TERT^{RM+}$) or in KGM-Gold ($N/TERT^{KGM}$) media. As shown in **Figure 2A**, PM1, HaCaT and RTS3b cells showed expression of Syntenin-2. However, compared to isogenic $N/TERT^{RM+}$ cells, Syntenin-2 was found to be downregulated in $N/TERT^{KGM}$. These data indicated that Syntenin-2 expression is culture media and differentiation dependent. To further confirm differentiation dependence, $N/TERT^{KGM}$ were exposed to high extracellular calcium concentrations (2 mM) for up to 8 days. Parallel to the induction of the differentiation marker loricrin, confirming the differentiation-inducing cell culture conditions, Syntenin-2

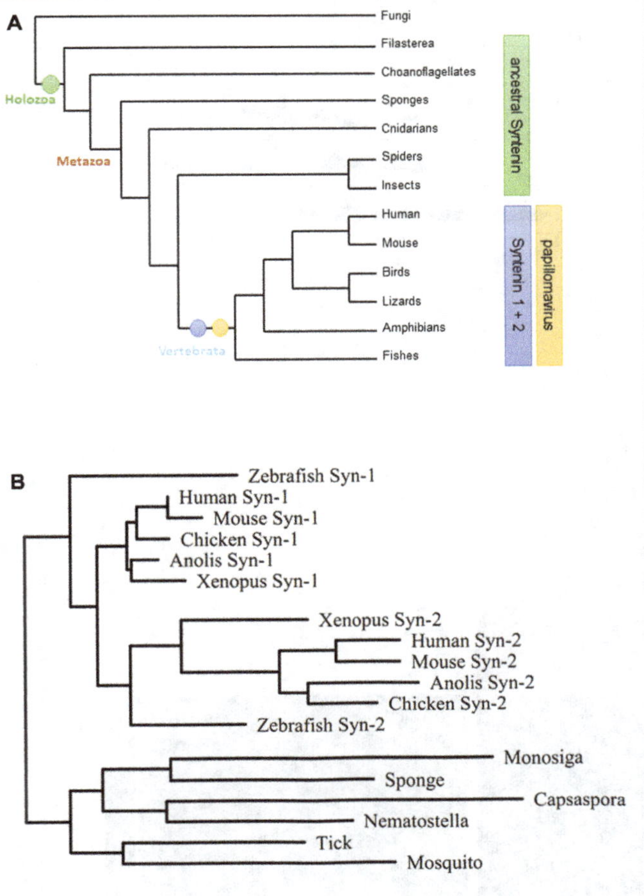

FIGURE 1 | Evolution of the Syntenin gene family. **(A)** Phylogram of major opisthokont lineages [tree simplified after (Torruella et al., 2015)]. Host range of papillomaviruses corresponds to Syntenin-1/Syntenin-2 evolutionary split. **(B)** Maximum likelihood tree for the Syntenin gene family. Representative Syntenin sequences were obtained from UniProt (The UniProt Consortium, 2017), aligned by the L-Ins-I algorithm of the MAFFT package (Katoh et al., 2002), and subjected to tree calculation by the T-Rex server (Boc et al., 2012) using the RAxML method (Stamatakis, 2006) (Syn-1: Syntenin-1; Syn-2: Syntenin-2).

was found to be upregulated in a calcium- and time-dependent manner (**Figure 2B**).

To further evaluate the expression pattern of Syntenin-2 in skin tumors induced by betaPV infection, we stained HPV8 positive skin tumors of EV patients. Staining against the viral E4 protein, which can have both a nuclear and cytoplasmic staining pattern in betaPV-induced tumors was used as surrogate marker for betaPV infection. To visualize E4, a broadly cross-reactive polyclonal antibody raised against the E4 protein of HPV5 and HPV8 was used (Borgogna et al., 2012). As demonstrated in **Figure 2C**, Syntenin-2 is expressed in the cytoplasm and nuclei of suprabasal keratinocytes in E4 negative EV skin and is absent in E4 positive lesional skin. Taken together, these findings implicated that Syntenin-2 expression is dependent on cell differentiation and is downregulated in skin with productive betaPV infection.

HPV8-E6 Represses Syntenin-2 Expression in Keratinocytes with a Basal Cell Phenotype

Given that HPV8-E6 mediated Syntenin-2 repression was previously identified in primary human keratinocytes (Lazic et al., 2012), we next tested whether E6 may also interfere with Syntenin-2 regulation in keratinocyte cell lines. As shown in **Figure 3A**, E6 mediated repression of Syntenin-2 transcription was only found to be significant in N/TERT^{KGM} and was not observed in HPV8-E6 positive N/TERT^{RM+}, RTS3b, HaCaT and PM1 cells. Immunocytochemical analysis revealed nuclear and cytoplasmic localization of Syntenin-2 in empty vector transduced N/TERT^{KGM} keratinocytes and a marked reduction of mainly cytoplasmic Syntenin-2 in HPV8-E6 positive cells (**Figure 3B**). To further elucidate the role of conserved amino acids in HPV8-E6 involved in regulation of Syntenin-2 expression, seven mutants of E6 were generated. To test whether repression of Syntenin-2 is a direct consequence of the previously described function of E6 to inhibit Mastermind-like protein 1 (MAML1) dependent differentiation processes (Brimer et al., 2012; Tan et al., 2012; Meyers et al., 2013), the mutants L61A, W63A and L61A/W63A were used. We could show in another study, that the E6 mutants L61A and W63A are still able to bind to MAML1 whereas the double mutant L61A/W63A is deficient in MAML1 binding (own unpublished data). Based on previously published data on HPV5-E6 mutants, the HPV8-E6 mutants V68A, D96A and D126A represent functional mutants, which are still able to inhibit UV-induced apoptosis but are incapable to induce proteasomal degradation of the pro-apoptotic protein Bak (Simmonds and Storey, 2008). The HPV8-E6-K136N mutant is, in contrast to wild type E6, deficient in inhibiting UV-induced DNA damage repair (Hufbauer et al., 2015). In line with wild type E6, the mutants L61A, W63A and the double mutant L61A/W63A (all positions are located within the first zinc-finger) were able to repress Syntenin-2 expression, whereas mutations located near the C-terminus (V68A, D96A, D126A, K136N) failed to inhibit Syntenin-2 expression (**Figures 3C,D**). This data provided evidence that E6 mediated downregulation of Syntenin-2, is a mechanism that is independent of E6 mediated blockade of MAML1 dependent differentiation processes.

Syntenin-2 Gene Repression in HPV8-E6 Cells Is Released by 5-Aza-2′-deoxycytidine

Hypermethylation of promoter regions can be involved in transcriptional regulation of cellular genes and E6 mediated promoter hypermethylation has previously been described for HPV16-E6 (D'Costa et al., 2012; Schütze et al., 2015; Yin et al., 2017). To test the hypothesis that Syntenin-2 promoter activity may also be methylation-dependent, the effect of 5-Aza-2′-deoxycytidine (5-Aza) mediated inhibition of DNA methylation on Syntenin-2 promoter regulation was measured in the presence and absence of HPV8-E6. E6 expression in cells used for these assays was confirmed by qRT-PCR (**Supplementary Figure S1**).

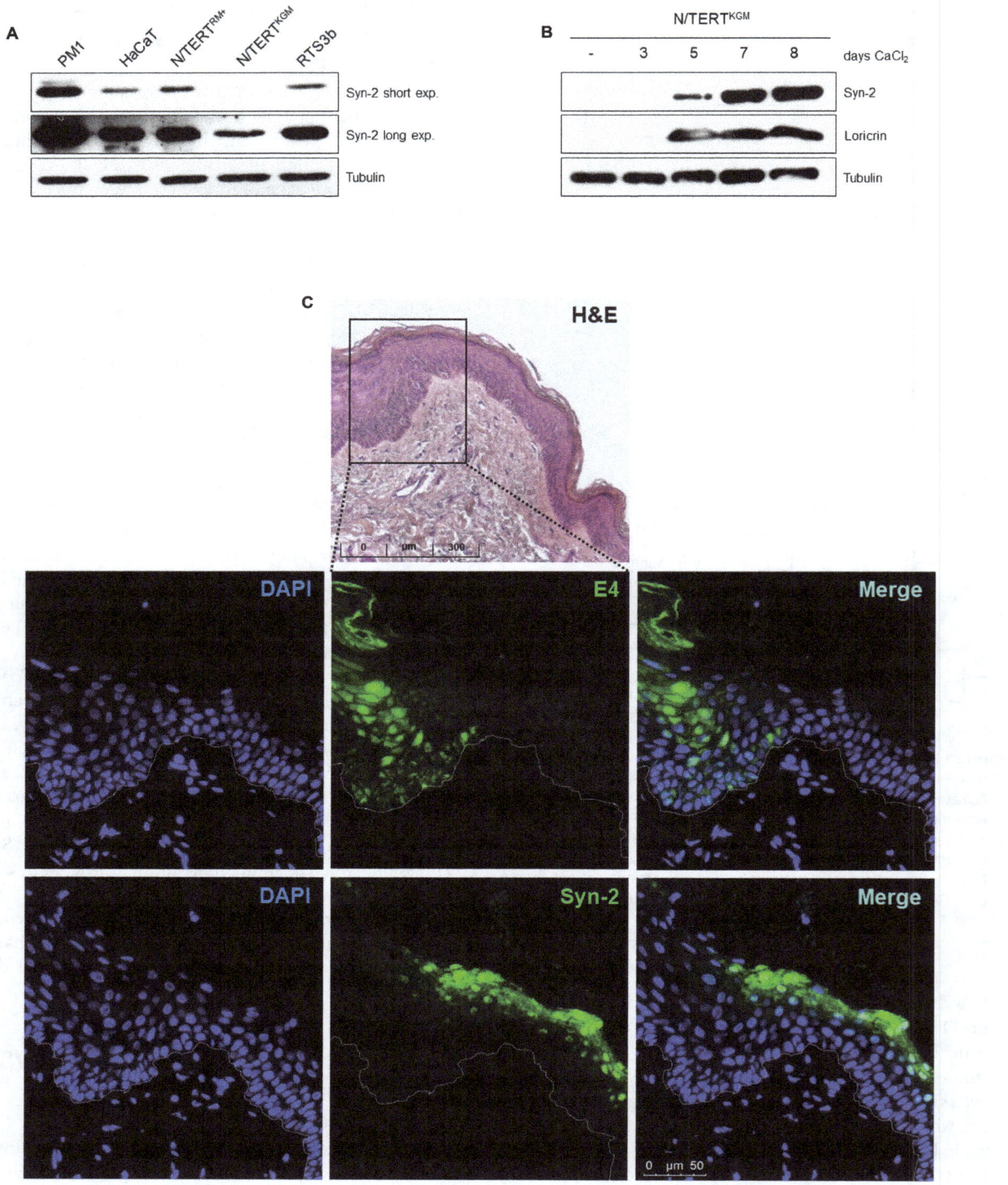

FIGURE 2 | Differentiation dependent expression of Syntenin-2 in skin keratinocytes. **(A)** Representative Western blot showing Syntenin-2 levels in total cell extracts of the keratinocyte cell lines PM1, HaCaT, RTS3b and isogenic N/TERT cells either cultured in RM+ (N/TERT^{RM+}) or in KGM-Gold (N/TERT^{KGM}). Equal loading was confirmed by immunoblotting for Tubulin. **(B)** Representative Western blot of Syntenin-2 levels in total cell extracts of N/TERT^{KGM} treated with 2 mM $CaCl_2$ for up to 8 days. Calcium induced keratinocyte differentiation was confirmed by Western blotting for Loricrin. Equal loading was confirmed by immunoblotting for Tubulin. **(C)** Representative immunofluorescence staining images detecting Syntenin-2 in EV-derived skin lesions. The skin area with productive betaPV infection was identified by anti-E4 staining. Nuclear counterstain was performed using DAPI. Syntenin-2 expression is present in suprabasal keratinocytes of non-lesional/E4-negative EV skin and absent in an E4-positive skin tumor. Top lane: H&E staining of the EV tissue analyzed.

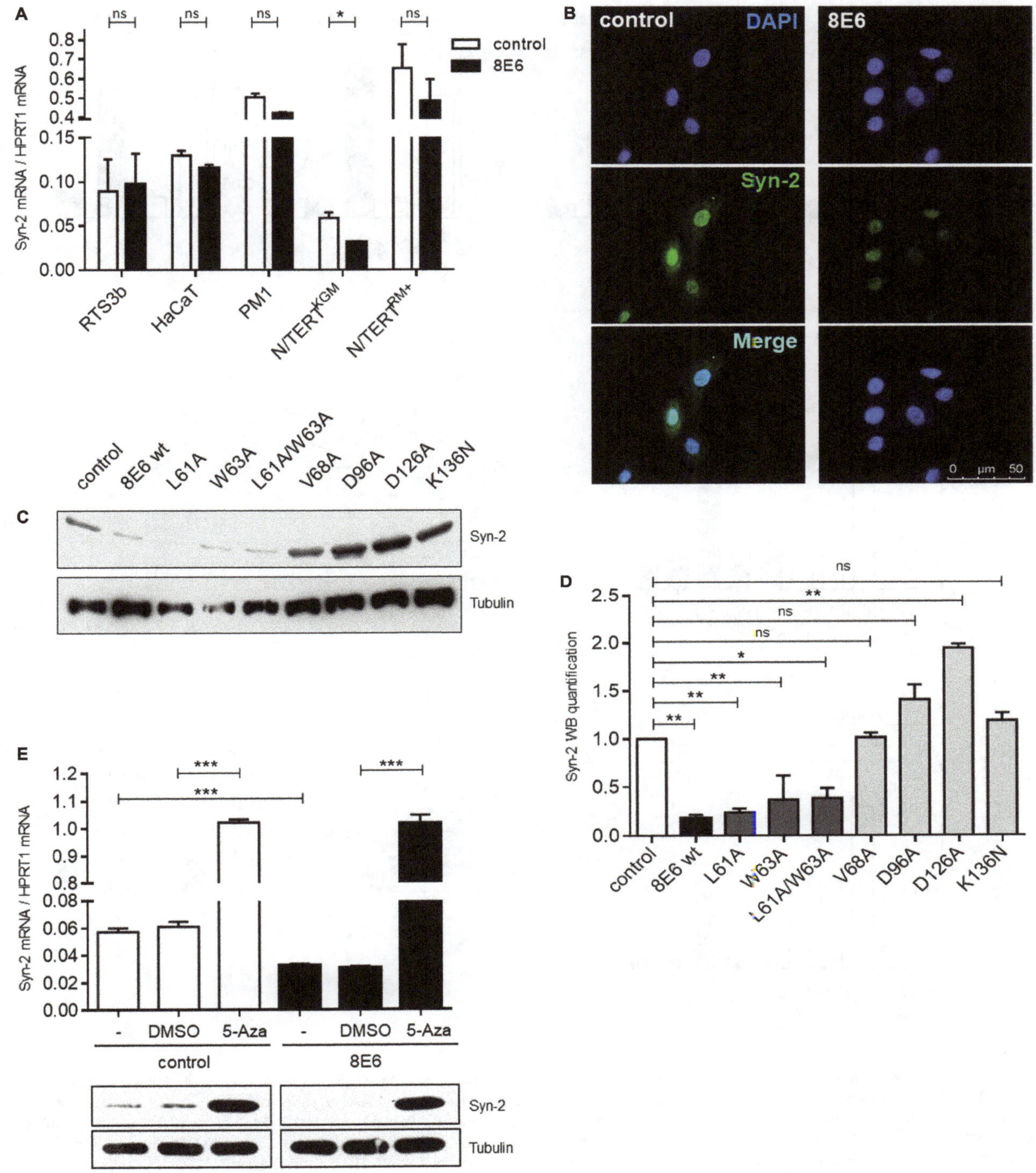

FIGURE 3 | Syntenin-2 expression is repressed by HPV8-E6 in keratinocytes with basal cell characteristics through promoter hypermethylation. **(A)** Quantification of Syntenin-2 mRNA expression by qRT-PCR in empty vector and HPV8-E6 expressing RTS3b, HaCaT, PM1 and isogenic N/TERT keratinocytes cultured either in RM− or KGM. **(B)** Representative immunocytochemical staining of Syntenin-2 in N/TERT^{KGM}-control (Left) and N/TERT^{KGM}-8E6 (Right) demonstrating reduction of mainly cytoplasmic Syntenin-2 in HPV8-E6 positive cells (blue: DAPI; green: Syntenin-2). **(C)** Representative Western blot showing Syntenin-2 in total cell extracts of N/TERT^{KGM} expressing either HPV8-E6 wild type or the E6 mutants L61A, W63A, L61A/W63A, V68A, D96A, D126A or K136N. Loading was confirmed by immunoblotting for Tubulin. **(D)** Quantification of Syntenin-2 protein levels from **(C)** normalized to Tubulin protein levels. **(E)** Quantification of Syntenin-2 mRNA expression in N/TERT^{KGM}-control and N/TERT^{KGM}-8E6 cells after treatment with 10 μM 5-Aza or DMSO ($n = 3$ independent experiments, measured in duplicate, Upper). Data are presented as mean ± SEM (***$p < 0.001$). Western blot analysis of Syntenin-2 in extracts from cells treated with 5-Aza. Equal loading was confirmed by immunoblotting for Tubulin (Lower).

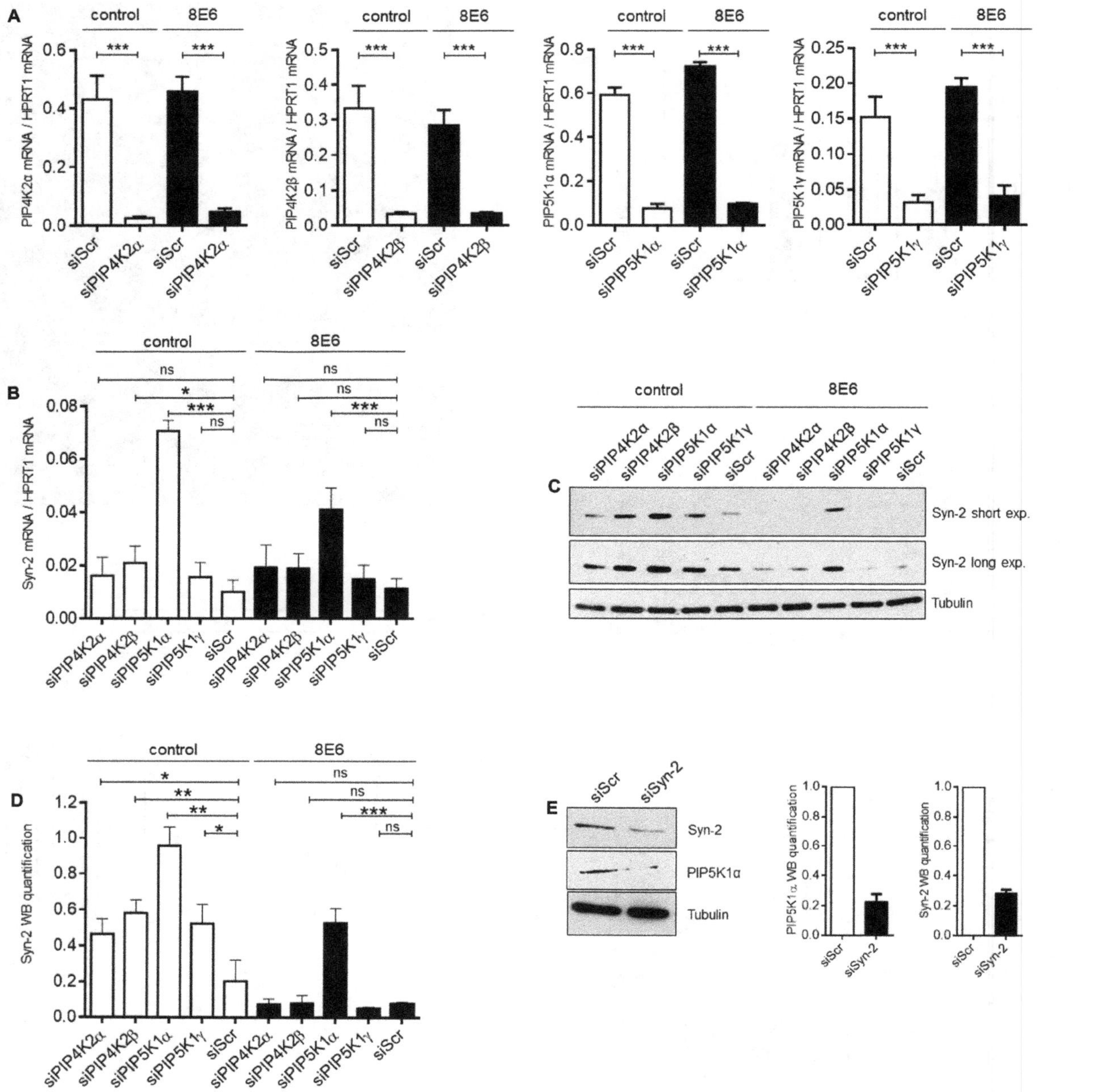

FIGURE 4 | $PI(4,5)P_2$ generating kinases are involved in control of Syntenin-2 expression. **(A)** Control (siScr), siPIP4KIIα, siPIP4KIIβ, siPIP5KIα or siPIP5KIγ transfected N/TERT[KGM]-control and N/TERT[KGM]-8E6 cells were harvested 48 h post transfection and mRNA expression of kinase isoforms was determined by qRT-PCR ($n = 3$ independent experiments, measured in duplicate). Data are presented as mean ± SEM (***$p < 0.001$). **(B)** Quantification of Syntenin-2 mRNA expression by qRT-PCR in N/TERT[KGM]-control and N/TERT[KGM]-8E6, in which the kinase isoforms PIP4KIIα, PIP4KIIβ, PIP5KIα and PIP5KIγ were silenced by siRNA transfection. **(C)** Representative Western blot showing Syntenin-2 expression in total cell extracts from N/TERT[KGM]-control and N/TERT[KGM]-8E6, in which kinase isoforms were silenced by siRNA transfection. Equal loading was confirmed by immunoblotting for Tubulin. **(D)** Quantification of Syntenin-2 protein levels in cells treated with siRNAs for specific kinase isoforms ($n = 3$ independent experiments). Data are presented as mean ± SEM. **(E)** Representative Western blot demonstrating downregulation of PIP5KIα protein levels in cells transfected with specific siRNA against Syntenin-2 (Left). Bars presenting the quantification of PIP5KIα and Syntenin-2 protein levels are shown in the Middle and Right ($n = 3$ independent experiments). Data are presented as mean ± SEM.

Syntenin-2 mRNA levels were low in DMSO treated cells but significantly increased following treatment with 5-Aza in control cells. This increase in mRNA was also mirrored on the protein level (**Figure 3E**). Syntenin-2 mRNA levels were lower in HPV8-E6 expressing cells compared to empty vector positive and DMSO treated keratinocytes. Syntenin-2 transcription levels were increased about 30-fold following 5-Aza treatment in E6 positive cells, restoring them to the same level that was detected in

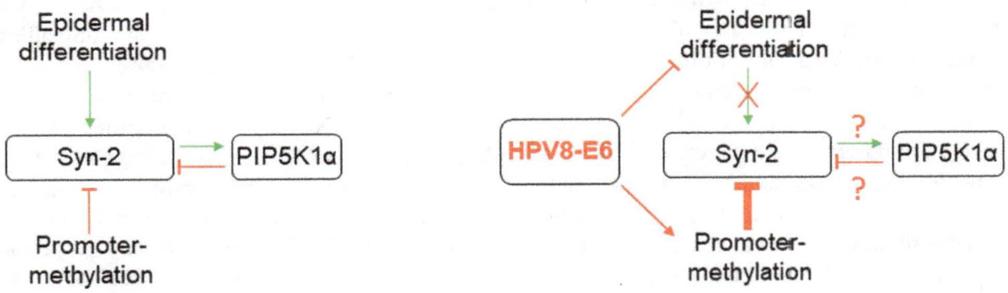

FIGURE 5 | Graphical summary of the regulatory pathways identified in this study controlling Syntenin-2 expression n normal keratinocytes (Left). Known HPV8-E6 mediated interference with these mechanisms is shown on the Right.

5-Aza treated control cells (**Figure 3E**). This complete restoration supports hyper-methylation dependent regulation of Syntenin-2 expression by HPV8-E6.

Phosphatidylinositol Metabolic Pathway Controls Syntenin-2 Gene Expression

It has been shown by Mortier et al. (2005), that nuclear $PI(4,5)P_2$ is required for the sub-nuclear enrichment of Syntenin-2. $PI(4,5)P_2$ generating kinases are present in the nucleus and have an impact on gene expression by contributing to chromatin unfolding and transcriptional regulation (Delage et al., 2013). In principle, $PI(4,5)P_2$ is synthesized by either the phosphorylation of phosphatidylinositol-4-phosphate (PI4P) by the lipid kinase phosphatidylinositol-4-phosphate-5-kinase type I (PIP5KI) or by the phosphorylation of phosphatidylinositol-5-phosphate (PI5P) through phosphatidylinositol-5-phosphate-4-kinase type II (PIP4KII) (van den Bout and Divecha, 2009). Each of these kinases comprises three isoforms, given the designations α, β and γ. To evaluate the functional correlation between the $PI(4,5)P_2$ pathway and Syntenin-2 gene expression, we next analyzed the impact of $PI(4,5)P_2$ generating kinases on Syntenin-2 expression through silencing of the single kinase isoforms. The kinase isoform PIP4KIIγ is not a nuclear protein and was therefore not studied (Itoh et al., 1998; Clarke et al., 2008) in addition to PIP5KIβ, which is not expressed in N/TERT^{KGM} (data not shown). A strong knockdown of the kinase isoforms could be achieved for all four tested enzymes using kinase specific siRNA pools in E6 negative and positive cells (**Figure 4A**). The expression of HPV8-E6 in these cells was confirmed by qRT-PCR and was not significantly changed in all siRNA treated cells (**Supplementary Figure S2**). Knockdown of PIP4KIIβ and particularly PIP5KIα led to a significant upregulation of Syntenin-2 mRNA expression in wild type keratinocytes. Interestingly, HPV8-E6 was able to counteract siPIP4KIIβ and siPIP5KIα mediated re-activation of Syntenin-2 transcription (**Figure 4B**). On protein level, kinase silencing led to the induction of Syntenin-2 expression in siPIP4KIIα, siPIP4KIIβ, siPIP5KIα and siPIP5KIγ transfected cells with siPIP5KIα showing the strongest effect in empty vector positive N/TERT^{KGM} cells. HPV8-E6 blocked Syntenin-2 protein re-expression in siPIP4KIIα, siPIP4KIIβ and siPIP5KIγ treated cells and counteracted siPIP5KIα-mediated re-expression of Syntenin-2 by 50% (**Figures 4C,D**). To further determine whether, on the other hand, Syntenin-2 is a regulator of PIP5K1α expression, we also measured protein levels in keratinocytes treated with Syntenin-2 specific siRNA. Unexpectedly, knockdown of Syntenin-2 led to a strong downregulation of PIP5K1α protein expression (**Figure 4E**).

DISCUSSION

We recently identified Syntenin-2 as the first PDZ protein to be targeted by HPV8-E6 on transcriptional level in primary keratinocytes cultured in low calcium media (Lazic et al., 2012). In this study we elucidated the mechanisms controlling Syntenin-2 gene expression. We now could show that Syntenin-2 is expressed in different keratinocyte cell lines cultured in RM+ media. It was, however, significantly downregulated in N/TERT cells grown in KGM media, under cell culture conditions in which keratinocytes do not differentiate and phenotypically resemble basal epidermal cells. Using N/TERT^{KGM} keratinocytes as a cell line model, we demonstrate that HPV8-E6 is capable of suppressing Syntenin-2 expression only in these keratinocytes. We previously demonstrated, that Syntenin-2 is absent in three-dimensional organotypic skin cultures of HPV8-E6 positive keratinocytes, which show loss of normal stratification and the absence of stratum corneum formation. In addition, downregulation of Syntenin-2 through shRNA expression inhibited differentiation of normal keratinocytes in skin cultures (Lazic et al., 2012). The interference of E6 with normal keratinocyte differentiation represents an oncogenic mechanism that has recently been linked to the ability of HPV8-E6 to bind to MAML1 and thus blocks NOTCH-dependent differentiation regulation (Brimer et al., 2012; Tan et al., 2012; Meyers et al., 2013). HPV8-E6 is also known to prevent pro-Caspase-14 cleavage, which is involved in the regulation of late terminal differentiation of keratinocytes (Kazem et al., 2011). We now show, that Syntenin-2 expression is absent in suprabasal cell layers of HPV8 positive EV skin tumors. The fact that the L61A/W63A mutant, which is not able to bind to MAML1 still represses Syntenin-2 indicated that Syntenin-2 downregulation is not linked to E6-mediated inhibition of MAML1/NOTCH-dependent differentiation. This led to the conclusion that reduction of Syntenin-2 by E6 may contribute to betaPV-mediated alteration of keratinocyte differentiation independent of MAML1 inhibition.

Another key observation is, that the Syntenin-2 promoter is regulated by DNA methylation. The observation, that Syntenin-2 mRNA and protein levels could completely be restored by 5-Aza treatment in HPV8-E6 expressing cells, led us to the conclusion, that E6 mediated suppression of Syntenin-2 is mediated through promoter hypermethylation. The exact mechanism how HPV8-E6 induces hypermethylation of cellular gene promoters and how the C-terminal part of E6 contributes to this needs still to be investigated.

Syntenin-2 is known to bind nuclear $PI(4,5)P_2$ with high affinity (Mortier et al., 2005). Phosphatidylinositides within the nucleus appear to influence many steps of transcriptional regulation, including reading and writing of the histone code, polymerase-dependent transcription, splicing and polyadenylation, and finally mRNA export (Lewis et al., 2011; Shah et al., 2013). In addition to our observation that differentiation and methylation pathways are involved in Syntenin-2 regulation, we also provide evidence, that Syntenin-2 is a target of the $PI(4,5)P_2$ metabolic pathway (**Figure 5**). Particularly, the downregulation of PIP5KIα resulted in re-expression of Syntenin-2 and this specific Syntenin-2 upregulation could only partially be counteracted by E6. Whether shortage of $PI(4,5)P_2$, accumulation of PI4P or PIP5KIα functions during keratinocyte differentiation (Xie et al., 2009; Shrestha et al., 2016) contribute to transcriptional repression of Syntenin-2 remains unclear. In addition, the observation that Syntenin-2 silencing using siRNAs resulted in inhibition of PIP5KIα protein expression points to a negative feedback loop between these two factors (**Figure 5**).

Known interaction partners of Syntenin-1 do not interact with Syntenin-2, which may imply that they are functionally not redundant (Koroll et al., 2001). Both Syntenins have evolved by gene duplication from an ancestral Syntenin gene during vertebrate evolution. Gene duplication has been linked to many aspects of genome evolution and is a potent way to create new biological functions (Wagner et al., 2007), which may also account for Syntenin proteins. Syntenin-1 is predominantly located in cell - cell adherens junctions and cytoplasm and is involved in diverse functions including human tumorigenesis (Beekman and Coffer, 2008; Friand et al., 2015; Philley et al., 2016). Interestingly, Syntenin-1 has been linked with the endocytic pathway controlling HPV entry into the host cell, controlling the delivery of internalized viral particles to endosomes and viral capsid disassembly in a CD63-Syntenin-1-ALIX dependent manner (Grassel et al., 2016). Although human Syntenin-2 is highly related to Syntenin-1 in its overall domain organization and sequence, both proteins show higher similarities with the homolog protein of other vertebrate species than to the variants expressed in an individual organism. It is tempting to speculate that during evolution Syntenin-1 may have provided the platform for virus-host specification of an ancestral papillomavirus as a key event in the evolution determinant of papillomaviruses (Gottschling et al., 2011; Van Doorslaer, 2013). However, at the same time, papillomaviruses may need to downregulate Syntenin-2 through E6 to achieve tissue dedifferentiation to enable efficient viral propagation.

CONCLUSION

We have advanced the understanding of Syntenin-2 gene regulation in normal cells and how HPV8-E6 can interfere with these mechanisms. Elucidation of the Syntenin-2 regulated pathways will provide further knowledge on its role in regulating keratinocyte differentiation.

AUTHOR CONTRIBUTIONS

Conceived and designed the experiments: BM and BA. Performed the experiments: BM, DM-L, KH, and MH. Analyzed the data: BM, DM-L, MH, and BA. Approved the final version of the manuscript: BM, DM-L, KH, SM, JD, MH, and BA. Contributed reagents/materials: SM and JD. Wrote the paper: BA.

ACKNOWLEDGMENTS

This work was funded by The German Research Foundation (Deutsche Forschungsgemeinschaft (DFG), grant nr. AK42/4-1) and by the Cologne Fortune Program (grant nr. 228/2016). MH was supported by the German Cancer Aid (Deutsche Krebshilfe, grant nr. 111087).

REFERENCES

Akgül, B., Bostanci, N., Westphal, K., Nindl, I., Navsaria, H., Storey, A., et al. (2010). Human papillomavirus 5 and 8 E6 downregulate interleukin-8 secretion in primary human keratinocytes. *J. Gen. Virol.* 91(Pt 4), 888–892. doi: 10.1099/vir.0.016527-0

Akgül, B., Cooke, J. C., and Storey, A. (2006). HPV-associated skin disease. *J. Pathol.* 208, 165–175. doi: 10.1002/path.1893

Akgül, B., Karle, P., Adam, M., Fuchs, P. G., and Pfister, H. J. (2003). Dual role of tumor suppressor p53 in regulation of DNA replication and oncogene E6-promoter activity of epidermodysplasia verruciformis-associated human papillomavirus type 8. *Virology* 308, 279–290. doi: 10.1016/S0042-6822(02)00133-2

Beekman, J. M., and Coffer, P. J. (2008). The ins and outs of syntenin, a multifunctional intracellular adaptor protein. *J. Cell Sci.* 121(Pt 9), 1349–1355. doi: 10.1242/jcs.026401

Boc, A., Diallo, A. B., and Makarenkov, V. (2012). T-REX: a web server for inferring, validating and visualizing phylogenetic trees and networks. *Nucleic Acids Res.* 40, W573–W579. doi: 10.1093/nar/gks485

Borgogna, C., Zavattaro, E., De Andrea, M., Griffin, H. M., Dell'Oste, V., Azzimonti, B., et al. (2012). Characterization of beta papillomavirus E4 expression in tumours from epidermodysplasia verruciformis patients and in experimental models. *Virology* 423, 195–204. doi: 10.1016/j.virol.2011.11.029

Boukamp, P., Petrussevska, R. T., Breitkreutz, D., Hornung, J., Markham, A., and Fusenig, N. E. (1988). Normal keratinization in a spontaneously immortalized aneuploid human keratinocyte cell line. *J. Cell Biol.* 106, 761–771. doi: 10.1083/jcb.106.3.761

Bravo, I. G., de Sanjose, S., and Gottschling, M. (2010). The clinical importance of understanding the evolution of papillomaviruses. *Trends Microbiol.* 18, 432–438. doi: 10.1016/j.tim.2010.07.008

Brimer, N., Lyons, C., Wallberg, A. E., and Vande Pol, S. B. (2012). Cutaneous papillomavirus E6 oncoproteins associate with MAML1 to repress transactivation and NOTCH signaling. *Oncogene* 31, 4639–4646. doi: 10.1038/onc.2011.589

Bultsma, Y., Keune, W. J., and Divecha, N. (2010). PIP4Kbeta interacts with and modulates nuclear localization of the high-activity PtdIns5P-4-kinase isoform PIP4Kalpha. *Biochem. J.* 430, 223–235. doi: 10.1042/BJ20100341

Chao, W. T., Ashcroft, F., Daquinag, A. C., Vadakkan, T., Wei, Z., Zhang, P., et al. (2010). Type I phosphatidylinositol phosphate kinase beta regulates focal adhesion disassembly by promoting beta1 integrin endocytosis. *Mol. Cell. Biol.* 30, 4463–4479. doi: 10.1128/MCB.01207-09

Clarke, J. H., Emson, P. C., and Irvine, R. F. (2008). Localization of phosphatidylinositol phosphate kinase IIgamma in kidney to a membrane trafficking compartment within specialized cells of the nephron. *Am. J. Physiol. Renal Physiol.* 295, F1422–F1430. doi: 10.1152/ajprenal.90310.2008

Couchman, J. R. (2003). Syndecans: proteoglycan regulators of cell-surface microdomains? *Nat. Rev. Mol. Cell Biol.* 4, 926–937. doi: 10.1038/nrm1257

D'Costa, Z. J., Jolly, C., Androphy, E. J., Mercer, A., Matthews, C. M., and Hibma, M. H. (2012). Transcriptional repression of E-cadherin by human papillomavirus type 16 E6. *PLOS ONE* 7:e48954. doi: 10.1371/journal.pone.0048954

Delage, E., Puyaubert, J., Zachowski, A., and Ruelland, E. (2013). Signal transduction pathways involving phosphatidylinositol 4-phosphate and phosphatidylinositol 4,5-bisphosphate: convergences and divergences among eukaryotic kingdoms. *Prog. Lipid Res.* 52, 1–14. doi: 10.1016/j.plipres.2012.08.003

Dickson, M. A., Hahn, W. C., Ino, Y., Ronfard, V., Wu, J. Y., Weinberg, R. A., et al. (2000). Human keratinocytes that express hTERT and also bypass a p16^{INK4a}-enforced mechanism that limits life span become immortal yet retain normal growth and differentiation characteristics. *Mol. Cell. Biol.* 20, 1436–1447. doi: 10.1128/MCB.20.4.1436-1447.2000

Egea-Jimenez, A. L., Gallardo, R., Garcia-Pino, A., Ivarsson, Y., Wawrzyniak, A. M., Kashyap, R., et al. (2016). Frizzled 7 and PIP2 binding by syntenin PDZ2 domain supports Frizzled 7 trafficking and signalling. *Nat. Commun.* 7:12101. doi: 10.1038/ncomms12101

Fares, J., Kashyap, R., and Zimmermann, P. (2016). Syntenin: key player in cancer exosome biogenesis and uptake? *Cell Adh. Migr.* 11, 124–126. doi: 10.1080/19336918.2016.1225632

Friand, V., David, G., and Zimmermann, P. (2015). Syntenin and syndecan in the biogenesis of exosomes. *Biol. Cell* 107, 331–341. doi: 10.1111/boc.201500010 doi: 10.1111/boc.201500010

Ganti, K., Broniarczyk, J., Manoubi, W., Massimi, P., Mittal, S., Pim, D., et al. (2015). The human papillomavirus E6 PDZ binding motif: from life cycle to malignancy. *Viruses* 7, 3530–3551. doi: 10.3390/v7072785

Gottschling, M., Goker, M., Stamatakis, A., Bininda-Emonds, O. R., Nindl, I., and Bravo, I. G. (2011). Quantifying the phylodynamic forces driving papillomavirus evolution. *Mol. Biol. Evol.* 28, 2101–2113. doi: 10.1093/molbev/msr030

Grassel, L., Fast, L. A., Scheffer, K. D., Boukhallouk, F., Spoden, G. A., Tenzer, S., et al. (2016). The CD63-Syntenin-1 complex controls post-endocytic trafficking of oncogenic human papillomaviruses. *Sci. Rep.* 6:32337. doi: 10.1038/srep32337

Grootjans, J. J., Zimmermann, P., Reekmans, G., Smets, A., Degeest, G., Durr, J., et al. (1997). Syntenin, a PDZ protein that binds syndecan cytoplasmic domains. *Proc. Natl. Acad. Sci. U.S.A.* 94, 13683–13688. doi: 10.1073/pnas.94.25.13683

Heuser, S., Hufbauer, M., Marx, B., Tok, A., Majewski, S., Pfister, H., et al. (2016). The levels of epithelial anchor proteins beta-catenin and zona occludens-1 are altered by E7 of human papillomaviruses 5 and 8. *J. Gen. Virol.* 97, 463–472. doi: 10.1099/jgv.0.000363

Howley, P. M., and Pfister, H. J. (2015). Beta genus papillomaviruses and skin cancer. *Virology* 47, 290–296. doi: 10.1016/j.virol.2015.02.004

Hübbers, C. U., and Akgül, B. (2015). HPV and cancer of the oral cavity. *Virulence* 6, 244–248. doi: 10.1080/21505594.2014.999570

Hufbauer, M., Biddle, A., Borgogna, C., Gariglio, M., Doorbar, J., Storey, A., et al. (2013). Expression of betapapillomavirus oncogenes increases the number of keratinocytes with stem cell-like properties. *J. Virol.* 87, 12158–12165. doi: 10.1128/JVI.01510-13

Hufbauer, M., Cooke, J., van der Horst, G. T., Pfister, H., Storey, A., and Akgül, B. (2015). Human papillomavirus mediated inhibition of DNA damage sensing and repair drives skin carcinogenesis. *Mol. Cancer* 14, 183. doi: 10.1186/s12943-015-0453-7

Itoh, T., Ijuin, T., and Takenawa, T. (1998). A novel phosphatidylinositol-5-phosphate 4-kinase (phosphatidylinositol-phosphate kinase IIgamma) is phosphorylated in the endoplasmic reticulum in response to mitogenic signals. *J. Biol. Chem.* 273, 20292–20299. doi: 10.1074/jbc.273.32.20292

James, C. D., and Roberts, S. (2016). Viral interactions with PDZ domain-containing proteins-an oncogenic trait? *Pathogens* 5:E8. doi: 10.3390/pathogens5010008

Katoh, K., Misawa, K., Kuma, K., and Miyata, T. (2002). MAFFT: a novel method for rapid multiple sequence alignment based on fast Fourier transform. *Nucleic Acids Res.* 30, 3059–3066. doi: 10.1093/nar/gkf436

Kazem, S., van der Meijden, E., Struijk, L., de Gruijl, F. R., and Feltkamp, M. C. (2011). Human papillomavirus 8 E6 disrupts terminal skin differentiation and prevents pro-caspase-14 cleavage. *Virus Res.* 163, 609–616. doi: 10.1016/j.virusres.2011.12.015

Koroll, M., Rathjen, F. G., and Volkmer, H. (2001). The neural cell recognition molecule neurofascin interacts with syntenin-1 but not with syntenin-2, both of which reveal self-associating activity. *J. Biol. Chem.* 276, 10646–10654. doi: 10.1074/jbc.M010647200

Lazic, D., Alborzi, F., Marcuzzi, G. P., Angel, P., Hess, J., Pfister, H., et al. (2011). Enhanced StefinA and Sprr2 expression during papilloma formation in HPV8 transgenic mice. *J. Dermatol. Sci.* 62, 84–90. doi: 10.1016/j.jdermsci.2011.02.006

Lazic, D., Hufbauer, M., Zigrino, P., Buchholz, S., Kazem, S., Feltkamp, M. C., et al. (2012). Human papillomavirus type 8 E6 oncoprotein inhibits transcription of the PDZ protein syntenin-2. *J. Virol.* 86, 7943–7952. doi: 10.1128/JVI.00132-12

Lewis, A. E., Sommer, L., Arntzen, M. O., Strahm, Y., Morrice, N. A., Divecha, N., et al. (2011). Identification of nuclear phosphatidylinositol 4,5-bisphosphate-interacting proteins by neomycin extraction. *Mol. Cell. Proteomics* 10:M110003376. doi: 10.1074/mcp.M110.003376

Lopez-Bueno, A., Mavian, C., Labella, A. M., Castro, D., Borrego, J. J., Alcami, A., et al. (2016). Concurrence of iridovirus, polyomavirus, and a unique member of a new group of fish papillomaviruses in lymphocystis disease-affected gilthead Sea Bream. *J. Virol.* 90, 8768–8779. doi: 10.1128/JVI.01369-16

Majewski, S., and Jablonska, S. (2006). Current views on the role of human papillomaviruses in cutaneous oncogenesis. *Int. J. Dermatol.* 45, 192–196. doi: 10.1111/j.1365-4632.2006.02758.x

Meyers, J. M., Spangle, J. M., and Munger, K. (2013). The human papillomavirus type 8 E6 protein interferes with NOTCH activation during keratinocyte differentiation. *J. Virol.* 87, 4762–4767. doi: 10.1128/JVI.02527-12

Mortier, E., Wuytens, G., Leenaerts, I., Hannes, F., Heung, M. Y., Degeest, G., et al. (2005). Nuclear speckles and nucleoli targeting by PIP2-PDZ domain interactions. *EMBO J.* 24, 2556–2565. doi: 10.1038/sj.emboj.7600722

Nicolaides, L., Davy, C., Raj, K., Kranjec, C., Banks, L., and Doorbar, J. (2011). Stabilization of HPV16 E6 protein by PDZ proteins, and potential implications for genome maintenance. *Virology* 414, 137–145. doi: 10.1016/j.virol.2011.03.017

Philley, J. V., Kannan, A., and Dasgupta, S. (2016). MDA-9/syntenin control. *J. Cell. Physiol.* 231, 545–550. doi: 10.1002/jcp.25136

Pim, D., Bergant, M., Boon, S. S., Ganti, K., Kranjec, C., Massimi, P., et al. (2012). Human papillomaviruses and the specificity of PDZ domain targeting. *FEBS J.* 279, 3530–3537. doi: 10.1111/j.1742-4658.2012.08709.x

Proby, C. M., Purdie, K. J., Sexton, C. J., Purkis, P., Navsaria, H. A., Stables, J. N., et al. (2000). Spontaneous keratinocyte cell lines representing early and advanced stages of malignant transformation of the epidermis. *Exp. Dermatol.* 9, 104–117. doi: 10.1034/j.1600-0625.2000.009002104.x

Purdie, K. J., Sexton, C. J., Proby, C. M., Glover, M. T., Williams, A. T., Stables, J. N., et al. (1993). Malignant transformation of cutaneous lesions in renal allograft patients: a role for human papillomavirus. *Cancer Res.* 53, 5328–5333.

Quint, K. D., Genders, R. E., de Koning, M. N., Borgogna, C., Gariglio, M., Bouwes Bavinck, J. N., et al. (2015). Human Beta-papillomavirus infection and keratinocyte carcinomas. *J. Pathol.* 235, 342–354. doi: 10.1002/path.4425

Rector, A., and Van Ranst, M. (2013). Animal papillomaviruses. *Virology* 445, 213–223. doi: 10.1016/j.virol.2013.05.007

Schütze, D. M., Kooter, J. M., Wilting, S. M., Meijer, C. J., Quint, W., Snijders, P. J., et al. (2015). Longitudinal assessment of DNA methylation changes during HPVE6E7-induced immortalization of primary keratinocytes. *Epigenetics* 10, 73–81. doi: 10.4161/15592294.2014.990787

Shah, Z. H., Jones, D. R., Sommer, L., Foulger, R., Bultsma, Y., D'Santos, C., et al. (2013). Nuclear phosphoinositides and their impact on nuclear functions. *FEBS J.* 280, 6295–6310. doi: 10.1111/febs.12543

Shrestha, C., Tang, Y., Fan, H., Li, L., Zeng, Q., Pennypacker, S. D., et al. (2016). Phosphoprotein phosphatase 1 is required for extracellular calcium-induced keratinocyte differentiation. *Biomed. Res. Int.* 2016:3062765. doi: 10.1155/2016/3062765

Simmonds, M., and Storey, A. (2008). Identification of the regions of the HPV 5 E6 protein involved in Bak degradation and inhibition of apoptosis. *Int. J. Cancer* 123, 2260–2266. doi: 10.1002/ijc.23815

Stamatakis, A. (2006). RAxML-VI-HPC: maximum likelihood-based phylogenetic analyses with thousands of taxa and mixed models. *Bioinformatics* 22, 2688–2690. doi: 10.1093/bioinformatics/btl446

Tan, M. J., White, E. A., Sowa, M. E., Harper, J. W., Aster, J. C., and Howley, P. M. (2012). Cutaneous beta-human papillomavirus E6 proteins bind mastermind-like coactivators and repress notch signaling. *Proc. Natl. Acad. Sci. U.S.A.* 109, E1473–E1480. doi: 10.1073/pnas.1205991109

The UniProt Consortium (2017). UniProt: the universal protein knowledgebase. *Nucleic Acids Res.* 45, D158–D169. doi: 10.1093/nar/gkw1099

Torruella, G., de Mendoza, A., Grau-Bove, X., Anto, M., Chaplin, M. A., del Campo, J., et al. (2015). Phylogenomics reveals convergent evolution of lifestyles in close relatives of animals and fungi. *Curr. Biol.* 25, 2404–2410. doi: 10.1016/j.cub.2015.07.053

van den Bout, I., and Divecha, N. (2009). PIP5K-driven PtdIns(4,5)P2 synthesis: regulation and cellular functions. *J. Cell Sci.* 122(Pt 21), 3837–3850. doi: 10.1242/jcs.056127

Van Doorslaer, K. (2013). Evolution of the papillomaviridae. *Virology* 445, 11–20. doi: 10.1016/j.virol.2013.05.012

Wagner, G. P., Pavlicev, M., and Cheverud, J. M. (2007). The road to modularity. *Nat. Rev. Genet.* 8, 921–931. doi: 10.1038/nrg2267

Wallace, N. A., and Galloway, D. A. (2015). Novel functions of the human papillomavirus E6 oncoproteins. *Annu. Rev. Virol.* 2, 403–423. doi: 10.1146/annurev-virology-100114-055021

Xie, Z., Chang, S. M., Pennypacker, S. D., Liao, E. Y., and Bikle, D. D. (2009). Phosphatidylinositol-4-phosphate 5-kinase 1alpha mediates extracellular calcium-induced keratinocyte differentiation. *Mol. Biol. Cell* 20, 1695–1704. doi: 10.1091/mbc.E08-07-0756

Yin, F., Wang, N., Wang, S., Yu, F., Sun, X., Yu, X., et al. (2017). HPV16 oncogenes E6 or/and E7 may influence the methylation status of RASSFIA gene promoter region in cervical cancer cell line HT-3. *Oncol. Rep.* 37, 2324–2334. doi: 10.3892/or.2017.5465

Yugawa, T., and Kiyono, T. (2009). Molecular mechanisms of cervical carcinogenesis by high-risk human papillomaviruses: novel functions of E6 and E7 oncoproteins. *Rev. Med. Virol.* 19, 97–113. doi: 10.1002/rmv.605

Zimmermann, P., and David, G. (1999). The syndecans, tuners of transmembrane signaling. *FASEB J.* 13(Suppl.), S91–S100.

16

Single-Molecule RNA Sequencing Reveals IFNγ-Induced Differential Expression of Immune Escape Genes in Merkel Cell Polyomavirus–Positive MCC Cell Lines

Tatjana Sauerer[1†‡], Christopher Lischer[2†‡], Adrian Weich[2], Carola Berking[3], Julio Vera[2§] and Jan Dörrie[1*§]*

[1] *RNA-based Immunotherapy, Hautklinik, Comprehensive Cancer Center Erlangen European Metropolitan Area of Nuremberg, Deutsches Zentrum Immuntherapie, Universitätsklinikum Erlangen, Friedrich-Alexander-Universität Erlangen-Nürnberg, Erlangen, Germany,* [2] *Systems Tumor Immunology, Hautklinik, Universitätsklinikum Erlangen, Friedrich-Alexander-Universität Erlangen-Nürnberg, Comprehensive Cancer Center Erlangen European Metropolitan Area of Nuremberg, Deutsches Zentrum Immuntherapie, Erlangen, Germany,* [3] *Hautklinik, Universitätsklinikum Erlangen, Friedrich-Alexander-Universität Erlangen-Nürnberg, Comprehensive Cancer Center Erlangen European Metropolitan Area of Nuremberg, Deutsches Zentrum Immuntherapie, Erlangen, Germany*

***Correspondence:**
Julio Vera
Julio.Vera-Gonzalez@uk-erlangen.de
Jan Dörrie
Jan.Doerrie@uk-erlangen.de

[†] *These authors have contributed equally to this work and share first authorship*

[‡] *The present work was performed in fulfilment of the requirement for obtaining the degree Dr. rer. nat. at the Friedrich-Alexander-Universität Erlangen-Nürnberg*

[§] *These authors share last authorship*

Merkel cell carcinoma (MCC) is a rare and highly aggressive cancer, which is mainly caused by genomic integration of the Merkel cell polyomavirus and subsequent expression of a truncated form of its large T antigen. The resulting primary tumor is known to be immunogenic and under constant pressure to escape immune surveillance. Because interferon gamma (IFNγ), a key player of immune response, is secreted by many immune effector cells and has been shown to exert both anti-tumoral and pro-tumoral effects, we studied the transcriptomic response of MCC cells to IFNγ. In particular, immune modulatory effects that may help the tumor evade immune surveillance were of high interest to our investigation. The effect of IFNγ treatment on the transcriptomic program of three MCC cell lines (WaGa, MKL-1, and MKL-2) was analyzed using single-molecule sequencing *via* the Oxford Nanopore platform. A significant differential expression of several genes was detected across all three cell lines. Subsequent pathway analysis and manual annotation showed a clear upregulation of genes involved in the immune escape of tumor due to IFNγ treatment. The analysis of selected genes on protein level underlined our sequencing results. These findings contribute to a better understanding of immune escape of MCC and may help in clinical treatment of MCC patients. Furthermore, we demonstrate that single-molecule sequencing can be used to assess characteristics of large eukaryotic transcriptomes and thus contribute to a broader access to sequencing data in the community due to its low cost of entry.

Keywords: Merkel cell carcinoma (MCC), third generation sequencing, Interferon gamma (IFNγ), immune escape, transcriptome

INTRODUCTION

Merkel cell carcinoma (MCC) is a rare and frequently metastatic neuroendocrine skin cancer with increasing incidence and high mortality (Fitzgerald et al., 2015; Paulson et al., 2018). Risk factors are increased age, UV light exposure, immunosuppression, and infection with the human Merkel cell polyomavirus (MCPyV; Heath et al., 2008). About 80% of all MCC tumors contain a mutated MCPyV genome that expresses viral oncoproteins (T antigens) (Feng H. et al., 2008; Houben et al., 2010). For malignant transformation, the MCPyV DNA is clonally integrated into the MCC genome in a replication-deficient form and expresses a truncated oncoprotein, called the large T (LT) antigen (Shuda et al., 2008). As this protein contains several tumor suppressors targeting motifs such as the retinoblastoma binding site, it promotes cell cycle progression that leads to uncontrolled cell proliferation (Borchert et al., 2014; Hesbacher et al., 2016). MCC is also characterized by an increased expression of programmed cell death protein 1 (PD-1), which allows the tumor cells to escape the control of the immune system (Afanasiev et al., 2013). Since 2018, checkpoint inhibitors (targeting PD-1 and its ligand PD-L1) have been approved by the Food and Drug Administration for the treatment of advanced MCC and show impressive clinical results, albeit not all patients respond to this treatment (Kaufman et al., 2016; Nghiem et al., 2016). It is suggested that MCC, as an immunogenic tumor, exerts different strategies of immune escape because it is capable of disturbing cellular immune responses by upregulation of PD-1 and PD-L1 and reducing the human leukocyte antigen (HLA) class I expression, leading to decreased or absent T cell infiltration (Ritter et al., 2017). The exact mechanism of immune escape is of high clinical relevance especially regarding immunotherapy resistance; however, it is not fully understood yet.

Interferons (IFNs) are suggested to beneficially influence antiviral immune responses and possess anti-polyomavirus (Co et al., 2007; Willmes et al., 2012) and anti-MCC activity (Krasagakis et al., 2008; Willmes et al., 2012), which makes them an interesting study subject in MCC. The type II IFN gamma (IFNγ) is of special interest, as it is well known for its ambiguous effects: Both anti-tumoral and pro-tumoral functions of IFNγ have been reported.

A closer investigation of the anti-tumoral effects shows that IFNγ is produced by activated lymphocytes including $CD4^+$ and $CD8^+$ T cells (Kasahara et al., 1983; Matsushita et al., 2015), gamma delta T cells (Gao et al., 2003), natural killer (NK) cells (Cooper et al., 2001; Yu et al., 2006), and NK T cells (Leite-De-Moraes et al., 1998). IFNγ plays a key role in modulating the immune response toward these effector cells in the tumor microenvironment. Its anti-tumor activity has been shown for fibrosarcoma and melanoma by the induction of HLA-I and signal transducer and activator of transcription 1 (STAT1)–associated cyclin-dependent kinase, leading to apoptosis of the tumor cells and recognition by the immune system (Ikeda et al., 2002; Gao et al., 2016). For MCC cell lines, it was shown that incubation with IFNγ slightly inhibited cell viability, reduced the expression of the MCPyV LT antigen (Willmes et al., 2012), and increased HLA-I expression (Paulson et al., 2014).

In contrast, pro-tumoral effects of IFNγ have been observed in colon carcinoma and melanoma, leading to a loss of IFNγ signaling sensitivity, reduced antigen expression (Beatty and Paterson, 2001), and induction of key immune suppressive molecules such as indoleamine-2,3-dioxygenase (IDO1) (Spranger et al., 2013) and immune checkpoint proteins (Benci et al., 2016). Hence, the same IFNγ signaling processes that promote anti-tumor immunity can achieve the opposite effect by inducing feedback inhibition and tumor immune escape (Bald et al., 2014).

To better understand the biology of a tumor and improve targeted therapies, high-throughput sequencing has been highly beneficial. The analysis of gene expression profiles of melanoma patients with checkpoint inhibitor treatment detected IFNγ-related mRNA profiles, which predicted clinical response to PD-1 treatment, underlining the huge clinical benefit of transcriptome sequencing studies (Ayers et al., 2017). Nanopore sequencing by Oxford Nanopore Technologies (ONT) belongs to the third-generation sequencing methods and enables real-time DNA and RNA sequencing using small nanopores (Jain et al., 2015, 2016). In this system, the DNA or RNA strand is guided through the nanopore creating nucleotide sequence-specific disturbance of the flow of an electrical current (Ip et al., 2015). In this process, up to 2×10^6 bases can be read continuously (Payne et al., 2019). Nanopore sequencing shows increasing popularity in the field of cancer biology (Euskirchen et al., 2017) and virology (Quick et al., 2016). It is characterized by relatively low establishment and maintenance costs as well as rapid sequencing and real-time data acquisition for further analysis.

As the comprehensive investigation of the transcriptomic response of MCC to IFNγ is of high interest, we used the Nanopore sequencing platform to study differentially expressed genes in MCC. We hypothesized that IFNγ stimulation of MCC cell lines would lead to transcriptomic alterations that elucidate the ambiguous pro- and anti-tumoral activity of this cytokine and hence examined the effect of IFNγ on the transcriptomes of three MCPyV-positive cell lines (WaGa, MKL-1, and MKL-2). Our results confirm the Nanopore sequencing technology as a suitable tool to study these alterations and show a clear upregulation of genes involved in tumor immune escape mechanisms, suggesting that these factors could contribute to the immune escape of MCC cells.

MATERIALS AND METHODS

Cell Culture

The MCC cell lines WaGa (RRID:CVCL_E998) (Houben et al., 2010), MKL-1(RRID:CVCL_EQ70) (Rosen et al., 1987), and MKL-2 (RRID:CVCL_D027) (Martin et al., 1991) were grown in Roswell Park Memorial Institute 1640 medium (Lonza, Verviers, Belgium) supplemented with 10% fetal bovine serum (FBS) (Merck KGaA, Darmstadt, Germany), 2 mM L-glutamine (Lonza), gentamycin (20 mg/L; Lonza), 10 mM hydroxyethyl piperazineethanesulfonic acid (HEPES; PAA Labortechnik, Pasching, Austria), and 20 mM beta-mercaptoethanol (Gibco) and maintained at 37°C in 5% CO_2. All cells were kindly provided by Prof. Jürgen Becker (DKTK, Essen, Germany), and mycoplasma testing was performed immediately after arrival of the cells. Cells were frozen and then thawed for further experiments, whereby they were cultured for 1 to 3 weeks before the experiments were performed.

Interferon Gamma Incubation and RNA Isolation of Cell Lines

For RNA extraction, 5 × 10^6 cells of each cell lines were seeded at six-well plates, and IFNγ (3,000 U/ml; PeproTech, Hamburg, Germany) was added in each cell suspension. Cells incubated without IFNγ served as control. After 24 h of incubation, cell pellets were stored at −80°C until further analysis. For each cell line, the IFNγ incubation was performed three times on different days to obtain three replicates and exclude any daily fluctuation.

From frozen cell pellets, RNA isolation was performed using the AllPrep DNA/RNA micro kit (Qiagen, Venlo, Netherlands). RNA concentration was measured *via* Nanodrop and stored at −20°C until library preparation.

Flow Cytometry Detection of Intracellular and Extracellular Markers

For antibody staining, 1 × 10^6 cells of each MCC cell line were cultured in a six-well plate in the presence or absence of IFNγ (3,000 U/ml) for 72 h. Cells were washed with fluorescence-activated cell sorting (FACS) buffer (dulbecco's phosphate-buffered saline with 1% FBS and 0.2% sodium azide) and stained for the following markers: STAT1α/β, Indoleamine-2,3-dioxygenase (IDO), C-X-C motif chemokine 10 (CXCL10), PD-L1, bone marrow stromal antigen 2 (BST2), HLA class II histocompatibility antigen gamma chain (CD74), and HLA A, B, and C (HLA-ABC) with the following monoclonal antibodies: anti-human STAT1 (phycoerythine; PE, clone REA272, Miltenyi Biotec), anti-IDO1 (PE, clone eyedio, Invitrogen), anti-human CXCL10 (PE, clone REA334, Miltenyi Biotec), anti-CD274 (Pe-Cy7, clone MIH1, BD Biosciences), anti-human BST2 (PE, clone REA202, Miltenyi Biotec), anti-CD74 (PE, clone 5-329, Miltenyi Biotec), and anti–HLA-ABC (fluorescein-5-isothiocyanat, BD Biosciences). STAT1, IDO, CXCL10, and CD74 were stained intracellularly using the Cytofix/Cytoperm™ Fixation/Permeabilization Solution Kit (Thermo Fisher Scientific, Waltham, MA, United States). PD-L1, BST2, HLA-ABC, and CD74 were stained as surface molecule. Stained cells were analyzed using a FACSCanto II flow cytometer (BD Biosciences) and FlowJo software, version 10.5.3 (BD Biosciences). Geometric mean of the mean fluorescence intensity was compared between ± IFNγ-treated cell lines.

Preparation of Cell Lysates and Immunoblotting of the Merkel Cell Polyomavirus–Large T Antigen

Cell lysates were prepared out of 1 × 10^6 cells for each cell line (WaGa, MKL-1, and MKL-2), incubated with or without IFNγ (3,000 U/ml) for 72 h. Cell pellets were frozen at −80°C, thawed, and resuspended in 35 μl of lysis buffer [10% glycerol, 2 mM ethylenediaminetetraacetic acid (EDTA), 137 mM NaCl, 50 mM Tris (pH 8.0) (all from Carl Roth GmbH, Germany), 0.5% sodium deoxycholate (Merck KGaA, Darmstadt, Germany)] freshly supplemented with 2 mM phenylmethylsulfonyl fluoride (Carl Roth GmbH, Germany), 2 mM sodium orthovanadate (Merck KGaA, Darmstadt, Germany), 20 mM sodium fluoride (Merck KGaA, Darmstadt, Germany), 0.1 M $MgCl_2$ (Carl Roth GmbH, Germany), and 0.1 μl of benzonase (250 U/μl, Merck KGaA, Darmstadt, Germany) and lysed on ice for 20 min. Cells were then centrifuged at 13,500 × *g* at 4°C for 20 min, supernatants were harvested, and the protein concentration in each lysate was determined using Bradford protein determination. Protein lysates were mixed with 4× Roti-load 1 (Carl Roth GmbH, Germany), followed by a denaturation step at 95°C for 10 min.

Per lane, 20 μg of protein lysate of the three MCC cell lines were loaded onto 12% sodium dodecylsulfate (SDS) polyacrylamide gels and separated using SDS-polyacrylamide gel electrophoresis (PAGE). Afterward, proteins were transferred onto a nitrocellulose membrane by semi-dry blot transfer. After blocking the membrane in 1× Roti-block (Carl Roth GmbH, Germany) for 1 h at room temperature, the membrane was incubated with anti-MCPyV LT antigen (clone CM2B4, Merck KGaA) diluted 1:1,000 in 1× Roti-block overnight at 4°C and with the horseradish peroxidase-conjugated secondary antibody (polyclonal anti-mouse immunoglobulin G; Cell Signaling, 1:2,500) for 1 h. The antibodies were detected *via* enhanced chemoluminescence (ECL) using Amersham ECL Prime Western blotting detection reagent (GE Healthcare, Solingen, Germany) and documented and quantified *via* the Amersham ImageQuant system (GE Healthcare). glyceraldehyde-3-phosphate dehydrogenase (GAPDH) (anti-GAPDH mouse monoclonal Ab, clone 6C5, Merck KGaA, Darmstadt, Germany) was used as a loading control.

Library Preparation and Nanopore Sequencing

Reagents and equipment for preparation and sequencing were obtained from ONT, Oxford, United Kingdom, unless stated otherwise. Library preparation was performed according to the instructions of the manufacturer using the PCR-cDNA Barcoding Kit (SQK-PCB109, ONT). Polyadenylated mRNA was reversely transcribed into cDNA and fused to barcodes (BCs) to allow sample-specific attribution. Of each RNA sample, 50 ng were used for library preparation. In total, six samples were loaded onto one flow cell with three biological replicates for each condition. Assigned BCs used were 1 through 6 for MKL-1 and 1, 2, 4, 5, 6, and 7 for both MKL-2 and WaGa.

Libraries were run for 72 h according to the guidelines of the manufacturer using the MK1B-MinION sequencer and R9.4 flow cells (FLO-MIN106, ONT). For each cell line, six samples (three replicates incubated with IFNγ and three replicates incubated without IFNγ) were loaded on one flow cell. Sequencing run monitoring and real-time data acquisition were performed using the MinKNOW software suite (v19.2.5). After real-time data were gathered, a high-accuracy base calling was performed using the CPU version of Guppy (v.4.2.2) deployed on a dedicated server, using the following command:

```
guppy_basecaller -r -i „fast5" -s
"sample" --num-callers \
1 -trim-barcodes -cpu_threads_per_caller
64 \
-c dna_r9.4.1_450bps_hac.cfg \
--barcode-kits SQK-PCB109 -q 0
```

Data Processing

After a high-accuracy base calling was performed, generated FASTQ files were aggregated per sample and filtered for average Phred score quality above 7 (Q>7). In addition, primary quality assessment was done with the package pycoQC (Leger and Leonardi, 2019). For raw data processing, we made use of the snakemake pipeline provided by Oxford Nanopore (available at[1]). The pipeline performs read alignment, quantification, and differential expression analysis as well as abundance estimation in transcripts per million. For the detailed version of the environment used, see "**Supplementary Material 1 versions.txt**". As a reference genome, we used the transcriptome cDNA reference provided by ensemble (Homo_sapiens.GRCh38.cdna.all.fa.gz, release 103). To quantify LT antigen expression, we added the sequence of the LT cDNA (GenBank: LC148302.1) to the assembly. As annotation, we used the corresponding GTF file where the LT antigen was added as an additional entry. For detailed sequence information, see **Supplementary Figure 1** for the sequence.

Differential Expression and Pathway Enrichment Analysis

Raw counts of the expressed transcripts were collected from the output of the snakemake pipeline. Further analysis was performed using the Bioconductor Package DESeq2 in R (Love et al., 2014); the code and data to perform the analysis were deposited at Zenodo under the DOI: 10.5281/zenodo.5031363. Because an exploratory approach was taken, we choose to set significance threshold to adjusted p-value < 0.1. P-values were adjusted using false discovery rate correction. Pairwise comparisons were performed between conditions (untreated and per flow cell and once across flow cell and cell lines). Gene set enrichment analysis was performed using the Bioconductor package fgsea (Sergushichev, 2016) with the C7 immune signature hallmarks, gene set version 7.2, by the Molecular Signatures Database (Subramanian et al., 2005; Liberzon et al., 2015).

Mapping of Different Human Leukocyte Antigen Alleles

To quantify expression of the six known HLA alleles of each cell line, we implemented a two-pass quantification procedure, which quantifies transcriptome wide expression in the first pass and then uses prior knowledge to estimate allele specific HLA expression in the second pass. The data were then aggregated and analyzed. This allowed us to leverage the allele specific reference sequences (Robinson et al., 2019) and to mitigate the high error rates in nanopore data. In the first step, the known HLA alleles of each cell line were used separately to create a reference FASTA file, encompassing all described sequence variants of these alleles. We then mapped generated FASTQ files against this reference while also only counting primary alignments of a read. Afterward, read counting was performed for all reads with a sequence identity of 80% to the reference. This was done to achieve a conservative expression estimate and reduce false positive mappings. We further aggregated all reads mapping to the variants to a four-digit resolution, because higher genotyping resolutions are not known for the cell lines. In a second step, we gathered count data from previous mapping runs against the human genome reference and recalculated transcripts per million (TPM) with the counts generated in the first step. We thus arrive at a conservative estimate of the expression of HLA alleles in the investigated cell lines.

Statistical Analysis

All graphs and statistical analysis for flow cytometry experiments were created by GraphPad Prism, version 8 (GraphPad Software, La Jolla, United States). The paired student's t-test was used to compare intracellular and surface markers between cell lines treated with or without IFNγ as well as for the analysis of Western blot data. Data are reported as the median with standard error of the mean (SEM). Significance was determined as p-value ≤ 0.05.

RESULTS

Interferon Gamma Increases Human Leukocyte Antigen Class I and PD-L1 in all Cell Lines, but Not Indoleamine-2,3-dioxygenase

To investigate the effect of IFNγ on important key players of the immune response, we measured the expression of (i) the HLA class I, whose loss can be a primary immune escape mechanism; (ii) PD-L1 as an important target for checkpoint inhibitors; and (iii) IDO as a key immunosuppressive enzyme. Antibody staining and FACS analysis of all three MCC cell lines were performed after 72-h incubation with IFNγ and as control without IFNγ. HLA class I was significantly upregulated in all three cell lines, whereas WaGa and MKL-2 cells displayed a stronger increase of HLA-ABC than MKL-1 cells (**Figure 1**). An increased expression of PD-L1 due to IFNγ was observed in all cell lines, but only for MKL-1 and MKL-2 with statistical significance. Staining for IDO showed no changes of the IDO status between the cell lines with and without IFNγ treatment. This indicates that all three cell lines are responsive to the cytokine but react differently to the treatment.

Sequencing Runs

To comprehend the different transcriptional programs induced in the different cell lines by IFNγ, we sequenced RNA of the three MCC cell lines (MKL-1, MKL-2, and WaGa) *via* the Nanopore sequencing technology. Before RNA isolation, the cells

[1] https://github.com/nanoporetech/pipeline-transcriptome-de/commit/47c850bd320031ed1e2b36cd631f287e0d98e464

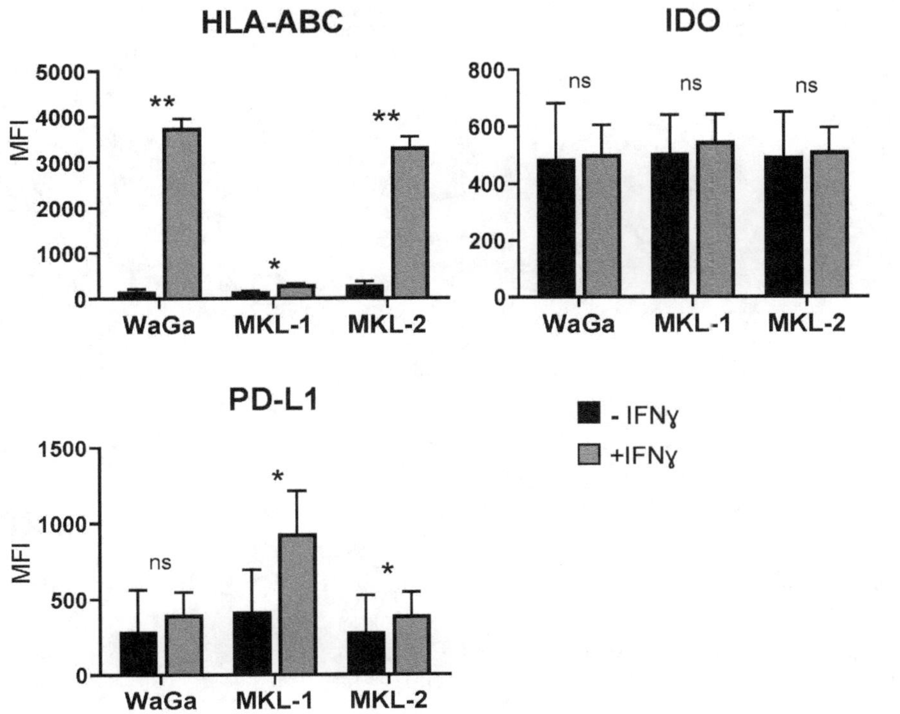

FIGURE 1 | Merkel cell carcinoma cell lines respond to IFNγ by upregulating different proteins. After 72 h of treatment with or without IFNγ (3,000 U/ml), the Merkel cell carcinoma cell lines MKL-1, MKL-2, and WaGa were stained for human leukocyte antigen A, B, and C (HLA-ABC), indoleamine-2,3-dioxygenase (IDO), and programmed cell death 1 ligand 1 (PD-L1) and analyzed by flow cytometry. The average mean fluorescent intensity (MFI) of three to four independent experiments ± standard error is indicated. *p*-values were determined using the paired student's *t*-test. **p* < 0.05; ***p* < 0.01; ns, not significant.

were incubated with or without IFNγ for 24 h. During the sequencing runs, MKL-1 and WaGa produced comparable base pair (bp) outputs with 11.68 Gigabases (Gb) and 9.40 Gb after high-accuracy base calling. The experiments had similar pore counts available, at sequencing start with 1,446 for MKL-1 and 1,489 for WaGa. The flow cell dedicated for MKL-2 performed worse with only producing 3.29 Gb in total although similar pores were available for sequencing (1,480) and all experimental parameters equal but age of flow cell (**Figure 2A**). Overall, all three experiments generated high-quality Phred scores and high read lengths over their runtime, with MKL-1 producing a median read length of 1,217 bp and a median Phred(Q) of 11.98, and MKL-2 producing median read length of 630 bp and a median Q of 11.59. Finally, WaGa produced median read lengths of 683 bp and a median Q of 11.49. BC read yield showed biases in efficiency of each multiplexing BC. As for MKL-1, we observed a failure of BC 3 with no reads being generated from this BC. Of the remaining BCs, BC 6 performed best in total output. In further runs, we skipped BC 3 and assigned no sample to it. For MKL-2, BCs 1, 2, and 4, all assigned to the control group, showed good performance with BC 1, producing the best yield. In the treated group (BCs 5, 6, and 7), however, BC 6 again produced most reads with BC 5 and BC 7 almost failing. WaGa showed similar results, with the first three BCs (1, 2, and 4) performing equally well with BC 5 and BC 7, producing only 1% of reads. In addition, in this experiment, we had about 0.3% of erroneously assigned BC 8 detected. Unclassified counts were consistently low for all samples ranging from 0.8 to 2.0% of reads passing principal quality control (**Figure 2B**). Overall, Nanopore sequencing allowed for the quick and robust gathering of transcriptomics data from our samples. However, it is of note that some aspects like differentially BC efficacy and flow cell sensitivity are still a considerable factor.

Differential Gene Expression

Our primary goal was to detect differentially expressed genes in the MCC cell lines after treatment with IFNγ. Therefore, we performed a differential expression analysis of the Nanopore sequencing data using raw counts produced by our referenced pipeline. First, we pooled counts of all three cell lines, treating them as biological replicates, and corrected for batch effects. At an adjusted p-value < 0.1 and an absolute fold change >2, we could detect 61 genes that were differentially expressed (**Supplementary Figure 1**). To check for plausibility and to further investigate the role of the differentially expressed genes in terms of cancer biology, we performed a pathway enrichment analysis. Several pathways such as the inflammatory response pathway and the interleukine 6-janus kinase-signal transducer and activator of transcription (IL6-JAK-STAT3) pathway were enriched in the presence of IFNγ. Seven hallmark pathways were slightly downregulated, but most importantly, genes involved in IFNγ and IFNα pathways were induced (**Figure 3A**). Because these two pathways overlap to a large degree, this indicates that the data are sound and plausible.

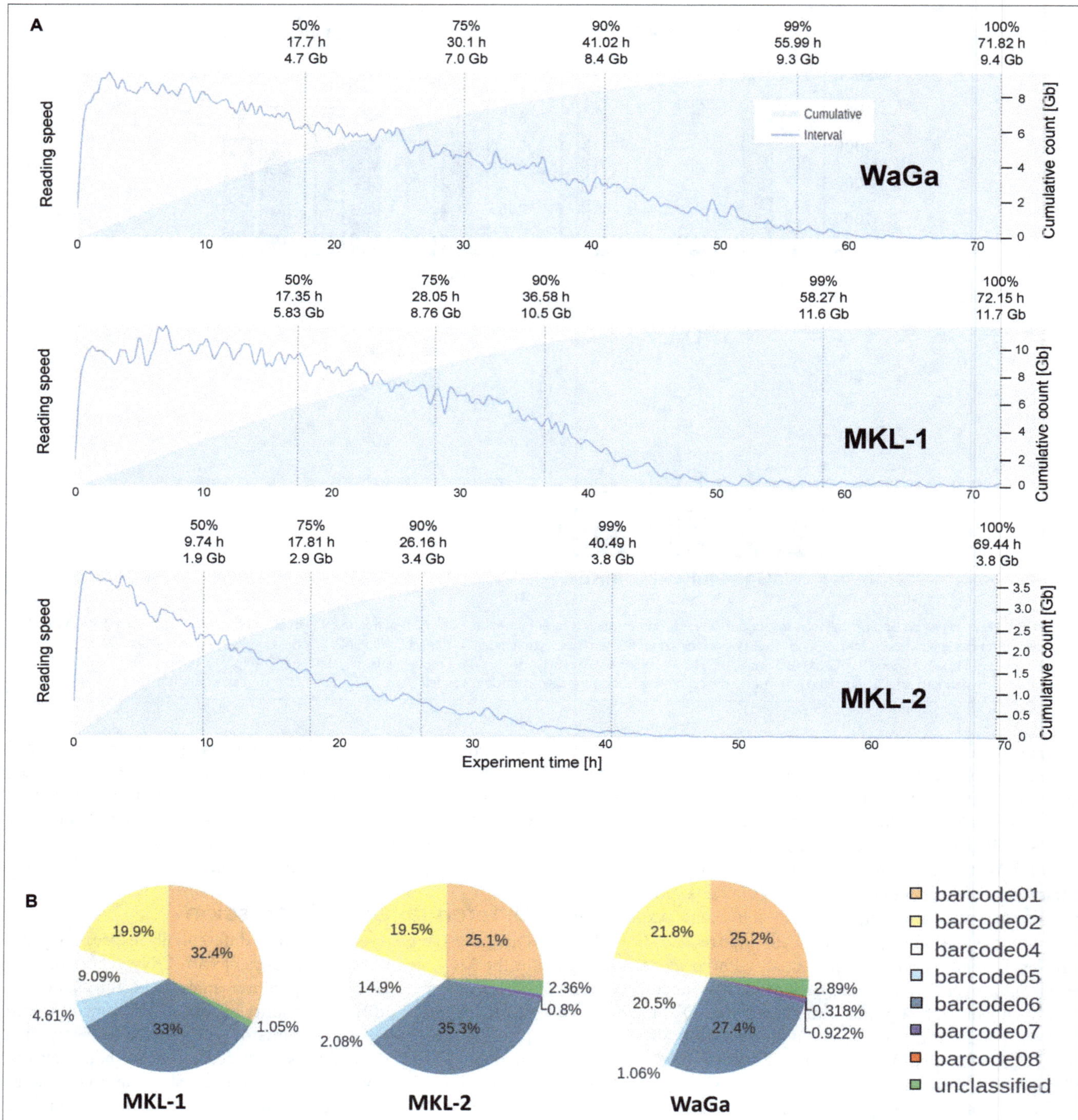

FIGURE 2 | Functional performance of the Nanopore flowcells and barcodes. **(A)** Depiction of output over time of MKL-1, MKL-2, and WaGa cells. For each cell line, a new flow cell was loaded with the multiplexed library. The sequencing run lasted 72 h. The blue line indicates relative reading speed, i.e., bases per time, the light blue area represents cumulative reading output. **(B)** Barcode distribution of detected barcodes during the sequencing run of the three cell lines MKL-1, MKL-2, and WaGa. Barcode 3 is not displayed as it failed in the first run of MKL-1 and was skipped for further experiments. In the run of WaGa, we additionally tested barcode 8, which failed similar as barcode 3. The other barcodes (1, 2, 4, 5, 6, and 7) could be used according to their performance for multiplexing studies.

To differentiate between the common IFNγ-induced program and a cell line-specific program, we investigated the cell lines individually and found 86 differentially expressed genes in cell line MKL-1, eight genes in MKL-2, and 10 genes in WaGa (**Figure 2B**). Six of these genes (UBE2L6, BST2, NLRC5, RARRES3, B2M, and STAT1) were differentially regulated in all

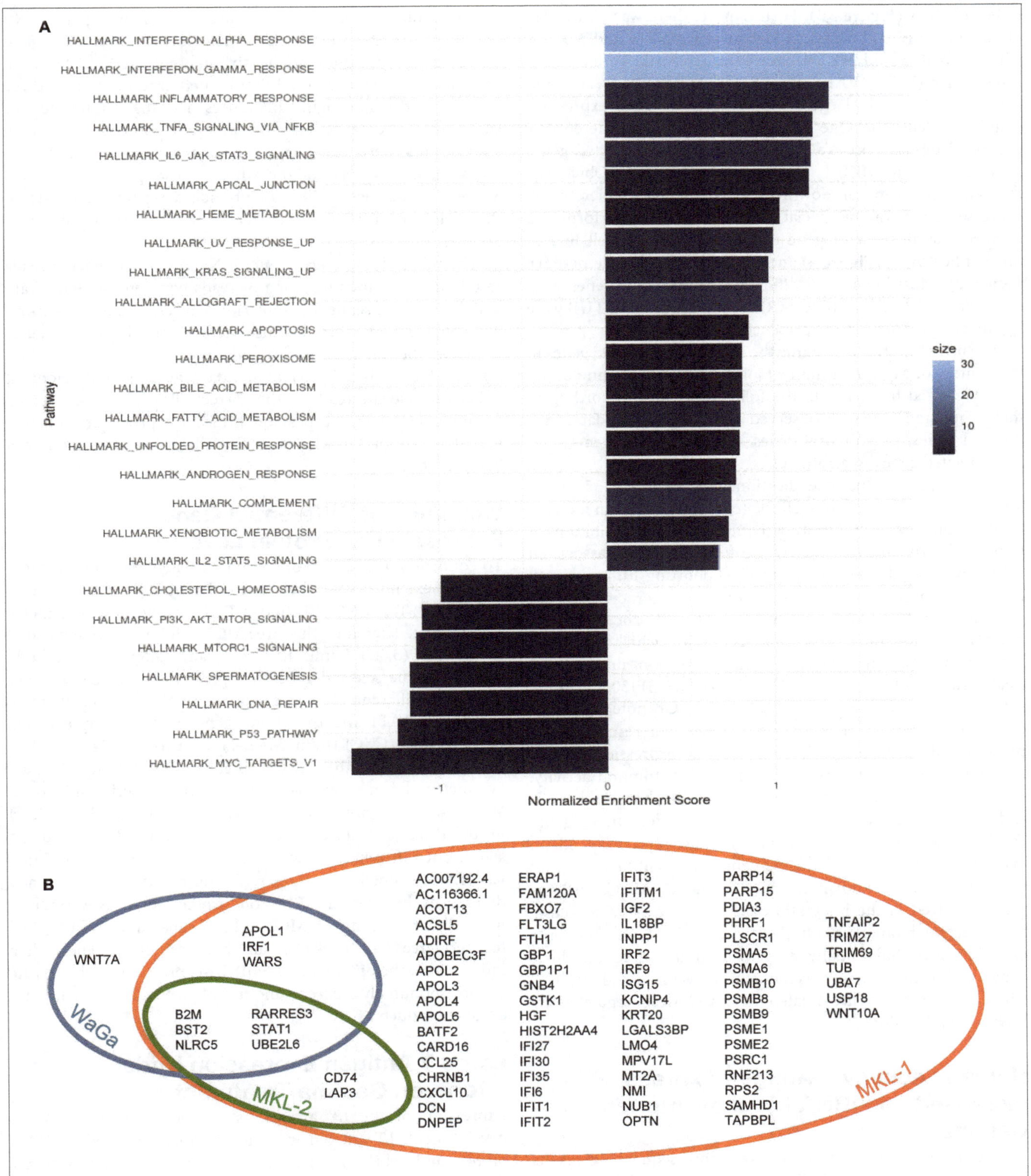

FIGURE 3 | Pathway annotation and distribution of differentially expressed genes. **(A)** Hallmark pathway enrichment analysis of all used MCC cell lines (MKL-1, MKL-2, and WaGa): Data were pooled for the three cell lines in one plot. Gene set enrichment analysis was performed using the Bioconductor package fgsea with the immune signature hallmarks by Molecular Signatures Database. Size corresponds to gene count of how many expressed genes from the input overlap with the pathway. **(B)** The Venn diagram of the three cell lines gives an overview over shared differentially expressed genes between the cell lines MKL-1 (red circle), MKL-2 (green circle), and WaGa (blue circle).

three cell lines (**Figure 3B**). Furthermore, there was an overlap of two genes (CD74 and LAP3) between MKL-1 and MKL-2, whereas WaGA and MKL-1 showed differential expression for three genes (IRF1, WARS, and APOL1). Between WaGa and MKL-2, no individual overlap of differential gene expression could be detected. One gene (WNT7A) was differentially expressed uniquely in WaGa, whereas 74 of all detected genes were unique in MKL-1 and none for MKL-2. Obviously, the regulation (up- or downregulation) of each differentially expressed gene was of special interest. Thus, we performed a detailed examination of gene expression for each cell line in form of heatmaps (**Figure 4**) and volcano plots (**Supplementary Figure 2**). Most but not all differentially expressed genes were upregulated; WNT7A, HGF, PARP15, FAM120A, and TUB were significantly reduced in the presence of IFNγ.

The next step was to examine the role of the identified genes in the context of MCC and tumor biology. By manual annotation, we categorized the genes in the following groups according to their regulation, which we observed in the sequencing data: anti-tumoral genes, pro-tumoral genes, immune escape genes, and MCC-related genes (see **Table 1**).

According to this classification, we detected 35 genes associated with anti-tumoral effects (e.g., resulting in an increase in the numbers of infiltrating lymphocytes or inhibition of tumor cell growth). In contrast, we found 49 genes associated with pro-tumoral effects (e.g., genes supporting tumor growth or increasing survival and migration of cancer cells). A lot of these pro-tumoral genes overlapped with the group of potential tumor immune escape genes, of which 11 genes showed significantly increased gene expression under IFNγ treatment: CD74, STAT1, B2M, IRF1, WARS, IFI30, TAPBPL, IFIT1, PDIA3, ERAP1, and LGALS3BP. Of note, in some cases, anti-tumoral genes were downregulated resulting in a pro-tumoral effect or, on the contrary, the expression of pro-tumoral genes was decreased leading to anti-tumoral activity. In addition, we found 14 genes, which could have both anti- and pro-tumoral activity. Which kind of effect these genes actually had was often cell-type or cancer-type dependent. With respect to the MCC-related genes, we identified 10 genes that were already known to play a role in MCC, such as genes involved in the integration site of the MCPyV or acting as predictive biomarker. Of these genes, B2M was the only one that was differentially expressed in all three cell lines while CD74 expression was altered in MKL-1 and MKL-2, whereas all other genes related to MCC were regulated by IFNγ to MKL-1 alone.

Human Leukocyte Antigen Expression Is Increased on mRNA Level by Interferon Gamma

The relatively high error rate of Nanopore sequencing results in poor mapping of the individual reads in the HLA regions of the reference genomes. Hence, we implemented a two-pass quantification procedure to exploit the up-front knowledge about the HLA-haplotypes of the used cell lines. With this two-pass quantification step, we were able to verify the upregulation of HLA-specific expression following an IFNγ treatment in the three MCC cell lines (**Figure 5**). The calculated TPM values of the six different HLA alleles were considerably higher for the IFNγ-treated group across all three cell lines, despite slight differences in single replicates or subtypes. However, because the different approaches on how read counts were generated, the data were not included in the statistical analysis of the whole transcriptomes described above. Instead, we decided to provide a separate estimate of the allele expression to make clear that these are two different avenues of analysis.

The relatively high error rate of Nanopore sequencing reads results in ubiquitous mapping of reads between loci that share a high degree of sequence similarity. This especially presents an issue with the HLA loci, because there is considerable sequence homology between the alleles and supertypes (HLA-A, B, and C). We found that, by using standard alignment methods, it is hard to allocate reads to the correct allele and thus decided to implement our two-pass quantification procedure, making use of the prior knowledge of the alleles present in our cell lines of interest.

Validation of Differential Gene Expression on Protein Level

To confirm our transcriptomic findings (**Figure 6A**) on protein level, we exemplarily studied four differentially expressed genes (STAT1, BST2, CXCL10, and CD74) using flow cytometry (**Figure 6B**). Therefore, the three MCC cell lines were incubated with IFNγ (3,000 U/ml) for 72 h, and, afterward, antibody staining of the selected genes was performed. We chose genes that were differentially expressed on mRNA level in all three cell lines (STAT1 and BST2) and genes that were upregulated in only one (CXCL10 in MKL-1) or two (CD74 in MKL-1 and MKL-2) of the MCC cell lines. Our findings in flow cytometry did mainly match with our transcriptomic data: We observed significantly increased STAT1 and BST2 level in all three cell lines. The molecule CXCL10 showed no significant differences between ± IFNγ in all tested cell lines. CD74 was stained as surface molecule but did not show any differences between ± IFNγ on protein level. Nevertheless, intracellular staining of MCC cells incubated with IFNγ led to an increase of CD74 in all three cell lines. These data indicate that the differences on mRNA-expression level translate to correspondingly different amounts of protein for most, but not all gene products.

Large T Antigen Expression Under Interferon Gamma Treatment

Expression of the LT antigen is a crucial factor for MCC development. LT antigen was shown to be regulated by IFNγ on protein level (Willmes et al., 2012); hence, we tested whether this regulation also takes place on mRNA level. TPM values were acquired from our sequencing output. The expression of the LT antigen was not substantially altered by IFNγ on mRNA level (**Figure 7A**). To study this result on protein level, we performed a Western Blot analysis with cell lysates treated with

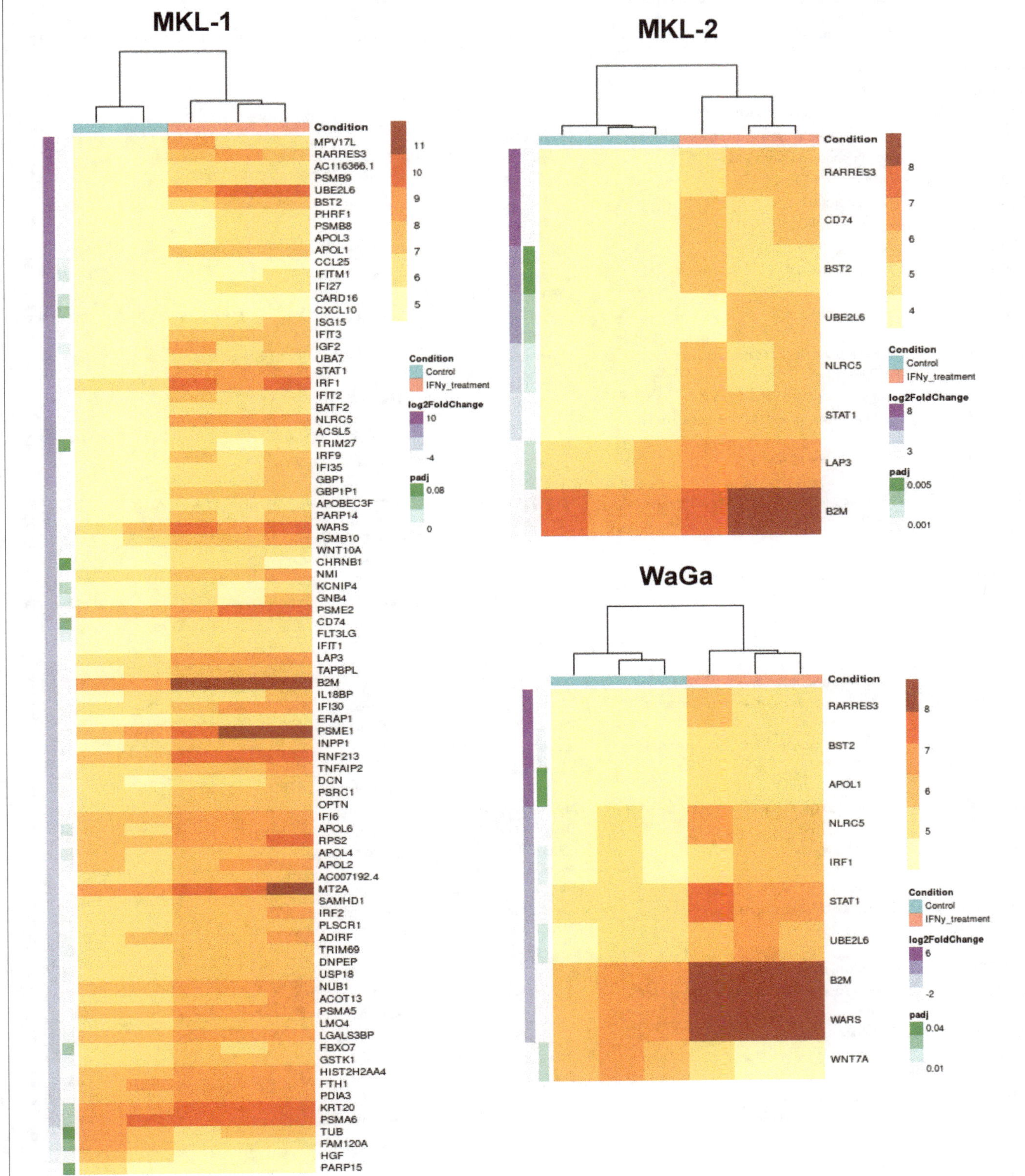

FIGURE 4 | Differentially expressed genes of the cell lines MKL-1, MKL-2, and WaGa illustrated in heatmaps. Cell lines were incubated with IFNγ (blue top labels) or without IFNγ (pink top labels). Adjusted *p*-values are indicated in green and $\log_2$ fold change in purple on the left side. Listed genes were differentially expressed with a false discovery rate-adjusted *p*-value < 0.1 and an absolute fold change >2. A total of 86 genes was detected in MKL-1, eight genes in MKL-2, and 10 genes in WaGa cells. Heat scale represents vst-normalized counts using DESeq2.

TABLE 1 | Overview of all differentially expressed genes categorized according to their activity in cancer biology.

Gene[1]	Protein name[2]	Anti-tumoral	Pro-tumoral	Immune escape	MCC related
AC007192.4 (↑)	Not annotated	–	–	–	–
AC116366.1	Not annotated	–	–	–	–
ACOT13 (↑)	Acyl–coenzyme A thioesterase 13	–	Liu et al., 2016	–	–
ACSL5 (↑)	Long-chain-fatty-acid–CoA ligase 5	Hung et al., 2017	–	–	–
ADIRF (↑)	Adipogenesis regulatory factor	–	–	–	–
APOBEC3F (↑)	DNA dC->dU-editing enzyme APOBEC-3F	Yen et al., 2017	–	–	–
APOL1 (↑)	Apolipoprotein L1	–	–	–	–
APOL2 (↑)	Apolipoprotein L2	–	–	–	–
APOL3 (↑)	Apolipoprotein L3	–	–	–	–
APOL4 (↑)	Apolipoprotein L4	–	–	–	–
APOL6 (↑)	Apolipoprotein L6	Yang et al., 2015	Liu et al., 2005	–	–
B2M (↑)	Beta-2-microglobulin	–	Maire et al., 2020	Maire et al., 2020	Zhang et al., 2021
BATF2 (↑)	Basic leucine zipper transcriptional factor ATF-like 2	Wen et al., 2014	–	–	–
BST2 (↑)	Bone marrow stromal antigen 2	–	Han et al., 2015	–	–
CARD16 (↑)	Caspase recruitment domain-containing protein 16	–	–	–	–
CCL25 (↑)	C-C motif chemokine 25	Liu et al., 2018	Chen et al., 2020; Niu et al., 2020	–	–
CD74 (↑)	HLA class II histocompatibility antigen gamma chain	Zhang et al., 2016	Greenwood et al., 2012; Zhang et al., 2014; Zeiner et al., 2018	Huang et al., 2013	Czech-Sioli et al., 2020
CHRNB1 (↑)	Acetylcholine receptor subunit beta	–	House et al., 2020	–	–
CXCL10 (↑)	C-X-C motif chemokine 10	Lo et al., 2010; Liu et al., 2011	Lo et al., 2010; Liu W. et al., 2020	–	Imaoka et al., 2019
DCN (↑)	Decorin	Järvinen and Prince, 2015	–	–	–
DNPEP (↑)	Aspartyl aminopeptidase	Geng et al., 2019	–	–	–
ERAP1 (↑)	Endoplasmic reticulum aminopeptidase 1	–	Stratikos, 2014; Steinbach et al., 2017	Steinbach et al., 2017	–
FAM120A (↓)	Constitutive coactivator of PPAR-gamma-like protein 1	Bartolomé et al., 2015	–	–	–
FBXO7 (↑)	F-box only protein 7	–	Lomonosov et al., 2011	–	–
FLT3LG (↑)	Fms-related tyrosine kinase 3 ligand	Abrahamsson et al., 2020; Pol et al., 2020	–	–	–
FTH1 (↑)	Ferritin heavy chain	Lobello et al., 2016; Aversa et al., 2017; Biamonte et al., 2018	Di Sanzo et al., 2011	–	–
GBP1 (↑)	Guanylate-binding protein 1	Lipnik et al., 2010; Britzen-Laurent et al., 2013	Mustafa et al., 2018; Ji et al., 2019; Wan et al., 2021	–	–
GBP1P1 (↑)	no protein, pseudogene	–	–	–	–
GNB4 (↑)	Guanine nucleotide-binding protein subunit beta-4	–	Wang B. et al., 2018; Gao et al., 2020a,b	–	–
GSTK1 (↑)	Glutathione S-transferase kappa 1	–	–	–	–
HGF (↓)	Hepatocyte growth factor	Owusu et al., 2017; Bonan et al., 2019	–	–	–
HIST2H2AA4 (↑)	Histone H2A type 2-A	–	–	–	–
IFI27 (↑)	Interferon alpha-inducible protein 27	–	Li et al., 2015; Wang H. et al., 2018; Chiang et al., 2019	–	–
IFI30 (↑)	Gamma-interferon-inducible lysosomal thiol reductase	–	Liu X. et al., 2020	Liu X. et al., 2020	–

(Continued)

TABLE 1 | (Continued)

Gene[1]	Protein name[2]	Anti-tumoral	Pro-tumoral	Immune escape	MCC related
IFI35 (↑)	Interferon-induced 35 kDa protein	–	–	–	–
IFI6 (↑)	Interferon alpha-inducible protein 6	–	Gupta et al., 2016; Liu Z. et al., 2020	–	–
IFIT1 (↑)	Interferon-induced protein with tetratricopeptide repeats 1	–	Pidugu et al., 2019	Pflügler et al., 2020	–
IFIT2 (↑)	Interferon-induced protein with tetratricopeptide repeats 2	Ohsugi et al., 2017	–	–	–
IFIT3 (↑)	Interferon induced protein with tetratricopeptide repeats 3	–	Niess et al., 2015	–	–
IFITM1 (↑)	Interferon-induced transmembrane protein 1	–	Yu et al., 2015; Yan et al., 2019		–
IGF2 (↑)	Insulin-like growth factor II	–	Kasprzak and Adamek, 2019	–	–
IL18BP (↑)	Interleukin-18-binding protein	–	Carbotti et al., 2013; Zhou et al., 2020	–	–
INPP1 (↑)	Inositol polyphosphate 1-phosphatase	–	Li et al., 2000; Li P. et al., 2019	–	–
IRF1 (↑)	Interferon regulatory factor 1	Bouker et al., 2005	–	Shao et al., 2019	–
IRF2 (↑)	Interferon regulatory factor 2	Kriegsman et al., 2019	–	–	–
IRF9 (↑)	Interferon regulatory factor 9	–	Luker et al., 2001; Brunn et al., 2021	–	–
ISG15 (↑)	Ubiquitin-like protein ISG15	D'Cunha et al., 1996; Zhou et al., 2017	Desai et al., 2006, 2012; Burks et al., 2014	–	–
KCNIP4 (↑)	Kv channel-interacting protein 4	–	–	–	Arora et al., 2020
KRT20 (↑)	Keratin, type I cytoskeletal 20	–	Wildi et al., 1999	–	–
LAP3 (↑)	Leucine aminopeptidase 3	–	Tian et al., 2014; Fang et al., 2019	–	–
LGALS3BP (↑)	Galectin-3-binding protein	–	Iacobelli et al., 1994; Rea et al., 1994	Läubli et al., 2014	Shao et al., 2013
LMO4 (↑)	LIM domain transcription factor LMO4	–	Sum et al., 2005; Wang W. et al., 2016	–	–
MPV17L (↑)	Mpv17-like protein	–	–	–	–
MT2A (↑)	Metallothionein-2	Pan et al., 2013	Jin et al., 2002; Kim et al., 2011	–	–
NLRC5 (↑)	NLR family CARD domain containing 5	Yoshihama et al., 2017, 2021	–	–	–
NMI (↑)	N-myc-interactor	Wang et al., 2017	Zhao et al., 2017	–	–
NUB1 (↑)	NEDD8 ultimate buster 1	Kito et al., 2001; Hosono et al., 2010; Zhang D. et al., 2020	–	–	–
OPTN (↑)	Optineurin	Liu et al., 2014	–	–	–
PARP14 (↑)	Protein mono-ADP-ribosyltransferase PARP14	–	Barbarulo et al., 2013; Yao et al., 2019	–	–
PARP15 (↓)	Protein mono-ADP-ribosyltransferase PARP15	–	–	–	–
PDIA3 (↑)	Protein disulfide-isomerase A3	–	Takata et al., 2016	Zhang H. et al., 2020	–
PHRF1 (↑)	PHD and RING finger domain-containing protein 1	Ettahar et al., 2013; Wang Y. et al., 2016	–	–	–
PLSCR1 (↑)	Phospholipid scramblase 1	–	Huang et al., 2020	–	–
PSMA5 (↑)	Proteasome subunit alpha type-5	–	Fu et al., 2019	–	–
PSMA6 (↑)	Proteasome subunit alpha type-6	–	Kakumu et al., 2017	–	–
PSMB10 (↑)	Proteasome subunit beta type-10	Rouette et al., 2016	–	–	–
PSMB8 (↑)	Proteasome subunit beta type-8	Kalaora et al., 2020	Kwon et al., 2016	–	Zhang et al., 2021
PSMB9 (↑)	Proteasome subunit beta type-9	Kalaora et al., 2020	Whitehead et al., 2005; Shoji et al., 2020	–	Zhang et al., 2021

(Continued)

TABLE 1 | (Continued)

Gene[1]	Protein name[2]	Anti-tumoral	Pro-tumoral	Immune escape	MCC related
PSME1 (↑)	Proteasome activator complex subunit 1	Wang et al., 2019	Sánchez-Martín et al., 2013	–	Kotowski et al., 2019
PSME2 (↑)	Proteasome activator complex subunit 2	–	Zheng et al., 2012	–	–
PSRC1 (↑)	Proline/serine-rich coiled-coil protein 1	–	–	–	–
RARRES3 (↑)	Retinoic acid receptor responder 3	Adelmann et al., 2016; Anderson et al., 2017	–	–	–
RNF213 (↑)	E3 ubiquitin-protein ligase RNF213	Wang et al., 2020	–	–	Yang et al., 2020
RPS2 (↑)	40S ribosomal protein S2	–	Chiao et al., 1992; Wang et al., 2009	–	–
SAMHD1 (↑)	Deoxynucleoside triphosphate triphosphohydrolase SAMHD1	Wang et al., 2014; Kodigepalli et al., 2017	Herold et al., 2017	–	–
STAT1 (↑)	Signal transducer and activator of transcription 1-alpha/beta	Meissl et al., 2017	Meissl et al., 2017; Zhang J. et al., 2020	Cerezo et al., 2018; Liu F. et al., 2020	–
TAPBPL (↑)	Tapasin-related protein	–	Lin et al., 2021	Hermann et al., 2015	–
TNFAIP2 (↑)	Tumor necrosis factor alpha-induced protein 2	–	Jia et al., 2016; Li et al., 2020	–	–
TRIM27 (↑)	Zinc finger protein RFP	–	Ma et al., 2016; Zhang et al., 2018; Xing et al., 2020	–	–
TRIM69 (↑)	E3 ubiquitin-protein ligase TRIM69	–	–	–	–
TUB (↓)	Tubby protein homolog	–	–	–	–
UBA7 (↑)	Ubiquitin-like modifier-activating enzyme 7	Feng Q. et al., 2008; Jiang et al., 2014; Lin et al., 2020	–	–	–
UBE2L6 (↑)	Ubiquitin conjugating enzyme E2 L6	–	Falvey et al., 2017	–	–
USP18 (↑)	Ubl carboxyl-terminal hydrolase 18	Hong et al., 2014	Tan et al., 2018; Diao et al., 2020	–	–
WARS (↑)	Tryptophanyl-tRNA synthetase	–	Adam et al., 2018	Adam et al., 2018	–
WNT10A (↑)	Protein Wnt-10a	–	Long et al., 2015; Li J. et al., 2019	–	Harms et al., 2013
WNT7A (↓)	Wnt family member 7A	Yoshioka et al., 2012; Wu et al., 2018	–	–	–

[1]*Genes with differential gene expression in form of upregulaton are marked with ↑, and downregulation is marked with ↓.*
[2]*Recommended protein name by UniProtKB (www.uniprot.org).*

or without IFNγ for 72 h (**Figures 7B,C**). We detected a small but significant decrease of LT antigen after IFNγ incubation in the cell lines WaGa and MKL-1, whereas LT antigen expression was not significantly altered in MKL-2.

DISCUSSION

In this study, single-molecule Nanopore sequencing has been used to analyze the transcriptome of MCC cells. Previously, whole transcriptome and genome studies of MCC using the second-generation sequencing could demonstrate distinct mutation spectra and expression profiles between virus-positive and virus-negative MCC (Starrett et al., 2017). Czech-Sioli et al. used genome sequencing *via* the Nanopore platform to perform high-resolution analysis of the genomic structure of the integration site of the MCPyV into the host genome of MCC cell lines and primary tumors. In addition, they employed the technology to reveal copy numbers and integration pattern of the MCPyV (Czech-Sioli et al., 2020), underlining the increasing popularity of Nanopore sequencing in cancer research. However, no studies on the transcriptome-wide response to key cytokines had been conducted so far.

Immune Escape Genes and Human Leukocyte Antigen Class I Upregulation

As shown for IFNγ in various other settings, our sequencing studies found numerous differentially expressed genes that have been associated with both anti-tumoral and pro-tumoral effects. These data indicate the different modes of action of IFNγ: On the one hand, it acts highly tumor suppressive; on the other hand, it dampens the immune response by synthesis of inhibitory molecules (John and Darcy, 2016). Furthermore, we detected 11 immune escape genes that were significantly increased by IFNγ, suggesting that these are involved in the formation of an immunosuppressive tumor microenvironment counteracting the inflammatory effect of IFNγ (Mojic et al., 2017). Targeting these genes could improve the responsiveness to checkpoint inhibitor therapy and increase immunosurveillance and survival of MCC patients.

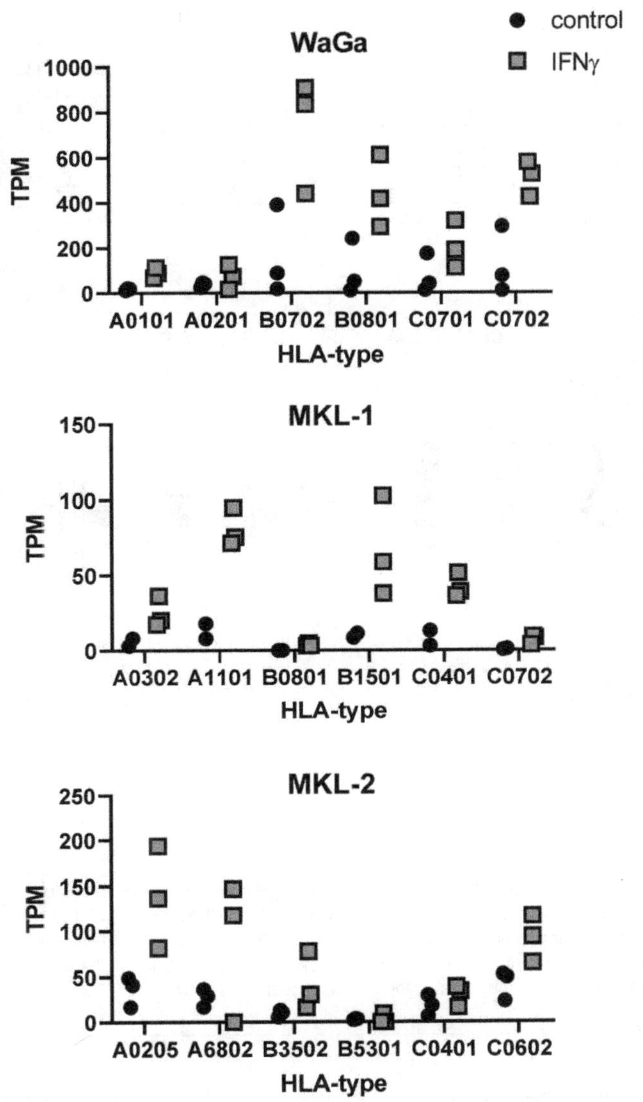

FIGURE 5 | Detection of HLA expression after IFNγ incubation on mRNA level. Transcripts per million (TPM) values of six different HLA alleles after IFNγ treatment (gray squares) or without IFNγ incubation (black dots) are depicted for each MCC cell line. TPM values were acquired from our sequencing output using a new two-pass quantification method. For each cell line, three independent experiments were performed (two for MKL-1 control), so that each symbol represents one replicate of the respective cell line.

Downregulation of HLA class I and upregulation of immune checkpoint proteins (PD-1, CTLA-4, and PD-L1) are known to help the tumor to escape the control of the immune system. Paulson et al. reported reduced expression of HLA class I in MCC cell lines, which was reversible by IFNγ treatment (Paulson et al., 2014). In our flow cytometry experiments, we could also detect a clear upregulation of HLA class I surface expression in the presence of IFNγ in MKL-2 and WaGa cells, whereas MKL-1 cells showed only a slight increase of HLA class I. This is noteworthy because MKL-1 had the highest number of differentially expressed genes after IFNγ treatment. Expression levels of HLA have previously been shown to be low in MKL-1 cells, intermediate in WaGa cells, and high in MKL-2 cells (Ritter et al., 2017). In our flow cytometry experiments, without the addition of IFNγ, we could detect only low levels of HLA in WaGa and MKL-1 cells and higher levels in MKL-2 cells. Increased HLA induced by IFNγ, which counteracts HLA downregulation by the tumor, could contribute to higher effectiveness of immunotherapies in MCC patients. In awareness of the high error rates of Nanopore sequencing and the variability of the HLA allele–specific expression, we were able to verify the changes in HLA expression behavior, previously detected by flow cytometry, in the sequencing data. This strengthens the usability of Nanopore sequencing for highly variable alleles and the measurement of transcriptome-wide response to key cytokines. However, without prior HLA-typing of the subject, we consider that the third-generation sequencing still has difficulties to identify and quantify expression of highly polymorphic HLA loci.

Immune Checkpoints Are Influenced by Interferon Gamma Treatment

We studied the effect of IFNγ on the immune checkpoint PD-L1 and the key immune suppressive molecule IDO. IDO is of special interest for MCC as it has been shown that IDO expression is associated with MCPyV status and prognosis (Wardhani et al., 2019). To date, the effect of IFNγ on IDO has not been studied in MCC. We could not detect any alteration of IDO in all cell lines neither on mRNA nor on protein level. In contrast, IDO has been reported to be upregulated by IFNγ in the tumor microenvironment of melanoma (Spranger et al., 2013) and several other cell types, such as dendritic cells (Jürgens et al., 2009). Interestingly, our sequencing data show that WARS, which can protect cancer cells from IDO-mediated tryptophan depletion (Adam et al., 2018), is highly upregulated on mRNA level in the presence of IFNγ in all cell lines, underlining the pro-inflammatory activity of IFNγ in this context.

Interferon gamma is known to contribute to tumor immune resistance by inducing the expression of immune checkpoint receptors and their ligands (Benci et al., 2016). We could demonstrate a slight upregulation of PD-L1 in MKL-1 and MKL-2 cells by flow cytometry analysis. Another interesting protein associated with inhibitory effects on T cells is Tapasin-related protein, encoded by the gene TAPBPL. TAPBPL was highly upregulated in IFNγ-exposed MKL-1 cells. Tapasin-related protein is a T cell co-inhibitory molecule identified in 2021 (Lin et al., 2021), which is expressed on cancer cells and antigen-presenting cells as well as the corresponding receptor on activated CD4 and CD8 T cells. As a new immune checkpoint molecule, it might be an interesting target for cancer therapy.

Alteration in Large T Antigen Expression on Protein but Not on mRNA Level

Large T antigen mRNA expression was not significantly altered by IFNγ treatment in all three MCC cell lines. However, our studies of the LT antigen on protein level showed small but

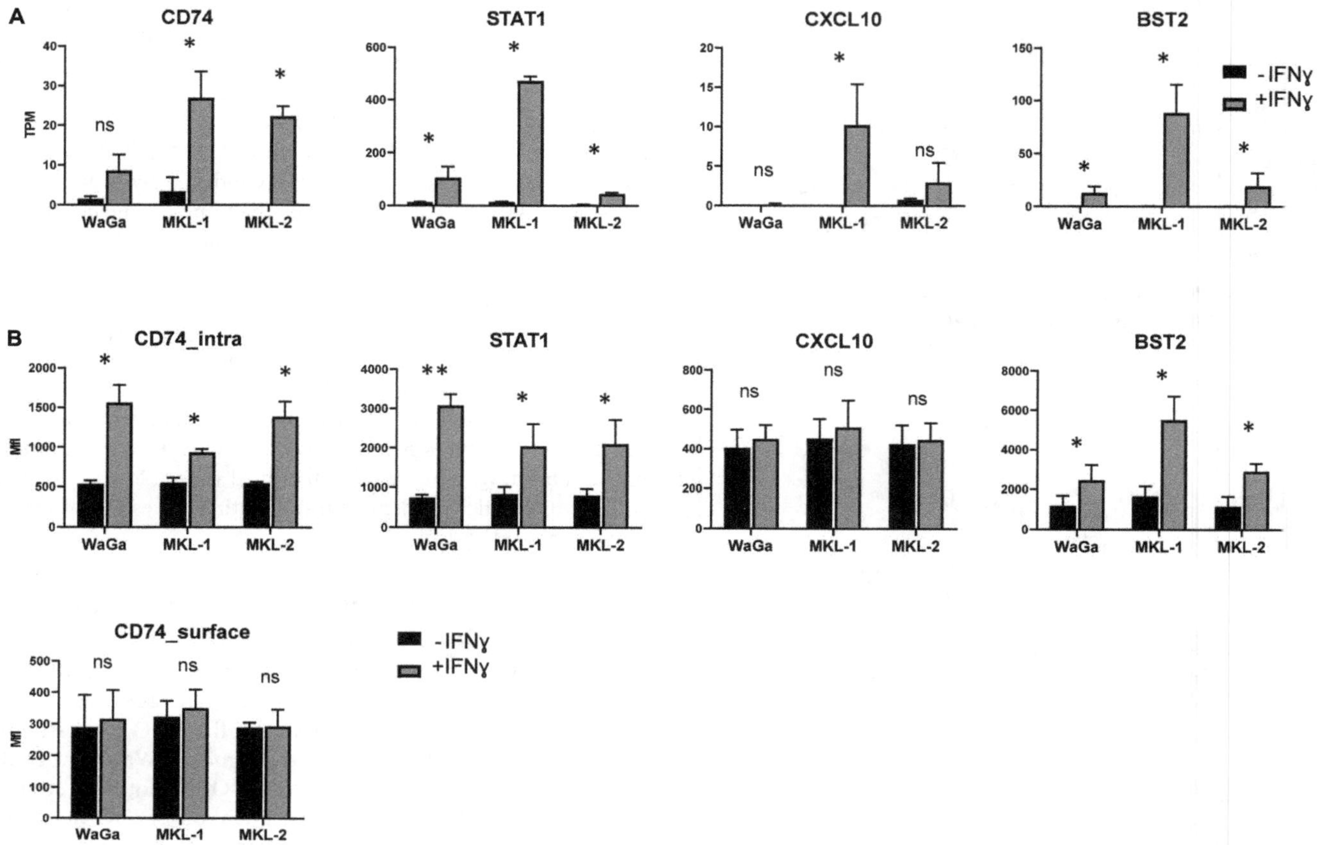

FIGURE 6 | Validation of differential gene expression in MCC cell lines on protein level and mRNA level. **(A)** TPM values were acquired from our sequencing output. The data represent mean values ± SEM from three independent experiments (two for MKL-1 control). **(B)** After 72 h of treatment with or without IFNγ (3,000 U/ml), the Merkel cell carcinoma cell lines MKL-1, MKL-2, and WaGa were stained for signal transducer and activator of transcription 1-alpha/beta (STAT1), bone marrow stromal antigen 2 (BST2), C-X-C motif chemokine 10 (CXCL10), and HLA class II histocompatibility antigen gamma chain (CD74) and analyzed by flow cytometry. The average MFI of three independent experiments ± standard error is indicated. *p*-values were determined using the paired student's *t*-test. *$p < 0.05$; **$p < 0.01$; ns, not significant.

significant decreased expression in WaGa and MKL-1, whereas no alteration could be detected in MKL-2. We hypothesize that IFNγ might have a destabilization effect only on protein level in WaGa and MKL-1 cells, which is not detectable in the mRNA profile. Interestingly, Willmes et al. described a clear reduction of the LT antigen on protein level in WaGa cells, whereas MKL-1 and MKL-2 cells showed no change in LT protein expression, when analyzed after 7 days of IFNγ treatment (Willmes et al., 2012). This discrepancy may be attributed to the kinetics of LT antigen regulation, which may yield different results at different time points.

Oxford Nanopore Sequencing for Transcriptomics

In this study, we strived to elucidate the biological response of MCC cell lines to IFNγ stimulation while also trying to ascertain whether the expression studies of large eukaryotic transcriptomes are sensible and feasible using the Nanopore platform. We especially were interested to produce reliable and reproducible data at the current stage of the yet relatively new Nanopore system. There have been several benchmarking studies on Nanopore sequencing in the context of cDNA or direct RNA sequencing that discuss the system in a benchmark-type situation (Workman et al., 2019; Chen et al., 2021). Our goal, however, was to test practicability, robustness, and reproducibility in an applied setting. We found that the Nanopore system offers great potential for researchers to get access to in-house-produced sequencing data with relatively low entry costs and virtually no maintenance costs. These advantages come, however, at the price of high hardware requirements, a necessity of sufficient bioinformatics infrastructure and a fast-evolving system, in which laboratory protocols, software versions, and specifications as well as the recommendations of the manufacturer change with higher frequency as compared to firmly established sequencing environments as Illumina. We especially had issues pinpointing specific points of failure in experimental procedures that were virtually identical but for the flow cell used. Documentation on troubleshooting was sparse and hard to find at the time of our experiments. It is, however, noteworthy that, since

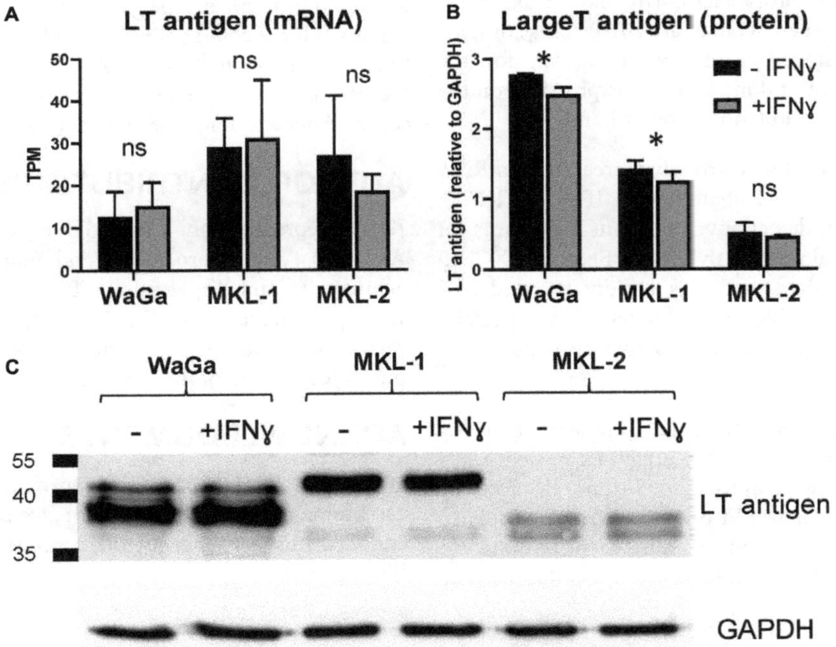

FIGURE 7 | Large T antigen expression before and after IFNγ treatment. **(A)** TPM values were acquired from our sequencing output. The data represent mean values ± SEM from three independent experiments (two for MKL-1 control). **(B)** LT antigen expression was analyzed on protein level *via* Western blot analysis. Expression levels are depicted relative to the loading control GAPDH. The average of three independent experiments ± standard error is indicated. *p*-values were determined using the paired student's *t*-test. *$p < 0.05$; **$p < 0.01$; ns, not significant. **(C)** Representative exposure of one western blot. Protein size standard is indicated in kilodalton.

then, Oxford Nanopore has greatly improved its available training resources.

Pore count at the beginning of an experiment appeared to be a good indicator of the possible total sequencing output for us; however, this was not true for flow cells that had been stored for longer periods and were approaching expiration date. In the experiment with MKL-2, we observed a rapid drop off of sequencing output after 24 h (**Figure 2A**) although the flow cell was older but still above warranty level and had ample pores available. In addition, BC performance widely varied. The good performance of BC 1 in terms of yield could be replicated across all three experiments, similar to BC 6. BC 3 failed completely—an issue the broader community was aware of, and we became aware of during troubleshooting. However, BC 5 and BC 7 bordered on failure as well over all three flow cells.

The MinION Sequencing platform by Oxford Nanopore is a rapidly evolving technology. Troubleshooting was challenging for us at times. The biological nature of embedded pores creates a necessity for stringent experiment planning, because extended storage times appeared to have a negative effect on yield. However, the access to sequencing data within 3 days from library prep to finished data is very attractive. In addition, long reads allow the accurate quantification of gene expression even at low sequencing depth because even in an cDNA assay, each reverse-transcribed molecule came from a native poly(A)-mRNA molecule with no fragmentation bias. Overall, the system is under active development and Q 20 chemistry (99% base call accuracy) has already been announced while constant improvements are made to hardware and protocols. The system offers a great entry point to sequencing, even for smaller laboratories, and allows rapid quantification of the expression landscape of a sample.

Validation of Transcriptomic Data on Protein Level

To validate our Nanopore sequencing data, we further analyzed the expression of STAT1, CXCL10, BST2, CD74, and the LT antigen on protein level. We detected a significant increase of STAT1 and BST2 in all three cell lines, as we had observed on mRNA level. STAT1 is itself involved in the IFNγ signaling pathway and both STAT1 and BST2 are known to be IFN inducible (Soler et al., 2003; Blasius et al., 2006; Krause et al., 2006; Yoo et al., 2011). In addition, CD74 significantly increased on protein level for all three cell lines. In our sequencing findings, increased CD74 was only significant for MKL-1 and MKL-2, whereas the observed upregulation in WaGa did not meet significance. Interestingly, CD74 showed significant regulation only when stained intracellularly; surface expression of CD74 on the MCC cell lines was, in general, lower and completely unaltered by IFNγ. The transcript of the CD74 gene forms invariant chain of the immature HLA class II complex. The cell surface form, in contrast, acts as receptor for macrophage migration inhibitory factor (Imaoka et al., 2019) and is involved in tumorigenesis (Liu et al., 2016). This complex post-translational processing is probably the reason for the discrepancy between mRNA and intracellular expression, on the one hand, and surface expression, on the other hand.

C-X-C motif chemokine 10 was strongly increased on mRNA level in one MCC cell line incubated with IFNγ (MKL-1); nevertheless, we could not detect any significant differences on protein level, and the signal was relatively low. Because CXCL10 is a chemokine, we speculate that it is rapidly secreted and does not accumulate to detectable levels intracellularly, especially because no secretion-blocking substances like brefeldin A or monensin were added.

In summary, we could demonstrate the complexity of IFNγ responses mirrored by numerous differentially expressed genes induced by IFNγ, mainly with anti- or pro-tumoral effects or even both. In this context, it would be interesting to sequence primary MCC cell cultures and to examine their response to IFNγ because this could better represent *in vivo* conditions. The identified immune escape genes are of special interest for further studies as these could deliver valuable information about how the tumor circumvents the control of the immune system. Targeting the genes involved in immune evasion and tumor progression could be beneficial for the clinical outcome of MCC patients.

AUTHOR CONTRIBUTIONS

JD: conceptualization. TS and JD: experimental procedures. CL, AW, and JV: data processing and analysis. JD and JV: funding acquisition and supervision. TS and CL: investigation and writing—original draft. CL, TS, AW, CB, JD, and JV: writing—review and editing. All authors have read and agreed to the published version of the manuscript.

ACKNOWLEDGMENTS

We thank Jürgen Becker for providing us the Merkel cell carcinoma cell lines. Furthermore, we thank Petra Mühl-Zürbes and Christina Draßner for their technical assistance in Western Blot preparation.

REFERENCES

Abrahamsson, H., Jensen, B. V., Berven, L. L., Nielsen, D. L., Šaltytė Benth, J., Johansen, J. S., et al. (2020). Antitumour immunity invoked by hepatic arterial infusion of first-line oxaliplatin predicts durable colorectal cancer control after liver metastasis ablation: 8-12 years of follow-up. *Int. J. Cancer* 146, 2019–2026. doi: 10.1002/ijc.32847

Adam, I., Dewi, D. L., Mooiweer, J., Sadik, A., Mohapatra, S. R., Berdel, B., et al. (2018). Upregulation of tryptophanyl-tRNA synthethase adapts human cancer cells to nutritional stress caused by tryptophan degradation. *Oncoimmunology* 7, e1486353–e1486353. doi: 10.1080/2162402X.2018.1486353

Adelmann, C. H., Ching, G., Du, L., Saporito, R. C., Bansal, V., Pence, L. J., et al. (2016). Comparative profiles of BRAF inhibitors: the paradox index as a predictor of clinical toxicity. *Oncotarget* 7, 30453–30460. doi: 10.18632/oncotarget.8351

Afanasiev, O. K., Yelistratova, L., Miller, N., Nagase, K., Paulson, K., Iyer, J. G., et al. (2013). Merkel polyomavirus-specific T cells fluctuate with Merkel cell carcinoma burden and express therapeutically targetable PD-1 and Tim-3 exhaustion markers. *Clin. Cancer Res.* 19, 5351–5360. doi: 10.1158/1078-0432.CCR-13-0035

Anderson, A. M., Kalimutho, M., Harten, S., Nanayakkara, D. M., Khanna, K. K., and Ragan, M. A. (2017). The metastasis suppressor RARRES3 as an endogenous inhibitor of the immunoproteasome expression in breast cancer cells. *Sci. Rep.* 7:39873. doi: 10.1038/srep39873

Arora, R., Choi, J. E., Harms, P. W., and Chandrani, P. (2020). Merkel cell polyomavirus in Merkel cell carcinoma: integration sites and involvement of the KMT2D tumor suppressor gene. *Viruses* 12:966. doi: 10.3390/v12090966

Aversa, I., Zolea, F., Ieranò, C., Bulotta, S., Trotta, A. M., Faniello, M. C., et al. (2017). Epithelial-to-mesenchymal transition in FHC-silenced cells: the role of CXCR4/CXCL12 axis. *J. Exp. Clin. Cancer Res.* 36:104. doi: 10.1186/s13046-017-0571-8

Ayers, M., Lunceford, J., Nebozhyn, M., Murphy, E., Loboda, A., Kaufman, D. R., et al. (2017). IFN-γ-related mRNA profile predicts clinical response to PD-1 blockade. *J. Clin. Invest.* 127, 2930–2940. doi: 10.1172/JCI91190

Bald, T., Landsberg, J., Lopez-Ramos, D., Renn, M., Glodde, N., Jansen, P., et al. (2014). Immune cell-poor melanomas benefit from PD-1 blockade after targeted type I IFN activation. *Cancer Discov.* 4, 674–687. doi: 10.1158/2159-8290.CD-13-0458

Barbarulo, A., Iansante, V., Chaidos, A., Naresh, K., Rahemtulla, A., Franzoso, G., et al. (2013). Poly(ADP-ribose) polymerase family member 14 (PARP14) is a novel effector of the JNK2-dependent pro-survival signal in multiple myeloma. *Oncogene* 32, 4231–4242. doi: 10.1038/onc.2012.448

Bartolomé, R. A., García-Palmero, I., Torres, S., López-Lucendo, M., Balyasnikova, I. V., and Casal, J. I. (2015). IL13 receptor α2 signaling requires a scaffold protein, FAM120A, to activate the FAK and PI3K pathways in colon cancer metastasis. *Cancer Res.* 75, 2434–2444. doi: 10.1158/0008-5472.CAN-14-3650

Beatty, G., and Paterson, Y. (2001). IFN-gamma-dependent inhibition of tumor angiogenesis by tumor-infiltrating CD4+ T cells requires tumor responsiveness to IFN-gamma. *J. Immunol.* 166, 2276–2282. doi: 10.4049/jimmunol.166.4.2276

Benci, J. L., Xu, B., Qiu, Y., Wu, T. J., Dada, H., Twyman-Saint Victor, C., et al. (2016). Tumor interferon signaling regulates a multigenic resistance program to immune checkpoint blockade. *Cell* 167, 1540–1554.e12. doi: 10.1016/j.cell.2016.11.022

Biamonte, F., Battaglia, A. M., Zolea, F., Oliveira, D. M., Aversa, I., Santamaria, G., et al. (2018). Ferritin heavy subunit enhances apoptosis of non-small cell lung cancer cells through modulation of miR-125b/p53 axis. *Cell Death Dis.* 9:1174. doi: 10.1038/s41419-018-1216-3

Blasius, A. L., Giurisato, E., Cella, M., Schreiber, R. D., Shaw, A. S., and Colonna, M. (2006). Bone marrow stromal cell antigen 2 is a specific marker of type I IFN-producing cells in the naive mouse, but a promiscuous cell surface antigen following IFN stimulation. *J. Immunol.* 177, 3260–3265. doi: 10.4049/jimmunol.177.5.3260

Bonan, N. F., Kowalski, D., Kudlac, K., Flaherty, K., Gwilliam, J. C., Falkenberg, L. G., et al. (2019). Inhibition of HGF/MET signaling decreases overall tumor burden and blocks malignant conversion in Tpl2-related skin cancer. *Oncogenesis* 8:1. doi: 10.1038/s41389-018-0109-8

Borchert, S., Czech-Sioli, M., Neumann, F., Schmidt, C., Wimmer, P., Dobner, T., et al. (2014). High-affinity Rb binding, p53 inhibition, subcellular localization, and transformation by wild-type or tumor-derived shortened Merkel cell polyomavirus large T antigens. *J. Virol.* 88, 3144–3160. doi: 10.1128/JVI.02916-13

Bouker, K. B., Skaar, T. C., Riggins, R. B., Harburger, D. S., Fernandez, D. R., Zwart, A., et al. (2005). Interferon regulatory factor-1 (IRF-1) exhibits tumor suppressor activities in breast cancer associated with caspase activation and induction of apoptosis. *Carcinogenesis* 26, 1527–1535. doi: 10.1093/carcin/bgi113

Britzen-Laurent, N., Lipnik, K., Ocker, M., Naschberger, E., Schellerer, V. S., Croner, R. S., et al. (2013). GBP-1 acts as a tumor suppressor in colorectal cancer cells. *Carcinogenesis* 34, 153–162. doi: 10.1093/carcin/bgs310

Brunn, D., Turkowski, K., Günther, S., Weigert, A., Muley, T., Kriegsmann, M., et al. (2021). Interferon regulatory factor 9 promotes lung cancer progression via regulation of versican. *Cancers (Basel)* 13:208. doi: 10.3390/cancers13020208

Burks, J., Reed, R. E., and Desai, S. D. (2014). ISGylation governs the oncogenic function of Ki-Ras in breast cancer. *Oncogene* 33, 794–803. doi: 10.1038/onc.2012.633

Carbotti, G., Barisione, G., Orengo, A. M., Brizzolara, A., Airoldi, I., Bagnoli, M., et al. (2013). The IL-18 antagonist IL-18-binding protein is produced in the human ovarian cancer microenvironment. *Clin. Cancer Res.* 19, 4611–4620. doi: 10.1158/1078-0432.CCR-13-0568

Cerezo, M., Guemiri, R., Druillennec, S., Girault, I., Malka-Mahieu, H., Shen, S., et al. (2018). Translational control of tumor immune escape via the eIF4F–STAT1–PD-L1 axis in melanoma. *Nat. Med.* 24, 1877–1886. doi: 10.1038/s41591-018-0217-1

Chen, H., Cong, X., Wu, C., Wu, X., Wang, J., Mao, K., et al. (2020). Intratumoral delivery of CCL25 enhances immunotherapy against triple-negative breast cancer by recruiting CCR9(+) T cells. *Sci. Adv.* 6:eaax4690–eaax4690. doi: 10.1126/sciadv.aax4690

Chen, Y., Davidson, N. M., Wan, Y. K., Patel, H., Yao, F., Low, H. M., et al. (2021). A systematic benchmark of nanopore long read RNA sequencing for transcript level analysis in human cell lines. *bioRxiv* [Preprint]. doi: 10.1101/2021.04.21.440736

Chiang, K.-C., Huang, S.-T., Wu, R.-C., Huang, S.-C., Yeh, T.-S., Chen, M.-H., et al. (2019). Interferon α-inducible protein 27 is an oncogene and highly expressed in cholangiocarcinoma patients with poor survival. *Cancer Manag. Res.* 11, 1893–1905. doi: 10.2147/CMAR.S196485

Chiao, P. J., Shin, D. M., Sacks, P. G., Hong, W. K., and Tainsky, M. A. (1992). Elevated expression of the ribosomal protein S2 gene in human tumors. *Mol. Carcinog.* 5, 219–231. doi: 10.1002/mc.2940050309

Co, J. K., Verma, S., Gurjav, U., Sumibcay, L., and Nerurkar, V. R. (2007). Interferon- alpha and - beta restrict polyomavirus JC replication in primary human fetal glial cells: implications for progressive multifocal leukoencephalopathy therapy. *J. Infect. Dis.* 196, 712–718. doi: 10.1086/520518

Cooper, M. A., Fehniger, T. A., Turner, S. C., Chen, K. S., Ghaheri, B. A., Ghayur, T., et al. (2001). Human natural killer cells: a unique innate immunoregulatory role for the CD56(bright) subset. *Blood* 97, 3146–3151. doi: 10.1182/blood.v97.10.3146

Czech-Sioli, M., Günther, T., Therre, M., Spohn, M., Indenbirken, D., Theiss, J., et al. (2020). High-resolution analysis of Merkel cell polyomavirus in Merkel cell carcinoma reveals distinct integration patterns and suggests NHEJ and MMBIR as underlying mechanisms. *PLoS Pathog.* 16:e1008562. doi: 10.1371/journal.ppat.1008562

D'Cunha, J., Knight, E. Jr., Haas, A. L., Truitt, R. L., and Borden, E. C. (1996). Immunoregulatory properties of ISG15, an interferon-induced cytokine. *Proc. Natl. Acad. Sci. U. S. A.* 93, 211–215. doi: 10.1073/pnas.93.1.211

Desai, S. D., Haas, A. L., Wood, L. M., Tsai, Y.-C., Pestka, S., Rubin, E. H., et al. (2006). Elevated expression of ISG15 in tumor cells interferes with the ubiquitin/26S proteasome pathway. *Cancer Res.* 66, 921–928. doi: 10.1158/0008-5472.CAN-05-1123

Desai, S. D., Reed, R. E., Burks, J., Wood, L. M., Pullikuth, A. K., Haas, A. L., et al. (2012). ISG15 disrupts cytoskeletal architecture and promotes motility in human breast cancer cells. *Exp. Biol. Med. (Maywood)* 237, 38–49. doi: 10.1258/ebm.2011.011236

Di Sanzo, M., Gaspari, M., Misaggi, R., Romeo, F., Falbo, L., De Marco, C., et al. (2011). H ferritin gene silencing in a human metastatic melanoma cell line: a proteomic analysis. *J. Proteome Res.* 10, 5444–5453. doi: 10.1021/pr200705z

Diao, W., Guo, Q., Zhu, C., Song, Y., Feng, H., Cao, Y., et al. (2020). USP18 promotes cell proliferation and suppressed apoptosis in cervical cancer cells via activating AKT signaling pathway. *BMC Cancer* 20:741. doi: 10.1186/s12885-020-07241-1

Ettahar, A., Ferrigno, O., Zhang, M.-Z., Ohnishi, M., Ferrand, N., Prunier, C., et al. (2013). Identification of PHRF1 as a tumor suppressor that promotes the TGF-β cytostatic program through selective release of TGIF-driven PML inactivation. *Cell Rep.* 4, 530–541. doi: 10.1016/j.celrep.2013.07.009

Euskirchen, P., Bielle, F., Labreche, K., Kloosterman, W. P., Rosenberg, S., Daniau, M., et al. (2017). Same-day genomic and epigenomic diagnosis of brain tumors using real-time nanopore sequencing. *Acta Neuropathol.* 134, 691–703. doi: 10.1007/s00401-017-1743-5

Falvey, C. M., O'Donovan, T. R., El-Mashed, S., Nyhan, M. J., O'Reilly, S., and McKenna, S. L. (2017). UBE2L6/UBCH8 and ISG15 attenuate autophagy in esophageal cancer cells. *Oncotarget* 8, 23479–23491. doi: 10.18632/oncotarget.15182

Fang, C., Zhang, J., Yang, H., Peng, L., Wang, K., Wang, Y., et al. (2019). Leucine aminopeptidase 3 promotes migration and invasion of breast cancer cells through upregulation of fascin and matrix metalloproteinases-2/9 expression. *J. Cell Biochem.* 120, 3611–3620. doi: 10.1002/jcb.27638

Feng, H., Shuda, M., Chang, Y , and Moore, P. S. (2008). Clonal integration of a polyomavirus in human Merkel cell carcinoma. *Science* 319, 1096–1100. doi: 10.1126/science.1152586

Feng, Q., Sekula, D., Guo, Y., Liu, X., Black, C. C., Galimberti, F., et al. (2008). UBE1L causes lung cancer growth suppression by targeting cyclin D1. *Mol. Cancer Ther.* 7, 3780–3788. doi: 10.1158/1535-7163.MCT-08-0753

Fitzgerald, T. L., Dennis, S., Kachare, S. D., Vohra, N. A., Wong, J. H., and Zervos, E. E. (2015). Dramatic increase in the incidence and mortality from Merkel cell carcinoma in the United States. *Am. Surg.* 81, 802–806. doi: 10.1177/000313481508100819

Fu, Z., Lu, C., Zhang, C., and Qiao, B. (2019). PSMA5 promotes the tumorigenic process of prostate cancer and is related to bortezomib resistance. *Anticancer Drugs* 30:e0773. doi: 10.1097/CAD.0000000000000773

Gao, J., Pan, H., Zhu, Z., Yu, T., Huang, B., and Zhou, Y. (2020a). Guanine nucleotide-binding protein subunit beta-4 promotes gastric cancer progression via activating Erk1/2. *Acta Biochim. Biophys. Sin. (Shanghai)* 52, 975–987. doi: 10.1093/abbs/gmaa084

Gao, J., Shi, L. Z., Zhao, H., Chen, J., Xiong, L., He, Q., et al. (2016). Loss of IFN-γ pathway genes in tumor cells as a mechanism of resistance to Anti-CTLA-4 therapy. *Cell* 167, 397–404.e9. doi: 10.1016/j.cell.2016.08.069

Gao, J., Yu, T., Xuan, Y., and Zhu, Z. (2020b). High expression of GNB4 predicts poor prognosis in patients with *Helicobacter* pylori -positive advanced gastric cancer. *Transl. Cancer Res.* 9, 4224–4238.

Gao, Y., Yang, W., Pan, M., Scully, E., Girardi, M., Augenlicht, L. H., et al. (2003). Gamma delta T cells provide an early source of interferon gamma in tumor immunity. *J. Exp. Med.* 198, 433–442. doi: 10.1084/jem.20030584

Geng, N., Zhang, W., Li, Y., and Li, F. (2019). Aspartyl aminopeptidase suppresses proliferation, invasion, and stemness of breast cancer cells via targeting CD44. *Anat. Rec.* 302, 2178–2185. doi: 10.1002/ar.24206

Greenwood, C., Metodieva, G., Al-Janabi, K., Lausen, B., Alldridge, L., Leng, L., et al. (2012). Stat1 and CD74 overexpression is co-dependent and linked to increased invasion and lymph node metastasis in triple-negative breast cancer. *J. Proteom.* 75, 3031–3040. doi: 10.1016/j.jprot.2011.11.033

Gupta, R., Forloni, M., Bisserier, M., Dogra, S. K., Yang, Q., and Wajapeyee, N. (2016). Interferon alpha-inducible protein 6 regulates NRASQ61K-induced melanomagenesis and growth. *eLife* 5:e16432. doi: 10.7554/eLife.16432

Han, T., Wang, Z., Yang, Y., Shu, T., Li, W., Liu, D., et al. (2015). The tumor-suppressive role of BATF2 in esophageal squamous cell carcinoma. *Oncol. Rep.* 34, 1353–1360. doi: 10.3892/or.2015.4090

Harms, P. W., Patel, R. M., Verhaegen, M. E., Giordano, T. J., Nash, K. T., Johnson, C. N., et al. (2013). Distinct gene expression profiles of viral- and nonviral-associated Merkel cell carcinoma revealed by transcriptome analysis. *J. Invest. Dermatol.* 133, 936–945. doi: 10.1038/jid.2012.445

Heath, M., Jaimes, N., Lemos, B., Mostaghimi, A., Wang, L. C., Penas, P. F., et al. (2008). Clinical characteristics of Merkel cell carcinoma at diagnosis in 195 patients: the AEIOU features. *J. Am. Acad. Dermatol.* 58, 375–381. doi: 10.1016/j.jaad.2007.11.020

Hermann, C., Trowsdale, J., and Boyle, L. H. (2015). TAPBPR: a new player in the MHC class I presentation pathway. *Tissue Antigens* 85, 155–166. doi: 10.1111/tan.12538

Herold, N., Rudd, S. G., Sanjiv, K., Kutzner, J., Bladh, J., Paulin, C. B. J., et al. (2017). SAMHD1 protects cancer cells from various nucleoside-based antimetabolites. *Cell Cycle* 16, 1029–1038. doi: 10.1080/15384101.2017.1314407

Hesbacher, S., Pfitzer, L., Wiedorfer, K., Angermeyer, S., Borst, A., Haferkamp, S., et al. (2016). RB1 is the crucial target of the Merkel cell polyomavirus large T antigen in Merkel cell carcinoma cells. *Oncotarget* 7, 32956–32968. doi: 10.18632/oncotarget.8793

Hong, B., Li, H., Lu, Y., Zhang, M., Zheng, Y., Qian, J., et al. (2014). USP18 is crucial for IFN-γ-mediated inhibition of B16 melanoma tumorigenesis and antitumor immunity. *Mol. Cancer* 13:132. doi: 10.1186/1476-4598-13-132

Hosono, T., Tanaka, T., Tanji, K., Nakatani, T., and Kamitani, T. (2010). NUB1, an interferon-inducible protein mediates anti-proliferative actions and apoptosis in renal cell carcinoma cells through cell-cycle regulation. *Br. J. Cancer* 102, 873–882. doi: 10.1038/sj.bjc.6605574

Houben, R., Shuda, M., Weinkam, R., Schrama, D., Feng, H., Chang, Y., et al. (2010). Merkel cell polyomavirus-infected Merkel cell carcinoma cells require expression of viral T antigens. *J. Virol.* 84, 7064–7072. doi: 10.1128/JVI.02 400-09

House, I. G., Savas, P., Lai, J., Chen, A. X. Y., Oliver, A. J., Teo, Z. L., et al. (2020). Macrophage-derived CXCL9 and CXCL10 are required for antitumor immune responses following immune checkpoint blockade. *Clin. Cancer Res.* 26, 487–504. doi: 10.1158/1078-0432.CCR-19-1868

Huang, M.-Y., Wang, J.-Y., and Lin, S.-R. (2013). CA9 and CHRNB1 were correlated with perineural invasion in Taiwanese colorectal cancer patients. *Biomark. Genom. Med.* 5, 84–86. doi: 10.1016/j.bgm.2013.07.001

Huang, P., Liao, R., Chen, X., Wu, X., Li, X., Wang, Y., et al. (2020). Nuclear translocation of PLSCR1 activates STAT1 signaling in basal-like breast cancer. *Theranostics* 10, 4644–4658. doi: 10.7150/thno.43150

Hung, J.-Y., Chiang, S.-R., Liu, K.-T., Tsai, M.-J., Huang, M.-S., Shieh, J.-M., et al. (2017). Overexpression and proliferation dependence of acyl-CoA thioesterase 11 and 13 in lung adenocarcinoma. *Oncol. Lett.* 14, 3647–3656. doi: 10.3892/ol. 2017.6594

Iacobelli, S., Sismondi, P., Giai, M., D'Egidio, M., Tinari, N., Amatetti, C., et al. (1994). Prognostic value of a novel circulating serum 90K antigen in breast cancer. *Br. J. Cancer* 69, 172–176. doi: 10.1038/bjc.1994.29

Ikeda, H., Old, L. J., and Schreiber, R. D. (2002). The roles of IFN gamma in protection against tumor development and cancer immunoediting. *Cytokine Growth Factor Rev.* 13, 95–109. doi: 10.1016/s1359-6101(01)00038-7

Imaoka, M., Tanese, K., Masugi, Y., Hayashi, M., and Sakamoto, M. (2019). Macrophage migration inhibitory factor-CD74 interaction regulates the expression of programmed cell death ligand 1 in melanoma cells. *Cancer Sci.* 110, 2273–2283. doi: 10.1111/cas.14038

Ip, C. L. C., Loose, M., Tyson, J. R., de Cesare, M., Brown, B. L., Jain, M., et al. (2015). MinION analysis and reference consortium: phase 1 data release and analysis. *F1000Res.* 4, 1075–1075. doi: 10.12688/f1000research.7201.1

Jain, M., Fiddes, I. T., Miga, K. H., Olsen, H. E., Paten, B., and Akeson, M. (2015). Improved data analysis for the MinION nanopore sequencer. *Nat. Methods* 12, 351–356. doi: 10.1038/nmeth.3290

Jain, M., Olsen, H. E., Paten, B., and Akeson, M. (2016). The Oxford Nanopore MinION: delivery of nanopore sequencing to the genomics community. *Genome Biol.* 17, 239–239.

Järvinen, T. A. H., and Prince, S. (2015). Decorin: a growth factor antagonist for tumor growth inhibition. *Biomed. Res. Int.* 2015, 654765–654765. doi: 10.1155/ 2015/654765

Ji, X., Zhu, H., Dai, X., Xi, Y., Sheng, Y., Gao, C., et al. (2019). Overexpression of GBP1 predicts poor prognosis and promotes tumor growth in human glioblastoma multiforme. *Cancer Biomark.* 25, 275–290. doi: 10.3233/CBM-171177

Jia, L., Zhou, Z., Liang, H., Wu, J., Shi, P., Li, F., et al. (2016). KLF5 promotes breast cancer proliferation, migration and invasion in part by upregulating the transcription of TNFAIP2. *Oncogene* 35, 2040–2051. doi: 10.1038/onc.2015.263

Jiang, A. P., Zhou, D. H., Meng, X. L., Zhang, A. P., Zhang, C., Li, X. T., et al. (2014). Down-regulation of epidermal growth factor receptor by curcumin-induced UBE1L in human bronchial epithelial cells. *J. Nutr. Biochem.* 25, 241–249. doi: 10.1016/j.jnutbio.2013.11.001

Jin, R., Chow, V. T., Tan, P. H., Dheen, S. T., Duan, W., and Bay, B. H. (2002). Metallothionein 2A expression is associated with cell proliferation in breast cancer. *Carcinogenesis* 23, 81–86. doi: 10.1093/carcin/23.1.81

John, L. B., and Darcy, P. K. (2016). The double-edged sword of IFN-γ-dependent immune-based therapies. *Immunol. Cell Biol.* 94, 527–528. doi: 10.1038/icb. 2016.37

Jürgens, B., Hainz, U., Fuchs, D., Felzmann, T., and Heitger, A. (2009). Interferon-γ-triggered indoleamine 2,3-dioxygenase competence in human monocyte-derived dendritic cells induces regulatory activity in allogeneic T cells. *Blood* 114, 3235–3243. doi: 10.1182/blood-2008-12-195073

Kakumu, T., Sato, M., Goto, D., Kato, T., Yogo, N., Hase, T., et al. (2017). Identification of proteasomal catalytic subunit PSMA6 as a therapeutic target for lung cancer. *Cancer Sci.* 108, 732–743. doi: 10.1111/cas.13185

Kalaora, S., Lee, J. S., Barnea, E., Levy, R., Greenberg, P., Alon, M., et al. (2020). Immunoproteasome expression is associated with better prognosis and response to checkpoint therapies in melanoma. *Nat. Commun.* 11:896. doi: 10.1038/s41467-020-14639-9

Kasahara, T., Hooks, J. J., Dougherty, S. F., and Oppenheim, J. J. (1983). Interleukin 2-mediated immune interferon (IFN-gamma) production by human T cells and T cell subsets. *J. Immunol.* 130, 1784–1789.

Kasprzak, A., and Adamek, A. (2019). Insulin-like growth factor 2 (IGF2) signaling in colorectal cancer-from basic research to potential clinical applications. *Int. J. Mol. Sci.* 20:4915. doi: 10.3390/ijms20194915

Kaufman, H. L., Russell, J., Hamid, O., Bhatia, S., Terheyden, P., D'Angelo, S. P., et al. (2016). Avelumab in patients with chemotherapy-refractory metastatic Merkel cell carcinoma: a multicentre, single-group, open-label, phase 2 trial. *Lancet Oncol.* 17, 1374–1385. doi: 10.1016/S1470-2045(16)30364-3

Kim, H. G., Kim, J. Y., Han, E. H., Hwang, Y. P., Choi, J. H., Park, B. H., et al. (2011). Metallothionein-2A overexpression increases the expression of matrix metalloproteinase-9 and invasion of breast cancer cells. *FEBS Lett.* 585, 421–428. doi: 10.1016/j.febslet.2010.12.030

Kito, K., Yeh, E. T., and Kamitani, T. (2001). NUB1, a NEDD8-interacting protein, is induced by interferon and down-regulates the NEDD8 expression. *J. Biol. Chem.* 276, 20603–20609. doi: 10.1074/jbc.M100920200

Kodigepalli, K. M., Li, M., Liu, S.-L., and Wu, L. (2017). Exogenous expression of SAMHD1 inhibits proliferation and induces apoptosis in cutaneous T-cell lymphoma-derived HuT78 cells. *Cell Cycle* 16, 179–188. doi: 10.1080/15384101. 2016.1261226

Kotowski, U., Erović, B. M., Schnöll, J., Stanek, V., Janik, S., Steurer, M., et al. (2019). Quantitative proteome analysis of Merkel cell carcinoma cell lines using SILAC. *Clin. Proteomics* 16:42. doi: 10.1186/s12014-019-9263-z

Krasagakis, K., Krüger-Krasagakis, S., Tzanakakis, G. N., Darivianaki, K., Stathopoulos, E. N., and Tosca, A. D. (2008). Interferon-alpha inhibits proliferation and induces apoptosis of Merkel cell carcinoma in vitro. *Cancer Invest.* 26, 562–568. doi: 10.1080/07357900701816477

Krause, C. D., He, W., Kotenko, S., and Pestka, S. (2006). Modulation of the activation of Stat1 by the interferon-γ receptor complex. *Cell Res.* 16, 113–123. doi: 10.1038/sj.cr.7310015

Kriegsman, B. A., Vangala, P., Chen, B. J., Meraner, P., Brass, A. L., Garber, M., et al. (2019). Frequent Loss of IRF2 in cancers leads to immune evasion through decreased MHC class I antigen presentation and increased PD-L1 expression. *J. Immunol.* 203, 1999–2010. doi: 10.4049/jimmunol.1900475

Kwon, C. H., Park, H. J., Choi, Y. R., Kim, A., Kim, H. W., Choi, J. H., et al. (2016). PSMB8 and PBK as potential gastric cancer subtype-specific biomarkers associated with prognosis. *Oncotarget* 7, 21454–21468. doi: 10. 18632/oncotarget.7411

Läubli, H., Alisson-Silva, F., Stanczak, M. A., Siddiqui, S. S., Deng, L., Verhagen, A., et al. (2014). Lectin galactoside-binding soluble 3 binding protein (LGALS3BP) is a tumor-associated immunomodulatory ligand for CD33-related Siglecs. *J. Biol. Chem.* 289, 33481–33491. doi: 10.1074/jbc.M114.593129

Leger, A., and Leonardi, T. (2019). pycoQC, interactive quality control for Oxford nanopore sequencing. *J. Open Source Softw.* 4:1236.

Leite-De-Moraes, M. C., Moreau, G., Arnould, A., Machavoine, F., Garcia, C., Papiernik, M., et al. (1998). IL-4-producing NK T cells are biased towards IFN-gamma production by IL-12. Influence of the microenvironment on the functional capacities of NK T cells. *Eur. J. Immunol.* 28, 1507–1515. doi: 10.1002/(SICI)1521-4141(199805)28:05<1507::AID-IMMU1507>3.0.CO;2-F

Li, J., Song, Y., Yu, B., and Yu, Y. (2020). TNFAIP2 promotes non-small cell lung cancer cells and targeted by miR-145-5p. *DNA Cell Biol.* 39, 1256–1263. doi: 10.1089/dna.2020.5415

Li, J., Zhang, Z., Wang, L., and Zhang, Y. (2019). The oncogenic role of Wnt10a in colorectal cancer through activation of canonical Wnt/β-catenin signaling. *Oncol. Lett.* 17, 3657–3664. doi: 10.3892/ol.2019.10035

Li, P., Zhang, Q., and Tang, H. (2019). INPP1 up-regulation by miR-27a contributes to the growth, migration and invasion of human cervical cancer. *J. Cell. Mol. Med.* 23, 7709–7716. doi: 10.1111/jcmm.14644

Li, S., Xie, Y., Zhang, W., Gao, J., Wang, M., Zheng, G., et al. (2015). Interferon alpha-inducible protein 27 promotes epithelial-mesenchymal transition and induces ovarian tumorigenicity and stemness. *J. Surg. Res.* 193, 255–264. doi: 10.1016/j.jss.2014.06.055

Li, S. R., Gyselman, V. G., Lalude, O., Dorudi, S., and Bustin, S. A. (2000). Transcription of the inositol polyphosphate 1-phosphatase gene (INPP1) is upregulated in human colorectal cancer. *Mol. Carcinog.* 27, 322–329. doi: 10. 1002/(sici)1098-2744(200004)27:4<322::aid-mc10>3.0.co;2-c

Liberzon, A., Birger, C., Thorvaldsdóttir, H., Ghandi, M., Mesirov, J. P., and Tamayo, P. (2015). The Molecular Signatures Database (MSigDB) hallmark gene set collection. *Cell Syst.* 1, 417–425. doi: 10.1016/j.cels.2015.12.004

Lin, M., Li, Y., Qin, S., Jiao, Y., and Hua, F. (2020). Ubiquitin-like modifier-activating enzyme 7 as a marker for the diagnosis and prognosis of breast cancer. *Oncol. Lett.* 19, 2773–2784. doi: 10.3892/ol.2020.11406

Lin, Y., Cui, C., Su, M., Silbart, L. K., Liu, H., Zhao, J., et al. (2021). Identification of TAPBPL as a novel negative regulator of T-cell function. *EMBO Mol. Med.* 13:e13404. doi: 10.15252/emmm.202013404

Lipnik, K., Naschberger, E., Gonin-Laurent, N., Kodajova, P., Petznek, H., Rungaldier, S., et al. (2010). Interferon gamma-induced human guanylate binding protein 1 inhibits mammary tumor growth in mice. *Mol. Med.* 16, 177–187. doi: 10.2119/molmed.2009.00172

Liu, F., Liu, J., Zhang, J., Shi, J., Gui, L., and Xu, G. (2020). Expression of STAT1 is positively correlated with PD-L1 in human ovarian cancer. *Cancer Biol. Ther.* 21, 963–971. doi: 10.1080/15384047.2020.1824479

Liu, M., Guo, S., and Stiles, J. K. (2011). The emerging role of CXCL10 in cancer (Review). *Oncol. Lett.* 2, 583–589. doi: 10.3892/ol.2011.300

Liu, W., Cao, Y., Guan, Y., and Zheng, C. (2018). BST2 promotes cell proliferation, migration and induces NF-κB activation in gastric cancer. *Biotechnol. Lett.* 40, 1015–1027. doi: 10.1007/s10529-018-2562-z

Liu, W., Kim, G. B., Krump, N. A., Zhou, Y., Riley, J. L., and You, J. (2020). Selective reactivation of STING signaling to target Merkel cell carcinoma. *Proc. Natl. Acad. Sci. U. S. A.* 117:13730. doi: 10.1073/pnas.1919690117

Liu, X., Song, C., Yang, S., Ji, Q., Chen, F., and Li, W. (2020). IFI30 expression is an independent unfavourable prognostic factor in glioma. *J. Cell. Mol. Med.* 24, 12433–12443. doi: 10.1111/jcmm.15758

Liu, Z., Chen, P., Gao, H., Gu, Y., Yang, J., Peng, H., et al. (2014). Ubiquitylation of autophagy receptor optineurin by HACE1 activates selective autophagy for tumor suppression. *Cancer Cell* 26, 106–120. doi: 10.1016/j.ccr.2014.05.015

Liu, Z., Chu, S., Yao, S., Li, Y., Fan, S., Sun, X., et al. (2016). CD74 interacts with CD44 and enhances tumorigenesis and metastasis via RHOA-mediated cofilin phosphorylation in human breast cancer cells. *Oncotarget* 7, 68303–68313. doi: 10.18632/oncotarget.11945

Liu, Z., Gu, S., Lu, T., Wu, K., Li, L., Dong, C., et al. (2020). IFI6 depletion inhibits esophageal squamous cell carcinoma progression through reactive oxygen species accumulation via mitochondrial dysfunction and endoplasmic reticulum stress. *J. Exp. Clin. Cancer Res.* 39:144. doi: 10.1186/s13046-020-01646-3

Liu, Z., Lu, H., Jiang, Z., Pastuszyn, A., and Hu, C. A. (2005). Apolipoprotein l6, a novel proapoptotic Bcl-2 homology 3-only protein, induces mitochondria-mediated apoptosis in cancer cells. *Mol. Cancer Res.* 3, 21–31.

Lo, B. K., Yu, M., Zloty, D., Cowan, B., Shapiro, J., and McElwee, K. J. (2010). CXCR3/ligands are significantly involved in the tumorigenesis of basal cell carcinomas. *Am. J. Pathol.* 176, 2435–2446. doi: 10.2353/ajpath.2010.081059

Lobello, N., Biamonte, F., Pisanu, M. E., Faniello, M. C., Jakopin, Ž, Chiarella, E., et al. (2016). Ferritin heavy chain is a negative regulator of ovarian cancer stem cell expansion and epithelial to mesenchymal transition. *Oncotarget* 7, 62019–62033. doi: 10.18632/oncotarget.11495

Lomonosov, M., Meziane el, K., Ye, H., Nelson, D. E., Randle, S. J., and Laman, H. (2011). Expression of Fbxo7 in haematopoietic progenitor cells cooperates with p53 loss to promote lymphomagenesis. *PLoS One* 6:e21165. doi: 10.1371/journal.pone.0021165

Long, A., Giroux, V., Whelan, K. A., Hamilton, K. E., Tétreault, M.-P., Tanaka, K., et al. (2015). WNT10A promotes an invasive and self-renewing phenotype in esophageal squamous cell carcinoma. *Carcinogenesis* 36, 598–606. doi: 10.1093/carcin/bgv025

Love, M. I., Huber, W., and Anders, S. (2014). Moderated estimation of fold change and dispersion for RNA-seq data with DESeq2. *Genome Biol.* 15:550. doi: 10.1186/s13059-014-0550-8

Luker, K. E., Pica, C. M., Schreiber, R. D., and Piwnica-Worms, D. (2001). Overexpression of IRF9 confers resistance to antimicrotubule agents in breast cancer cells. *Cancer Res.* 61, 6540–6547.

Ma, Y., Wei, Z., Bast, R. C., Wang, Z., Li, Y., Gao, M., et al. (2016). Downregulation of TRIM27 expression inhibits the proliferation of ovarian cancer cells in vitro and in vivo. *Lab. Invest.* 96, 37–48. doi: 10.1038/labinvest.2015.132

Maire, C. L., Mohme, M., Bockmayr, M., Fita, K. D., Riecken, K., Börnigen, D., et al. (2020). Glioma escape signature and clonal development under immune pressure. *J. Clin. Invest.* 130, 5257–5271. doi: 10.1172/JCI138760

Martin, E. M., Gould, V. E., Hoog, A., Rosen, S. T., Radosevich, J. A., and Deftos, L. J. (1991). Parathyroid hormone-related protein, chromogranin A, and calcitonin gene products in the neuroendocrine skin carcinoma cell lines MKL1 and MKL2. *Bone Miner.* 14, 113–120. doi: 10.1016/0169-6009(91)90088-h

Matsushita, H., Hosoi, A., Ueha, S., Abe, J., Fujieda, N., Tomura, M., et al. (2015). Cytotoxic T lymphocytes block tumor growth both by lytic activity and IFNγ-dependent cell-cycle arrest. *Cancer Immunol. Res.* 3, 26–36. doi: 10.1158/2326-6066.CIR-14-0098

Meissl, K., Macho-Maschler, S., Müller, M., and Strobl, B. (2017). The good and the bad faces of STAT1 in solid tumours. *Cytokine* 89, 12–20. doi: 10.1016/j.cyto.2015.11.011

Mojic, M., Takeda, K., and Hayakawa, Y. (2017). The dark side of IFN-γ: its role in promoting cancer immunoevasion. *Int. J. Mol. Sci.* 19:89. doi: 10.3390/ijms19010089

Mustafa, D. A. M., Pedrosa, R., Smid, M., van der Weiden, M., de Weerd, V., Nigg, A. L., et al. (2018). T lymphocytes facilitate brain metastasis of breast cancer by inducing guanylate-binding protein 1 expression. *Acta Neuropathol.* 135, 581–599. doi: 10.1007/s00401-018-1806-2

Nghiem, P. T., Bhatia, S., Lipson, E. J., Kudchadkar, R. R., Miller, N. J., Annamalai, L., et al. (2016). PD-1 blockade with pembrolizumab in advanced Merkel-cell carcinoma. *N. Engl. J. Med.* 374, 2542–2552. doi: 10.1056/NEJMoa1603702

Niess, H., Camaj, P., Mair, R., Renner, A., Zhao, Y., Jäckel, C., et al. (2015). Overexpression of IFN-induced protein with tetratricopeptide repeats 3 (IFIT3) in pancreatic cancer cellular "pseudoinflammation" contributing to an aggressive phenotype. *Oncotarget* 6, 3306–3318. doi: 10.18632/oncotarget.2494

Niu, Y., Tang, D., Fan, L., Gao, W., and Lin, H. (2020). CCL25 promotes the migration and invasion of non-small cell lung cancer cells by regulating VEGF and MMPs in a CCR9-dependent manner. *Exp. Ther. Med.* 19, 3571–3580. doi: 10.3892/etm.2020.8635

Ohsugi, T., Yamaguchi, K., Zhu, C., Ikenoue, T., and Furukawa, Y. (2017). Decreased expression of interferon-induced protein 2 (IFIT2) by Wnt/β-catenin signaling confers anti-apoptotic properties to colorectal cancer cells. *Oncotarget* 8, 100176–100186. doi: 10.18632/oncotarget.22122

Owusu, B. Y., Galemmo, R., Janetka, J., and Klampfer, L. (2017). Hepatocyte growth factor, a key tumor-promoting factor in the tumor microenvironment. *Cancers* 9:35. doi: 10.3390/cancers9040035

Pan, Y., Huang, J., Xing, R., Yin, X., Cui, J., Li, W., et al. (2013). Metallothionein 2A inhibits NF-κB pathway activation and predicts clinical outcome segregated with TNM stage in gastric cancer patients following radical resection. *J. Transl. Med.* 11:173. doi: 10.1186/1479-5876-11-173

Paulson, K. G., Park, S. Y., Vandeven, N. A., Lachance, K., Thomas, H., Chapuis, A. G., et al. (2018). Merkel cell carcinoma: current US incidence and projected increases based on changing demographics. *J. Am. Acad. Dermatol.* 78, 457–463.e2. doi: 10.1016/j.jaad.2017.10.028

Paulson, K. G., Tegeder, A., Willmes, C., Iyer, J. G., Afanasiev, O. K., Schrama, D., et al. (2014). Downregulation of MHC-I expression is prevalent but reversible in Merkel cell carcinoma. *Cancer Immunol. Res.* 2, 1071–1079. doi: 10.1158/2326-6066.CIR-14-0005

Payne, A., Holmes, N., Rakyan, V., and Loose, M. (2019). BulkVis: a graphical viewer for Oxford nanopore bulk FAST5 files. *Bioinformatics* 35, 2193–2198. doi: 10.1093/bioinformatics/bty841

Pflügler, S., Svinka, J., Scharf, I., Crncec, I., Filipits, M., Charoentong, P., et al. (2020). IDO1+ Paneth cells promote immune escape of colorectal cancer. *Commun. Biol.* 3:252. doi: 10.1038/s42003-020-0989-y

Pidugu, V. K., Wu, M.-M., Yen, A.-H., Pidugu, H. B., Chang, K.-W., Liu, C.-J., et al. (2019). IFIT1 and IFIT3 promote oral squamous cell carcinoma metastasis and contribute to the anti-tumor effect of gefitinib via enhancing p-EGFR recycling. *Oncogene* 38, 3232–3247. doi: 10.1038/s41388-018-0662-9

Pol, J. G., Le Naour, J., and Kroemer, G. (2020). FLT3LG – a biomarker reflecting clinical responses to the immunogenic cell death inducer oxaliplatin. *Oncoimmunology* 9, 1755214–1755214. doi: 10.1080/2162402X.2020.1755214

Quick, J., Loman, N. J., Duraffour, S., Simpson, J. T., Severi, E., Cowley, L., et al. (2016). Real-time, portable genome sequencing for Ebola surveillance. *Nature* 530, 228–232. doi: 10.1038/nature16996

Rea, A., Palmieri, G., Tinari, N., Natoli, C., Tagliaferri, P., Morabito, A., et al. (1994). 90k is a serum marker of poor-prognosis in non-hodgkins-lymphoma patients. *Oncol. Rep.* 1, 723–725. doi: 10.3892/or.1.4.723

Ritter, C., Fan, K., Paschen, A., Reker Hardrup, S., Ferrone, S., Nghiem, P., et al. (2017). Epigenetic priming restores the HLA class-I antigen processing machinery expression in Merkel cell carcinoma. *Sci. Rep.* 7:2290. doi: 10.1038/s41598-017-02608-0

Robinson, J., Barker, D. J., Georgiou, X., Cooper, M. A., Flicek, P., and Marsh, S. G. E. (2019). IPD-IMGT/HLA database. *Nucleic Acids Res.* 48, D948–D955.

Rosen, S. T., Gould, V. E., Salwen, H. R., Herst, C. V., Le Beau, M. M., Lee, I., et al. (1987). Establishment and characterization of a neuroendocrine skin carcinoma cell line. *Lab. Invest.* 56, 302–312.

Rouette, A., Trofimov, A., Haberl, D., Boucher, G., Lavallée, V.-P., D'Angelo, G., et al. (2016). Expression of immunoproteasome genes is regulated by cell-intrinsic and -extrinsic factors in human cancers. *Sci. Rep.* 6:34019. doi: 10.1038/srep34019

Sánchez-Martín, D. S., Martínez-Torrecuadrada, J., Teesalu, T., Sugahara, K. N., Alvarez-Cienfuegos, A., Ximénez-Embún, P., et al. (2013). Proteasome activator complex PA28 identified as an accessible target in prostate cancer by in vivo selection of human antibodies. *Proc. Natl. Acad. Sci. U. S. A.* 110, 13791–13796. doi: 10.1073/pnas.1300013110

Sergushichev, A. A. (2016). An algorithm for fast preranked gene set enrichment analysis using cumulative statistic calculation. *bioRxiv* [Preprint]. doi: 10.1101/060012

Shao, L., Hou, W., Scharping, N. E., Vendetti, F. P., Srivastava, R., Roy, C. N., et al. (2019). IRF1 inhibits antitumor immunity through the upregulation of PD-L1 in the tumor cell. *Cancer Immunol. Res.* 7, 1258–1266. doi: 10.1158/2326-6066.CIR-18-0711

Shao, Q., Byrum, S. D., Moreland, L. E., Mackintosh, S. G., Kannan, A., Lin, Z., et al. (2013). A proteomic study of human Merkel cell carcinoma. *J. Proteomics Bioinform.* 6, 275–282. doi: 10.4172/jpb.1000291

Shoji, T., Kikuchi, E., Kikuchi, J., Takashima, Y., Furuta, M., Takahashi, H., et al. (2020). Evaluating the immunoproteasome as a potential therapeutic target in cisplatin-resistant small cell and non-small cell lung cancer. *Cancer Chemother. Pharmacol.* 85, 843–853. doi: 10.1007/s00280-020-04061-9

Shuda, M., Feng, H., Kwun, H. J., Rosen, S. T., Gjoerup, O., Moore, P. S., et al. (2008). T antigen mutations are a human tumor-specific signature for Merkel cell polyomavirus. *Proc. Natl. Acad. Sci. U. S. A.* 105, 16272–16277. doi: 10.1073/pnas.0806526105

Soler, C., Felipe, A., García-Manteiga, J., Serra, M., Guillén-Gómez, E., Casado, F. J., et al. (2003). Interferon-gamma regulates nucleoside transport systems in macrophages through signal transduction and activator of transduction factor 1 (STAT1)-dependent and -independent signalling pathways. *Biochem. J.* 375, 777–783. doi: 10.1042/BJ20030260

Spranger, S., Spaapen, R. M., Zha, Y., Williams, J., Meng, Y., Ha, T. T., et al. (2013). Up-regulation of PD-L1, IDO, and T(regs) in the melanoma tumor microenvironment is driven by CD8(+) T cells. *Sci. Transl. Med.* 5:200ra116. doi: 10.1126/scitranslmed.3006504

Starrett, G. J., Marcelus, C., Cantalupo, P. G., Katz, J. P., Cheng, J., Akagi, K., et al. (2017). Merkel cell polyomavirus exhibits dominant control of the tumor genome and transcriptome in virus-associated Merkel cell carcinoma. *mBio* 8:e02079-16. doi: 10.1128/mBio.02079-16

Steinbach, A., Winter, J., Reuschenbach, M., Blatnik, R., Klevenz, A., Bertrand, M., et al. (2017). ERAP1 overexpression in HPV-induced malignancies: a possible novel immune evasion mechanism. *Oncoimmunology* 6, e1336594. doi: 10.1080/2162402X.2017.1336594

Stratikos, E. (2014). Modulating antigen processing for cancer immunotherapy. *Oncoimmunology* 3:e27568. doi: 10.4161/onci.27568

Subramanian, A., Tamayo, P., Mootha, V. K., Mukherjee, S., Ebert, B. L., Gillette, M. A., et al. (2005). Gene set enrichment analysis: a knowledge-based approach for interpreting genome-wide expression profiles. *Proc. Natl. Acad. Sci. U. S. A.* 102, 15545–15550. doi: 10.1073/pnas.0506580102

Sum, E. Y. M., Segara, D., Duscio, B., Bath, M. L., Field, A. S., Sutherland, R. L., et al. (2005). Overexpression of LMO4 induces mammary hyperplasia, promotes cell invasion, and is a predictor of poor outcome in breast cancer. *Proc. Natl. Acad. Sci. U. S. A.* 102, 7659–7664. doi: 10.1073/pnas.0502990102

Takata, H., Kudo, M., Yamamoto, T., Ueda, J., Ishino, K., Peng, W. X., et al. (2016). Increased expression of PDIA3 and its association with cancer cell proliferation and poor prognosis in hepatocellular carcinoma. *Oncol. Lett.* 12, 4896–4904. doi: 10.3892/ol.2016.5304

Tan, Y., Zhou, G., Wang, X., Chen, W., and Gao, H. (2018). USP18 promotes breast cancer growth by upregulating EGFR and activating the AKT/Skp2 pathway. *Int. J. Oncol.* 53, 371–383. doi: 10.3892/ijo.2018.4387

Tian, S.-Y., Chen, S.-H., Shao, B.-F., Cai, H.-Y., Zhou, Y., Zhou, Y.-L., et al. (2014). Expression of leucine aminopeptidase 3 (LAP3) correlates with prognosis and malignant development of human hepatocellular carcinoma (HCC). *Int. J. Clin. Exp. Pathol.* 7, 3752–3762.

Wan, Q., Qu, J., Li, L., and Gao, F. (2021). Guanylate-binding protein 1 correlates with advanced tumor features, and serves as a prognostic biomarker for worse survival in lung adenocarcinoma patients. *J. Clin. Lab. Anal.* 35:e23610. doi: 10.1002/jcla.23610

Wang, B., Li, D., Rodriguez-Juarez, R., Farfus, A., Storozynsky, Q., Malach, M., et al. (2018). A suppressive role of guanine nucleotide-binding protein subunit beta-4 inhibited by DNA methylation in the growth of anti-estrogen resistant breast cancer cells. *BMC Cancer* 18:817. doi: 10.1186/s12885-018-4711-0

Wang, H., Qiu, X., Lin, S., Chen, X., Wang, T., and Liao, T. (2018). Knockdown of IFI27 inhibits cell proliferation and invasion in oral squamous cell carcinoma. *World J. Surg. Oncol.* 16:64. doi: 10.1186/s12957-018-1371-0

Wang, J., Zou, K., Feng, X., Chen, M., Li, C., Tang, R., et al. (2017). Downregulation of NMI promotes tumor growth and predicts poor prognosis in human lung adenocarcinomas. *Mol. Cancer* 16:158. doi: 10.1186/s12943-017-0705-9

Wang, J. L., Lu, F. Z., Shen, X. Y., Wu, Y., and Zhao, L. T. (2014). SAMHD1 is down regulated in lung cancer by methylation and inhibits tumor cell proliferation. *Biochem. Biophys. Res. Commun.* 455, 229–233. doi: 10.1016/j.bbrc.2014.10.153

Wang, M., Hu, Y., and Stearns, M. E. (2009). RPS2: a novel therapeutic target in prostate cancer. *J. Exp. Clin. Cancer Res.* 28:6. doi: 10.1186/1756-9966-28-6

Wang, Q., Pan, F., Li, S., Huang, R., Wang, X., Wang, S., et al. (2019). The prognostic value of the proteasome activator subunit gene family in skin cutaneous melanoma. *J. Cancer* 10, 2205–2219. doi: 10.7150/jca.30612

Wang, W., Wu, S., Guo, M., and He, J. (2016). LMO4 is a prognostic marker involved in cell migration and invasion in non-small-cell lung cancer. *J. Thorac. Dis.* 8, 3682–3690. doi: 10.21037/jtd.2016.12.22

Wang, X., Ye, M., Wu, M., Fang, H., Xiao, B., Xie, L., et al. (2020). RNF213 suppresses carcinogenesis in glioblastoma by affecting MAPK/JNK signaling pathway. *Clin. Transl. Oncol.* 22, 1506–1516. doi: 10.1007/s12094-020-02286-x

Wang, Y., Wang, H., Pan, T., Li, L., Li, J., and Yang, H. (2016). Overexpression of PHRF1 attenuates the proliferation and tumorigenicity of non-small cell lung cancer cells. *Oncotarget* 7, 64360–64370. doi: 10.18632/oncotarget.11842

Wardhani, L. O., Matsushita, M., Iwasaki, T., Kuwamoto, S., Nonaka, D., Nagata, K., et al. (2019). Expression of the IDO1/TDO2-AhR pathway in tumor cells or the tumor microenvironment is associated with Merkel cell polyomavirus status and prognosis in Merkel cell carcinoma. *Hum. Pathol.* 84, 52–61. doi: 10.1016/j.humpath.2018.09.003

Wen, H., Chen, Y., Hu, Z., Mo, Q., Tang, J., and Sun, C. (2014). Decreased expression of BATF2 is significantly associated with poor prognosis in oral tongue squamous cell carcinoma. *Oncol. Rep.* 31, 169–174. doi: 10.3892/or.2013.2863

Whitehead, C. M., Nelson, R., Hudson, R., Gore, M., Marcelpoil, R., Morel, D., et al. (2005). Overexpression of the PSMB9 component of the proteasome in early stage, node negative breast cancer is prognostic for an increased risk of early relapse or death. *Cancer Res.* 65, 740–740.

Wildi, S., Kleeff, J., Maruyama, H., Maurer, C. A., Friess, H., Büchler, M. W., et al. (1999). Characterization of cytokeratin 20 expression in pancreatic and colorectal cancer. *Clin. Cancer Res.* 5, 2840–2847.

Willmes, C., Adam, C., Alb, M., Völkert, L., Houben, R., Becker, J. C., et al. (2012). Type I and II IFNs inhibit Merkel cell carcinoma via modulation of the Merkel cell polyomavirus T antigens. *Cancer Res.* 72, 2120–2128. doi: 10.1158/0008-5472.CAN-11-2651

Workman, R. E., Tang, A. D., Tang, P. S., Jain, M., Tyson, J. R., Razaghi, R., et al. (2019). Nanopore native RNA sequencing of a human poly(A) transcriptome. *Nat. Methods* 16, 1297–1305.

Wu, D.-j, Jiang, Y.-s, He, R.-z., Tao, L.-y., Yang, M.-w., Fu, X.-l., et al. (2018). High expression of WNT7A predicts poor prognosis and promote tumor metastasis in pancreatic ductal adenocarcinoma. *Sci. Rep.* 8:15792. doi: 10.1038/s41598-018-34094-3

Xing, L., Tang, X., Wu, K., Huang, X., Yi, Y., and Huan, J. (2020). TRIM27 functions as a novel oncogene in non-triple-negative breast cancer by blocking cellular senescence through p21 ubiquitination. *Mol. Ther. Nucleic Acids* 22, 910–923. doi: 10.1016/j.omtn.2020.10.012

Yan, J., Jiang, Y., Lu, J., Wu, J., and Zhang, M. (2019). Inhibiting of proliferation, migration, and invasion in lung cancer induced by silencing interferon-induced transmembrane protein 1 (IFITM1). *Biomed. Res. Int.* 2019:9085435. doi: 10.1155/2019/9085435

Yang, R. K., Qing, Y., Jelloul, F. Z., Routbort, M. J., Wang, P., Shaw, K., et al. (2020). Identification of biomarkers of immune checkpoint blockade efficacy in recurrent or refractory solid tumor malignancies. *Oncotarget* 11, 600–618. doi: 10.18632/oncotarget.27466

Yang, Z., Zhuang, L., Yu, Y., Zhou, W., Lu, Y., Xu, Q., et al. (2015). Overexpression of APOBEC3F in tumor tissues is potentially predictive for poor recurrence-free survival from HBV-related hepatocellular carcinoma. *Discov. Med.* 20, 349–356.

Yao, N., Chen, Q., Shi, W., Tang, L., and Fu, Y. (2019). PARP14 promotes the proliferation and gemcitabine chemoresistance of pancreatic cancer cells through activation of NF-κB pathway. *Mol. Carcinog.* 58, 1291–1302. doi: 10.1002/mc.23011

Yen, M. C., Kan, J. Y., Hsieh, C. J., Kuo, P. L., Hou, M. F., and Hsu, Y. L. (2017). Association of long-chain acyl-coenzyme A synthetase 5 expression in human breast cancer by estrogen receptor status and its clinical significance. *Oncol. Rep.* 37, 3253–3260. doi: 10.3892/or.2017.5610

Yoo, H., Park, S. H., Ye, S. K., and Kim, M. (2011). IFN-γ-induced BST2 mediates monocyte adhesion to human endothelial cells. *Cell. Immunol.* 267, 23–29. doi: 10.1016/j.cellimm.2010.10.011

Yoshihama, S., Cho, S. X., Yeung, J., Pan, X., Lizee, G., Konganti, K., et al. (2021). NLRC5/CITA expression correlates with efficient response to checkpoint blockade immunotherapy. *Sci. Rep.* 11:3258. doi: 10.1038/s41598-021-82729-9

Yoshihama, S., Vijayan, S., Sidiq, T., and Kobayashi, K. S. (2017). NLRC5/CITA: a key player in cancer immune surveillance. *Trends Cancer* 3, 28–38. doi: 10.1016/j.trecan.2016.12.003

Yoshioka, S., King, M. L., Ran, S., Okuda, H., MacLean, J. A. II, McAsey, M. E., et al. (2012). WNT7A regulates tumor growth and progression in ovarian cancer through the WNT/β-catenin pathway. *Mol. Cancer Res.* 10, 469–482. doi: 10.1158/1541-7786.MCR-11-0177

Yu, F., Xie, D., Ng, S. S., Lum, C. T., Cai, M.-Y., Cheung, W. K., et al. (2015). IFITM1 promotes the metastasis of human colorectal cancer via CAV-1. *Cancer Lett.* 368, 135–143. doi: 10.1016/j.canlet.2015.07.034

Yu, J., Wei, M., Becknell, B., Trotta, R., Liu, S., Boyd, Z., et al. (2006). Pro- and antiinflammatory cytokine signaling: reciprocal antagonism regulates interferon-gamma production by human natural killer cells. *Immunity* 24, 575–590. doi: 10.1016/j.immuni.2006.03.016

Zeiner, P. S., Zinke, J., Kowalewski, D. J., Bernatz, S., Tichy, J., Ronellenfitsch, M. W., et al. (2018). CD74 regulates complexity of tumor cell HLA class II peptidome in brain metastasis and is a positive prognostic marker for patient survival. *Acta Neuropathol. Commun.* 6:18. doi: 10.1186/s40478-018-0521-5

Zhang, D., Wu, P., Zhang, Z., An, W., Zhang, C., Pan, S., et al. (2020). Overexpression of negative regulator of ubiquitin-like proteins 1 (NUB1) inhibits proliferation and invasion of gastric cancer cells through upregulation of p27Kip1 and inhibition of epithelial-mesenchymal transition. *Pathol. Res. Pract.* 216:153002. doi: 10.1016/j.prp.2020.153002

Zhang, H., Cui, B., Zhou, Y., Wang, X., Wu, W., Wang, Z., et al. (2021). B2M overexpression correlates with malignancy and immune signatures in human gliomas. *Sci. Rep.* 11:5045. doi: 10.1038/s41598-021-84465-6

Zhang, H., Zhou, Y., Cheng, Q., Dai, Z., Wang, Z., Liu, F., et al. (2020). PDIA3 correlates with clinical malignant features and immune signature in human gliomas. *Aging (Albany NY)* 12, 15392–15413. doi: 10.18632/aging.103601

Zhang, J., Wang, F., Liu, F., and Xu, G. (2020). Predicting STAT1 as a prognostic marker in patients with solid cancer. *Ther. Adv. Med. Oncol.* 12:1758835920917558. doi: 10.1177/1758835920917558

Zhang, J.-F., Hua, R., Liu, D.-J., Liu, W., Huo, Y.-M., and Sun, Y.-W. (2014). Effect of CD74 on the prognosis of patients with resectable pancreatic cancer. *Hepatobiliary Pancreat. Dis. Int.* 13, 81–86. doi: 10.1016/s1499-3872(14)60011-4

Zhang, Y., Feng, Y., Ji, D., Wang, Q., Qian, W., Wang, S., et al. (2018). TRIM27 functions as an oncogene by activating epithelial-mesenchymal transition and p-AKT in colorectal cancer. *Int. J. Oncol.* 53, 620–632. doi: 10.3892/ijo.2018.4408

Zhang, Z., Sun, T., Chen, Y., Gong, S., Sun, X., Zou, F., et al. (2016). CCL25/CCR9 signal promotes migration and invasion in hepatocellular and breast cancer cell lines. *DNA Cell Biol.* 35, 348–357. doi: 10.1089/dna.2015.3104

Zhao, J., Dong, Q.-Z., Zhong, F., Cai, L.-L., Qin, Z.-Y., Liu, Y., et al. (2017). NMI promotes hepatocellular carcinoma progression via BDKRB2 and MAPK/ERK pathway. *Oncotarget* 8, 12174–12185. doi: 10.18632/oncotarget.14556

Zheng, D. L., Huang, Q. L., Zhou, F., Huang, Q. J., Lin, J. Y., and Lin, X. (2012). PA28β regulates cell invasion of gastric cancer via modulating the expression of chloride intracellular channel 1. *J. Cell. Biochem.* 113, 1537–1546. doi: 10.1002/jcb.24022

Zhou, M.-J., Chen, F.-Z., Chen, H.-C., Wan, X.-X., Zhou, X., Fang, Q., et al. (2017). ISG15 inhibits cancer cell growth and promotes apoptosis. *Int. J. Mol. Med.* 39, 446–452. doi: 10.3892/ijmm.2016.2845

Zhou, T., Damsky, W., Weizman, O.-E., McGeary, M. K., Hartmann, K. P., Rosen, C. E., et al. (2020). IL-18BP is a secreted immune checkpoint and barrier to IL-18 immunotherapy. *Nature* 583, 609–614. doi: 10.1038/s41586-020-2422-6

17

Epidermodysplasia Verruciformis: Inborn Errors of Immunity to Human Beta-Papillomaviruses

Sarah J. de Jong[1], Elias Imahorn[2], Peter Itin[2,3], Jouni Uitto[4,5], Gérard Orth[6], Emmanuelle Jouanguy[1,7,8], Jean-Laurent Casanova[1,7,8,9,10] and Bettina Burger[2]*

[1] St. Giles Laboratory of Human Genetics of Infectious Diseases, Rockefeller Branch, The Rockefeller University, New York, NY, United States, [2] Department of Biomedicine, University Hospital of Basel, University of Basel, Basel, Switzerland, [3] Department of Dermatology, University Hospital of Basel, Basel, Switzerland, [4] Department of Dermatology and Cutaneous Biology, Sidney Kimmel Medical College, Thomas Jefferson University, Philadelphia, PA, United States, [5] Jefferson Institute of Molecular Medicine, Thomas Jefferson University, Philadelphia, PA, United States, [6] Pasteur Institute, Paris, France, [7] INSERM UMR 1163, Laboratory of Human Genetics of Infectious Diseases, Necker Branch, Necker Hospital for Sick Children, Paris, France, [8] Imagine Institute, Paris Descartes University, Paris, France, [9] Pediatric Hematology and Immunology Unit, Necker Hospital for Sick Children, Paris, France, [10] Howard Hughes Medical Institute, New York, NY, United States

***Correspondence:**
Jean-Laurent Casanova
casanova@rockefeller.edu;
jean-laurent.casanova@mail.rockefeller.edu

Epidermodysplasia verruciformis (EV) is an autosomal recessive skin disorder with a phenotype conditional on human beta-papillomavirus (beta-HPV) infection. Such infections are common and asymptomatic in the general population, but in individuals with EV, they lead to the development of plane wart-like and red or brownish papules or pityriasis versicolor-like skin lesions, from childhood onwards. Most patients develop non-melanoma skin cancer (NMSC), mostly on areas of UV-exposed skin, from the twenties or thirties onwards. At least half of the cases of typical EV are caused by biallelic loss-of-function mutations of *TMC6/EVER1* or *TMC8/EVER2*. The cellular and molecular basis of disease in TMC/EVER-deficient patients is unknown, but a defect of keratinocyte-intrinsic immunity to beta-HPV is suspected. Indeed, these patients are not susceptible to other infectious diseases and have apparently normal leukocyte development. In contrast, patients with an atypical form of EV due to inborn errors of T-cell immunity invariably develop clinical symptoms of EV in the context of other infectious diseases. The features of the typical and atypical forms of EV thus suggest that the control of beta-HPV infections requires both EVER1/EVER2-dependent keratinocyte-intrinsic immunity and T cell-dependent adaptive immunity.

Keywords: epidermodysplasia verruciformis, beta-HPV, TMC/EVER, non-melanoma skin cancer, primary immunodeficiency

INTRODUCTION

Epidermodysplasia verruciformis (EV) is a rare skin disease characterized by persistent disseminated flat warts and pityriasis versicolor-like lesions, associated with a high risk of non-melanoma skin cancer (NMSC). About 501 patients have been reported worldwide (Burger and Itin, 2014; Imahorn et al., 2017). EV was first described in Lewandowsky and Lutz (1922) as a congenital skin disease. The observation of parental consanguinity and familial cases led to the suggestion that EV might be a genetic disease with autosomal recessive inheritance

(Cockayne, 1933; Rajagopalan et al., 1972). This notion was not confirmed until 70 years later, when inactivating mutations of the *EVER1/TMC6* and *EVER2/TMC8* genes accounting for about 50% of all known cases of EV were identified (Ramoz et al., 2002; Orth, 2006, 2008; Imahorn et al., 2017). Auto- and heteroinoculation experiments performed from 1946 onward showed that the phenotype of EV was dependent on a viral infection (Lutz, 1946; Jablonska and Milewski, 1957). Viral particles were then detected in EV lesions (Ruiter and van Mullem, 1966; Jablonska et al., 1968), and, subsequently, EV-specific human papillomaviruses (HPVs) were identified, some of which, such as HPV-5 in particular, were shown to be associated with the cancers observed in EV patients (reviewed in Orth et al., 1980; Orth, 2006). EV thus results from a genetically determined susceptibility to specific skin-tropic HPVs (Orth, 2006, 2008; Imahorn et al., 2017). These viruses belong to the beta-genus, and are almost ubiquitous and apparently benign in the general population. EV patients are not prone to other viral, bacterial, or fungal infections. NMSC is the only type of cancer presenting a higher incidence in these patients than in the general population (Orth, 2006, 2008). The EVER1 and EVER2 proteins are thought to govern keratinocyte-intrinsic immunity to beta-HPVs. However, patients with cutaneous clinical symptoms of beta-HPV infection and other infectious manifestations caused by profound T-cell defects have been reported. This clinical picture is referred to as "atypical EV." The cumulative findings of almost a century of studies of typical and atypical EV suggest that both keratinocytes and T cells are required for the control of beta-HPVs. We review here the various facets of EV.

CLINICAL MANIFESTATIONS AND HISTOPATHOLOGY OF EV

EV manifests as multiple polymorphic skin lesions, which begin to appear during infancy or early childhood and persist throughout the individual's life. Flat-topped papular lesions resembling verrucae planae typically develop on the extremities. The lesions may also present as red or red-brownish papules or pityriasis versicolor-like lesions, mostly on the trunk, neck, and face (Lewandowsky and Lutz, 1922). In addition, verruca-like papillomatous or seborrheic keratosis-like lesions may develop. The frequency of verruca vulgaris is no higher in these patients than in the general population. In many patients, isomorphic lesions develop preferentially at sites of traumas (the Koebner phenomenon) (de Oliveira et al., 2003). Some patients have persistent palmar lesions similar to palmar pits and dermatoscopically consistent with plane warts (Imahorn et al., 2017). Over the course of the patient's lifetime, the phenotype of a particular skin area may change, and lesions may progress to NMSC. There is currently no cure for EV. The development of EV lesions cannot be prevented, but frequent examinations of skin lesions that might develop into skin cancers and appropriate treatment of these lesions are recommended, such as surgical removal and cryotherapy. Patients with typical EV are otherwise healthy and are not particularly susceptible to any other unusually severe infectious diseases. Provided that cancers are treated appropriately, life expectancy is similar to that in the general population; multifocal carcinomas might, however, be fatal if untreated. Histological examinations of lesions typically reveal hyperkeratosis and parakeratosis, mild acanthosis, and the presence of koilocytes, keratinocytes with pale-stained cytoplasm in the upper epidermis associated with high levels of intranuclear viral replication. On hematoxylin-eosin staining, the cytoplasm of the affected cells stains pale blue (so-called "blue cells") and numerous round basophilic keratohyalin granules are visible. This histological finding is pathognomonic for infections with HPV (Orth, 2006). Possible immune infiltration has not been comprehensively characterized in EV lesions. A number of atypical EV cases have been reported, which will be reviewed below.

CLINICAL MANIFESTATIONS OF ATYPICAL EV

Patients with atypical EV have a broader clinical phenotype than those with typical EV. The phenotype of EV, as described above, is undistinguishable between patients with typical and atypical forms. Indeed, the skin lesions develop early in life and are caused by the same beta-HPV subtypes that are found in patients with typical EV (see **Table 1**) The other clinical phenotypes, mostly infectious and auto-immune, differ between patients (Crequer et al., 2012a,b; Sanal et al., 2012; Stray-Pedersen et al., 2014; Stepensky et al., 2015; Li et al., 2016; Platt et al., 2017; Tahiat et al., 2017). The clinical features of patients with atypical EV are reviewed in **Table 1**. Some patients have growth retardation or mild developmental delay. Others present auto-immune features, which may be clinically overt and affect various tissues and organs, or covert, with detectable auto-antibodies but no clinical signs. Bacterial infections, including skin abscesses, pneumonia, and ear infections, are frequent. Infections with cutaneous herpes viruses, molluscum, mucocutaneous candidiasis, and non-beta-HPV infections have also been documented. Moreover, some patients display recurrent respiratory and gastrointestinal infections. Cancers, such as Burkitt lymphoma and EBV-lymphoma, have been reported in some patients. Finally, a few patients have been reported to display clinical manifestations of beta- and alpha-HPV co-infections in different lesions (Azzimonti et al., 2005; Borgogna et al., 2014; Landini et al., 2014). These patients display cutaneous alpha- and beta-HPV- (Borgogna et al., 2014) or genital (Landini et al., 2014) alpha-HPV-driven infections, but no broad susceptibility to infections. These cases suggest that covert immunological abnormalities might favor the development of beta- and alpha-HPV-induced cutaneous and mucosal lesions in other individuals. Based on these clinical observations, the molecular and cellular basis of typical and atypical EV phenotype appear to be different. The typical EV phenotype is, in itself, suggestive of a keratinocyte-intrinsic defect, whereas the atypical EV phenotype, with its myriad of infections and auto-immune features, is more consistent with an adaptive T-cell defect.

TABLE 1 | Immunological parameters of patients with typical and atypical EV.

Disease	Genetic etiology*	Clinical phenotypes (affected/total no. of patients)	Expression pattern	T cell counts	T cell function	Other immunological features	Reference
Typical EV	AR TMC6/EVER1	EV	Broad (including keratinocytes and T cells)	Normal	Normal	None	Orth, 2006, 2008; Imahorn et al., 2017
	AR TMC8/EVER2	EV	Broad (including keratinocytes and T cells)	Normal with slightly high proportions for skin-homing subsets	Normal	None	
Atypical EV	AR RHOH deficiency (2 siblings)	Cutaneous viral infections, bronchopulmonary disease, Burkitt lymphoma, **disseminated EV-like flat warts (histologically consistent with EV, HPV-3, -12, and -20 on Southern blotting and PCR)**	Lymphoid lineage	Naïve CD4+ T-cell lymphopenia, high memory CD4+ and CD8+ T-cell counts, low proportions of skin-homing T-cell subsets	Mildly impaired antigen-induced T-cell proliferation, no anti-CD3-induced proliferation	Normal B cell number and function, normal NK cells	Crequer et al., 2012a
	AR MST1 deficiency # (1 patient)	Recurrent respiratory infections, candidiasis, **disseminated EV-like flat warts (HPV-5 and -15 positive by Southern blotting and PCR)**, cervical adenopathy, growth retardation	Broad (including keratinocytes and T cells)	Profound CD4+ T-cell lymphopenia (naïve low, memory high), modest naïve and central memory CD8+ lymphopenia, revertant memory CD8+ T-cell counts high	Impaired mitogen (PHA, PMA/Ionomycin)- and antigen (candida, tetanus toxoid, tuberculin)-induced proliferation	Normal B and NK cells, cANCA autoantibodies, high IgA and IgE levels, poor antibody response to several vaccines	Crequer et al., 2012b
	AR CORO1A deficiency # (2 siblings)	Bronchiectasis; fatal EBV-positive lymphoma (1/2); mucocutaneous immunodeficiency syndrome with molluscum contagiosum, oral-cutaneous herpetic (HSV-1) ulcers, **disseminated EV-like HPV infection (HPV-5 and -17 positive by PCR)** and tuberculoid leprosy (1/2)	Broad (including keratinocytes and T cells)	Complete deficiency of naïve CD4+ T cells, high level of double-negative (CD3+CD4-CD8-) gd T cells	Impaired mitogen-induced proliferation, normal antigen-induced proliferation (candida and tetanus toxoid)	T-B+NK+ SCID; absent memory B cells; low NK cell counts, elevated serum IgE, normal serum IgG	Stray-Pedersen et al., 2014
	AR ARTEMIS # p.Leu123Ser (hypomorphic) (1 patient)	Recurrent respiratory and gastrointestinal infections, **persistent disseminated flat warts (histologically consistent with EV, no HPV confirmation)**	broad (including keratinocytes and T cells)	CD4+ T-cell lymphopenia, CD8+ T-cell counts normal	Impaired mitogen- and antigen-induced proliferation	T low B- leaky SCID, IgM levels normal, IgG levels high, IgA absent, normal NK cell counts	Tahiat et al., 2017
	AR DOCK8 deficiency # (4 families)	Recurrent or severe viral infections associated with cancer, atopic dermatitis, recurrent respiratory or gastrointestinal tract infections, disseminated Molluscum contagiosum; disseminated **flat-topped warts (histologically consistent with EV, HPV-5 positive by PCR),** eczema, hyperpigmentation, and folliculitis	Broad (including keratinocytes and T cells)	CD4+ T-cell lymphopenia	Normal mitogen-induced proliferation	IgM levels low, IgE levels high, variably impaired specific antibody production, normal CD8+ T-cell and B-cell numbers	Sanal et al., 2012; Liu et al., 2017

(Continued)

TABLE 1 | Continued

Disease	Genetic etiology*	Clinical phenotypes (affected/total no. of patients)	Expression pattern	T cell counts	T cell function	Other immunological features	Reference
	AR RASGRP1 # deficiency (1 patient)	Recurrent ear infections, skin abscesses, chronic non-bloody diarrhea, **disseminated warts (histologically consistent with EV, no HPV confirmation)**, severe failure to thrive, splenomegaly, diffuse lymphadenopathy, fatal EBV-positive B cell lymphoma	Broad (including keratinocytes and T cells)	CD4+ T-cell lymphopenia, CD8+ T-cell counts high	Impaired proliferation in response to mitogen (PHA) and antigen (candida and tetanus toxoid)	Normal NK cell number with reduced function, IgG levels low, IgM levels high	Platt et al., 2017
	AR LCK # c.188-2A>G (3 siblings)	Recurrent bacterial pneumonia; **pityriasis-versicolor-like lesions and flat warts on hands, abdomen, legs (histologically consistent with EV, HPV-5, -20, -38 positive by PCR)** and histologically confirmed squamous cell carcinomas, fatal in 1 sibling; genital warts (HPV-6 positive by PCR)	Lymphoid lineage	CD4+ T-cell lymphopenia	Not tested	Not tested	Li et al., 2016
	AR TPP2 deficiency (2 siblings)	Evans syndrome (immune thrombocytopenic purpura and autoimmune hemolytic anemia) (2/2); progressive leukopenia (2/2); mild viral infections (1/2); **flat, hypopigmented warts (HPV-15 positive by PCR) (1/2)**, mild developmental delay (1/2)	Broad (including keratinocytes and T cells)	Normal or slightly low CD4+ T lymphocyte counts	Senescent CD8+ T cells (impaired proliferation, enhanced staurosporine-induced apoptosis)	Premature immunosenescence (T and B cells) and antinuclear antibodies; normal IgA and IgE levels; IgG and IgM levels high	Stepensky et al., 2015

Unless the specific mutation is listed, complete deficiency has been verified experimentally. #Other cases with the same genetic etiology but without EV-like symptoms and beta-HPV infections have been described. AR, autosomal recessive+; SCID, severe combined immunodeficiency.

SKIN CANCER

Patients with EV have a higher than normal risk of developing actinic keratosis and NMSC, particularly cutaneous squamous cell carcinoma (cSCC), cSCC *in situ* (Bowen's disease) and, to a lesser extent basal cell carcinoma (BCC) (Lewandowsky and Lutz, 1922; Rajagopalan et al., 1972; Orth et al., 1979; Mitsuishi et al., 2008). About two third of EV patients develop NMSC, with an onset during their twenties or thirties (Lewandowsky and Lutz, 1922; Rajagopalan et al., 1972; Orth et al., 1978; Majewski and Jablonska, 1997; de Oliveira et al., 2003). NMSC typically occurs in lesions exposed to the sun, about 20 years after the appearance of the first lesions, suggesting that UV irradiation and HPV are cocarcinogens for the development of this cancer. EV patients should, therefore, pay particular attention to protecting their skin against exposure to the sun. The role of HPVs in carcinogenesis is well established. The first evidence for the oncogenic behavior of HPVs was actually documented in a study of EV (Orth et al., 1980). EV has long served as a human model for studies of viral cutaneous oncogenesis (Jablonska et al., 1972; Casanova and Abel, 2004). This oncogenic behavior of beta-HPVs led to speculations that these viruses might also contribute to the development of cSCC in the general population. However, in cases of cSCC in the general population, less than one viral genome per cell is generally detected; by contrast, viral load is very high in cSCC of EV patients, indicating that different mechanisms of cancer initiation and maintenance are probably at work (Howley and Pfister, 2015). In particular, oncogenic HPV-5 and HPV-8 have been found in EV-associated NMSC, leading to their classification, by the WHO, as possible carcinogens in EV patients (Bouvard et al., 2009). The detection of high loads of HPV-5 E6 and E7 transcripts suggested a role in the cancer induction or maintenance, although the underlying mechanism remains unclear (Orth, 1987). Radiotherapy for cSCC treatment can be effective in the general population, but is counterproductive in EV patients, as the development of more aggressive tumors after treatment has been reported (Rajabi et al., 2014; de Oliveira et al., 2015). Patients should undergo frequent physical examinations, to facilitate the identification of precancerous and cancer lesions as early as possible. However, it has been shown that infection with oncogenic HPVs known to be associated with a high risk of skin cancer is not sufficient, in itself, to cause cancer. Environmental and genetic factors thus contribute to the inter-individual variability of outcome for HPV infection.

VIRAL ETIOLOGY

More than half a century ago, EV was recognized as a virus-induced disease, based on several experimental observations. Inoculation experiments showed EV to be transmissible (Lutz, 1946; Jablonska and Milewski, 1957; Jablonska et al., 1966). The first viral particles were then detected in lesions by electron microscopy (Ruiter and van Mullem, 1966; Jablonska et al., 1968) and, several years later, the first EV-specific HPV types, all from genus beta-HPV, were isolated from EV lesions (Orth et al., 1978;

Orth, 1986). EV patients not only have high HPV loads in their lesions, they also have a high serum antibody reactivity to beta-HPVs (Michael et al., 2010). At least 25 different beta-HPV genotypes have been found in patients with EV, and patients are usually infected with multiple EV-HPV types, HPV-5 being the most prevalent genotype (Orth, 2006). HPV-5 is also the most common genotype in cases of malignant conversion (Orth, 1986; Imahorn et al., 2017). Beta-HPVs are also frequently found in the skin of healthy individuals of the general population, but mostly at low copy numbers, and they do not cause clinical disease. This suggests that beta-HPVs are commensals of the skin (Antonsson et al., 2003a,b). However, it remains a matter of debate whether these beta-HPVs are really non-pathogenic in individuals without EV, as some studies have associated EV-HPV seropositivity and viral DNA load in the eyebrow with the risk of cSCC in the general population (Neale et al., 2013; Iannacone et al., 2014). The mechanisms of persistent, asymptomatic EV-HPV infection remain largely unknown. It has been suggested that beta-HPVs lack an essential growth-promoting function, limiting their pathogenicity. Indeed, unlike the alpha- and gamma-HPVs responsible for cutaneous warts, cervical cancers, and laryngeal papillomatosis, beta-HPVs do not possess the *E5* or *E8* (also reported as E10[1]) open-reading frames typically found in pathogenic non-beta HPVs and shown to be a growth-promoting factor for keratinocytes *in vivo* (Danos et al., 1983; Giri et al., 1985; Hu et al., 2002; Nonnenmacher et al., 2006; Orth, 2006, 2008). Beta-HPVs can overcome this lack of a growth-promoting function and attain full pathogenicity, only in genetically predisposed individuals, implying that these patients have a specific cutaneous immune defect (reviewed by Orth, 2006, 2008).

HUMAN GENETICS OF TYPICAL EV

Typical EV is a Mendelian condition that is transmitted as an autosomal recessive trait and shows complete penetrance in the first decade of life, across different ethnic groups (Orth, 2006). An autosomal recessive mode of inheritance was initially proposed in Cockayne (1933), confirmed in 1974 (Rajagopalan et al., 1972) and subsequently supported by a study of 147 EV cases, in which 11% of patients were the offspring of consanguineous marriages, and 10% came from multiplex families in which 25% of the siblings were affected, with an equal sex ratio (Lutzner, 1978). Shortly after the mapping of two susceptibility loci for EV to chromosomes 17q25 (EV1) and 2p21-p24 (EV2) (Ramoz et al., 1999, 2000), bi-allelic loss-of-function mutations of two adjacent genes termed *TMC6* and *TMC8*, also named *EVER1* and *EVER2*, respectively, located within the EV1 locus, were identified (Ramoz et al., 2002). Eight different mutations of *TMC6/EVER1* and 11 mutations of *TMC8/EVER2* have been described to date, in a total of 32 patients from 19 families and 5 ethnicities reviewed in Burger and Itin (2014) and Imahorn et al. (2017). These mutations are nonsense, frameshift, or splice-site mutations with full clinical penetrance for EV in homozygotes and compound heterozygotes. The effects of these mutations on mRNA and protein levels have not been investigated in most patients. Nonsense-mediated RNA decay and undetectable TMC8/EVER2 protein have been reported in two patients with premature stop codons (Ramoz et al., 2002; Landini et al., 2012). However, splice-site mutations of *TMC8/EVER2* have been identified that have no effect on mRNA levels, despite the detection of aberrantly spliced, shorter transcripts (Miyauchi et al., 2016; Imahorn et al., 2017). Nevertheless, all mutations are assumed to be loss-of-function. By contrast, the missense polymorphisms found in the general population are not predicted to be deleterious and are too common to account for EV. Despite these genetic analyses, more than 40% of the EV families identified to date have no mutations of the genes known to be associated with this disease (Zuo et al., 2006; Arnold et al., 2011; Imahorn et al., 2017) suggesting that high-throughput sequencing studies are required to identify the causal genes in these families.

HUMAN GENETICS OF ATYPICAL EV

Inactivating mutations of *RHOH* (Crequer et al., 2012b), *STK4* (encoding the MST1 protein) (Crequer et al., 2012a), *CORO1A* (Stray-Pedersen et al., 2014), *DCLRE1C (encoding the Artemis protein)* (Tahiat et al., 2017), *DOCK8* (Sanal et al., 2012; Liu et al., 2017), *RASGRP1* (Platt et al., 2017), *LCK* (Li et al., 2016), and *TPP2* (Stepensky et al., 2015) have been reported in patients with atypical EV. Interestingly, the clinical penetrance of these genetic disorders for EV lesions is low, as only a few patients present with manifestations of EV. This is at odds with the findings for typical EV, which is a fully penetrant Mendelian trait. A complete loss of function has been reported for all mutations, except those for Artemis (hypomorphic) and Lck (no functional investigation). All these patients suffer from a classic T-cell primary immunodeficiency. Some also display impaired mitogen- and/or antigen-induced T-cell proliferation. NK cells counts are normal in all these diseases, except for CORO1A. Hyper-IgM and hyper-IgE are observed in RASGRP1 and in CORO1A and DOCK8, respectively. Autoimmunity has been reported for STK4 and TPP2 deficiencies. T-cell senescence has been reported for RHOH and TPP2 deficiencies. It remains unclear whether these observations are the cause or consequence of severe, disseminated, chronic, life-long beta-HPV and other recurrent acute and chronic infections in these patients. Few studies have addressed the specific responses of leukocytes, but a lack of autologous T-cell response to HPV-infected keratinocytes has been described (Cooper et al., 1990). Most of these genes are broadly expressed (including in T cells and other types of skin-resident cells), with the exception of *RHOH* and *LCK*, which are expressed exclusively in the lymphoid linage (**Table 1**). An additional contribution of cells other than T lymphocytes, including other types of skin-resident cells, to the pathogenesis of atypical EV cannot, therefore, be ruled out. Nevertheless, the T-cell defects underlying atypical EV are likely to be specific, as most inherited and acquired forms of T-cell deficiency do not cause clinically apparent infections with beta-HPVs.

[1] http://PAVE.niaid.nih.gov

LEUKOCYTE IMMUNITY

Atypical EV is associated with T-cell deficiency. The only immunological feature common to all known etiologies is CD4$^+$ lymphopenia. More detailed immunological studies have been performed only in RhoH-deficient patients. These patients had impaired tissue-homing T-cells marker expression, with a small decreased in the number of memory skin-homing (CLA$^+$) CD4$^+$ T cells and a large decrease in the number of integrin beta7$^+$ CD4$^+$ T cells. Broad immunological evaluations of patients with typical EV have proved difficult, due to the rarity of the disease, and the data available are therefore highly patchy. *TMC6/EVER1* and *TMC8/EVER2*, which are mutated in patients with typical EV, are widely expressed, including in lymphocytes and the skin (Lazarczyk et al., 2012). Patients with typical EV have normal humoral immunity and antibody responses (Jablonska et al., 1979), their Langerhans cells have normal alloantigen presentation capacity (Majewski and Jablonska, 1992), and they have largely normal NK cell activity (Majewski et al., 1986). They have been reported to display impairments of cellular immunity, including low T-cell counts, CD4$^+$/CD8$^+$ T-cell ratios, a lack of responsiveness to T-cell mitogens, anergy to skin antigens and sensitization to dinitrochlorobenzene (Glinski et al., 1976, 1981; Prawer et al., 1977; Majewski et al., 1986; Majewski and Jablonska, 1992; Majewski et al., 1997; de Oliveira et al., 2003), but these defects were inconsistent and further complicated the assessment of immunological dysfunction in EV patients. All these observations suggest that a role for TMC6/EVER1 and TMC8/EVER2 in skin-intrinsic immunity.

KERATINOCYTE IMMUNITY

Keratinocytes contribute to protective immunity in the skin in at least three ways. First, they form a physical barrier. Second, they secrete and respond to cytokines, chemokines, and growth factors, participating in leukocyte-mediated operations (Kupper and Fuhlbrigge, 2004). Third, keratinocyte-intrinsic mechanisms are thought to contribute to the control of keratinocyte-tropic viruses. TMC6/EVER1 and TMC8/EVER2 thus provide us a unique opportunity to study the role of keratinocytes in host defense against HPV infection. TMC6/EVER1 and TMC8/EVER2 belong to a large family of highly conserved transmembrane channel-like (TMC) proteins that are expressed in the endoplasmic reticulum, where they act as or modulate the activity of transmembrane channels (Keresztes et al., 2003; Kurima et al., 2003). It has been suggested that these two proteins interact with the zinc transporter ZnT-1, influencing intracellular Zn^{2+} concentration, and, thus, the activity of the transcription factors, such as AP-1, a key activator in the HPV life cycle and cellular proliferation (Lazarczyk et al., 2008). It has also been suggested that TMC8/EVER2 influences the cellular response to TNF-α by promoting apoptosis rather than NF-κB activation and pro-survival signaling pathways (Gaud et al., 2013; Vuillier et al., 2014). TMC6/EVER1 and TMC8/EVER2 are thus thought to serve as restriction factors for beta-HPVs in keratinocytes, through the limitation of viral replication and gene expression. Studies of TMC6/EVER1 and TMC8/EVER2 have proved technically difficult, partly due to problems raising robust antibodies against these highly hydrophobic proteins, which have 10 and 8 transmembrane domains, respectively. Known molecular functions/mechanism of TMC6/EVER1 and TMC8/EVER2 are reviewed in Orth (2008) and Lazarczyk et al. (2009). The cellular and molecular bases of beta-HPV-driven lesions in TMC6/EVER1 and TMC8/EVER2-deficient patients with EV remain unknown. The genetic defects prevent patients from controlling beta-HPV in keratinocytes (Akgul et al., 2006). The patients are susceptible to skin infections with these particular types of HPV (Boxman et al., 1999). In addition, some patients with severe combined immunodeficiency (SCID) caused by mutations of *IL2RG* or *JAK3* may develop EV. These patients develop EV only after successful bone marrow transplantation, indicating that disease development in these patients is related to a keratinocyte defect (Laffort et al., 2004).

A CLASSIFICATION OF EV INTO TWO MAJOR TYPES

In the past, EV patients rarely underwent immunological follow-up, and typical and atypical cases were treated as the same diagnostic entity. This has led to conflicting reports about the impairment of immunity in only some patients. Patients with typical EV probably have a keratinocyte-intrinsic defect allowing beta-HPVs to persist in the skin, leading to the development of clinically apparent lesions. Consistent with this notion, three TMC8/EVER2-deficient EV patients have been reported to display a largely normal partitioning of circulating T cells, possibly even with slightly larger than normal skin-homing T-cell populations (Crequer et al., 2013). These normal numbers of circulating T cells do not exclude the possibility of an impaired recognition of and response to HPV-infected keratinocytes by these cells (Cooper et al., 1990). Once it became clear that these patients had a selective susceptibility to beta-HPV infections and TMC6/EVER1 and TMC8/EVER2 deficiencies had been described as a genetic etiology, EV was identified as a primary immunodeficiency (Notarangelo et al., 2004; Orth, 2008; Casanova, 2015). It has been suggested that the TMC/EVER proteins function as antiviral restriction factors in keratinocytes, and that they control constitutive intrinsic immunity (Orth, 2008). Consistent with this hypothesis, patients with acquired or treatment-induced immunosuppression do not normally develop EV, despite the commensal nature of beta-HPVs (Antonsson et al., 2003a,b). This contrasts with common warts due to alpha-HPVs, which are more common in immunosuppressed individuals (Wieland et al., 2014). Rare cases of EV-like syndromes developing in previously unaffected adults, and known as "acquired EV," have been described in patients with suppressed cell-mediated immunity. The clinical presentations of these patients and proposed treatments have been reviewed in detail elsewhere (Zampetti et al., 2013; Ovits et al., 2017). The rarity of atypical EV in patients with broad and severe genetic T-cell deficiencies and in immunocompromised individuals suggests that immunosuppression *per se* is not sufficient for the development of this disease. This is the case for most infectious diseases striking patients with such T-cell disorders, and it suggests that other host and environmental factors are involved in pathogenesis.

CONCLUDING REMARKS

In summary, both keratinocytes and T cells probably contribute to immunity to beta-HPV. Genetic defects affecting one or, potentially, both cell types lead to the EV-defining clinical manifestations of beta-HPV infection. All individuals with severe, recurrent, and persistent flat warts and with a diagnosis of typical or atypical EV should be tested for genetic etiologies of typical and atypical EV. The presence and extent of a systemic T-cell defect determines the spectrum of other clinical manifestations of an infectious, autoimmune, or allergic nature. Future studies should provide more conclusive demonstrations of the keratinocyte-intrinsic nature of EVER-dependent immunity to beta-HPVs. The identification of new genes associated with typical and atypical EV will pave the way for analyses of the molecular and cellular bases of EV, including studies of the respective contributions of keratinocytes and T cells to anti-beta-HPV immunity. The highly restricted susceptibility to beta-HPV observed in patients with EV has important clinical and biological implications in the fields of HPV, mucocutaneous immunology, and cell-intrinsic immunity. Elucidation of the genetic and immunological bases of EV will facilitate studies of the virulence mechanisms of other HPVs, including the role of E5 and E8 proteins produced by alpha- and gamma-HPVs, respectively. These studies will also facilitate the development of novel approaches for the diagnosis and management of patients with various conditions due to HPVs.

AUTHOR CONTRIBUTIONS

SdJ, EI, PI, GO, EJ, J-LC, and BB wrote the manuscript. SdJ, EI, PI, JU, GO, EJ, J-LC, and BB reviewed and edited the manuscript.

FUNDING

The Laboratory of Human Genetics of Infectious Diseases was supported by grants from the National Institutes of Health (NIH, Grant No: 5 R21 AI107508-02), the French National Cancer Institute (Grant No. 2013-1-PL BIO-11-1), and the French National Research Agency (ANR) under the "Investissements d'Avenir" program (Grant No. ANR-10-IAHU-01). SdJ was supported by the German Research Foundation (Jo 1151-1), funds from the Women & Science Fellowship program at The Rockefeller University, the National Institute of Allergy and Infectious Diseases of the NIH (Grant No. R21AI107508), and the NIH Clinical and Translational Science Award (CTSA) program (Grant No. UL1TR000043).

REFERENCES

Akgul, B., Cooke, J. C., and Storey, A. (2006). HPV-associated skin disease. *J. Pathol.* 208, 165–175. doi: 10.1002/path.1893

Antonsson, A., Erfurt, C., Hazard, K., Holmgren, V., Simon, M., Kataoka, A., et al. (2003a). Prevalence and type spectrum of human papillomaviruses in healthy skin samples collected in three continents. *J. Gen. Virol.* 84, 1881–1886.

Antonsson, A., Karanfilovska, S., Lindqvist, P. G., and Hansson, B. G. (2003b). General acquisition of human papillomavirus infections of skin occurs in early infancy. *J. Clin. Microbiol.* 41, 2509–2514.

Arnold, A. W., Burger, B., Kump, E., Rufle, A., Tyring, S. K., Kempf, W., et al. (2011). Homozygosity for the c.917A?T (p.N306l) polymorphism in the EVER2/TMC8 gene of two sisters with epidermodysplasia verruciformis Lewandowsky-Lutz originally described by Wilhelm Lutz. *Dermatology* 222, 81–86. doi: 10.1159/000322536

Azzimonti, B., Mondini, M., De Andrea, M., Gioia, D., Dianzani, U., Mesturini, R., et al. (2005). CD8+ T-cell lymphocytopenia and lack of EVER mutations in a patient with clinically and virologically typical epidermodysplasia verruciformis. *Arch. Dermatol.* 141, 1323–1325.

Borgogna, C., Landini, M. M., Lanfredini, S., Doorbar, J., Bouwes Bavinck, J. N., Quint, K. D., et al. (2014). Characterization of skin lesions induced by skin-tropic alpha- and beta-papillomaviruses in a patient with epidermodysplasia verruciformis. *Br. J. Dermatol.* 171, 1550–1554. doi: 10.1111/bjd.13156

Bouvard, V., Baan, R., Straif, K., Grosse, Y., Secretan, B., El Ghissassi, F., et al. (2009). A review of human carcinogens–Part B: biological agents. *Lancet Oncol.* 10, 321–322. doi: 10.1016/S1470-2045(09)70096-8

Boxman, I. L., Mulder, L. H., Russell, A., Bouwes Bavinck, J. N., Green, A., and Ter Schegget, J. (1999). Human papillomavirus type 5 is commonly present in immunosuppressed and immunocompetent individuals. *Br. J. Dermatol.* 141, 246–249. doi: 10.1046/j.1365-2133.1999.02972.x

Burger, B., and Itin, P. H. (2014). Epidermodysplasia verruciformis. *Curr. Probl. Dermatol.* 45, 123–131. doi: 10.1159/000356068

Casanova, J. L. (2015). Severe infectious diseases of childhood as monogenic inborn errors of immunity. *Proc. Natl. Acad. Sci. U.S.A.* 112, E7128–E7137. doi: 10.1073/pnas.1521651112

Casanova, J. L., and Abel, L. (2004). The human model: a genetic dissection of immunity to infection in natural conditions. *Nat. Rev. Immunol.* 4, 55–66. doi: 10.1038/nri1264

Cockayne, E. (1933). *Inherited Abnormalities of the Skin and its Appendages.* London: Oxford University Press.

Cooper, K. D., Androphy, E. J., Lowy, D., and Katz, S. I. (1990). Antigen presentation and T-cell activation in epidermodysplasia verruciformis. *J. Invest. Dermatol.* 94, 769–776. doi: 10.1111/1523-1747.ep12874631

Crequer, A., Picard, C., Patin, E., D'Amico, A., Abhyankar, A., Munzer, M., et al. (2012a). Inherited MST1 deficiency underlies susceptibility to EV-HPV infections. *PLoS One* 7:e44010. doi: 10.1371/journal.pone.0044010

Crequer, A., Picard, C., Pedergnana, V., Lim, A., Zhang, S. Y., Abel, L., et al. (2013). EVER2 deficiency is associated with mild T-cell abnormalities. *J. Clin. Immunol.* 33, 14–21. doi: 10.1007/s10875-012-9749-1

Crequer, A., Troeger, A., Patin, E., Ma, C. S., Picard, C., Pedergnana, V., et al. (2012b). Human RHOH deficiency causes T cell defects and susceptibility to EV-HPV infections. *J. Clin. Invest.* 122, 3239–3247. doi: 10.1172/JCI62949

Danos, O., Engel, L., Chen, E., Yaniv, M., and Howley, P. (1983). Comparative analysis of the human type 1a and bovine type 1 papillomavirus genomes. *J. Virol.* 46, 557–566.

de Oliveira, W. R., da Cruz Silva, L. L., Neto, C. F., and Tyring, S. (2015). Deleterious effect of radiation therapy on epidermodysplasia verruciformis patients. *J. Cutan. Med. Surg.* 19, 416–421. doi: 10.1177/1203475415576859

de Oliveira, W. R., Festa Neto, C., Rady, P. L., and Tyring, S. K. (2003). Clinical aspects of epidermodysplasia verruciformis. *J. Eur. Acad. Dermatol. Venereol.* 17, 394–398. doi: 10.1046/j.1468-3083.2003.00703.x

Gaud, G., Guillemot, D., Jacob, Y., Favre, M., and Vuillier, F. (2013). EVER2 protein binds TRADD to promote TNF-alpha-induced apoptosis. *Cell Death Dis.* 4:e499. doi: 10.1038/cddis.2013.27

Giri, I., Danos, O., and Yaniv, M. (1985). Genomic structure of the cottontail rabbit (Shope) papillomavirus. *Proc. Natl. Acad. Sci. U.S.A.* 82, 1580–1584. doi: 10.1073/pnas.82.6.1580

Glinski, W., Jablonska, S., Langner, A., Obalek, S., Haftek, M., and Proniewska, M. (1976). Cell-mediated immunity in epidermodysplasia verruciformis. *Dermatologica* 153, 218–227. doi: 10.1159/000251060

Glinski, W., Obalek, S., Jablonska, S., and Orth, G. (1981). T cell defect in patients with epidermodysplasia verruciformis due to human papillomavirus type 3 and 5. *Dermatologica* 162, 141–147. doi: 10.1159/000250262

Howley, P. M., and Pfister, H. J. (2015). Beta genus papillomaviruses and skin cancer. *Virology* 479–480, 290–296. doi: 10.1016/j.virol.2015.02.004

Hu, J., Han, R., Cladel, N. M., Pickel, M. D., and Christensen, N. D. (2002). Intracutaneous DNA vaccination with the E8 gene of Cottontail Rabbit Papillomavirus induces protective immunity against virus challenge in Rabbits. *J. Virol.* 76, 6453–6459. doi: 10.1128/JVI.76.13.6453-6459.2002

Iannacone, M. R., Gheit, T., Pfister, H., Giuliano, A. R., Messina, J. L., Fenske, N. A., et al. (2014). Case-control study of genus-beta human papillomaviruses in plucked eyebrow hairs and cutaneous squamous cell carcinoma. *Int. J. Cancer* 134, 2231–2244. doi: 10.1002/ijc.28552

Imahorn, E., Yuksel, Z., Spoerri, I., Gurel, G., Imhof, C., Saracoglu, Z. N., et al. (2017). Novel TMC8 splice site mutation in epidermodysplasia verruciformis and review of HPV infections in patients with the disease. *J. Eur. Acad. Dermatol. Venereol.* 31, 1722–1726. doi: 10.1111/jdv.14431

Jablonska, S., Biczysko, W., Jakubowicz, K., and Dabrowski, J. (1968). On the viral etiology of epidermodysplasia verruciformis Lewandowsky-Lutz. Electron microscope studies. *Dermatologica* 137, 113–125. doi: 10.1159/000254038

Jablonska, S., Dabrowski, J., and Jakubowicz, K. (1972). Epidermodysplasia verruciformis as a model in studies on the role of papovaviruses in oncogenesis. *Cancer Res.* 32, 583–589.

Jablonska, S., Fabjanska, L., and Formas, I. (1966). On the viral etiology of epidermodysplasia verruciformis. *Dermatologica* 132, 369–385. doi: 10.1159/000254437

Jablonska, S., and Milewski, B. (1957). Information on epidermodysplasia verruciformis Lewandowsky-Lutz; positive results of auto- and heteroinoculation. *Dermatologica* 115, 1–22. doi: 10.1159/000255982

Jablonska, S., Orth, G., Jarzabek-Chorzelska, M., Glinski, W., Obalek, S., Rzesa, G., et al. (1979). Twenty-one years of follow-up studies of familial epidermodysplasia verruciformis. *Dermatologica* 158, 309–327. doi: 10.1159/000250775

Keresztes, G., Mutai, H., and Heller, S. (2003). TMC and EVER genes belong to a larger novel family, the TMC gene family encoding transmembrane proteins. *BMC Genomics* 4:24. doi: 10.1186/1471-2164-4-24

Kupper, T. S., and Fuhlbrigge, R. C. (2004). Immune surveillance in the skin: mechanisms and clinical consequences. *Nat. Rev. Immunol.* 4, 211–222. doi: 10.1038/nri1310

Kurima, K., Yang, Y., Sorber, K., and Griffith, A. J. (2003). Characterization of the transmembrane channel-like (TMC) gene family: functional clues from hearing loss and epidermodysplasia verruciformis. *Genomics* 82, 300–308. doi: 10.1016/S0888-7543(03)00154-X

Laffort, C., Le Deist, F., Favre, M., Caillat-Zucman, S., Radford-Weiss, I., Debre, M., et al. (2004). Severe cutaneous papillomavirus disease after haemopoietic stem-cell transplantation in patients with severe combined immune deficiency caused by common gammac cytokine receptor subunit or JAK-3 deficiency. *Lancet* 363, 2051–2054. doi: 10.1016/S0140-6736(04)16457-X

Landini, M. M., Borgogna, C., Peretti, A., Colombo, E., Zavattaro, E., Boldorini, R., et al. (2014). alpha- and beta-papillomavirus infection in a young patient with an unclassified primary T-cell immunodeficiency and multiple mucosal and cutaneous lesions. *J. Am. Acad. Dermatol.* 71, 108.e1–115.e1. doi: 10.1016/j.jaad.2014.01.859

Landini, M. M., Zavattaro, E., Borgogna, C., Azzimonti, B., De Andrea, M., Colombo, E., et al. (2012). Lack of EVER2 protein in two epidermodysplasia verruciformis patients with skin cancer presenting previously unreported homozygous genetic deletions in the EVER2 gene. *J. Invest. Dermatol.* 132, 1305–1308. doi: 10.1038/jid.2011.399

Lazarczyk, M., Cassonnet, P., Pons, C., Jacob, Y., and Favre, M. (2009). The EVER proteins as a natural barrier against papillomaviruses: a new insight into the pathogenesis of human papillomavirus infections. *Microbiol. Mol. Biol. Rev.* 73, 348–370. doi: 10.1128/MMBR.00033-08

Lazarczyk, M., Dalard, C., Hayder, M., Dupre, L., Pignolet, B., Majewski, S., et al. (2012). EVER proteins, key elements of the natural anti-human papillomavirus barrier, are regulated upon T-cell activation. *PLoS One* 7:e39995. doi: 10.1371/journal.pone.0039995

Lazarczyk, M., Pons, C., Mendoza, J. A., Cassonnet, P., Jacob, Y., and Favre, M. (2008). Regulation of cellular zinc balance as a potential mechanism of EVER-mediated protection against pathogenesis by cutaneous oncogenic human papillomaviruses. *J. Exp. Med.* 205, 35–42. doi: 10.1084/jem.20071311

Lewandowsky, F., and Lutz, W (1922). Ein Fall einer bisher nicht beschriebenen hauterkrankung (Epidermodysplasia verruciformis). *Arch. Dermatol. Syphilol.* 141, 193–203. doi: 10.1007/BF01938833

Li, S. L., Duo, L. N., Wang, H. J., Dai, W., Zhou, E. H., Xu, Y. N., et al. (2016). Identification of LCK mutation in a family with atypical epidermodysplasia verruciformis with T-cell defects and virus-induced squamous cell carcinoma. *Br. J. Dermatol.* 175, 1204–1209. doi: 10.1111/bjd.14679

Liu, Y. Q., Zhang, G. L., Mo, X. H., Wang, B., Wu, F., Chen, J., et al. (2017). A novel homozygous DOCK8 mutation associated with unusual coexistence of gross molluscum contagiosum and epidermodysplasia verruciformis in a DOCK8 deficiency patient. *J. Eur. Acad. Dermatol. Venereol.* 31, e504–e505. doi: 10.1111/jdv.14344

Lutz, W. (1946). A propos de l'épidermodysplasie verruciforme. *Dermatologica* 92, 30–43. doi: 10.1159/000255805

Lutzner, M. A. (1978). Epidermodysplasia verruciformis. An autosomal recessive disease characterized by viral warts and skin cancer. A model for viral oncogenesis. *Bull. Cancer* 65, 169–182.

Majewski, S., and Jablonska, S. (1992). Epidermodysplasia verruciformis as a model of human papillomavirus-induced genetic cancers: the role of local immunosurveillance. *Am. J Med. Sci.* 304, 174–179. doi: 10.1097/00000441-199209000-00006

Majewski, S., and Jablonska, S. (1997). Skin autografts in epidermodysplasia verruciformis: human papillomavirus-associated cutaneous changes need over 20 years for malignant conversion. *Cancer Res.* 57, 4214–4216.

Majewski, S., Jablonska, S., and Orth, G. (1997). Epidermodysplasia verruciformis. Immunological and nonimmunological surveillance mechanisms: role in tumor progression. *Clin. Dermatol.* 15, 321–334. doi: 10.1016/S0738-081X(96)00169-1

Majewski, S., Skopinska-Rozewska, E., Jablonska, S., Wasik, M., Misiewicz, J., and Orth, G. (1986). Partial defects of cell-mediated immunity in patients with epidermodysplasia verruciformis. *J. Am. Acad. Dermatol.* 15, 966–973. doi: 10.1016/S0190-9622(86)70258-2

Michael, K. M., Waterboer, T., Pfister, H., Gariglio, M., Majewski, S., Favre, M., et al. (2010). Seroreactivity of 38 human papillomavirus types in epidermodysplasia verruciformis patients, relatives, and controls. *J. Invest. Dermatol.* 130, 841–848. doi: 10.1038/jid.2009.356

Mitsuishi, T., Ohara, K., Suzuki, T., Mochizuki, T., Kaneko, T., and Kawana, S. (2008). Epidermodysplasia verruciformis with keratoacanthoma, Bowen's disease and squamous cell carcinoma: isolation of high-risk types of HPV 5 and unknown type of human papillomavirus. *J. Eur. Acad. Dermatol. Venereol.* 22, 1126–1127. doi: 10.1111/j.1468-3083.2007.02526.x

Miyauchi, T., Nomura, T., Suzuki, S., Takeda, M., Shinkuma, S., Arita, K., et al. (2016). Genetic analysis of a novel splice-site mutation in TMC8 reveals the in vivo importance of the transmembrane channel-like domain of TMC8. *Br. J. Dermatol.* 175, 803–806. doi: 10.1111/bjd.14569

Neale, R. E., Weissenborn, S., Abeni, D., Bavinck, J. N., Euvrard, S., Feltkamp, M. C., et al. (2013). Human papillomavirus load in eyebrow hair follicles and risk of cutaneous squamous cell carcinoma. *Cancer Epidemiol. Biomarkers Prev.* 22, 719–727. doi: 10.1158/1055-9965.EPI-12-0917-T

Nonnenmacher, M., Salmon, J., Jacob, Y., Orth, G., and Breitburd, F. (2006). Cottontail rabbit papillomavirus E8 protein is essential for wart formation and provides new insights into viral pathogenesis. *J. Virol.* 80, 4890–4900. doi: 10.1128/JVI.80.10.4890-4900.2006

Notarangelo, L., Casanova, J. L., Fischer, A., Puck, J., Rosen, F., Seger, R., et al. (2004). Primary immunodeficiency diseases: an update. *J. Allergy Clin. Immunol.* 114, 677–687. doi: 10.1016/j.jaci.2004.06.044

Orth, G. (1986). Epidermodysplasia verruciformis: a model for understanding the oncogenicity of human papillomaviruses. *Ciba Found. Symp.* 120, 157–174.

Orth, G. (1987). "Epidermodysplasia verruciformis," in *The Papovaviridae. The Papillomaviruses*, Vol. 2, eds P. M. Howley and N. P. Salzman (New York, NY: Plenum Press Inc.), 199–243.

Orth, G. (2006). Genetics of epidermodysplasia verruciformis: insights into host defense against papillomaviruses. *Semin. Immunol.* 18, 362–374. doi: 10.1016/j.smim.2006.07.008

Orth, G. (2008). Host defenses against human papillomaviruses: lessons from epidermodysplasia verruciformis. *Curr. Top. Microbiol. Immunol.* 321, 59–83. doi: 10.1007/978-3-540-75203-5_3

Orth, G., Favre, M., Breitburd, F., Croissant, O., Jablonska, M., Obalek, S., et al. (1980). "Epidermodysplasia verruciformis: a model for the role of papillomavirus in human cancer," in *Viruses in Naturally Occurring Cancers*, eds M. Essex, G. Todaro, and H. Hausen (Cold Spring Harbor, NY: Cold Spring Harbor Laboratory Press), 259.

Orth, G., Jablonska, S., Favre, M., Croissant, O., Jarzabek-Chorzelska, M., and Rzesa, G. (1978). Characterization of two types of human papillomaviruses in lesions of epidermodysplasia verruciformis. *Proc. Natl. Acad. Sci. U.S.A.* 75, 1537–1541. doi: 10.1073/pnas.75.3.1537

Orth, G., Jablonska, S., Jarzabek-Chorzelska, M., Obalek, S., Rzesa, G., Favre, M., et al. (1979). Characteristics of the lesions and risk of malignant conversion associated with the type of human papillomavirus involved in epidermodysplasia verruciformis. *Cancer Res.* 39, 1074–1082.

Ovits, C. G., Amin, B. D., and Halverstam, C. (2017). Acquired epidermodysplasia verruciformis and its relationship to immunosuppressive therapy: report of a case and review of the literature. *J. Drugs Dermatol.* 16, 701–704.

Platt, C. D., Fried, A. J., Hoyos-Bachiloglu, R., Usmani, G. N., Schmidt, B., Whangbo, J., et al. (2017). Combined immunodeficiency with EBV positive B cell lymphoma and epidermodysplasia verruciformis due to a novel homozygous mutation in RASGRP1. *Clin. Immunol.* 183, 142–144. doi: 10.1016/j.clim.2017.08.007

Prawer, S. E., Pass, F., Vance, J. C., Greenberg, L. J., Yunis, E. J., and Zelickson, A. S. (1977). Depressed immune function in epidermodysplasia verruciformis. *Arch. Dermatol.* 113, 495–499. doi: 10.1001/archderm.1977.01640040103018

Rajabi, M. T., Ghasemi, H., Safizadeh, M., Jamshidi, S., Asadi-Amoli, F., Abrishami, Y., et al. (2014). Conjunctival squamous cell carcinoma with intraocular invasion after radiotherapy in epidermodysplasia verruciformis. *Can. J. Ophthalmol.* 49, e43–e46. doi: 10.1016/j.jcjo.2013.12.009

Rajagopalan, K., Bahru, J., Loo, D. S., Tay, C. H., Chin, K. N., and Tan, K. K. (1972). Familial epidermodysplasia verruciformis of Lewandowsky and Lutz. *Arch. Dermatol.* 105, 73–78. doi: 10.1001/archderm.1972.01620040045008

Ramoz, N., Rueda, L. A., Bouadjar, B., Favre, M., and Orth, G. (1999). A susceptibility locus for epidermodysplasia verruciformis, an abnormal predisposition to infection with the oncogenic human papillomavirus type 5, maps to chromosome 17qter in a region containing a psoriasis locus. *J. Invest. Dermatol.* 112, 259–263. doi: 10.1046/j.1523-1747.1999.00536.x

Ramoz, N., Rueda, L. A., Bouadjar, B., Montoya, L. S., Orth, G., and Favre, M. (2002). Mutations in two adjacent novel genes are associated with epidermodysplasia verruciformis. *Nat. Genet.* 32, 579–581. doi: 10.1038/ng1044

Ramoz, N., Taieb, A., Rueda, L. A., Montoya, L. S., Bouadjar, B., Favre, M., et al. (2000). Evidence for a nonallelic heterogeneity of epidermodysplasia verruciformis with two susceptibility loci mapped to chromosome regions 2p21-p24 and 17q25. *J. Invest. Dermatol.* 114, 1148–1153. doi: 10.1046/j.1523-1747.2000.00996.x

Ruiter, M., and van Mullem, P. J. (1966). Demonstration by electronmicroscopy of an intranuclear virus in epidermodysplasia verruciformis. *J. Invest. Dermatol.* 47, 247–252. doi: 10.1038/jid.1966.137

Sanal, O., Jing, H., Ozgur, T., Ayvaz, D., Strauss-Albee, D. M., Ersoy-Evans, S., et al. (2012). Additional diverse findings expand the clinical presentation of DOCK8 deficiency. *J. Clin. Immunol.* 32, 698–708. doi: 10.1007/s10875-012-9664-5

Stepensky, P., Rensing-Ehl, A., Gather, R., Revel-Vilk, S., Fischer, U., Nabhani, S., et al. (2015). Early-onset Evans syndrome, immunodeficiency, and premature immunosenescence associated with tripeptidyl-peptidase II deficiency. *Blood* 125, 753–761. doi: 10.1182/blood-2014-08-593202

Stray-Pedersen, A., Jouanguy, E., Crequer, A., Bertuch, A. A., Brown, B. S., Jhangiani, S. N., et al. (2014). Compound heterozygous CORO1A mutations in siblings with a mucocutaneous-immunodeficiency syndrome of epidermodysplasia verruciformis-HPV, molluscum contagiosum and granulomatous tuberculoid leprosy. *J. Clin. Immunol.* 34, 871–890. doi: 10.1007/s10875-014-0074-8

Tahiat, A., Badran, Y. R., Chou, J., Cangemi, B., Lefranc, G., Labgaa, Z. M., et al. (2017). Epidermodysplasia verruciformis as a manifestation of ARTEMIS deficiency in a young adult. *J. Allergy Clin. Immunol.* 139, 372.e4–375.e4. doi: 10.1016/j.jaci.2016.07.024

Vuillier, F., Gaud, G., Guillemot, D., Commere, P. H., Pons, C., and Favre, M. (2014). Loss of the HPV-infection resistance EVER2 protein impairs NF-kappaB signaling pathways in keratinocytes. *PLoS One* 9:e89479. doi: 10.1371/journal.pone.0089479

Wieland, U., Kreuter, A., and Pfister, H. (2014). Human papillomavirus and immunosuppression. *Curr. Probl. Dermatol.* 45, 154–165. doi: 10.1159/000357907

Zampetti, A., Giurdanella, F., Manco, S., Linder, D., Gnarra, M., Guerriero, G., et al. (2013). Acquired epidermodysplasia verruciformis: a comprehensive review and a proposal for treatment. *Dermatol. Surg.* 39, 974–980. doi: 10.1111/dsu.12135

Zuo, Y. G., Ma, D., Zhang, Y., Qiao, J., and Wang, B. (2006). Identification of a novel mutation and a genetic polymorphism of *EVER1* gene in two families with epidermodysplasia verruciformis. *J. Dermatol. Sci.* 44, 153–159. doi: 10.1016/j.jdermsci.2006.08.013

18

The Role of Human Papillomaviruses and Polyomaviruses in BRAF-Inhibitor Induced Cutaneous Squamous Cell Carcinoma and Benign Squamoproliferative Lesions

*Karin J. Purdie[1], Charlotte M. Proby[2], Hasan Rizvi[3], Heather Griffin[4], John Doorbar[4], Mary Sommerlad[5], Mariet C. Feltkamp[6], Els Van der Meijden[6], Gareth J. Inman[2], Andrew P. South[7], Irene M. Leigh[8] and Catherine A. Harwood[1,5]**

Centre for Cell Biology and Cutaneous Research, Blizard Institute, Barts and the London School of Medicine and Dentistry, Queen Mary University of London, London, United Kingdom, [2] Division of Cancer Research, School of Medicine, University of Dundee, Dundee, United Kingdom, [3] Department of Pathology, Barts Health NHS Trust, London, United Kingdom, Division of Virology, Department of Pathology, University of Cambridge, Cambridge, United Kingdom, [5] Department of Dermatology, Barts Health NHS Trust, London, United Kingdom, [6] Department of Medical Microbiology, Leiden University Medical Center, Leiden, Netherlands, [7] Department of Dermatology and Cutaneous Biology, Thomas Jefferson University, Philadelphia, PA, United States, [8] Institute of Dentistry, Barts and the London School of Medicine and Dentistry, Queen Mary University of London, London, United Kingdom

***Correspondence:**
Catherine A. Harwood
caharwood@doctors.org.uk

Background: Human papillomavirus (HPV) has long been proposed as a cofactor in the pathogenesis of cutaneous squamous cell carcinoma (cSCC). More recently, the striking clinico-pathological features of cSCCs that complicate treatment of metastatic melanoma with inhibitors targeting BRAF mutations (BRAFi) has prompted speculation concerning a pathogenic role for oncogenic viruses. Here, we investigate HPV and human polyomaviruses (HPyV) and correlate with clinical, histologic, and genetic features in BRAFi-associated cSCC.

Materials and Methods: Patients receiving BRAFi treatment were recruited at Barts Health NHS Trust. HPV DNA was detected in microdissected frozen samples using reverse line probe technology and degenerate and nested PCR. HPV immunohistochemistry was performed in a subset of samples. Quantitative PCR was performed to determine the presence and viral load of HPyVs with affinity for the skin (HPyV6, HPyV7, HPyV9, MCPyV, and TSPyV). These data were correlated with previous genetic mutational analysis of H, K and NRAS, NOTCH1/2, TP53, CDKN2A, CARD11, CREBBP, TGFBR1/2. Chromosomal aberrations were profiled using single nucleotide polymorphism (SNP) arrays.

Results: Forty-five skin lesions from seven patients treated with single agent vemurafenib in 2012–2013 were analyzed: 12 cSCC, 19 viral warts (VW), 2 actinic keratosis (AK), 5 verrucous keratosis/other squamoproliferative (VK/SP) lesions, one melanocytic lesion and 6 normal skin samples. Significant histologic features of viral infection were seen in 10/12 (83%) cSCC. HPV DNA was detected in 18/19 (95%) VW/SP, 9/12 (75%) cSCC, 4/5 (80%) SP, and 3/6 (50%) normal skin samples and in 1/12 cases assessed by immunohistochemistry. HPyV was co-detected in 22/30 (73%) of samples, usually at low viral load, with MCPyV and HPyV7 the most common. SNP arrays confirmed low levels of chromosomal abnormality and there was no significant correlation between HPV or HPyV detection and individual gene mutations or overall mutational burden.

Conclusion: Despite supportive clinicopathologic evidence, the role for HPV and HPyV infection in the pathogenesis of BRAFi-induced squamoproliferative lesions remains uncertain. Synergistic oncogenic mechanisms are plausible although speculative. Nonetheless, with the prospect of a significant increase in the adjuvant use of these drugs, further research is justified and may provide insight into the pathogenesis of other BRAFi-associated malignancies.

Keywords: human polyomaviruses, human papillomaviruses, cutaneous squamous cell carcinomas, BRAF inhibitors, melanoma

INTRODUCTION

Human papillomaviruses (HPV), particularly those of the beta genus (beta-PV), have long been proposed as cofactors with ultraviolet radiation in the pathogenesis of cutaneous squamous cell carcinoma (cSCC), especially those associated with the rare genodermatosis, epidermodysplasia verruciformis and with immune suppression (Wang et al., 2014; Howley and Pfister, 2015; Quint et al., 2015; Harwood et al., 2017). Over the past decade, 13 human polyomaviruses (HPyV) have been identified and classified (Calvignac-Spencer et al., 2016) and those with affinity for the skin include HPyV6, HPyV7, HPyV9, the trichodysplasia spinulosa-associated polyomavirus (TSPyV), the Merkel cell polyomavirus (MCPyV) (DeCaprio and Garcea, 2013; Feltkamp et al., 2013; van der Meijden et al., 2010, 2013; Nguyen et al., 2017) and the Lyon IARC polyomavirus (LIPyV) (Gheit et al., 2017). MCPyV was the first to be associated with malignancy - the aggressive cutaneous neuroendocrine cancer Merkel cell carcinoma (Feng et al., 2008; Shuda et al., 2008) - and has also been investigated in the context of cSCC (Dworkin et al., 2009; Scola et al., 2012). More recently, the clinical and histologic features of cSCCs and other squamoproliferative lesions that complicate treatment for metastatic melanoma with oral small molecule *BRAF* inhibitors (BRAFi) have raised the possibility of significant viral involvement in their pathogenesis (Boussemart et al., 2013). Both HPV and HPyV have been investigated, but studies have to date provided conflicting evidence for their role. With the prospect of future widespread adjuvant use of these drugs (Long et al., 2017; Maio et al., 2018), a more detailed understanding of the pathogenesis of BRAFi-induced cSCC (BRAFi-SCC) remains important.

Oncogenic mutations in the oncoprotein *BRAF*, which encodes the growth signal transduction serine/threonine protein kinase B-Raf, are found in approximately 50% of melanomas and result in constitutive activation of the RAS/mitogen-activated protein kinase (MAPK) pathway. The most common BRAF mutation results in a substitution of a valine (V) residue to glutamic acid (E) at amino acid position 600 (V600E) (Long et al., 2011). This locks the kinase into the active conformation and results in melanocyte hyperproliferation. BRAF inhibitors have been developed that exploit this mutation and competitively bind to the active conformation of the kinase (Zhang et al., 2009; Ribas and Flaherty, 2011) Vemurafenib and dabrafenib are two such selective small molecule inhibitors of oncogenic *BRAF* and are associated with high response rates and improved progression-free survival and overall survival compared with chemotherapy in patients with BRAFV600 mutated melanoma (Chapman et al., 2017). However, responses are generally temporary, with a median time to relapse of approximately 6 months. Vemurafenib entered routine clinical use in 2011/2012 and has been associated with various cutaneous adverse effects. These include rashes, photosensitivity, hyperkeratosis and development of *de novo* squamoproliferative lesions in 16–26.7% of patients, ranging from benign VW and squamous papillomas/verrucous keratoses (VK) to keratoacanthomas (KA) and cSCC (Flaherty et al., 2010; Sosman et al., 2012; Anforth et al., 2013; Blank et al., 2017; Chapman et al., 2017). The median time to presentation for BRAFi-SCC is 8–12 weeks and it is argued that this rapid timeframe points to pre-existing mutations being given a selective advantage due to BRAFi treatment, rather than mutations arising *de novo* due to therapy. Consistent with this mechanism, there is evidence for paradoxical hyperactivation of the MAPK pathway in cells with wild-type BRAF but mutated RAS through allosteric and catalytic mechanisms that relieve the auto-inhibition of wild-type RAF kinase (Hatzivassiliou et al., 2010; Heidorn et al., 2010; Poulikakos et al., 2010). Indeed, many of these BRAFi features overlap with the cutaneous manifestations of RASopathies - genetic diseases such as cardiofaciocutaneous and Costello syndromes characterized by activating germ line mutations in RAS (Rinderknecht et al., 2013; Sfecci et al., 2017). Also consistent with this, 18–60% of BRAFi-cSCC have somatic mutations in HRAS or KRAS, which is significantly higher than in sporadic cSCC (Oberholzer et al., 2012; Su et al., 2012; South et al., 2014). Nevertheless, many BRAFi-cSCC are RAS wild type, and RAS mutations have been also been detected in benign epithelial skin lesions (South et al., 2014; Hassel et al., 2015), suggesting that accelerated oncogenesis of RAS-mutated cells is not the only aetiologic mechanism and that additional cofactors may be involved. Attention has focused on infectious agents, particularly oncogenic viruses. HPV has been the main candidate given its previous proposed role in EV and immune suppression-associated cSCCs, coupled with evidence in BRAFi-cSCC of clinical and histological patterns of viral wart-like features and overexpression of p16 (Boussemart et al., 2013). Human polyomaviruses, particularly MCPyV, have also been investigated but, to date, the available evidence for both HPV and HPyV remains inconclusive (Anforth et al., 2012; Chu et al., 2012; Boussemart et al., 2013; Ganzenmueller et al., 2013; Falchook et al., 2013, 2016; Ko et al., 2013; Frouin et al., 2014; Holderfield et al., 2014; Schrama et al., 2014; Cohen et al., 2015; Dika et al., 2015; Viarisio et al., 2017a,b).

Single agent BRAFi therapy has generally been replaced by combination BRAFi and MEK inhibition (MEKi): phase III studies demonstrated improved clinical outcomes and significantly delayed resistance compared with BRAFi alone and BRAFi-MEKi combination therapy (vemurafenib/cobimetanib and dabrafenib/trametinib) is now the standard of care for BRAF mutated metastatic melanoma (Flaherty et al., 2012; Larkin et al., 2014). Combination therapy also results in decreased incidence of BRAFi-SCC to around 4%, which may be due to the fact that MEKi bypasses the point of paradoxical RAF activation (Dummer et al., 2012). Although rates of BRAFi-SCC are consequently reduced with combination therapy, these drugs are now being introduced as adjuvant treatment in high-risk, non-metastatic primary melanoma (stages IIC–IIIA–IIIB–IIIC). In the recent BRIM-8 study of adjuvant vemurafenib in BRAF-mutated melanoma, 16% of patients treated with adjuvant vemurafenib had BRAFi-cSCC or KA (Maio et al., 2018). This incidence is considerably lower with BRAFi-MEKi combination adjuvant therapy (Long et al., 2017), but with approval for adjuvant treatment comes the prospect of a huge increase in the numbers of patients receiving these agents in the near future. The need to better understand the pathogenesis of their associated cSCC therefore remains important.

In this study we have examined HPV and HPyV status in a series of benign and malignant BRAFi-associated skin lesions and correlated these data with key clinical, histologic and genetic parameters in order to further investigate the contribution of these viruses to the pathogenesis of BRAFi-induced skin tumors.

MATERIALS AND METHODS

Patients and Samples

Patients were recruited from the melanoma clinic at Barts Health NHS Trust. Punch biopsies were taken after surgical excision of lesions or from bisected shave biopsies. They were immediately snap-frozen in liquid nitrogen and stored at −80°C. The remainder of the tissue was sent for formalin fixation and histologic diagnosis. In order to enrich for tumor cell populations, fresh-frozen samples were laser-capture microdissected using the Zeiss Palm Microbeam microscope (Zeiss, Cambridge, United Kingdom). Depending on sample size and purity, as estimated from a reference hematoxylin and eosin slide, between 30 and 60 sections of 8 mm thickness were cut onto 1.0 mm PEN membrane slides (Zeiss), stained in 0.05% acid fuchsin (Acros Organics, Morris Plains, NJ, United States) in distilled water and 0.05% toluidine blue O (Acros Organics, Morris Plains, NJ, United States) in 70% ethanol, and microdissected, with tumor cells collected into 180 μl ATL buffer (Qiagen, Crawley, United Kingdom). All sections were cut using a fresh microtome to prevent cross-contamination. DNA extraction was performed using the QIAamp DNA micro kit (Qiagen, Crawley, United Kingdom) according to the manufacturer's instructions. To provide a source of germline DNA, paired venous blood samples were obtained concomitantly with lesional tissue and stored at −80°C before DNA extraction using the QIAamp DNA blood mini kit (Qiagen, Crawley, United Kingdom). The quality of the extracted DNA was assessed by β-globin reference gene PCR.

Histopathology

Histology sections were prepared from formalin-fixed paraffin-embedded tissue and stained with hematoxylin and eosin under standard conditions. All diagnoses were confirmed after review by an experienced dermatopathologist (HR). Samples were scored as having features consistent with viral infection if koilocytosis was observed in conjunction with at least three of the following five features: acanthosis, hypergranulosis, parakeratosis, hyperkeratosis, and typical papillomatous architecture. Consensus scoring of viral features was reached with two additional observers (KP, CH).

HPV Detection and Genotyping

Beta, gamma, alpha, mu, nu, and novel HPV types were detected using a comprehensive panel of HPV detection and typing methodologies. The presence of beta-HPV was investigated using RHA kit skin (beta) HPV detection system (de Koning et al., 2006) according to the manufacturer's instructions (Diassay, Rijswijk, The Netherlands). In addition, the RHA kit HPV SPF10-LiPA25 (Labo Bio-medical products BV, Rijswijk, The Netherlands) was used to detect the presence of 25 high- and low-risk mucosotropic alpha-HPVs, according to the manufacturer's instructions. Degenerate nested PCR protocols were used to investigate the presence of cutaneous alpha-HPV and mu and nu genera (Harwood et al., 1999) and the gamma genus (Forslund et al., 1999; Antonsson et al., 2000).

Polyomavirus Detection and Genotyping

In lesional samples for which sufficient DNA was available, quantitative PCR was performed as previously described (van der Meijden et al., 2014, 2017), to determine the presence and load of HPyV9, MCPyV, and TSPyV. For HPyV6 and HPyV7 quantitative PCR the following primers and probes located in VP1 were used: 5′-GTAGGGTATGCTGGTAAC-3′ (HPyV6 sense), 5′-CAGGAATTGTCTAAACATCATATC-3′ (HPyV6 antisense), 5′-CTCTCCTCTGTCTGAAGTGAACTC-TAA-3′ (HPyV6 probe), 5′-GTGCTGATATGGTTGGAA-3′ (HPyV7 sense), 5′-TCTGCAGTGGACTCTAAA-3′ (HPyV7 antisense), 5′-AGCCTGTACTGTTCTCTGGTTACT-3′ (HPyV7 probe). Input cell equivalents were determined by normalization to beta-globin.

All DNA extractions and PCRs for both HPV and HPyV were performed using standard operating procedures designed to reduce the possibility of contamination (Harwood et al., 1999). DNA extraction, water and buffer PCR controls were used to exclude contamination and these were consistently negative.

Immunohistochemistry

Immunofluorescence analysis was carried out using polyclonal antibodies raised against the E4 proteins of HPV 5, 8, and 23 (beta-PV types), or the E4 protein of HPV2 and 57 (alpha-PV types) using the protocols previously described (Griffin and Doorbar, 2016). In the double staining experiments, a monoclonal antibody (8H3) prepared against the HPV 8 E4 protein was used in place of the beta-PV E4 polyclonal antibodies. Polyclonal and monoclonal antibodies were prepared against GST-E4 fusion proteins (Doorbar et al., 1997; Borgogna et al., 2012). Techniques for the overlay of fluorescence staining patterns onto the hematoxylin and eosin sections have been described previously (Griffin et al., 2015). All tissue sections were formalin fixed prior to staining. Sections were counterstained with DAPI to visualize cell nuclei.

SNP Array Analysis of Gross Chromosomal Aberrations

Cutaneous squamous cell carcinoma and paired venous blood DNA samples were subjected to the GeneChip Genome-Wide Human SNP Array 6.0 assay (Affymetrix Inc., Santa Clara, CA, United States) according to the manufacturer's protocol. Processing was performed as previously described (Teh et al., 2005) using the Genome Oriented Laboratory File (GOLF) system for the analysis and display of single nucleotide polymorphism (SNP) signal data. Copy number profiles of vemurafenib-associated cSCC were compared with those observed in a previous study of sporadic cSCC (Purdie et al., 2009).

Genetic Mutational Analysis

Targeted genetic analysis of all samples was undertaken using 454 pyrosequencing performed using the GS Junior system (Roche/454 Life Sciences, Branford, CT, United States) and Fluidigm (Fluidigm Corporation, San Francisco, CA, United States) PCR amplicon libraries as template. In addition to *H, K,* and *NRAS,* we also analyzed the genes *NOTCH1, NOTCH2, TP53, CDKN2A, CARD11, CREBBP, TGFBR1,* and *2,* all of which our previous research has implicated in the pathogenesis of cSCC (Brown et al., 2004; South et al., 2014; Cammareri et al., 2016; Watt et al., 2015, 2016). Primers were designed and validated by Fluidigm (Fluidigm Corporation, San Francisco, CA, United States) as per recommended guidelines for Roche Titanium sequencing (Roche, Mannheim, Germany). Variant detection required a minimum of four supporting reads and a minimum variant allele frequency threshold of 0.1. Detailed genetic analysis of these samples has previously been reported (South et al., 2014; Cammareri et al., 2016).

Ethical Approval

This study was carried out in accordance with the recommendations of East London and City Health Authority local ethics committee. The protocol was approved by the East London and City Health Authority local ethics committee. All subjects gave written informed consent in accordance with the Declaration of Helsinki.

RESULTS

Patients

A total of seven patients with 45 skin lesions were recruited (**Figures 1, 2** and **Table 1**). They included 4 men (mean age 61.25 years, range 35–87 years) and 3 women (mean age 56.3 years, range 33–82 years). All patients had metastatic melanoma with V600E BRAF mutations. All were treated in 2012–2013 with single agent vemurafenib. For all patients, samples were collected at first presentation with skin lesions after starting vemurafenib. The mean time to either disease progression (n = 3 patients) or death from melanoma whilst receiving vemurafenib (n = 4 patients) was 7.7 months (range 3–17 months).

Samples (Table 1)

Samples consisted of 12 SCC, 19 VW, 2 actinic keratoses (AK), one melanocytic lesion and 6 non-lesional skin samples (3 normal skin and 3 normal skin perilesional to cSCC), 4 verrucous keratoses (VK – squamous papillomas, some with viral features but without evidence of dysplasia) and one squamoproliferative (SP) lesion with viral features and dysplasia but no clear invasion (SP). Lesions were from both chronically sun-exposed (SE) and non-chronically sun-exposed (NSE) sites. SE sites included head and neck, arms, and lower legs in females. NSE included all other sun-protected sites. Lesions from SE sites included 6/12 (50%) cSCCs, 5/5 VKs, 9/19 (47%) VWs, and 1/2 AKs. The normal skin samples comprised 2 SE, one NSE and 3 perilesional to SCCs on SE sites.

The mean time to development of biopsy-proven lesions after initiation of vemurafenib was 8.75 weeks for AK (range 6–11.25), 9.7 weeks for VK/SP (range 8–12), 9.9 weeks for VW (range 6–13), and 11.25 weeks for cSCC (range 8–16 weeks). For 2 patients, additional samples were collected at more than one further time point: for patient 1, samples were collected at 9, 13, 14, 18, and 34 weeks; for patient 2, at 9 and 28 weeks.

Histopathology

Significant histological features of viral infection (i.e., koilocytosis and at least three of acanthosis, hypergranulosis, parakeratosis, hyperkeratosis or typical papillomatous architecture) were seen in all VW and AKs, 10/12 (83%) SCC, but no normal skin or VK samples (**Figure 3** and **Table 1**).

Detection of Human Papillomavirus and Human Polyomaviruses

Human Papillomavirus Detection

Human papillomavirus DNA was detected in 18/19 (95%) VW, 9/12 (75%) SCC, 2/2 AK, 4/5 (80%) VK/SPs, and 3/6 (50%) normal skin samples (**Table 1**). HPV positivity was significantly higher in VW compared to normal skin (Fisher's exact test: p = 0.0312,) but not in cSCC (Fisher's exact test: p = 0.344). Multiple HPV types were detected in 28/37 (76%) of HPV positive samples, with a median number of 4 in VW and 3 in SCC compared with 0.5 in normal skin (two-sided Mann–Whitney U-test: p = 0.007 for VW and 0.13 for SCC).

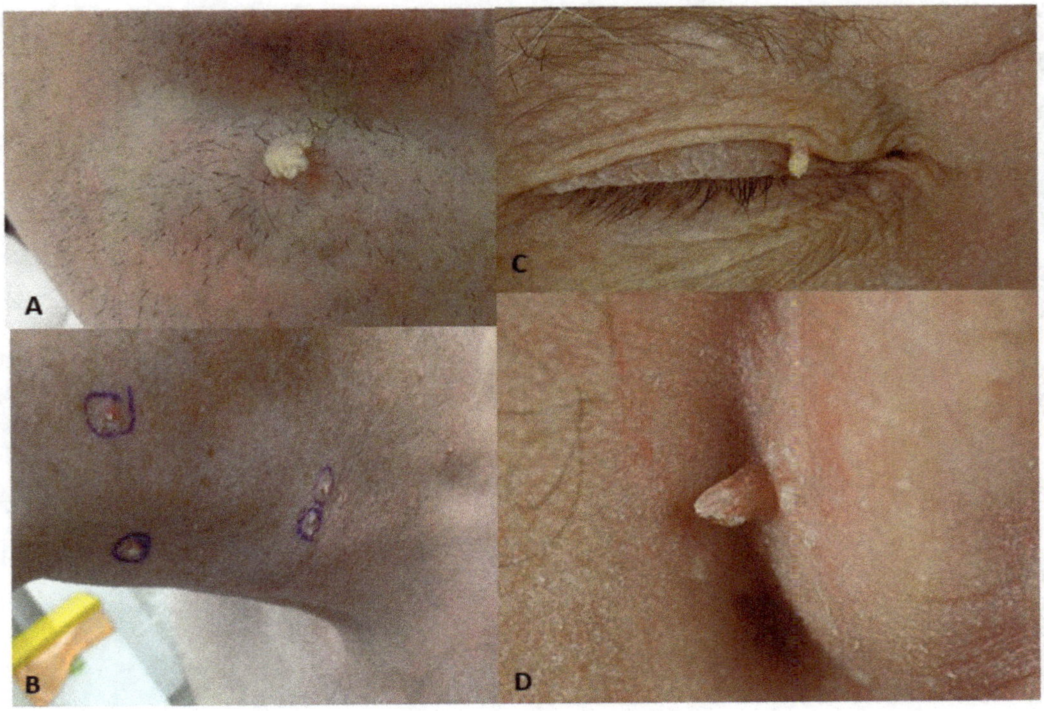

FIGURE 1 | Viral-wart like lesions developing after BRAFi exposure. **(A)** Lesion V10, viral wart on chin of patient 2; **(B)** Viral warts on the neck and chin of patient 1; **(C)** Viral wart on the eyelid of patient 5; **(D)** Lesion V22, post-auricular viral wart in patient 3.

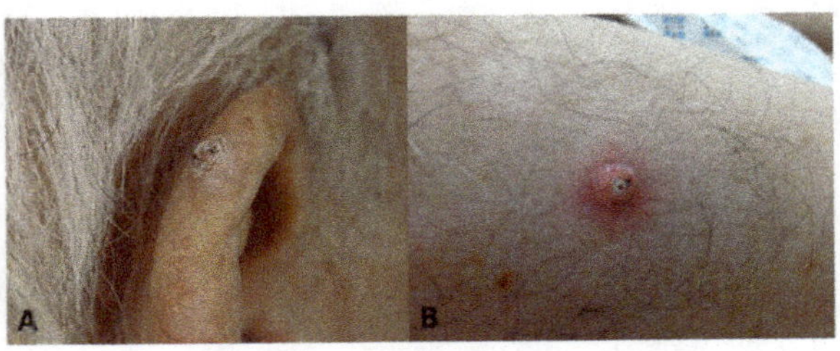

FIGURE 2 | Cutaneous squamous cell carcinomas developing after BRAFi exposure. **(A)** Well-differentiated SCC on the ear of patient 1; **(B)** Lesion V4, well-differentiated SCC on the arm of patient 1.

Cutaneous beta-PV were detected in all HPV positive lesions, with HPV-8, 12, 24, 36, and 92 the most frequent types. Alpha genus HPV types (alpha-PV) were found VW only (4/19, 21%) and were mucocutaneous alpha-PVs (HPV28 and HPV57), but not low or high-risk mucosal alpha-PVs. One cSCC contained a gamma HPV type. Although the RHA detection methodology used for beta and alpha-PV detection is not strictly quantitative, band intensity provides a surrogate read-out for predicted viral load. Analysis of these data suggested that the majority of HPV positive samples were likely to be associated with low viral load: the bands identified were faint or very faint in all cases, with the exception of samples V10, V18, V20, V29, V44 in which strongly positive bands were obtained for HPV types 57, 12, and 80. Four of these five lesions were VWs.

In all patients except one, multiple lesions were analyzed. Clear patterns of HPV carriage for each individual emerged. For example, beta-PVs 8, 12, 24, 36, 92, 93, and 111 were detected in patient 1 across both benign and malignant lesions at different body sites; this patient's normal, non-sun exposed skin sample also harbored HPV92 in addition to HPV5. Patient 2 had a spectrum of HPV types (HPV8, 12, 76, 80, and 57) that were concordant in VW at two separate body sites. Three other patients with more than one HPV positive lesion also had similar individual repertoires of HPV types across at least 2 lesions (patient 3, HPVs 22, 107; patient 4, HPV9; patient 7, HPV80). In the case of patient 6, all samples were negative, including two normal skin samples.

Only a minority of the 36 lesions with significant viral features on histological assessment had high levels of HPV DNA indicative of active infection. However, the 9 samples with no histological evidence of viral change (one cSCC, 2 VKs and 6 normal/perilesional skin samples) had significantly fewer HPV types detected compared to lesions with histological evidence of viral change (2-tailed Mann–Whitney U-test: $p = 0.0114$).

Immunohistochemistry was used to further investigate HPV DNA detection in a subset of 12 lesions. Although all had been HPV positive with multiple types detected, HPV protein expression was detected in only a single sample, a viral wart that had been strongly positive for both HPV57 and HPV80:

TABLE 1 | Clinical, histologic, viral, and genetic features of the seven patients and 45 lesions analyzed.

Pt	Sex/ age (years)	Lesion code	Weeks on BRAFi[1] (weeks)	Body site	SE/ NSE[2]	Diagnosis[3]	Viral features[4]	Mutations[5]	Beta-PV[6]	Alpha-PV	Gamma-PV	IHC[7]	HPyV6[8]	HPyV7[8]	HPyV9[8]	TSPyV[8]	MCPyV[8]
1	M/67	V1	9	Scalp	SE	VW	Y	NOTCH1, CREBBP	8, 9, 36, 38, 111	28		ND	7.5×10^{-6}	3.6×10^{-2}	Neg	Neg	1.7×10^{-2}
		V2	9	Suprapubic	NSE	V K	Y	NOTCH1, HRAS, CARD11	8, 24, 36, 92, 111			ND	ND	ND	ND	ND	ND
		V3	9	Post-auricular	SE	VW	Y	TGFBR2, CDKN2a, CARD11, NOTCH2, CREBBP	8, 36			ND	ND	ND	ND	ND	ND
		V4	9	Arm	SE	SCC	Y	TGFBR1, NOTCH1, HRAS	8, 12, 24, 36, 111, FA51			ND	Neg	1.7×10^{-4}	Neg	Neg	4.6×10^{-2}
		V5	9	Inner Thigh	NSE	VW	Y	NOTCH1, NOTCH2, HRAS, CREBBP	8, 12, 36, 111			ND	2.9×10^{-4}	Neg	Neg	Neg	2.8×10^{-2}
		V6	9	Lower Back	NSE	SCC	Y	TP53, HRAS	12, 36, 92			ND	5.12×10^{-5}	1.3×10^{-1}	Neg	Neg	3.9×10^{-3}
		V7	9	Shoulder	NSE	SCC	Y	NOTCH1, TP53, TGFBR1, CREBBP	15, 24, 36, 76, 92, 107, FA84			Neg	Neg	3.9×10^{-5}	Neg	Neg	1.8×10^{-2}
		V8	9	Posterior neck	SE	VK	Y	NOTCH1, CARD11, TGFBR1	8, 24, 36, 93			Neg	4.6×10^{-5}	4.8×10^{-4}	Neg	Neg	2.3×10^{-1}
		V9	9	Cheek	SE	VW	Y	HRAS, TP53*, NOTCH1,* NOTCH2*	8, 12, 24, 36, 76, 92 93	28		ND	ND	ND	ND	ND	ND
		V11	13	Scalp	SE	VW	Y	NOTCH1, TGFBR2, CARD11, CREBBP	8,23, 36, 92, 93			Neg	Neg	2.2×10^{-4}	Neg	Neg	1×10^{-1}
		V12	13	Abdomen	NSE	N-NSE	N	NOTCH1	5, 92			ND	ND	ND	ND	ND	ND
		V13	13	Lower back	NSE	SCC	Y	Nil	8, 24, 92, 107, 111, FA14			Neg	3.9×10^{-5}	2.4×10^{-4}	Neg	Neg	5.9×10^{-3}
		V14	13	Popliteal Fossa	NSE	VW	Y	NOTCH1, CREBBP	12, 24, 36			ND	Neg	1.3×10^{-2}	Neg	Neg	1.7×10^{-3}
		V15	13	Post-auricular	SE	VW	Y	CARD11	93			ND	Neg	1.6×10^{-3}	Neg	Neg	5.6×10^{-2}
		V16	13	Abdomen	NSE	VW	Y	TP53, HRAS	8, 36, 92, 93			ND	Neg	$6, \times 10^{-4}$	Neg	Neg	9.9×10^{-3}

(Continued)

TABLE 1 | Continued

Pt	Sex/ age (years)	Lesion code	Weeks on BRAFi[1] (weeks)	Body site	SE/ NSE[2]	Diagnosis[3]	Viral features[4]	Mutations[5]	Beta-PV[6]	Alpha-PV	Gamma-PV	IHC[7]	HPyV6[8]	HPyV7[8]	HPyV9[8]	TSPyV[8]	MCPyV[8]
		V17	13	Abdomen	NSE	VW	Y	NOTCH1, CDKN2a	8, 36, 92, 113			ND	Neg	1.4×10^{-1}	Neg	Neg	6.2×10^{-4}
		V18	14	Chest	NSE	VW	Y	NOTCH1, HRAS, KRAS	8**, 12, 24, 76, 92**, 111			Neg	1.12×10^{-5}	$5, \times 10^{-5}$	Neg	Neg	5.8×10^{-3}
		V19	14	Groin	NSE	SCC	Y	HRAS, NOTCH1	8, 12, 24, 36, 92			Neg	3.93×10^{-6}	1.4×10^{-4}	Neg	Neg	3.6×10^{-3}
		V20	14	Chest	SE	SCC	Y	Nil	8, 12, 24, 92**, 93			Neg	1.29×10^{-5}	2.4×10^{-4}	Neg	Neg	1.2×10^{-2}
		V25	18	Arm	SE	N-P V27	N	NOTCH1	Neg			ND	ND	ND	ND	ND	ND
		V26	18	Abdomen	NSE	VW	Y	CARD11, NOTCH1, HRAS, CREBBP	8, 92			Neg	Neg	5.9×10^{-5}	Neg	Neg	5.3×10^{-3}
		V27	18	Upper arm	SE	SCC	Y	HRAS, CARD11, CREBBP, NOTCH1 NOTCH2* KRAS* TP53*	Novel			Neg	Neg	Neg	Neg	Neg	Neg
		V28	18	Lower abdomen	NSE	SCC	Y	NOTCH2, NOTCH1*	Neg			Neg	ND	ND	ND	ND	ND
		V31	34	Cheek	SE	VK	N	Nil	Novel			ND	3.66×10^{-6}	2.4×10^{-4}	Neg	Neg	7.6×10^{-3}
		V32	34	Upper Arm	SE	VW	Y	NOTCH1, NOTCH2, HRAS, CREBBP, TP53*	24**, 36, 92, 93			ND	ND	ND	ND	ND	ND
2	M/35	V10	13	Chin	SE	VW	Y	Nil	8, 12, 80**, 76	57**		57, beta	ND	ND	ND	ND	ND
		V29	28	Scapula	NSE	VW	Y	NOTCH2, CREBBP	12**, 8, 20, 23, 36,76, 80, 92, 90	57		ND	ND	D	ND	ND	ND
3	M/56	V21	8	Neck	SE	VK	N	HRAS, CARD11, NOTCH1 * NOTCH2*	22, 115, 150			ND	3.73×10^{-5}	6.4×10^{-5}	Neg	Neg	Neg
		V22	14	Post-auricular	SE	VW	Y	TGFBR1, HRAS NOTCH2*	22, 107			ND	ND	ND	ND	ND	ND
		V23	14	Upper arm	SE	SCC	Y	CREBBP, CARD11, TGFBR1, NOTCH2*	2, 14D, 22, 38, 107, 115			Neg	Neg	Neg	Neg	Neg	1.3×10^{-4}
		V24	14	Upper Arm	SE	N-P to V23	N	NOTCH1	Novel			ND	ND	ND	ND	ND	ND

(Continued)

TABLE 1 | Continued

Pt	Sex/ age (years)	Lesion code	Weeks on BRAFi[1] (weeks)	Body site	SE/ NSE[2]	Diagnosis[3]	Viral features[4]	Mutations[5]	Beta-PV[6]	Alpha-PV	Gamma -PV	IHC[7]	HPyV6[8]	HPyV7[8]	HPyV9[8]	TSPyV[8]	MCPyV[8]
4	F/33	V30	16	Abdomen	NSE	SCC	N	TP53, HRAS, NOTCH1* NOTCH2*	Neg		FA49	ND	Neg	Neg	Neg	Neg	Neg
5	M/87	V33	6	Ear	SE	VW	Y	NOTCH1, TP53	9			ND	Neg	Neg	Neg	Neg	Neg
		V34	6	Chin	SE	AK	Y	Nil	9, 38			ND	Neg	1.5×10^{-5}	Neg	Neg	Neg
6	F/82	V35	12	Neck	SE	SCC	Y	TGFBR1, TGFBR2, NOTCH1, TP53, KRAS, NOTCH2, CARD11, CREBBP	Neg			ND	Neg	Neg	Neg	Neg	Neg
		V36	12	Neck	SE	N-P V35	N	Nil	Neg			ND	ND	ND	ND	ND	ND
		V37	12	Neck	SE	N -SE	N	NOTCH1, CARD11	Neg			ND	ND	ND	ND	ND	ND
		V38	12	Shoulder	NSE	VW	Y	TGFBR1, TGFBR2, TP53, KRAS, NRAS, CARD11, CREBBP	Neg			ND	ND	ND	ND	ND	ND
		V39	12	Lower Leg	SE	SP	Y	TGFBR1, NOTCH1, NOTCH2,, TP53, CREBBP	Neg			ND	Neg	Neg	Neg	Neg	1.5×10^{-3}
		V40	12	Arm	SE	SCC	Y	TGFBR2, CREBBP	Neg			ND	Neg	Neg	4×10^{-4}	Neg	2.9×10^{-3}
7	F/54	V41	11.5	Neck	SE	N-SE	N	NOTCH2, CREBBP	Novel			ND	ND	ND	ND	ND	ND
		V42	11.5	Back	NSE	VW	Y	TP53	80			ND	Neg	Neg	Neg	Neg	Neg
		V43	11.5	Back	NSE	M		NOTCH1, NOTCH2, NRAS, CARD11, CREBBP	80			ND	Neg	Neg	Neg	Neg	9×10^{-4}
		V44	11.5	Back	NSE	VW	Y	CARD11	80**			ND	Neg	Neg	Neg	Neg	Neg
		V45	11.5	Back	NSE	AK	Y	NOTCH1, TP53	80			ND	Neg	Neg	Neg	Neg	1.4×10^{-4}

[1]*Weeks on BRAFi: number of weeks on vemurafenib at the time lesion was removed.* [2]*SE/NSE: Sun exposed or non-sun exposed body site.* [3]*Diagnosis: SCC – well differentiated SCC; V, viral wart; VK, verrucous keratosis; AK, actinic keratosis; N-P, normal skin perilesional to; N-SE, normal skin sun exposed; N-NSE – normal skin non sun exposed; M, benign melanocytic; SP, squamoproliferative lesion with viral features and dysplasia but no clear evidence of invasion.* [4]*Viral features: Y, yes; N, no: yes if koilocytosis was observed in conjunction with at least 3 of the following 5 features: acanthosis, hypergranulosis, parakeratosis, hyperkeratosis and typical papillomatous architecture.* [5]*Mutations: these have previously been published (South, 2014; Cammareri, 2016). * indicates lesion bisected and results represent total mutations found across both portions.* [6]*Beta-PV: beta HPV types. Beta-PV types associated with strong bands on the RH assay are recorded as **; neg, negative.* [7] *IHC; immunohistochemistry – performed on 12 selected lesions.* [8]*HPyV6, -7, -9, TSPyV and MCPyV: neg, negative; N/D, not done; values recorded are viral copies per cell.*

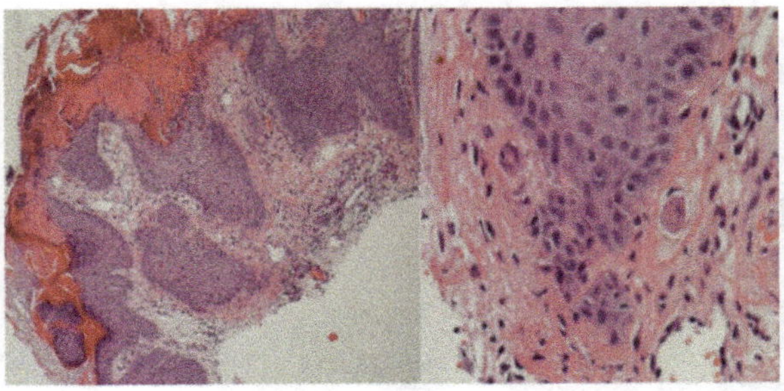

FIGURE 3 | Histology of lesion V4: Micro invasion in an SCC from patient 1 with features of viral infection in overlying and adjacent epidermis.

both HPV57 and beta-PV were detected, but were expressed in spatially distinct cells within the lesion (**Figure 4**).

Human Polyomavirus Detection

Thirty lesional samples from 5 individuals were tested for the presence of HPyV (VW, n = 12; SCC, n = 11; VK/SP, n = 4; AK, n = 2; melanocytic, n = 1). Normal skin was not examined. The majority of samples were positive for at least one HPyV, albeit at low levels and independent of the presence or absence of significant histological viral features (**Table 1**). Individual HPyV positivity ranged from 0% positivity for TSPyV; 3.3% for HPyV9 (SCC, n = 1); 33% for HPyV6 (VW, n = 3, 25%; SCC, n = 4, 36%; VK, n = 3, 36%); 60% for HPyV7 (VW, n = 8, 67%; SCC, n = 6, 54%; VK, n = 3, 25%; AK, n = 1, 50%) to 73% positivity for MCPyV (VW, n = 9, 75%; SCC, n = 8, 73%; VK, n = 3, 75%; AK, n = 1, 50%; melanocytic, n = 1, 100%). For all viruses, the difference in positivity between BRAFi-cSCC and VW was not significant (Fisher's exact test: $p = 1$ for HPyV9, HPyV6, MCPyV; $p = 0.68$ for HPyV7). Viral loads were generally less than one copy per thousand cells. The exceptions were four HPyV7-positive benign samples with viral loads ranging from 1 copy per 100 cells to one copy per seven cells and eight MCPyV-positive samples (two cSCC with viral loads of 2–5 copies per 100 cells and six benign lesions with viral loads from 1 copy per 100 cells to 1 copy per 4 cells).

Co-detection of HPV and HPyV

At least one HPV type and one HPyV type were co-detected in 22/30 (73%) of lesions. There was no significant correlation between specific HPV and HPyV types. However, it was noteworthy that lesions from patient 6, which were all negative for HPV, were also largely negative for HPyV, despite having significant histological features of viral infection. Similarly, the cSCC for patient 4 was negative for all beta-PV and HPyV types tested.

Virus Status and Chromosomal Changes

In order to examine gross chromosomal aberrations in vemurafenib-associated sSCC, we analyzed six well-differentiated cSCC from patient 1 using SNP array analysis to determine the signal values in tumor and paired non-tumor DNA at 250,000 SNPs throughout the genome. A comparison of tumor: non-tumor signal value ratios from vemurafenib-associated cSCC plotted according to chromosomal position with those from sporadic well-differentiated SCC analyzed in a previous study (Purdie et al., 2009) revealed that the patterns of gross chromosomal aberrations were significantly different: none of these 6 cSCC had gross chromosomal aberrations and there were significantly fewer chromosomal changes compared with sporadic well differentiated SCC (**Figure 5**). There were no clear correlations with virus status identified.

Virus Status and Association With Specific Genetic Mutations

We have reported gene mutations identified by targeted sequencing in these 45 samples for *H, K* and *NRAS, NOTCH1 and 2, TP53, CDKN2A, CARD11, CREBBP, TGFBR1/2* and this has previously been presented in detail (South et al., 2014; Cammareri et al., 2016). In the current study we analyzed the association between these mutations and the presence of HPV and HPyV. HRAS mutations were identified in 5/12 (42%) SCC and 5/19 (31%) VW. Mutation did not correlate with sun-exposed sites or lesion type and no mutations were detected in normal skin samples (**Table 1**). There was no significant difference between HRAS mutated vs. HRAS wild type lesions and HPV or HPyV status. The same was true for virus status and mutations in each of the other genes examined. Although it was noteworthy that v35 – the most highly mutated SCC – was negative for all viruses tested, there was no evidence of a significant correlation between overall mutational burden and virus status.

Virus Status and Clinical Response to Vemurafenib

There was no clear evidence of a significant association between virus status of lesions tested and prognosis in terms of disease progression and death from melanoma (data not shown).

DISCUSSION

We report HPV and HPyV analysis of 45 benign and malignant BRAFi-induced skin lesions from 7 individuals, including BRAFi-SCC and correlate this with clinical, histologic and genetic features. A high proportion of BRAFi-cSCCs had histologic viral wart-like features on histology, consistent with virus-driven processes, and the majority were positive for beta-PV, HPyV7 and MCPyV, which were co-detected in 73% of lesions tested. HPyV6 was found in one third of cases, but HPyV9 and TSPyV were rarely detected. As expected from previous studies of normal skin and hair follicles (Harwood et al., 2004; Bouwes Bavinck et al., 2010, 2017; Proby et al., 2011), normal skin samples also harbored beta-PV, but the HPV burden of individual types detected was significantly fewer than in lesional skin. Histologic evidence of virus infection appeared to correlate with HPV burden. However, viral loads were low in the majority of lesions and validation by immunohistochemistry for HPV was negative in all but one of 12 cases. Gross chromosomal changes characterized by SNP arrays in BRAFi-cSCC indicated that these tumors have

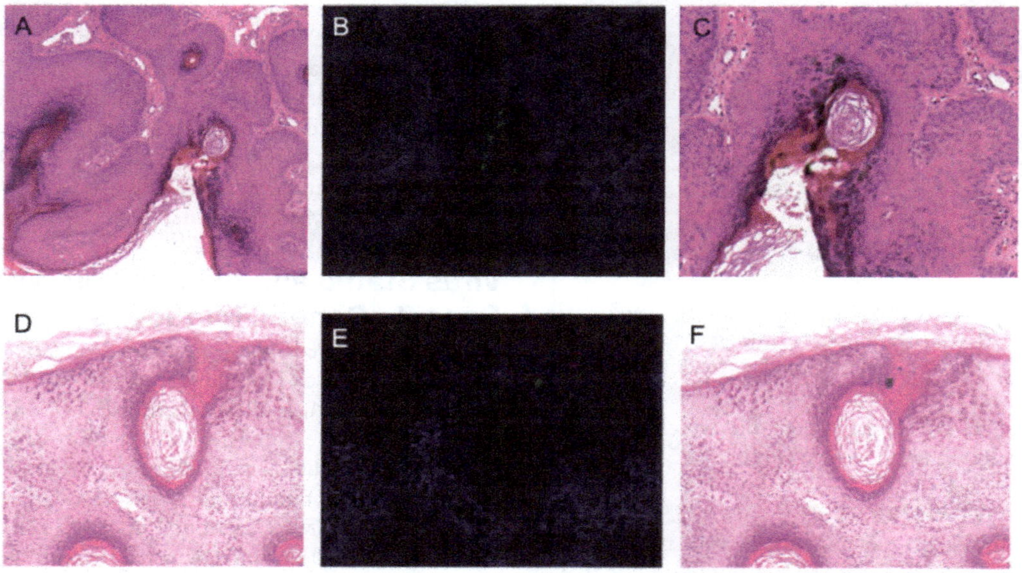

FIGURE 4 | Human papillomavirus immunohistochemistry. **(A,D)** Hematoxylin and eosin stained sections of 2 different areas of lesion V10 (strongly PCR positive for beta-PV types 8, 12, 76, 80, and alpha-PV 57); **(B,E)** double staining immunofluorescence with antibodies to the E4 protein of HPV8 (green) and HPV2/57 (red) **(C,F)** H&E stained sections overlaid with the images from immunofluorescence microscopy to identify cells with productive HPV infection.

significantly fewer chromosomal aberrations than non-BRAFi-cSCC, providing a further indication that additional cofactors may be involved. However, we were unable to establish clear correlations between the presence of either HPV or HPyV and specific genetic mutations or total mutational burden.

Human Papillomaviruses and BRAFi-cSCC

Human papillomaviruses has been investigated as a potential viral carcinogen in BRAFi-cSCC since these drugs were first approved in 2011/2012: the rapid onset of skin lesions, their clinical morphology and viral wart-like histology all point to a possible role for HPV (Boussemart et al., 2013). Initial studies designed to detect alpha-PV infection by immunohistochemistry reported negative results (Anforth et al., 2012; Chu et al., 2012; Ko et al., 2013). A surrogate for alpha-PV infection in mucosal sites is p16 immunoreactivity and in two studies the majority of BRAFi-cSCC were found to strongly express p16 (Anforth et al., 2012; Boussemart et al., 2013), but this is not a consistent finding (Frouin et al., 2014). Both approaches are less sensitive than PCR-based detection methodologies that have been used in other studies, although the latter are often limited by the use of formalin-fixed paraffin-embedded tissue (FFPE) and/or PCR primers detecting a limited range of HPV types. Using an alpha-PV specific PCR/line probe assay method, Dika et al failed to detect alpha-PV in 9 FFPE VK samples (Dika et al., 2015). Using the same assay together with a degenerate PCR methodology (FAP59/64) capable of detecting cutaneous HPV types, HPV was not detected in 8 BRAFi-cSCC/KA FFPE samples (Frouin et al., 2014). Holderfield et al used the FPA 59/64 primers and additional degenerate primers (CP65/CP70 and CP66/CP69) and found 2/13 (15%) FFPE BRAFi-cSCC (Holderfield et al., 2014). Schrama et al. (2014) used E1 primers originally tested for alpha-PV types but theoretically capable of detecting any HPV type; in FFPE samples from 14 cSCC, 3 KA and one acanthoma, all were HPV positive, although the specific types detected were not reported. Subsequently, Cohen et al. (2015) used the most comprehensive degenerate PCR-based methodology in 69 FFPE BRAFi-cSCC and found all samples to be positive with predominantly beta-PV types of which HPV-17, HPV-38 and HPV-111 were the most common. Falchook et al. (2016) found 6/12 (50%) FFPE BRAFi-cSCCs to be positive, almost exclusively with beta-PV types including 12, 17, 24, 47, 124 and novel types but, as in our study, HPV positivity was not significantly different when compared to normal skin. However, we found a significant difference in HPV burden between lesional and normal skin in terms of the numbers of HPV types detected and it is possible that the total burden of HPV types as well as the specific types detected is relevant to potential pathogenic processes.

Against the background of these previous studies, our HPV detection methodology has notable strengths, although the data are still limited by small sample size. We have used a more comprehensive and sensitive approach to detecting HPV from alpha, beta, mu, nu, gamma genera with RHA and degenerate PCR/sequencing. We have also used fresh frozen tissue samples in order to reduce the likelihood of false negative results, which may occur with use of FFPE-derived DNA. Laser capture micro dissection allowed enrichment for lesional tissue and reduces the possibility of contamination by virus carriage in non-lesional tissue. Neither strategy for optimizing viral detection has been used in these previous studies. In addition, we used

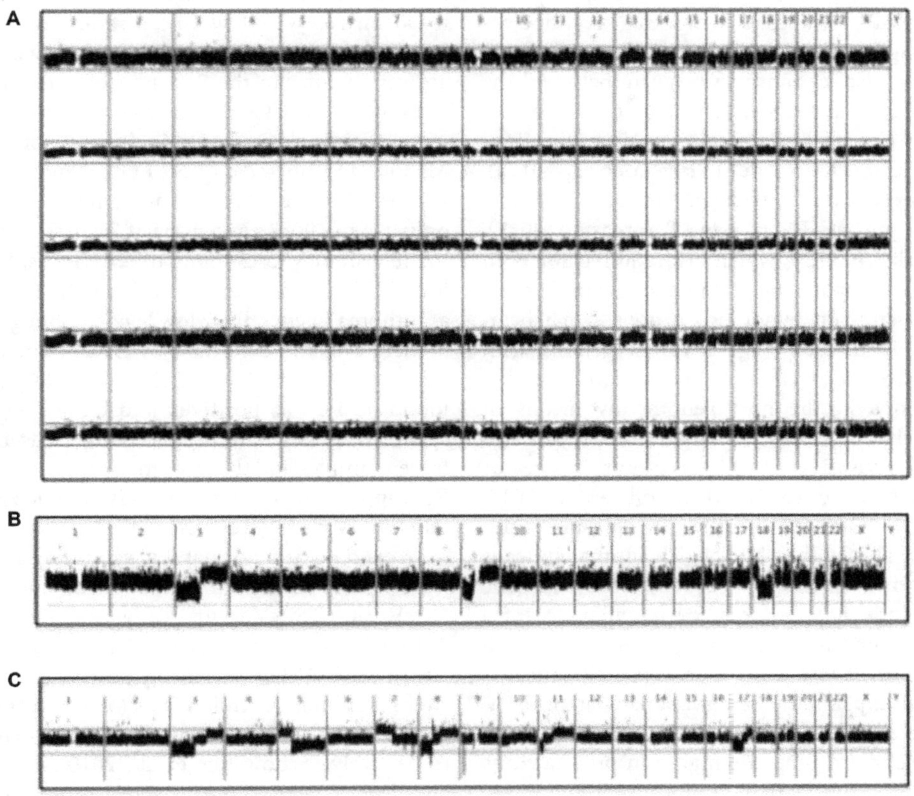

FIGURE 5 | SNP microarray analysis of vemurafenib-associated cSCC. BRAFi-SCC did not display the gross chromosomal aberrations typically observed in sporadic cSCC (Purdie et al., 2009). A running average of 2 consecutive tumor: non-tumor signal value ratios is plotted on a log2 scale according to chromosomal position. Upper line represents log2(2) and lower represents log2(0.5). **(A)** Copy number profiles of 5 vemurafenib-associated cSCC **(B)** Comparison with copy number profile from a sporadic cSCC showing 3p and 9p loss: these changes were characteristic of well-differentiated cSCC (Purdie et al., 2009). Although chromosome 18 loss is also seen in this particular tumor, chromosome 18 aberrations were not as common as 3p and 9p changes in other sporadic well-differentiated cSCC (Purdie et al., 2009). **(C)** More extensive allelic imbalance in a sporadic moderately-differentiated cSCC (Purdie et al., 2009).

immunohistochemistry to try and understand the nature and significance of multiple HPV detection using a double staining technique not used in previous studies of BRAFi lesions.

Our study was not designed to address the functional significance of HPV detection in BRAFi-associated squamoproliferative skin lesions. To date, this has been attempted in only a few other studies. Ganzenmueller et al. (2013) used next-generation sequencing to look for viral transcripts indicative of active HPV infection: none were identified in 4 BRAFi-associated VK. Although this small study arguably calls into question a role for HPV, it is important to note that BRAFi-cSCC were not examined and the presence of very low abundance transcripts cannot be entirely excluded. In a compelling experimental approach, exposure to vemurafenib in a transgenic murine model (K14-HPV16 mice) of alpha-PV-driven cSCC was associated with an upregulation of the MAPK pathway and an increase in cSCC incidence from 22 to 70%. More than half of these tumors were *RAS* wild type, suggesting that vemurafenib and HPV may be cooperating to promote tumorigenesis in both the presence and absence of RAS mutations (Holderfield et al., 2014). Data from a more recent beta-PV transgenic mouse model provides evidence of significant synergism between beta-PV, UV, and BRAFi (Viarisio et al., 2017a). The K14-HPV38 E6/E7 transgenic mouse expresses the beta-PV HPV38 E6 andE7 oncogenes in the basal layer of the epidermis under the control of the cytokeratin K14 promoter and requires UV exposure for AK and cSCC development (Viarisio et al., 2011). Vemurafenib increased the number and size of UV-induced cSCC. All BRAFi-treated transgenic mice developed cSCC by 34 weeks in contrast to none of the wild-type mice and only one-third of untreated transgenic mice. Ras mutations were not detected, but MAPK upregulation was evident in HPV38 E6/E7 over-expressing keratinocytes (Viarisio et al., 2017a).

The mechanisms responsible for the synergism between HPV and BRAFi are speculative. However, experimental data indicate that upregulation of the MAPK pathway enhances alpha-PV replication, stability, and infectivity (Wang et al., 2009; Bowser et al., 2011). If this is also the case for other HPV types, then it is possible that BRAFi-induced paradoxical upregulation of MAPK in the keratinocytes of normal skin – which is likely to harbor beta-PV HPV (Harwood et al., 2004; Bouwes Bavinck et al., 2010, 2017; Proby et al., 2011) – also leads to enhanced replication and stability of these beta-PV. The resulting increased beta-PV viral load in normal keratinocytes may drive not only benign squamoproliferative lesions associated with BRAFi, but may also enhance synergism between the oncogenic effects of beta-PV and UV, independent of RAS status, which ultimately leads to increased carcinogenesis in the K14-HPV38-E6/7 transgenic murine model (Viarisio et al., 2017a). Consistent with this, experimental evidence increasingly points to a "hit and run" role for beta-PV in skin (Tommasino, 2017). In contrast to high-risk alpha-PV which are required for both initiation and maintenance of a malignant phenotype in mucosal carcinogenesis, the hit-and-run hypothesis proposes that beta-PVs are required only at an early stage of carcinogenesis, with beta-PV E6 and E7 oncogenes facilitating accumulation of UV-induced DNA mutations in the host genome by means of multiple mechanisms that, for example, target DNA repair and apoptosis leading to inactivation of cellular tumor suppressor proteins or activation of oncoproteins (Connolly et al., 2014; Howley and Pfister, 2015; Quint et al., 2015; Tommasino, 2017; Viarisio et al., 2017b). This is the "hit," which ultimately leads to cellular transformation (Viarisio et al., 2017b). Viral oncogene expression is subsequently not required for maintenance of a malignant phenotype, rendering the viral genome dispensible and without consequence if lost from an established cancer – the "run." This would explain the observations that beta-PV DNA loads are always significantly less than one viral genome copy per cell in cSCC and are generally higher in precancerous AK (Weissenborn et al., 2005), that viral transciptomes are absent from BRAFi and non-BRAFi-cSCC (Arron et al., 2011; Ganzenmueller et al., 2013), and are supported by together with findings in the recent murine K14-HPV38E6/7 transgenic models (Viarisio et al., 2018). However, although biologically plausible, this hypothesis remains to be definitively confirmed in human studies.

Such a hit-and-run role for beta-PV may also potentiate the deleterious effects of cSCC cofactors such as immune suppression and contribute to the higher susceptibility to cSCC of immune suppressed individuals such as solid organ transplant recipients (Harwood et al., 2017). We and others have previously shown that beta-PV carriage is significantly more common in the normal skin and hair follicles of immune suppressed individuals (Weissenborn et al., 2012) and, particularly in the presence of concordant beta-PV seropositivity, is associated with cSCC risk in both OTR (Proby et al., 2011; Bouwes Bavinck et al., 2017) and immunocompetent individuals (Bouwes Bavinck et al., 2010; Chahoud et al., 2016). Although detailed comparison of virus status in BRAFi- and non-BRAFi-associated cSCC might provide insight into the effects of BRAFi on the biological activity of beta-PV in skin, the small numbers of published studies in BRAFi-cSCC and the wide variations in HPV analyses used in these studies limit the power of such an analysis.

Human Polyomaviruses and BRAFi-cSCC

We detected HPyV6 in one third of all 30 lesions tested, HPyV7 in 60% and MCPyV in 73%, with no significant differences seen between benign and malignant lesions. In most cases the loads for all viruses were low. In our series HPyV9 was negative in all cases and TSPyV positive in just one cSCC. Our data for MCPyV are very similar to the 72% positivity reported in a series of 18 FFPE BRAFi-cSCCs (Schrama et al., 2014) and 75% of 12 BRAFi-cSCC (Falchook et al., 2016). In contrast, Cohen et al detected MCPyV in only 22% of 58 FFPE benign and malignant FFPE lesions (Cohen et al., 2015) and a fourth study found MCPyV in only two of 19 VKs and none of 7 cSCCs (Frouin et al., 2014). Of the few studies to examine other HPyVs, Schrama et al. (2014) found HPyV6 and 7 in all FFPE samples (14 cSCC, 3 KA, and one acanthoma), generally at low levels, although HPyV6 was present at high level and detectable by IHC in one cSCC. In contrast, in FFPE samples of 19 VKs, 1KA and 7 cSCC, Frouin et al. (2014) found no HPyV6 positivity and HPyV7 in one VK only. Once again, in all previous studies samples were FFPE rather than frozen samples and this, together with the tumor enrichment and PCR approaches used in our study, may account for some of these differences in HPyV detection.

We did not test normal skin samples, but MCPyV, HPyV6 and 7 are well-established members of the normal skin virome, with HPyV9 and TSPyV significantly less common (Schowalter et al., 2010; Foulongne et al., 2012; Kazem et al., 2012; Wieland et al., 2014). MCPyV has previously been detected in 40–62% of skin swabs from normal individuals (Wieland et al., 2009; Schowalter et al., 2010) and HPyV6 and 7 have been detected in 14 and 11%, respectively (Schowalter et al., 2010). In comparison, HPyV9 and TSPyV were found in skin swabs from only 1/111 (0.9%) and 6/249 (2%) healthy individuals, respectively (Sauvage et al., 2011; Kazem et al., 2012). A previous study analyzed MCPyV in 9 FFPE normal skin biopsies from patients with BRAFi-associated proliferative skin lesions and found all to be negative, whereas 5/9 (56%) were positive for HPV of predominantly beta-PV types (Falchook et al., 2016). A case report by the same authors also failed to detect MCPyV in a normal skin of a patient with BRAFi-cSCC (Falchook et al., 2013). Other HPyV have not been analyzed in normal skin from BRAFi-exposed individuals. These data provide a possible signal that HPyV6 and 7 are overrepresented in BRAFi-cSCC, with our findings of 36 and 54% positivity, respectively. However, as normal skin is frequently positive for MCPyV, our findings in BRAFi-cSCC are less convincing. However, this interpretation is speculative and needs to be confirmed in future studies that specifically include matched normal skin samples from BRAFi-exposed individuals.

To date, there have been no functional studies specifically addressing the role of HPyVs in BRAFi-cSCC. The oncogenic potential of MCPyV is well established in MCC (Church and Nghiem, 2015; Paulson et al., 2017) and it is plausible that the large and small T-antigen oncoproteins may be relevant in BRAFi-cSCC. To date, none of the 12 other HPyVs have been implicated in causing cancer (Church and Nghiem, 2015). However, recent *in vitro* studies have indicated that MCPyV, HPyV6, and TSPyV can all induce cellular MAPK pathways (Wu et al., 2016, 2017a,b). It is therefore, plausible that such activity may act synergistically with BRAFi-induced MAPK upregulation and contribute to driving squamoproliferative lesions.

Co-detection of HPV and HPyV

Human papillomavirus and HPyV were co-detected in the majority of virus positive lesions, usually at low copy number. There were no clear associations of specific types, although beta-PVs and MCPyV were most commonly co-detected, as previously reported (Falchook et al., 2013, 2016; Cohen et al., 2015). Our interpretation of these data is limited by the fact we have only examined normal skin for HPVs and not for HPyVs. However, co-detection of these potentially oncogenic viruses in BRAFi-cSCC remains an important observation. Although it is not possible from these data to conclude whether one virus type is biologically more relevant than another in either driving the virus features seen histologically, the potential for their interaction in playing an oncogenic role merits further functional investigation. In particular, it is plausible that the ability of HPyV to upregulate MAPK and the effects of MAPK upregulation on HPV replication, infectivity and stability may act synergistically in enhancing the oncogenic potential of both in contributing to the pathogenesis of BRAFi-associated squamoproliferative lesions.

Virus Status and Genetic Alterations

We have previously used SNP array analysis to show that UV-associated well-differentiated cSCC have significantly different patterns of chromosomal aberrations compared with moderately and poorly differentiated cSCC (Purdie et al., 2009). Although BRAFi-cSCCs are histologically similar to well- differentiated sporadic cSCC, we have shown that they do not display the characteristic gross chromosomal aberrations typically associated with well-differentiated cSCC. This possibly reflects the shorter time course and more prominent role for MAPK upregulation induced by BRAFi, rather than through lifetime accumulated UVR-induced DNA damage, as seen in sporadic UV-associated cSCC (Lambert et al., 2014). Arguably, however, it also provides circumstantial evidence for alternative etiological agents such as oncogenic viruses.

At the individual gene level, as previously reported, we found a significantly higher level of HRAS mutations in BRAFi-cSCC compared with non-BRAFi-cSCC (South et al., 2014). In the current study, we specifically sought a possible association with virus status in HRAS mutated compared with HRAS wild type lesions. This may provide insights into the mechanisms underlying carcinogenesis in BRAFi-cSCC that are additional to mutant HRAS-associated upregulation of the MAPK pathway and, for example, related to viral oncogenes. However, no clear correlation emerged between virus and HRAS status. We also specifically looked for evidence of an inverse association between the detection of virus and mutational burden in terms of the numbers of mutated genes, as is seen in MCC (Harms et al., 2015; Wong et al., 2015; Goh et al., 2016; Becker et al., 2017; Starrett et al., 2017; Carter et al., 2018). Once again, no clear association emerged, although this study may have been underpowered to detect such an association.

CONCLUSION

Despite the suggestive clinical and histologic evidence, a compelling experimental murine model and genetic evidence that HRAS mutations are absent in a significant proportion of BRAFi-induced squamoproliferative skin lesions, the contribution of HPVs and HPyVs to the development of these lesions suggested by results from previous studies remains inconclusive. The data presented here provide further circumstantial evidence for a possible role for HPV and HPyV. They also point to possible synergistic interactions between these potentially oncogenic skin viruses. Given the major increase predicted in adjuvant use of these agents in the near future, further research into the role of these and possibly other existing or novel members of the human skin virome is justified and may provide insights into the pathogenesis of other BRAF-induced skin disorders and malignancies.

AUTHOR CONTRIBUTIONS

CH, KP, CP, and IL conceived and designed the study. CH, KP, HR, EM, MF, JD, HG, AS, GI, IL, and CP developed the methodology. CH, KP, HR, EM, MF, JD, HG, MS, GI, and AS acquired the data. CH, KP, HR, EM, MF, JD, HG, MS, AS, GI, and CP analyzed and interpreted the data. CH, KP, JD, MF, HR, IL, and CP wrote, reviewed, and revised the manuscript. CH, CP, and IL supervised the study.

REFERENCES

Anforth, R., Fernandez-Peñas, P., and Long, G. V. (2013). Cutaneous toxicities of RAF inhibitors. *Lancet Oncol.* 14:e11-8. doi: 10.1016/S1470-2045(12)70413-8

Anforth, R. M., Blumetti, T. C., Kefford, R. F., Sharma, R., Scolyer, R. A., Kossard, S., et al. (2012). Cutaneous manifestations of dabrafenib (GSK2118436): a selective inhibitor of mutant BRAF in patients with metastatic melanoma. *Br. J. Dermatol.* 167, 1153–1160. doi: 10.1111/j.1365-2133.2012.11155.x

Antonsson, A., Forslund, O., Ekberg, H., Sterner, G., and Hansson, B. G. (2000). The ubiquity and impressive genomic diversity of human skin papillomaviruses suggest a commensalic nature of these viruses. *J. Virol.* 74, 11636–11641. doi: 10.1128/JVI.74.24.11636-11641.2000

Arron, S. T., Ruby, J. G., Dybbro, E., Ganem, D., and Derisi, J. L. (2011). Transcriptome sequencing demonstrates that human papillomavirus is not active in cutaneous squamous cell carcinoma. *J. Invest. Dermatol.* 131, 1745–1753. doi: 10.1038/jid.2011.91

Becker, J. C., Stang, A., DeCaprio, J. A., Cerroni, L., Lebbé, C., Veness, M., et al. (2017). Merkel cell carcinoma. *Nat. Rev. Dis. Primers* 3:17077. doi: 10.1038/nrdp.2017.77

Blank, C. U., Larkin, J., Arance, A. M., Hauschild, A., Queirolo, P., Del Vecchio, M., et al. (2017). Open-label, multicentre safety study of vemurafenib in 3219 patients with BRAFV600 mutation-positive metastatic melanoma: 2-year follow-up data and long-term responders' analysis. *Eur. J. Cancer* 79, 176–184. doi: 10.1016/j.ejca.2017.04.007

Borgogna, C., Zavattaro, E., De Andrea, M., Griffin, H., Dell'Oste, V., Azzimonti, B., et al. (2012). Characterization of beta papillomavirus E4 expression in tumours from epidermodysplasia verruciformis patients and in experimental models. *Virology* 423, 195–204. doi: 10.1016/j.virol.2011.11.029

Boussemart, L., Routier, E., Mateus, C., Opletalova, K., Sebille, G., Kamsu-Kom, N., et al. (2013). Prospective study of cutaneous side-effects associated with the BRAF inhibitor vemurafenib: a study of 42 patients. *Ann. Oncol.* 24, 1691–1697. doi: 10.1093/annonc/mdt015

Bouwes Bavinck, J. N., Feltkamp, M. C. W., Green, A. C., Fiocco, M., Euvrard, S., Harwood, C. A., et al. (2017). Human papillomavirus and posttransplantation cutaneous squamous cell carcinoma: a multicenter, prospective cohort study. *Am. J. Transplant.* doi: 10.1111/ajt.14537 [Epub ahead of print].

Bouwes Bavinck, J. N., Neale, R. E., Abeni, D., Euvrard, S., Green, A. C., Harwood, C. A., et al. (2010). Multicenter study of the association between betapapillomavirus infection and cutaneous squamous cell carcinoma. *Cancer Res.* 70, 9777–9786. doi: 10.1158/0008-5472.CAN-10-0352

Bowser, B. S., Alam, S., and Meyers, C. (2011). Treatment of a human papillomavirus type 31b-positive cell line with benzo[a]pyrene increases viral titer through activation of the Erk1/2 signaling pathway. *J. Virol.* 85, 4982–4992. doi: 10.1128/JVI.00133-11

Brown, V. L., Harwood, C. A., Crook, T. Cronin, J. G., Kelsell, D. P., and Proby, C. M. (2004). p16INK4a and p14ARF tumor suppressor genes are commonly inactivated in cutaneous squamous cell carcinoma. *J. Invest. Dermatol.* 122, 1284–1292. doi: 10.1111/j.0022-202X.2004.22501.x

Calvignac-Spencer, S., Feltkamp, M. C. W., Daugherty, M. D., Moens, U., Ramqvist, T., Johne, R., et al. (2016). A taxonomy update for the family Polyomaviridae. *Arch. Virol.* 161, 1739–1750. doi: 10.1007/s00705-016-2794-y

Cammareri, P., Rose, A. M., Vincent, D. F., Wang, J., Nagano, A., Libertini, S., et al. (2016). Frequent loss of function mutations in TGFβR1 and TGFβ implicate hair follicle bulge stem cells as a cell of origin of cutaneous squamous cell carcinoma. *Nat. Commun.* 7:12493. doi: 10.1038/ncomms12493

Carter, M. D., Gaston, D., Huang, W. Y., Greer, W. L., Pasternak, S., Ly, T. Y., et al. (2018). Genetic profiles of different subsets of Merkel cell carcinoma show links between combined and pure MCPyV-negative tumors. *Hum. Pathol.* 117–125. doi: 10.1016/j.humpath.2017.10.014

Chahoud, J., Semaan, A., Chen, Y., Cao, M., Rieber, A. G., Rady, P., et al. (2016). Association between beta-genus human papillomavirus and cutaneous squamous cell carcinoma in immunocompetent individuals – a meta-analysis. *JAMA Dermatol.* 152, 1354–1364. doi: 10.1001/jamadermatol.2015.4530

Chapman, P. B., Robert, C., Larkin, J., Haanen, J. B., Ribas, A., Hogg, D., et al. (2017). Vemurafenib in patients with BRAFV600 mutation-positive metastatic melanoma: final overall survival results of the randomized BRIM-3 study. *Ann. Oncol.* 28, 2581–2587. doi: 10.1093/annonc/mdx339

Chu, E. Y., Wanat, K. A., Miller, C. J., Amaravadi, R. K., Fecher, L. A., Brose, M. S., et al. (2012). Diverse cutaneous side effects associated with BRAF inhibitor therapy: a clinicopathologic study. *J. Am. Acad. Dermatol.* 67, 1265–1272. doi: 10.1016/j.jaad.2012.04.008

Church, C. D., and Nghiem, P. (2015). How does the Merkel polyomavirus lead to a lethal cancer? Many answers, many questions, and a new mouse model. *J. Invest. Dermatol.* 135, 1221–1224. doi: 10.1038/jid.2015.4

Cohen, D. N., Lawson, S. K., Shaver, A. C., Du, L., Nguyen, H. P., He, Q., et al. (2015). Contribution of beta-HPV infection and UV damage to rapid-onset cutaneous squamous cell carcinoma during BRAF-inhibition therapy. *Clin. Cancer Res.* 21, 2624–2634. doi: 10.1158/1078-0432.CCR-14-2667

Connolly, K., Manders, P., Earls, P., and Epstein, R. J. (2014). Papillomavirus-associated squamous skin cancers following transplant immunosuppression: one Notch closer to control. *Cancer Treat. Rev.* 40, 205–214. doi: 10.1016/j.ctrv.2013.08.005

de Koning, M., Quint, W., Struijk, L., Kleter, B., Wanningen, P., van Doorn, L. J., et al. (2006). Evaluation of a novel highly sensitive, broad-spectrum PCR-reverse hybridization assay for detection and identification of beta-papillomavirus DNA. *J. Clin. Microbiol.* 44, 1792–1800. doi: 10.1128/JCM.44.5.1792-1800.2006

DeCaprio, J. A., and Garcea, R. L. (2013). A cornucopia of human polyomaviruses. *Nat. Rev. Microbiol.* 11, 264–276. doi: 10.1038/nrmicro2992

Dika, E., Patrizi, A., Venturoli, S., Fanti, P. A., Barbieri, D., Strammiello, R., et al. (2015). Human papillomavirus evaluation of vemurafenib induced skin epithelial tumors: a case series. Human papillomavirus evaluation of vemurafenib-induced skin epithelial tumors: a case series. *Br. J. Dermatol.* 172, 540–542. doi: 10.1111/bjd.13275

Doorbar, J. C., Foo, N., Coleman, E., Medcalf, O., Hartley, T., Prospero, S., et al. (1997). Characterization of events during the late stages of HPV16 infection in vivo using high affinity synthetic Fabs to E4. *Virology* 238, 40–52. doi: 10.1006/viro.1997.8768

Dummer, R., Tsao, H., and Robert, C. (2012). How cutaneous eruptions help to understand the mode of action of kinase inhibitors. *Br. J. Dermatol.* 167, 965–967. doi: 10.1111/bjd.12080

Dworkin, A. M., Tseng, S. Y., Allain, D. C., Iwenofu, O. H., Peters, S. B., and Toland, A. E. (2009). Merkel cell polyomavirus in cutaneous squamous cell carcinoma of immunocompetent individuals. *J. Invest. Dermatol.* 129, 2868–2874. doi: 10.1038/jid.2009.183

Falchook, G. S., Rady, P., Hymes, S., Nguyen, H. P., Tyring, S. K., Prieto, V. G., et al. (2013). Merkel cell polyomavirus and HPV-17 associated with cutaneous squamous cell carcinoma arising in a patient with melanoma treated with the BRAF inhibitor dabrafenib. *JAMA Dermatol.* 149, 322–326. doi: 10.1001/jamadermatol.2013.2023

Falchook, G. S., Rady, P., Konopinski, J. C., Busaidy, N., Hess, K., Hymes, S., et al. (2016). Merkel cell polyomavirus and human papilloma virus in proliferative skin lesions arising in patients treated with BRAF inhibitors. *Arch. Dermatol. Res.* 308, 357–365. doi: 10.1007/s00403-016-1650-y

Feltkamp, M. C., Kazem, S., van der Meijden, E., Lauber, C., and Gorbalenya, A. E. (2013). From Stockholm to Malawi: recent developments in studying human polyomaviruses. *J. Gen. Virol.* 94(Pt 3), 482–496. doi: 10.1099/vir.0.048462-0

Feng, H., Shuda, M., Chang, Y., and Moore, P. S. (2008). Clonal integration of a polyomavirus in human Merkel cell carcinoma. *Science* 319, 1096–1100. doi: 10.1126/science.1152586

Flaherty, K. T., Infante, J. R., Daud, A., Gonzalez, R., Kefford, R. F., Sosman, J., et al. (2012). Combined BRAF and MEK inhibition in melanoma with BRAF V600 mutations. *N. Engl. J. Med.* 367, 1694–703. doi: 10.1056/NEJMoa1210093

Flaherty, K. T., Puzanov, I., Kim, K. B., Ribas, A., McArthur, G. A., Sosman, J. A., et al. (2010). Inhibition of mutated, activated BRAF in metastatic melanoma. *N. Engl. J. Med.* 363, 809–819. doi: 10.1056/NEJMoa1002011

Forslund, O., Antonsson, A., Nordin, P., Stenquist, B., and Hansson, B. G. (1999). A broad range of human papillomavirus types detected with a general PCR method suitable for analysis of cutaneous tumours and normal skin. *J. Gen. Virol.* 80, 2437–2443. doi: 10.1099/0022-1317-80-9-2437

Foulongne, V., Sauvage, V., Hebert, C., Dereure, O., Cheval, J., Gouilh, M. A., et al. (2012). Human skin microbiota: high diversity of DNA viruses identified on the human skin by high throughput sequencing. *PLoS One* 7:e38499. doi: 10.1371/journal.pone.0038499

Frouin, E., Guillot, B., Larrieux, M., Tempier, A., Boulle, N., Foulongne, V., et al. (2014). Cutaneous epithelial tumors induced by vemurafenib involve the MAPK and Pi3KCA pathways but not HPV nor HPyV viral infection. *PLoS One* 9:e110478. doi: 10.1371/journal.pone.0110478

Ganzenmueller, T., Hage, E., Yakushko, Y., Kluba, J., Woltemate, S., Schacht, V., et al. (2013). No human virus sequences detected by next-generation sequencing in benign verrucous skin tumors occurring in BRAF-inhibitor-treated patients. *Exp. Dermatol.* 22, 725–729. doi: 10.1111/exd.12249

Gheit, T., Dutta, S., Oliver, J., Robitaille, A., Hampras, S., Combes, J. D., et al. (2017). Isolation and characterization of a novel putative human polyomavirus. *Virology* 506, 45–54. doi: 10.1016/j.virol.2017.03.007

Goh, G., Walradt, T., Markarov, V., Blom, A., Riaz, N., Doumani, R., et al. (2016). Mutational landscape of MCPyV-positive and MCPyV-negative Merkel cell carcinomas with implications for immunotherapy. *Oncotarget* 7, 3403–3415. doi: 10.18632/oncotarget.6494

Griffin, H., and Doorbar, J. (2016). Detection of papillomavirus gene expression patterns in tissue sections. *Curr. Protoc.* 41, 14B.7.1–14B.7.20. doi: 10.1002/cpmc.6

Griffin, H., Soneji, Y., Van Baars, R., Arora, R., Jenkins, D., van de Sandt, M., et al. (2015). Stratification of HPV-induced cervical pathology using the virally encoded molecular marker E4 in combination with p16 or MCM. *Mod. Pathol.* 28, 977–993. doi: 10.1038/modpathol.2015.52

Harms, P. W., Vats, P., Verhaegen, M. E., Robinson, D. R., Wu, Y. M., Dhanasekaran, S. M., et al. (2015). The distinctive mutational spectra of polyomavirus-negative merkel cell carcinoma. *Cancer Res.* 75, 3720–3727. doi: 10.1158/0008-5472.CAN-15-0702

Harwood, C. A., Spink, P. J., Surentheran, T., Leigh, I. M., de Villiers, E.-M., McGregor, J., et al. (1999). Degenerate and nested PCR: a highly sensitive and specific method for detection of human papillomavirus in cutaneous warts. *J. Clin. Microbiol.* 37, 3545–3555.

Harwood, C. A., Surentheran, T., Sasieni, P., Proby, C. M., Bordea, C., Leigh, I. M., et al. (2004). Increased risk of skin cancer associated with the presence of EV HPV types in normal skin. *Br. J. Dermatol.* 150, 949–952. doi: 10.1111/j.1365-2133.2004.05847.x

Harwood, C. A., Toland, A. E., Proby, C. M., Euvrard, S., Hofbauer, G. F. L., Tommasino, M., et al. (2017). The pathogenesis of cutaneous squamous cell carcinoma in organ transplant recipients. *Br. J. Dermatol.* 177, 1217–1224. doi: 10.1111/bjd.15956

Hassel, J. C., Groesser, L., Herschberger, E., Weichert, W., and Hafner, C. (2015). RAS mutations in benign epithelial tumors associated with BRAF inhibitor treatment of melanoma. *J. Invest. Dermatol.* 135, 636–639. doi: 10.1038/jid.2014.360

Hatzivassiliou, G., Song, K., Yen, I., Brandhuber, B. J., Anderson, D. J., Alvarado, R., et al. (2010). RAF inhibitors prime wild-type RAF to activate the MAPK pathway and enhance growth. *Nature* 464, 431–435. doi: 10.1038/nature08833

Heidorn, S. J., Milagre, C., Whittaker, S., Nourry, A., Niculescu-Duvas, I., Dhomen, N., et al. (2010). Kinase-dead BRAF and oncogenic RAS cooperate to drive tumor progression through CRAF. *Cell* 140, 209–221. doi: 10.1016/j.cell.2009.12.040

Holderfield, M., Lorenzana, E., Weisburd, B., Lomovasky, L., Boussemart, L., Lacroix, L., et al. (2014). Vemurafenib cooperates with HPV to promote initiation of cutaneous tumors. *Cancer Res.* 74, 2238–2245. doi: 10.1158/0008-5472.CAN-13-1065-T

Howley, P. M., and Pfister, H. J. (2015). Beta genus papillomaviruses and skin cancer. *Virology* 479–480, 290–296. doi: 10.1016/j.virol.2015.02.004

Kazem, S., van der Meijden, E., Kooijman, S., Rosenberg, A. S., Hughey, L. C., Browning, J. C., et al. (2012). *Trichodysplasia spinulosa* is characterized by active polyomavirus infection. *J. Clin. Virol.* 53, 225–230. doi: 10.1016/j.jcv.2011.11.007

Ko, C. J., McNiff, J. M., Iftner, A., Iftner, T., and Choi, J. N. (2013). Vemurafenib (PLX-4032)-induced keratoses: verrucous but not verrucae. *J. Am. Acad. Dermatol.* 69:e95-6. doi: 10.1016/j.jaad.2012.03.027

Lambert, S. R., Mladkova, N., Gulati, A., Hamoudi, R., Purdie, K., Cerio, R., et al. (2014). Key differences identified between actinic keratosis and cutaneous squamous cell carcinoma by transcriptome profiling. *Br. J. Cancer* 110, 520–529. doi: 10.1038/bjc.2013.760

Larkin, J., Ascierto, P. A., Dréno, B., Atkinson, V., Liszkay, G., Maio, M., et al. (2014). Combined vemurafenib and cobimetinib in BRAF-mutated melanoma. *N. Engl. J. Med.* 371, 1867–1876. doi: 10.1056/NEJMoa1408868

Long, G. V., Hauschild, A., Santinami, M., Atkinson, V., Mandalà, M., Chiarion-Sileni, V., et al. (2017). Adjuvant dabrafenib plus trametinib in stage III BRAF-mutated melanoma. *N. Engl. J. Med.* 377, 1813–1823. doi: 10.1056/NEJMoa1708539

Long, G. V., Menzies, A. M., Nagrial, A. M., Haydu, L. E., Hamilton, A. L., Mann, G. J., et al. (2011). Prognostic and clinicopathologic associations of oncogenic BRAF in metastatic melanoma. *J. Clin. Oncol.* 29, 1239–1246. doi: 10.1200/JCO.2010.32.4327

Maio, M., Lewis, K., Demidov, L., Mandalà, M., Bondarenko, I., Ascierto, P. A., et al. (2018). Adjuvant vemurafenib in resected, $BRAF^{V600}$ mutation-positive melanoma (BRIM8): a randomised, double-blind, placebo-controlled, multicentre, phase 3 trial. *Lancet Oncol.* 19, 510–520. doi: 10.1016/S1470-2045(18)30106-2

Nguyen, K. D., Lee, E. E., Yue, Y., Stork, J., Pock, L., North, J. P., et al. (2017). Human polyomavirus 6 and 7 are associated with pruritic and dyskeratotic dermatoses. *J. Am. Acad. Dermatol.* 76, 932–940.e3. doi: 10.1016/j.jaad.2016.11.035

Oberholzer, P. A., Kee, D., Dziunycz, P., Sucker, A., Kamsukom, N., Jones, R., et al. (2012). RAS mutations are associated with the development of cutaneous squamous cell tumors in patients treated with RAF inhibitors. *J. Clin. Oncol.* 30, 316–321. doi: 10.1200/JCO.2011.36.7680

Paulson, K. G., Lewis, C. W., Redman, M. W., Simonson, W. T., Lisberg, A., Ritter, D., et al. (2017). Viral oncoprotein antibodies as a marker for recurrence of Merkel cell carcinoma: a prospective validation study. *Cancer* 123, 1464–1474. doi: 10.1002/cncr.30475

Poulikakos, P. I., Zhang, C., Bollag, G., Shokat, K. M., and Rosen, N. (2010). RAF inhibitors transactivate RAF dimers and ERK signalling in cells with wild-type BRAF. *Nature* 464, 427–430. doi: 10.1038/nature08902

Proby, C. M., Harwood, C. A., Neale, R. E., Green, A. C., Euvrard, S., Naldi, L., et al. (2011). A case-control study of Betapapillomavirus infection and cutaneous squamous cell carcinoma in organ transplant recipients. *Am. J. Transplant.* 11, 1498–1508. doi: 10.1111/j.1600-6143.2011.03589.x

Purdie, K. J., Harwood, C. A., Gulati, A., Chaplin, T., Lambert, S. R., Cerio, et al. (2009). SNP array analysis defines a specific genetic fingerprint for well-differentiated SCC. *J. Invest. Dermatol.* 129, 1562–1568. doi: 10.1038/jid.2008.408

Quint, K. D., Genders, R. E., de Koning, M. N., Borgogna, C., Gariglio, M., Bouwes Bavinck, J. N., et al. (2015). Human Betapapillomavirus infection and keratinocyte carcinomas. *J. Pathol.* 235, 342–354. doi: 10.1002/path.4425

Ribas, A., and Flaherty, K. T. (2011). BRAF targeted therapy changes the treatment paradigm in melanoma. *Nat. Rev. Clin. Oncol.* 8, 426–433. doi: 10.1038/nrclinonc.2011.69

Rinderknecht, J. D., Goldinger, S. M., Rozati, S., Kamarashev, J., Kerl, K., French, L. E., et al. (2013). RASopathic skin eruptions during vemurafenib therapy. *PLoS One* 8:e58721. doi: 10.1371/journal.pone.0058721

Sauvage, V., Foulongne, V., Cheval, J., Ar Gouilh, M., Pariente, K., Dereure, O., et al. (2011). Human polyomavirus related to African green monkey lymphotropic polyomavirus. *Emerg. Infect. Dis.* 17, 1364–1370. doi: 10.3201/eid1708.110278

Schowalter, R. M., Pastrana, D. V., Pumphrey, K. A., Moyer, A. L., and Buck, C. B. (2010). Merkel cell polyomavirus and two previously unknown polyomaviruses are chronically shed from human skin. *Cell Host Microbe* 7, 509–515. doi: 10.1016/j.chom.2010.05.006

Schrama, D., Groesser, L., Ugurel, S., Hafner, C., Pastrana, D. V., Buck, C. B., et al. (2014). Presence of human polyomavirus 6 in mutation-specific BRAF inhibitor-induced epithelial proliferations. *JAMA Dermatol.* 150, 1180–1186. doi: 10.1001/jamadermatol.2014.1116

Scola, N., Wieland, U., Silling, S., Altmeyer, P., Stücker, M., and Kreuter, A. (2012). Prevalence of human polyomaviruses in common and rare types of non-Merkel cell carcinoma skin cancer *Br. J. Dermatol.* 167, 1315–1320. doi: 10.1111/j.1365-2133.2012.11141.x

Sfecci, A., Dupuy, A., Dinulescu, M., Droitcourt, C., Adamski, H., Hadj-Rabia, S., et al. (2017). Do the side effects of BRAF inhibitors mimic RASopathies? *J. Invest. Dermatol.* 137, 805–809. doi: 10.1016/j.jid.2016.12.012

Shuda, M., Feng, H., Kwun, H. J., Rosen, S. T., Gjoerup, O., Moore, P. S., et al. (2008). Antigen mutations are a human tumor-specific signature for Merkel cell polyomavirus. *Proc. Natl. Acad. Sci. U.S.A.* 105, 16272–16277. doi: 10.1073/pnas.0806526105

Sosman, J. A., Kim, K. B., Schuchter, L., Gonzalez, R., Pavlick, A. C., Weber, J. S., et al. (2012). Survival in BRAF V600-mutant advanced melanoma treated with vemurafenib. *N. Engl. J. Med.* 366, 707–714. doi: 10.1056/NEJMoa1112302

South, A. P., Purdie, K. J., Watt, S. A., Haldenby, S., den Breems, N., Dimon, M., et al. (2014). NOTCH1 mutations occur early during cutaneous squamous cell carcinogenesis. *J. Invest. Dermatol.* 134, 2630–2638. doi: 10.1038/jid.2014.154

Starrett, G. J., Marcelus, C., Cantalupo, P. G., Katz, J. P., Cheng, J., Akagi, K., et al. (2017). Merkel cell polyomavirus exhibits dominant control of the tumor genome and transcriptome in virus-associated Merkel cell carcinoma. *mBio* 8:e02079-16. doi: 10.1128/mBio.02079-16

Su, F., Viros, A., Milagre, C., Trunzer, K., Bollag, G., and Spleiss, O. (2012). RAS mutations in cutaneous squamous-cell carcinomas in patients treated with BRAF inhibitors. *N. Engl. J. Med.* 366, 207–215. doi: 10.1056/NEJMoa1105358

Teh, M. T., Blaydon, D., Chaplin, T., Foot, N. J., Skoulakis, S., Raghavan, M., et al. (2005). Genomewide single nucleotide polymorphism microarray mapping in basal cell carcinomas unveils uniparental disomy as a key somatic event. *Cancer Res.* 65, 8597–8603. doi: 10.1158/0008-5472.CAN-05-0842

Tommasino, M. (2017). The biology of beta human papillomaviruses. *Virus Res.* 231, 128–138. doi: 10.1016/j.virusres.2016.11.013

van der Meijden, E., Bialasiewicz, S., Rockett, R. J., Tozer, S. J., Sloots, T. P., and Feltkamp, M. C. (2013). Different serologic behavior of MCPyV, TSPyV, HPyV6, HPyV7 and HPyV9 polyomaviruses found on the skin. *PLoS One* 8:e81078. doi: 10.1371/journal.pone.0081078

van der Meijden, E., Horváth, B., Nijland, M., de Vries, K., Rácz, E. K., Diercks, G. F., et al. (2017). Primary polyomavirus infection, not reactivation, as the cause of *Trichodysplasia Spinulosa* in immunocompromised patients. *J. Infect. Dis.* 215, 1080–1084.

van der Meijden, E., Janssens, R. W., Lauber, C., Bouwes Bavinck, J. N., Gorbalenya, A. E., and Feltkamp, M. C. (2010). Discovery of a new human polyomavirus associated with *Trichodysplasia spinulosa* in an immunocompromized patient. *PLoS Pathog.* 6:e1001024. doi: 10.1371/journal.ppat.1001024

van der Meijden, E., Wunderink, H. F., van der Blij-de Brouwer, C. S., Zaaijer, H. L., Rotmans, J. I., et al. (2014). Human polyomavirus 9 infection in kidney transplant patients. *Emerg. Infect. Dis.* 20, 991–999. doi: 10.3201/eid2006.140055

Viarisio, D., Gissmann, L., and Tommasino, M. (2017a). Human papillomaviruses and carcinogenesis: well-established and novel models. *Curr. Opin. Virol.* 26, 56–62. doi: 10.1016/j.coviro.2017.07.014

Viarisio, D., Müller-Decker, K., Hassel, J. C., Alvarez, J. C., Flechtenmacher, C., Pawlita, M., et al. (2017b). The BRAF inhibitor vemurafenib enhances UV-induced skin carcinogenesis in beta HPV38 E6 and E7 transgenic mice. *J. Invest. Dermatol.* 137, 261–264. doi: 10.1016/j.jid.2016.08.030

Viarisio, D., Mueller-Decker, K., Kloz, U., Aengeneyndt, B., Kopp-Schneider, A., Gröne, H. J., et al. (2011). E6 and E7 from beta HPV38 cooperate with ultraviolet light in the development of actinic keratosis-like lesions and squamous cell carcinoma in mice. *PLoS Pathog.* 7:e1002125. doi: 10.1371/journal.ppat.1002125

Viarisio, D., Müller-Decker, K., Accardi, R., Robitaille, A., Dürst, M., Beer, K., et al. (2018). Beta HPV38 oncoproteins act with a hit-and-run mechanism in ultraviolet radiation-induced skin carcinogenesis in mice. *PLoS Pathog.* 14:e1006783. doi: 10.1371/journal.ppat.1006783

Wang, J., Aldabagh, B., Yu, J., and Tuttleton, A. S. (2014). Role of human papillomavirus in cutaneous squamous cell carcinoma: a meta-analysis. *J. Am. Acad. Dermatol.* 70, 621–629. doi: 10.1016/j.jaad.2014.01.857

Wang, Q., Kennedy, A., Das, P., McIntosh, P. B., Howell, S. A., Isaacson, E. R., et al. (2009). Phosphorylation of the human papillomavirus type 16 E1–E4 protein at T57 by ERK triggers a structural change that enhances keratin binding and protein stability. *J. Virol.* 83, 3668–3683. doi: 10.1128/JVI.02063-08

Watt, S. A., Purdie, K. J., den Breems, N. Y., Dimon, M., Arron, S. T., McHugh, A., et al. (2015). Novel CARD11 mutations in human cutaneous squamous cell carcinoma lead to aberrant NF-κB regulation. *Am. J. Pathol.* 185, 2354–2363. doi: 10.1016/j.ajpath.2015.05.018

Watt, S. A., Purdie, K. J., den Breems, N. Y., Dimon, M., Tucker, S., Arron, S. T., et al. (2016). CREBBP mutation in human cutaneous squamous cell carcinoma. *Exp. Dermatol.* 25, 650–651. doi: 10.1111/exd.13044

Weissenborn, S., Neale, R. E., Waterboer, T., Abeni, D., Bavinck, J. N., Green, A. C., et al. (2012). Beta-papillomavirus DNA loads in hair follicles of immunocompetent people and organ transplant recipients. *Med. Microbiol. Immunol.* 201, 117–125. doi: 10.1007/s00430-011-0212-3

Weissenborn, S. J., Nindl, I., Purdie, K., Harwood, C., Proby, C., Breuer, J., et al. (2005). Human papillomavirus-DNA-loads in actinic keratoses exceed those in non-melanoma skin cancers. *J. Invest. Dermatol.* 125, 93–97. doi: 10.1111/j.0022-202X.2005.23733.x

Wieland, U., Mauch, C., Kreuter, A., Krieg, T., and Pfister, H. (2009). Merkel cell polyomavirus DNA in persons without Merkel cell carcinoma. *Emerg. Infect. Dis.* 15, 1496–1498. doi: 10.3201/eid1509.081575

Wieland, U., Silling, S., Hellmich, M., Potthoff, A., Pfister, H., and Kreuter, A. (2014). Human polyomaviruses 6, 7, 9, 10 and *Trichodysplasia spinulosa*-associated polyomavirus in HIV-infected men. *J. Gen. Virol.* 95(Pt 4), 928–932. doi: 10.1099/vir.0.061259-0

Wong, S. Q., Waldeck, K., Vergara, I. A., Schröder, J., Madore, J., Wilmott, J. S., et al. (2015). UV-associated mutations underlie the etiology of MCV-negative merkel cell carcinomas. *Cancer Res.* 75, 5228–5234. doi: 10.1158/0008-5472.CAN-15-1877

Wu, J. H., Narayanan, D., Simonette, R. A., Rady, P. L., Tyring, S. K. (2017a). Dysregulation of the MEK/ERK/MNK1 signalling cascade by middle T antigen of the trichoydsplasia spinulosa polyomavirus. *J. Eur. Acad. Dermatol. Venereol.* 31, 1338–1341. doi: 10.1111/jdv.14326

Wu, J. H., Simonette, R. A., Nguyen, H. P., Rady, P. L., and Tyring, S. K. (2017b). Molecular mechanisms supporting a pathogenic role for human polyomavirus 6 small T antigen: protein phosphatase 2A targeting and MAPK cascade activation. *J. Med. Virol.* 89, 742–747. doi: 10.1002/jmv.24688

Wu, J. H., Simonette, R. A., Nguyen, H. P., Rady, P. L., and Tyring, S. K. (2016). Small T-antigen of the TS-associated polyomavirus activates factors implicated in the MAPK pathway. *J. Eur. Acad. Dermatol. Venereol.* 30, 1061–1062. doi: 10.1111/jdv.13111

Zhang, J., Yang, P. L., and Gray, N. S. (2009). Targeting cancer with small molecule kinase inhibitors. *Nat. Rev. Cancer* 9, 28–39. doi: 10.1038/nrc2559

Permissions

All chapters in this book were first published by Frontiers; hereby published with permission under the Creative Commons Attribution License or equivalent. Every chapter published in this book has been scrutinized by our experts. Their significance has been extensively debated. The topics covered herein carry significant findings which will fuel the growth of the discipline. They may even be implemented as practical applications or may be referred to as a beginning point for another development.

The contributors of this book come from diverse backgrounds, making this book a truly international effort. This book will bring forth new frontiers with its revolutionizing research information and detailed analysis of the nascent developments around the world.

We would like to thank all the contributing authors for lending their expertise to make the book truly unique. They have played a crucial role in the development of this book. Without their invaluable contributions this book wouldn't have been possible. They have made vital efforts to compile up to date information on the varied aspects of this subject to make this book a valuable addition to the collection of many professionals and students.

This book was conceptualized with the vision of imparting up-to-date information and advanced data in this field. To ensure the same, a matchless editorial board was set up. Every individual on the board went through rigorous rounds of assessment to prove their worth. After which they invested a large part of their time researching and compiling the most relevant data for our readers.

The editorial board has been involved in producing this book since its inception. They have spent rigorous hours researching and exploring the diverse topics which have resulted in the successful publishing of this book. They have passed on their knowledge of decades through this book. To expedite this challenging task, the publisher supported the team at every step. A small team of assistant editors was also appointed to further simplify the editing procedure and attain best results for the readers.

Apart from the editorial board, the designing team has also invested a significant amount of their time in understanding the subject and creating the most relevant covers. They scrutinized every image to scout for the most suitable representation of the subject and create an appropriate cover for the book.

The publishing team has been an ardent support to the editorial, designing and production team. Their endless efforts to recruit the best for this project, has resulted in the accomplishment of this book. They are a veteran in the field of academics and their pool of knowledge is as vast as their experience in printing. Their expertise and guidance has proved useful at every step. Their uncompromising quality standards have made this book an exceptional effort. Their encouragement from time to time has been an inspiration for everyone.

The publisher and the editorial board hope that this book will prove to be a valuable piece of knowledge for researchers, students, practitioners and scholars across the globe.

List of Contributors

Luisa Bopp
Institute of Virology, National Reference Center for Papilloma- and Polyomaviruses, University of Cologne, Faculty of Medicine and University Hospital of Cologne, Cologne, Germany
Department of Dermatology and Venereology, University of Cologne, Cologne, Germany

Ulrike Wieland, Herbert Pfister and Steffi Silling
Institute of Virology, National Reference Center for Papilloma- and Polyomaviruses, University of Cologne, Faculty of Medicine and University Hospital of Cologne, Cologne, Germany

Martin Hellmich
Institute of Medical Statistics and Computational Biology, Faculty of Medicine and University Hospital Cologne, University of Cologne, Cologne, Germany

Alexander Kreuter
Department of Dermatology, Venereology, and Allergology, Helios St. Elisabeth Hospital Oberhausen, University Witten-Herdecke, Witten, Germany

Lisa M. Hillen, Dorit Rennspiess, Ernst-Jan Speel, Véronique Winnepenninckx and Axel zur Hausen
Department of Pathology and GROW-School for Oncology and Developmental Biology, Maastricht University Medical Center, Maastricht, Netherlands

Anke M. Haugg
Department of Gynaecology, University Hospital RWTH Aachen, Aachen, Germany

Daniel Hasche and Frank Rösl
Division of Viral Transformation Mechanisms, Research Program "Infection, Inflammation and Cancer", German Cancer Research Center, Heidelberg, Germany

Sabrina E. Vinzón
Laboratory of Molecular and Cellular Therapy, Fundación Instituto Leloir, IIBBA-CONICET, Buenos Aires, Argentina

Carlotta Olivero
Virology Unit, Department of Translational Medicine, Novara Medical School, University of Eastern Piedmont, Novara, Italy
European Cancer Stem Cell Research Institute, Cardiff School of Biosciences, Cardiff University, Cardiff, United Kingdom

Simone Lanfredini and Girish K. Patel
European Cancer Stem Cell Research Institute, Cardiff School of Biosciences, Cardiff University, Cardiff, United Kingdom

Cinzia Borgogna and Marisa Gariglio
Virology Unit, Department of Translational Medicine, Novara Medical School, University of Eastern Piedmont, Novara, Italy

Federica Calati
Virology Unit, Department of Translational Medicine, Novara Medical School, University of Eastern Piedmont, Novara, Italy

Marco De Andrea
Virology Unit, Department of Translational Medicine, Novara Medical School, University of Eastern Piedmont, Novara, Italy
Virology Unit, Department of Public Health and Pediatric Sciences, Turin Medical School, University of Turin, Turin, Italy

Elisa Zavattaro and Paola Savoia
Dermatology Unit, Department of Health Sciences, Novara Medical School, Novara, Italy

Elena Trisolini and Renzo Boldorini
Pathology Unit, Department of Health Sciences, Novara Medical School, Novara, Italy

Matthias Kirschberg, Adnan Shahzad Syed, Sandra Heuser, Martin Hufbauer and Baki Akgül
Medical Faculty and University Hospital Cologne, Institute of Virology, University of Cologne, Cologne, Germany

Hanife Güler Dönmez
Medical Faculty and University Hospital Cologne, Institute of Virology, University of Cologne, Cologne, Germany
Department of Biology, Hacettepe University, Ankara, Turkey

Astrid Wilbrand-Hennes
Cologne Excellence Cluster on Cellular Stress Responses in Aging-Associated Diseases (CECAD) and Center for Molecular Medicine (CMMC), University of Cologne, Cologne, Germany

Angel Alonso
German Cancer Research Center (DKFZ), Heidelberg, Germany

Sebastian O. Wendel and Nicholas A. Wallace
Division of Biology, Kansas State University, Manhattan, KS, United States

Marta Podgórska, Anna Marthaler, Alina Fingerle, Barbara Walch-Rückheim, Stefan Lohse, Artur Wnorowski and Sigrun Smola
Institute of Virology, Saarland University Medical Center, Homburg, Germany

Monika Ołdak
Institute of Virology, Saarland University Medical Center, Homburg, Germany
Department of Histology and Embryology, Center of Biostructure Research, Medical University of Warsaw, Warsaw, Poland

Cornelia S. L. Müller and Thomas Vogt
Department of Dermatology, Saarland University Medical Center, Homburg, Germany

Mart Ustav
Icosagen Cell Factory OÜ, Institute of Technology, University of Tartu, Tartu, Estonia

Magdalena Malejczyk
Diagnostic Laboratory of STDs, Department of Dermatology and Venereology, Medical University of Warsaw, Warsaw, Poland

Sławomir Majewski
Department of Dermatology and Venereology, Medical University of Warsaw, Warsaw, Poland

Nathan A. Krump and Jianxin You
Department of Microbiology, Perelman School of Medicine, University of Pennsylvania, Philadelphia, PA, United States

Stefanie Taute, Herbert J. Pfister and Gertrud Steger
Institute of Virology, University of Cologne, Cologne, Germany

Lisett Liblekas, Alla Piirsoo, Annika Laanemets, Eva-Maria Tombak, Airiin Laaneväli, Ene Ustav and Marko Piirsoo
Institute of Technology, University of Tartu, Tartu, Estonia

Celestino Velásquez and Alexis Harold
Cancer Virology Program, University of Pittsburgh Medical Center Hillman Cancer Center, Pittsburgh, PA, United States

Yutaka Amako and Masahiro Shuda
Cancer Virology Program, University of Pittsburgh Medical Center Hillman Cancer Center, Pittsburgh, PA, United States
Department of Microbiology and Molecular Genetics, University of Pittsburgh, Pittsburgh, PA, United States

Tuna Toptan and Yuan Chang
Cancer Virology Program, University of Pittsburgh Medical Center Hillman Cancer Center, Pittsburgh, PA, United States
Department of Pathology, University of Pittsburgh, Pittsburgh, PA, United States

Els van der Meijden and Mariet Feltkamp
Department of Medical Microbiology, Leiden University Medical Center, Leiden, Netherlands

Jordan M. Meyers
Program in Virology, Harvard Medical School, Boston, MA, United States
Department of Developmental, Molecular and Chemical Biology, Tufts University School of Medicine, Boston, MA, United States

Miranda Grace and Karl Munger
Department of Developmental, Molecular and Chemical Biology, Tufts University School of Medicine, Boston, MA, United States

Aayushi Uberoi and Paul F. Lambert
McArdle Laboratory for Cancer Research, Department of Oncology, School of Medicine and Public Health, University of Wisconsin–Madison, Madison, WI, United States

Benjamin Marx and Daliborka Miller-Lazic
Institute of Virology, University of Cologne, Cologne, Germany

Slawomir Majewski
Department of Dermatology and Venereology, Medical University of Warsaw, Warsaw, Poland

Kay Hofmann
Institute for Genetics, University of Cologne, Cologne, Germany

Tatjana Sauerer and Jan Dörrie
RNA-based Immunotherapy, Hautklinik, Comprehensive Cancer Center Erlangen European Metropolitan Area of Nuremberg, Deutsches Zentrum Immuntherapie, Universitätsklinikum Erlangen, Friedrich-Alexander-Universität Erlangen-Nürnberg, Erlangen, Germany

Christopher Lischer, Adrian Weich and Julio Vera
Systems Tumor Immunology, Hautklinik, Universitätsklinikum Erlangen, Friedrich-Alexander-Universität Erlangen-Nürnberg, Comprehensive Cancer Center Erlangen European Metropolitan Area of Nuremberg, Deutsches Zentrum Immuntherapie, Erlangen, Germany

Carola Berking
Hautklinik, Universitätsklinikum Erlangen, Friedrich-Alexander-Universität Erlangen-Nürnberg, Comprehensive Cancer Center Erlangen European Metropolitan Area of Nuremberg, Deutsches Zentrum Immuntherapie, Erlangen, Germany

Sarah J. de Jong
St. Giles Laboratory of Human Genetics of Infectious Diseases, Rockefeller Branch, The Rockefeller University, New York, NY, United States

Elias Imahorn and Bettina Burger
Department of Biomedicine, University Hospital of Basel, University of Basel, Basel, Switzerland

Peter Itin
Department of Biomedicine, University Hospital of Basel, University of Basel, Basel, Switzerland
Department of Dermatology, University Hospital of Basel, Basel, Switzerland

Jouni Uitto
Department of Dermatology and Cutaneous Biology, Sidney Kimmel Medical College, Thomas Jefferson University, Philadelphia, PA, United States
Jefferson Institute of Molecular Medicine, Thomas Jefferson University, Philadelphia, PA, United States

Gérard Orth
Pasteur Institute, Paris, France

Emmanuelle Jouanguy
St. Giles Laboratory of Human Genetics of Infectious Diseases, Rockefeller Branch, The Rockefeller University, New York, NY, United States
INSERM UMR 1163, Laboratory of Human Genetics of Infectious Diseases, Necker Branch, Necker Hospital for Sick Children, Paris, France
Imagine Institute, Paris Descartes University, Paris, France

Jean-Laurent Casanova
St. Giles Laboratory of Human Genetics of Infectious Diseases, Rockefeller Branch, The Rockefeller University, New York, NY, United States
INSERM UMR 1163, Laboratory of Human Genetics of Infectious Diseases, Necker Branch, Necker Hospital for Sick Children, Paris, France
Imagine Institute, Paris Descartes University, Paris, France
Pediatric Hematology and Immunology Unit, Necker Hospital for Sick Children, Paris, France
Howard Hughes Medical Institute, New York, NY, United States

Karin J. Purdie
Centre for Cell Biology and Cutaneous Research, Blizard Institute, Barts and the London School of Medicine and Dentistry, Queen Mary University of London, London, United Kingdom

Charlotte M. Proby and Gareth J. Inman
Division of Cancer Research, School of Medicine, University of Dundee, Dundee, United Kingdom

Hasan Rizvi
Department of Pathology, Barts Health NHS Trust, London, United Kingdom,

Heather Griffin and John Doorbar
Division of Virology, Department of Pathology, University of Cambridge, Cambridge, United Kingdom

Mary Sommerlad
Department of Dermatology, Barts Health NHS Trust, London, United Kingdom

Andrew P. South
Department of Dermatology and Cutaneous Biology, Thomas Jefferson University, Philadelphia, PA, United States

Irene M. Leigh
Institute of Dentistry, Barts and the London School of Medicine and Dentistry, Queen Mary University of London, London, United Kingdom

Catherine A. Harwood
Centre for Cell Biology and Cutaneous Research, Blizard Institute, Barts and the London School of Medicine and Dentistry, Queen Mary University of London, London, United Kingdom
Department of Dermatology, Barts Health NHS Trust, London, United Kingdom

Index

R

S

T

V

www.ingramcontent.com/pod-product-compliance
Lightning Source LLC
LaVergne TN
LVHW082217200926
848484LV00008B/2271